DERMATOLOGY
SECRETS PLUS
TH EDITION

E. Fitzpatrick, MD
Professor
ent of Dermatology
School of Medicine
Aurora, Colorado

ph G. Morelli, MD
iatric Dermatology
Children's Hospital
ogy and Pediatrics
ent of Dermatology
School of Medicine
Aurora, Colorado

ELSEVIER
MOSBY

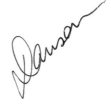

ELSEVIER
MOSBY

1600 John F. Kennedy Blvd.
Ste 1800
Philadelphia, PA 19103-2899

DERMATOLOGY SECRETS PLUS, FOURTH EDITION   ISBN: 978-0-323-07154-3

Notices

Knowledge and best practice in this field are constantly changing. As new research and experience broaden our understanding, changes in research methods, professional practices, or medical treatment may become necessary.

 Practitioners and researchers must always rely on their own experience and knowledge in evaluating and using any information, methods, compounds, or experiments described herein. In using such information or methods they should be mindful of their own safety and the safety of others, including parties for whom they have a professional responsibility.

 With respect to any drug or pharmaceutical products identified, readers are advised to check the most current information provided (i) on procedures featured or (ii) by the manufacturer of each product to be administered, to verify the recommended dose or formula, the method and duration of administration, and contraindications. It is the responsibility of practitioners, relying on their own experience and knowledge of their patients, to make diagnoses, to determine dosages and the best treatment for each individual patient, and to take all appropriate safety precautions.

 To the fullest extent of the law, neither the Publisher nor the authors, contributors, or editors, assume any liability for any injury and/or damage to persons or property as a matter of products liability, negligence or otherwise, or from any use or operation of any methods, products, instructions, or ideas contained in the material herein.

Library of Congress Cataloging-in-Publication Data

Dermatology secrets plus / [edited by] James E. Fitzpatrick, Joseph G.
Morelli. — 4th ed.
 p. ; cm. — (Secrets)
 Rev. ed. of: Dermatology secrets in color. 3rd ed. c2007.
 Includes bibliographical references and index.
 ISBN 978-0-323-07154-3 (pbk. : alk. paper)
 1. Dermatology--Miscellanea. I. Fitzpatrick, James E., 1948- II.
Morelli, Joseph G. III. Dermatology secrets in color. IV. Series:
Secrets series.
 [DNLM: 1. Skin Diseases—Examination Questions. 2. Skin
Diseases—Handbooks. WR 18.2]

 RL72.D466 2011
 616.5—dc22

              2010030467

Senior Acquisitions Editor: James Merritt
Developmental Editor: Andrea Vosburgh
Publishing Services Manager: Patricia Tannian
Senior Project Manager: Kristine Feeherty
Design Direction: Steven Stave
Marketing Manager: Jason Oberacker

Printed in China

Last digit is the print number: 9 8 7 6 5 4 3 2 1

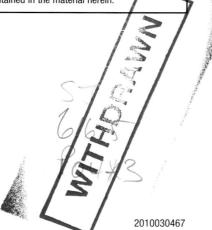

This book is dedicated to my supportive wife, Lois Fitzpatrick (JEF),
and Nonna Morelli and Grammy Costlow (JGM).

CONTRIBUTORS

John L. Aeling, MD
Professor, Department of Dermatology, University of Colorado School of Medicine, Aurora, Colorado

H. Alan Arbuckle, MD, FAAP, FAAD
Assistant Professor of Pediatrics and Dermatology, Department of Dermatology, University of Colorado School of Medicine; Director, Epidermolysis Bullosa Center of Excellence, Department of Dermatology, The Children's Hospital, Aurora, Colorado; Assistant Chief, Dermatology Service, VA Medical Center, Denver, Colorado

Scott D. Bennion, MS, MD
Central Wyoming Skin Clinic, Casper, Wyoming

Paul M. Benson, MD, COL (Ret), MC, USA
Private Practice, Johnson City, Tennessee

Carl F. Bigler, MD
Private Practice, Northern Arizona Dermatology Center, Flagstaff, Arizona

Sylvia L. Brice, MD
Associate Professor of Dermatology, University of Colorado, Denver, Aurora, Colorado

Mariah Ruth Brown, MD
Fellow, Department of Dermatology, University of Colorado School of Medicine, Aurora, Colorado

Joanna M. Burch, MD
Associate Professor, Departments of Dermatology and Pediatrics, University of Colorado, Denver, Denver, Colorado; Clinic Director, Department of Pediatric Dermatology, The Children's Hospital, Denver; Department of Dermatology, University Hospital, Aurora, Colorado

Michael R. Campoli, MD, PhD
Resident, Department of Dermatology, University of Colorado Denver, Aurora, Colorado

T. Minsue Chen, MD
Private Practice, Skin and Laser Surgery Associates, Pasadena, Texas; Private Practice, Laser and Cosmetic Surgery Center of Houston, Houston, Texas; Adjunct Faculty, Lecturer, Program in Histotechnology, School of Health Sciences, Adjunct Faculty, Lecturer, School of Health Professions, University of Texas M.D. Anderson Cancer Center, Houston, Texas

Donna M. Corvette, MD
Dermatology Center of Williamsburg, Williamsburg, Virginia

Daniel C. Dapprich, MD
Clinical Assistant Professor, Department of Internal Medicine, Michigan State University College of Human Medicine, East Lansing, Michigan; Attending Physician, Department of Dermatology, Spectrum Health; Attending Physician, Department of Dermatology, St. Mary's Hospital, Grand Rapids, Michigan

Kathleen M. David-Bajar, MD
Aurora, Colorado

Carl W. Demidovich, MD
Assistant Clinical Professor, Department of Dermatology, University of Colorado; Dermatologist and Mohs Surgeon, Dermatology and Laser Center at Harvard Park, Denver, Colorado

Genevieve L. Egnatios, MD
Resident, Department of Dermatology, Mayo Clinic Arizona, Phoenix, Arizona

Stephen W. Eubanks, MD
Assistant Professor, University of Colorado School of Medicine; Dermatology and Laser Center at Harvard Park, Denver, Colorado

James E. Fitzpatrick, MD
Professor, Department of Dermatology, University of Colorado School of Medicine, Aurora, Colorado

Shayla Francis, MD
Resident Physician, Department of Dermatology, University of Colorado School of Medicine, Denver, Colorado

Brian J. Gerondale, MD
Partner and Physician, Dermatology Associates of West Michigan; Department Chief, Dermatology, St. Mary's Health Services; Department of Dermatology, Spectrum Health, Grand Rapids, Michigan

Martin B. Giandoni, MD
Mountain View Dermatology, El Paso, Texas

Heidi Gilchrist, MD
Dermatopathology Fellow, Department of Pathology, University of Virginia Health System, Charlottesville, Virginia

Loren E. Golitz, MD
Clinical Professor of Pathology and Dermatology, Department of Dermatology, University of Colorado School of Medicine, Denver, Colorado

Nadja Y. Grammer-West, MD, COL, MC, USA
Commander, Womack Army Medical Center, Fort Bragg,
North Carolina

Clayton B. Green, MD, PhD
Department of Dermatology, Marshfield Clinic, Marshfield,
Wisconsin

Ronald E. Grimwood, MD
Division of Dermatology, University of Texas Health Sciences
Center at San Antonio, San Antonio, Texas

Anne R. Halbert, MB BS (Hons), FACD
Clinical Lecturer, School of Pediatrics and Child Health,
University of Western Australia; Head, Department of
Pediatric Dermatology, Princess Margaret Hospital of
Children, Perth, Western Australia

Deborah B. Henderson, MD, MPH
Chief Resident, Division of Dermatology and Cutaneous
Surgery, University of Texas Health Science Center at San
Antonio, San Antonio, Texas

Whitney A. High, MD, JD, MEng
Department of Dermatology, University of Colorado, Denver,
Colorado

Simone A. Ince, MD
Physician, Department of Dermatology, Virginia Mason
Medical Center, Seattle, Washington

William D. James, MD
Paul R. Gross Professor, Department of Dermatology,
University of Pennsylvania, Philadelphia, Pennsylvania

Rohit K. Katial, MD
Professor, Department of Medicine, National Jewish Health,
Denver, Colorado

Richard A. Keller, MD
Clinical Professor, Division of Dermatology and Cutaneous
Surgery, University of Texas Health Science Center; Chief
of Dermatologic Surgery, Department of Dermatology,
Audie L. Murphy Veterans Hospital, South Texas Veterans
Health Care System, San Antonio, Texas

Alison S. Klenk, MD
Assistant Professor of Dermatology, Director, Adult
Outpatient Center, Department of Dermatology, Indiana
University School of Medicine, Indianapolis, Indiana

Todd T. Kobayashi, MD, Lt Col, USAF, MC
Fellow, Dermatopathology, Department of Dermatology,
University of Colorado at Denver, Aurora, Colorado;
Instructor of Dermatology, Department of Dermatology,
Uniformed Services University of the Health Sciences,
Bethesda, Maryland

Kehua Li, MD
Assistant Professor, Departments of Dermatology and Cuta-
neous Biology, Thomas Jefferson University; Assistant
Professor, Department of Dermatology, Thomas Jefferson
University Hospital, Philadelphia, Pennsylvania; Medical
Director, Advanced Dermatology, PC, Sewell, New Jersey

Lori Lowe, MD
Professor of Dermatology and Pathology, Director of
Dermatopathology, University of Michigan Medical
School, Ann Arbor, Michigan

Lisa E. Maier, MD
Assistant Clinical Professor, Department of Dermatology,
University of Michigan; Staff Physician, Department of
Dermatology, Veterans Administration Ann Arbor Health-
care System, Ann Arbor, Michigan

Thomas W. McGovern, MD
Volunteer Assistant Professor, Department of Dermatology,
University of Indiana School of Medicine, Indianapolis,
Indiana; Fort Wayne Dermatology Consultants, Fort
Wayne, Indiana

Jeffrey J. Meffert, MD
Associate Clinical Professor, Department of Dermatology,
University of Texas Health Science Center, San Antonio,
Texas

J. Ramsey Mellette, MD
Professor of Dermatology, Department of Dermatology,
University of Colorado Denver; Director of Dermatologic
Surgery, Department of Dermatology, University of
Colorado Hospital, Aurora, Colorado

Misha D. Miller, MD, FACOG
Resident Physician, Department of Dermatology, University
of Colorado School of Medicine, Denver, Colorado

Joseph G. Morelli, MD
Professor of Dermatology and Pediatrics, Department of
Dermatology, University of Colorado School of Medicine,
Aurora, Colorado

Margaret E. Muldrow, MD
HM Medical Consultants, Denver, Colorado

Scott A. Norton, MD, MPH, COL, MC, USA
Dermatology Division, Department of Medicine, Georgetown
University; Dermatology Division, Department of Medi-
cine, Georgetown University Hospital, Washington, DC

Christina S. O'Hara, 2LT MC (HPSP, CPT MI (HD)), USA
Medical Student (third year), East Tennessee State University Quillen College of Medicine, Johnson City, Tennessee

Theresa R. Pacheco, MD
Associate Professor, Department of Dermatology, University
of Colorado Denver, Denver, Colorado

James W. Patterson, MD
Professor of Pathology and Dermatology, Director of
Dermatopathology, Department of Pathology, University
of Virginia, Charlottesville, Virginia

Renata Prado, MD
Resident, Department of Dermatology, University of
Colorado Denver, Aurora, Colorado

Lori D. Prok, MD
Assistant Professor, Department of Pediatric Dermatology
and Dermatopathology, University of Colorado Denver
and the Children's Hospital, Denver, Colorado

Barbara R. Reed, MD
Clinical Professor, Courtesy Staff, Department of Dermatol-
ogy, University of Colorado Hospital; Courtesy Staff,
Department of Medicine, Rose Medical Center, Denver,
Colorado

Curt P. Samlaska, MD, FACP, FAAD
Assistant Professor of Medicine, Department of Medicine, University of Nevada School of Medicine, Las Vegas, Nevada

C. Paul Sayers, MD
Clinical Instructor, Department of Dermatology, University of Colorado Medical Center, Fort Collins, Colorado

Milton J. Schleve, MD
Private Practice, Denver, Colorado

Dieter K.T. Schmidt, MD, FAAD, FACMS
Dermatologist and Mohs Micrographic Surgeon, Department of Dermatology, Providence Everett Medical Center, Everett, Washington; Dermatologist and Mohs Micrographic Surgeon, Private Practice, North Sound Dermatology, Mill Creek, Washington

Elizabeth R. Shurnas, MD
Assistant Clinical Professor, Department of Internal Medicine, University of Colorado School of Medicine, Denver, Colorado

Stephen Thomas Spates, MD
Director, Mohs Surgery Center, The Dermatology Group, PC, West Orange, New Jersey; Department of Medicine, The Mountainside Hospital, Montclair, New Jersey; Department of Medicine, Clara Maass Medical Center, Belleville, New Jersey; Department of Medicine, Chilton Memorial Hospital, Pompton Plains, New Jersey

Larisa S. Speetzen, MD
Resident, Department of Dermatology, Mayo Clinic Arizona, Scottsdale, Arizona

Leonard C. Sperling, MD
Professor and Chair, Department of Dermatology, Uniformed Services University of the Health Sciences, Bethesda, Maryland

Leslie A. Stewart, MD
Clinical Assistant Professor of Dermatology, University of Colorado School of Medicine, Denver, Colorado; Private Practice, Greenwood Village, Colorado

Alexandra Theriault, MD
House Staff, Department of Dermatology, Rose Hospital, Denver, Colorado

Paul B. Thompson, MD
Chief, Department of Dermatology, Olympic Memorial Hospital, Port Angeles, Washington

Jeffrey B. Travers, MD, PhD
Kampen-Nornis Professor and Chair of Department, Department of Dermatology, Indiana University School of Medicine, Indianapolis, Indiana

George W. Turiansky, MD, COL, MC
Professor, Department of Dermatology, Uniformed Services University of the Health Sciences; Program Director, National Capital Consortium Dermatology Residency Dermatology; Dermatology Department, National Naval Medical Center, Bethesda, Maryland; Dermatology Service, Walter Reed Army Medical Center; Dermatology Consultant, DiLorenzo TRICARE Health Clinic, The Pentagon, Washington, DC

Patrick Walsh, MD
Clinical Associate Professor, Department of Dermatology, University of Texas Southwestern Medical School, Dallas, Texas

Karen E. Warschaw, MD
Associate Professor, Department of Dermatology, Mayo Clinic Arizona, Scottsdale, Arizona

William L. Weston, MD
Professor Emeritus, Department of Dermatology, University of Colorado School of Medicine, Aurora, Colorado

Joseph Yohn, MD
Dermatology Section, Intercoastal Medical Group, Sarasota, Florida

PREFACE

Socrates
Greek philosopher (470 BC – 399 BC)

It is only fitting to preface the fourth edition of *Dermatology Secrets Plus* with a quote from the great Athenian philosopher Socrates, since the entire *Secrets* series of medical textbooks is based on the Socratic method of teaching, which involves asking and answering questions to stimulate critical thinking. The Socratic method (*elenchus*) in medicine is primarily taught on medical rounds or even at the patient's bedside and has been used for centuries to challenge the minds of medical trainees. It is the goal of this textbook to simulate the kinds of questions that might be used on dermatology patient rounds as the senior attending physician applies the Socratic method of teaching to medical students, interns, and residents.

The fourth edition once again finds me working with my friend and colleague, Dr. Joseph Morelli, a renowned pediatric dermatologist, who continues to bring his outstanding insight, hard work, and expertise to this book. This edition brings many changes—every chapter has been revised with the addition of numerous new questions and tables. We have paid particular attention to the length of the answers to questions, believing that more concise answers will enhance the reader's learning. Since dermatology is a largely visual medical specialty, we have also added 99 new or replacement clinical color photographs to tie the questions to a visual experience. Many of the new photographs have come from the JLA Collection, which was donated to the University of Colorado by Dr. John L. Aeling, a former editor of this book; the WLW Collection, donated to the University of Colorado by Dr. William L. Weston, the former chairman of the Department of Dermatology at the University of Colorado; and the JB Collection, donated to the University of Colorado by Dr. Joanna Burch, who is currently one of our pediatric dermatologists. Finally, we have added a much needed new chapter, "Disorders of the Female Genitalia."

Finally, I would like to acknowledge the special contribution of Nicole Brevik from CU Dermatopathology, who in addition to providing administrative support, also designed and developed two new figures for this textbook. I would also like to thank all of the editorial staff at Elsevier, especially Andrea Vosburgh, who patiently worked with us and allowed this textbook to come to fruition, as well as Cassie Carey at Graphic World Publishing Services for her patience and support.

—James E. Fitzpatrick, MD

CONTENTS

TOP 100 SECRETS   1

I   GENERAL   5

CHAPTER 1   STRUCTURE AND FUNCTION OF THE SKIN   6
Scott D. Bennion, MS, MD

CHAPTER 2   MORPHOLOGY OF PRIMARY AND SECONDARY SKIN LESIONS   14
Donna M. Corvette, MD

CHAPTER 3   DIAGNOSTIC TECHNIQUES   22
Stephen Thomas Spates, MD

II   INHERITED DISORDERS   29

CHAPTER 4   DISORDERS OF KERATINIZATION   30
H. Alan Arbuckle, MD, FAAP, FAAD, and Lori D. Prok, MD

CHAPTER 5   NEUROCUTANEOUS DISORDERS   37
Anne R. Halbert, MB BS (Hons), FACD

CHAPTER 6   MECHANOBULLOUS DISORDERS   43
H. Alan Arbuckle, MD, FAAP, FAAD, and Ronald E. Grimwood, MD

III   INFLAMMATORY DISORDERS   49

CHAPTER 7   PAPULOSQUAMOUS SKIN ERUPTIONS   50
Alison S. Klenk, MD, and Jeffrey B. Travers, MD, PhD

CHAPTER 8   DERMATITIS (ECZEMA)   57
Thomas W. McGovern, MD

CHAPTER 9   CONTACT DERMATITIS   64
Leslie A. Stewart, MD

CHAPTER 10   VESICULOBULLOUS DISORDERS   70
Todd T. Kobayashi, MD, Lt Col, USAF, MC, and Kathleen M. David-Bajar, MD

CHAPTER 11   PUSTULAR ERUPTIONS   78
James E. Fitzpatrick, MD

CHAPTER 12   LICHENOID SKIN ERUPTIONS   84
Whitney A. High, MD, JD, MEng

CHAPTER 13   GRANULOMATOUS DISEASES OF THE SKIN   90
James E. Fitzpatrick, MD

CHAPTER 14   DRUG ERUPTIONS   97
Alexandra Theriault, MD

CHAPTER 15   VASCULITIS   105
Curt P. Samlaska, MD, and James E. Fitzpatrick, MD

CHAPTER 16   DEPOSITION DISORDERS   112
Lisa E. Maier, MD, and Lori Lowe, MD

CHAPTER 17   PHOTOSENSITIVE DERMATITIS   118
Todd T. Kobayashi, MD, Lt Col, USAF, MC, and Kathleen M. David-Bajar, MD

CHAPTER 18   DISORDERS OF PIGMENTATION   126
Joseph Yohn, MD

CHAPTER 19   PANNICULITIS   135
Heidi Gilchrist, MD, and James W. Patterson, MD

CHAPTER 20   ALOPECIA   143
Leonard C. Sperling, MD

CHAPTER 21   ACNE AND ACNEIFORM ERUPTIONS   148
Joanna M. Burch, MD, and John L. Aeling, MD

CHAPTER 22   AUTOIMMUNE CONNECTIVE TISSUE DISEASES   156
Todd T. Kobayashi, MD, Lt Col, USAF, MC, and Kathleen M. David-Bajar, MD

CHAPTER 23   URTICARIA AND ANGIOEDEMA   166
Rohit K. Katial, MD

IV   INFECTIONS AND INFESTATIONS   171

CHAPTER 24   VIRAL EXANTHEMS   172
William L. Weston, MD

CHAPTER 25   BULLOUS VIRAL ERUPTIONS   175
Sylvia L. Brice, MD

CHAPTER 26   WARTS AND MOLLUSCUM CONTAGIOSUM   182
Barbara R. Reed, MD

CHAPTER 27   BACTERIAL INFECTIONS   188
James E. Fitzpatrick, MD

CHAPTER 28 SYPHILIS 195
Clayton B. Green, MD, PhD, and
James E. Fitzpatrick, MD

CHAPTER 29 HANSEN'S DISEASE (LEPROSY) 201
Kehua Li, MD, and Loren E. Golitz, MD

CHAPTER 30 MYCOBACTERIAL INFECTIONS 207
Genevieve L. Egnatios, MD, and
Karen E. Warschaw, MD

CHAPTER 31 SUPERFICIAL FUNGAL INFECTIONS 216
Richard A. Keller, MD, and
Deborah B. Henderson, MD, MPH

CHAPTER 32 DEEP FUNGAL INFECTIONS 224
Larisa S. Speetzen, MD, and
Karen E. Warschaw, MD

CHAPTER 33 PARASITIC INFESTATIONS 234
Jeffrey J. Meffert, MD

CHAPTER 34 ARTHROPOD BITES AND STINGS 241
C. Paul Sayers, MD

V **CUTANEOUS MANIFESTATIONS
OF INTERNAL DISEASES** **251**

CHAPTER 35 CUTANEOUS MANIFESTATIONS OF INTERNAL
MALIGNANCY 252
Simone A. Ince, MD, and John L. Aeling, MD

CHAPTER 36 CUTANEOUS MANIFESTATIONS OF
ENDOCRINOLOGIC DISEASE 260
Shayla Francis, MD, and Carl F. Bigler, MD

CHAPTER 37 SKIN SIGNS OF GASTROINTESTINAL DISEASE 267
Christina S. O'Hara, MSIII, 2LT MC, and
Paul M. Benson, MD, COL (Ret), MC

CHAPTER 38 CUTANEOUS MANIFESTATIONS OF RENAL
DISEASE 274
Todd T. Kobayashi, MD, Lt Col, USAF, MC,
and Kathleen M. David-Bajar, MD

CHAPTER 39 CUTANEOUS MANIFESTATIONS OF AIDS 280
George W. Turiansky, MD, COL, MC, USA,
and William D. James, MD

CHAPTER 40 CUTANEOUS SIGNS OF NUTRITIONAL
DISTURBANCES 287
Carl W. Demidovich, MD

VI **BENIGN TUMORS OF THE SKIN** **293**

CHAPTER 41 BENIGN MELANOCYTIC TUMORS 294
Michael R. Campoli, MD, PhD, and
Patrick Walsh, MD

CHAPTER 42 VASCULAR AND LYMPHATIC NEOPLASMS 301
Joseph G. Morelli, MD

CHAPTER 43 FIBROUS TUMORS OF THE SKIN 305
James E. Fitzpatrick, MD

VII **MALIGNANT TUMORS OF THE SKIN** **311**

CHAPTER 44 COMMON CUTANEOUS MALIGNANCIES 312
Mariah Ruth Brown, MD, and
Milton J. Schleve, MD

CHAPTER 45 MALIGNANT MELANOMA 319
Michael R. Campoli, MD, PhD, and
Patrick Walsh, MD

CHAPTER 46 LEUKEMIC AND LYMPHOMATOUS INFILTRATES
OF THE SKIN 331
Theresa R. Pacheco, MD

CHAPTER 47 UNCOMMON MALIGNANT TUMORS OF
THE SKIN 339
Renata Prado, MD, and
J. Ramsey Mellette, MD

CHAPTER 48 CUTANEOUS METASTASES 346
Martin B. Giandoni, MD, and
James E. Fitzpatrick, MD

VIII **TREATMENT OF SKIN DISORDERS** **351**

CHAPTER 49 SUNSCREENS AND PREVENTION OF
SKIN CANCER 352
Joseph Yohn, MD

CHAPTER 50 TOPICAL STEROIDS 358
T. Minsue Chen, MD

CHAPTER 51 FUNDAMENTALS OF CUTANEOUS SURGERY 364
Dieter K.T. Schmidt, MD, FAAD, FACMS

CHAPTER 52 CRYOSURGERY 371
Mariah Ruth Brown, MD, and
Milton J. Schleve, MD

CHAPTER 53 MOHS SURGERY 374
Mariah Ruth Brown, MD, and
J. Ramsey Mellette, MD

CHAPTER 54 LASERS IN DERMATOLOGY 378
Stephen W. Eubanks, MD

CHAPTER 55 THERAPEUTIC PHOTOMEDICINE 386
Todd T. Kobayashi, MD, Lt Col, USAF, MC,
and Paul B. Thompson, MD

CHAPTER 56 RETINOIDS 393
James E. Fitzpatrick, MD

IX **SPECIAL PATIENT POPULATIONS** **399**

CHAPTER 57 NEONATAL INFECTIONS 400
Elizabeth R. Shurnas, MD

CHAPTER 58 PEDIATRIC DERMATOLOGY 404
            Joseph G. Morelli, MD

CHAPTER 59 GERIATRIC DERMATOLOGY 409
            James E. Fitzpatrick, MD

CHAPTER 60 DERMATOSES OF PREGNANCY 416
            Misha D. Miller, MD, FACOG

CHAPTER 61 DISORDERS OF THE FEMALE GENITALIA 422
            Misha D. Miller, MD, FACOG

CHAPTER 62 SPECIAL CONSIDERATIONS IN SKIN OF COLOR 427
            Whitney A. High, MD, JD, MEng, and Nadja Y.
            Grammer-West, MD, COL, MC, USA

CHAPTER 63 CULTURAL DERMATOLOGY 435
            Scott A. Norton, MD, MPH, COL, MC, USA,
            and James E. Fitzpatrick, MD

X EMERGENCIES AND MISCELLANEOUS
   PROBLEMS 441

CHAPTER 64 DERMATOLOGIC EMERGENCIES 442
            Scott D. Bennion, MS, MD

CHAPTER 65 OCCUPATIONAL DERMATOLOGY 452
            Leslie A. Stewart, MD

CHAPTER 66 PSYCHOCUTANEOUS DISEASES 456
            Margaret E. Muldrow, MD, and
            James E. Fitzpatrick, MD

CHAPTER 67 APPROACHING THE PRURITIC PATIENT 461
            Theresa R. Pacheco, MD

CHAPTER 68 NAIL DISORDERS 467
            Brian J. Gerondale, MD, and
            Daniel C. Dapprich, MD

CHAPTER 69 DERMATOLOGIC TRIVIA 473
            James E. Fitzpatrick, MD

TOP 100 SECRETS

These secrets are 100 of the top board alerts. They summarize the concepts, principles, and most salient details of dermatologic pathology, diagnosis, and therapy.

1. Langerhans cells are antigen-presenting cells found in the epidermis; they are responsible for immune surveillance.
2. Apocrine glands, which are found in the highest concentration in the axillae and genital regions, produce odorless sweat that is acted on by bacteria to produce body odor.
3. Meissner corpuscles (touch) and Pacinian corpuscles (vibration) are the two primary encapsulated nerve receptors in the skin.
4. The Koebner phenomenon is produced by superficial trauma to the epidermis, causing certain preexisting skin diseases (e.g., psoriasis, lichen planus, lichen nitidus) to form at the site of trauma.
5. Lichen simplex chronicus is a secondary lesion consisting of a focal area of thickened skin with accentuated skin markings produced by chronic scratching or rubbing.
6. Maculopapular eruptions are most commonly seen with viral exanthems and drug-induced reactions.
7. In experienced hands, microscopic examination of KOH-treated clinical material (epidermal scale, hair, nails) is more sensitive than cultures for establishing the diagnosis of a dermatophyte infection.
8. Tzanck preparations are useful for quickly establishing the diagnosis of either varicella-zoster virus or herpes simplex virus infection but cannot distinguish between the two.
9. Nontreponemal test antibody titers (e.g., Venereal Disease Research Laboratory [VDRL]) are reported in the form of a titer and correlate with disease activity in syphilis. Adequately treated patients demonstrate low or negative titers. Treponemal tests (e.g., fluorescent treponemal antibody–absorption [FTA-ABS]) can be positive in both treated and untreated patients with syphilis. The test may revert to negative in some patients after treatment or remain positive indefinitely.
10. Topical emollients containing glycolic acid, lactic acid, urea, and glycerin are the mainstay of therapy in mild disorders of keratinization. In severe disorders of keratinization, oral retinoids are the most effective therapy.
11. Multiple Lisch nodules are pathognomonic of neurofibromatosis type 1 (NF-1). Multiple café-au-lait macules are the earliest skin sign of NF-1, occurring in approximately 80% of affected babies by the end of the first year of life. Neurofibromatosis type 2 most commonly presents with deafness or tinnitus related to underlying vestibular schwannomas.
12. Hypomelanotic macules are a useful diagnostic skin sign for tuberous sclerosis in infants with seizures.
13. Psoriasis classically has symmetrical red plaques with silver-white scale on elbows, and knees. Nail changes in psoriasis can mimic those seen with a dermatophyte fungal infection. Guttate psoriasis is more common in childhood than in later life.
14. Pityriasis rubra pilaris is characterized by large areas of orange-red–colored plaques with islands of sparing and thickened skin of the hands and feet.
15. Seborrheic dermatitis can be found not only on the scalp, but also on the face around the nares, on the central chest, in the axillae, and even on the genitalia.
16. Pityriasis rosea has oval papules and plaques that tend to arise along skin lines ("Christmas tree" pattern) with trailing scale (scale does not reach the end of the lesion).
17. The "two-pajama" treatment brings rapid relief to children with severe atopic dermatitis.
18. Eighty percent of contact dermatitis reactions are due to irritation, and 20% are due to allergic causes. Location of the dermatitis can help identify the causative agent. Patch testing is the only way to distinguish between allergic and irritant contact dermatitis.
19. Naproxen is the drug most commonly associated with pseudoporphyria. Vancomycin is the drug most commonly associated with drug-induced linear IgA bullous dermatosis.
20. Erythema toxicum neonatorum, a common pustular eruption of the neonate, is associated with peripheral eosinophilia in 20% of cases.
21. Cephalosporins are the most common drugs that produce generalized pustular drug eruptions (acute generalized exanthematous pustulosis).
22. The primary lesion of lichen planus is a flat-topped, pruritic, purple polygonal papule. Lichen planus may be clinically and histologically mimicked by numerous drugs (lichenoid drug eruptions).
23. In localized granuloma annulare, the lesions spontaneously resolve in 50% to 80% of patients within 2 years.
24. Rheumatoid nodules occur in 25% of patients with rheumatoid arthritis. Pseudorheumatoid nodules (deep granuloma annulare) most commonly occur as subcutaneous nodules in children and are not associated with rheumatoid arthritis.
25. Wegener's granulomatosis is strongly associated (up to 90% of cases) with antibodies cytoplasmic antineutrophil cytoplasmic antibody (c-ANCA) directed against serine proteinase 3, an enzyme found in the cytoplasm of neutrophils. High titers correlate with increased disease activity.
26. The four primary functions of the skin are: 1) barrier function and prevention of desiccation, 2) immune surveillance, 3) temperature control, and 4) cutaneous sensation.

27. "Pinch purpura," caused by amyloid deposition in blood vessel walls, is seen in systemic amyloidosis. Macroglossia may also be associated with systemic amyloidosis.

28. Thick plaques on the anterior shin in a patient with Graves' disease is a typical finding in pretibial myxedema.

29. Calciphylaxis should be considered in the differential diagnosis of painful infarctive ulcerations in a patient with chronic renal failure.

30. In patients with erythropoietic protoporphyria, the red blood cells demonstrate fleeting fluorescence when examined with direct immunofluorescence. In patients with porphyria cutanea tarda, urine fluoresces a coral red color when examined under a Wood's light.

31. Oculocutaneous albinism–1 (OCA-1) is due to inactive or missing melanocyte tyrosinase. It is characterized by a complete lack of cutaneous pigmentation, depigmented iris and retina, foveal hypoplasia, misrouted optic chiasm nerve fibers, and nystagmus.

32. Vitiligo is characterized by enlarging depigmented patches on the hands, elbows, and knees. Skin biopsy of a depigmented area reveals normal histology except for complete absence of epidermal melanocytes.

33. Tinea versicolor (TV) is characterized by hyper- or hypopigmented scaly patches on the chest and back. Microscopic analysis of lesional scales reveals multiple, short, blunt hyphae, and yeast. TV is due to overgrowth of normal flora, *Pityrosporum* (*Malassezia globosa*) yeast. It is often aggravated by heat and humidity.

34. Erythema ab igne is characterized by hyperpigmentation due to repeated heat exposure of the skin. No treatment is necessary as long as the patient stops using the heating pad. The hyperpigmentation will resolve in several months to a year.

35. Panniculitis is inflammation of the fat due to a wide variety of causes. Clinical clues, such as duration and location of the lesions, presence of ulcers, and association with systemic disease, can help in the initial evaluation. A deep incisional biopsy, including a wide base of fat, may be a critical evaluative tool.

36. Congenital ichthyosiform erythroderma and lamellar ichthyosis are the two disorders of keratinization that are most likely to present as a collodion baby.

37. In acne, the pilosebaceous unit is the target of disease. The microcomedone is the earliest lesion. Comedonal lesions should be treated with a topical retinoid. For inflammatory acne (red papules, pustules, or nodules), a topical or oral antibiotic should be used with a keratolytic and a benzoyl peroxide gel to minimize antibiotic resistance. Do not use antibiotics alone for acne vulgaris.

38. Perioral dermatitis is often caused by the inappropriate use of topical corticosteroids; always obtain a history of topical medication use.

39. Rosacea is common in fair-skinned caucasian adults. Reassure patients that treatment is available and that rhinophyma (W.C. Fields nose) is rare, especially in women. Fifty percent of rosacea patients will have some eye involvement; always obtain a history of eye symptoms and examine this area.

40. Dermatomyositis may present with normal muscle findings. This uncommon presentation is called amyopathic dermatomyositis or dermatomyositis sine myositis. Adult patients with dermatomyositis should have age-appropriate cancer screening, and women should be screened for ovarian carcinoma. Cancer screening is not necessary for pediatric-aged patients.

41. Acute urticaria is usually from a secondary cause such as an allergic reaction to food, drugs, insect stings, or infection. Chronic urticaria is most often idiopathic and not due to an allergic etiology but has an autoimmune basis in up to 50% of cases. The most common physical urticaria is dermographism, but in chronic urticaria, screen for physical stimuli such as pressure, cold, and heat.

42. For angioedema without urticaria, screen for both hereditary and acquired angioedema by obtaining a C4 level.

43. The STAR complex is a viral infection presenting as rash, pharyngitis, and monoarticular arthritis (**s**ore **t**hroat, **a**rthritis, and **r**ash).

44. Parvovirus B19 is the cause of slapped cheeks (Fifth's disease), and purpuric gloves and socks syndrome.

45. Most people with genital herpes do not know that they have it. Herpes simplex virus (HSV) infection may involve and recur at any location on the mucocutaneous surface.

46. Most human papillomavirus (HPV) infections are not carcinogenic, but persistent infections with some genotypes, especially HPV-16 and HPV-18, are associated with a high risk of epithelial neoplasia.

47. Epidermolysis bullosa is an inherited group of disorders characterized by genetic defects of structural proteins needed for the normal attachment and integrity of the epidermis.

48. The Jarisch-Herxheimer reaction is an acute febrile reaction, associated with shaking, chills, malaise, sore throat, myalgia, headache, and localized inflammation of infected mucocutaneous sites. It may occur 6 to 8 hours after penicillin treatment for infection, especially syphilis.

49. Leprosy is a chronic granulomatous infection caused by *Mycobacterium leprae*, affecting primarily skin and peripheral nerves. The nine-banded armadillo (*Dasypus novemcinctus*) carries *Mycobacterium leprae* and probably serves as the source of some cases of leprosy in Texas and parts of Louisiana.

50. Cutaneous tuberculosis has a broad clinical spectrum depending on the route of infection, virulence of the organism, and immune status of the host. Lupus vulgaris and scrofuloderma, although rare, are the two most common forms of cutaneous tuberculosis. *M. tuberculosis* can be diagnosed using acid-fast bacilli stains, culture, or polymerase chain reaction.

51. Deep fungal infections can be divided into subcutaneous (localized), systemic, and opportunistic categories. Localized fungal infections are due to local injury and implantation of the organism. Opportunistic fungal infections are increasingly common because of the rise in the number of organ transplant patients and human immunodeficiency virus (HIV) infection.

52. Creeping eruption (cutaneous larva migrans) occurs when the larvae of dog and cat hookworms (*Ancylostoma caninum* and *A. braziliense*) penetrate intact, exposed skin and begin migrating through the epidermis.

53. Attached ticks are best removed with traction, using blunt-angled forceps applied to the tick parts closest to the skin.
54. Patients with biopsy-proven Sweet's syndrome should have a complete blood count to evaluate for an underlying hematologic malignancy.
55. Acanthosis nigricans is a common condition, and most cases are associated with obesity and insulin resistance.
56. Any refractory eczematous eruption on the breast should be biopsied to exclude mammary Paget's disease. The diagnosis of extramammary Paget's disease should prompt a careful evaluation for underlying gastrointestinal and genitourinary adenocarcinoma.
57. The presence of one or more xanthomas on the skin usually indicates an abnormality of lipid metabolism or, less commonly, a monoclonal gammopathy. The presence of eruptive xanthomas always indicates high levels of triglycerides. Patients with eruptive xanthomas are at increased risk to develop pancreatitis.
58. Bilirubin has a strong affinity for elastic-rich tissue, which accounts for its preferential accumulation in the sclera of the eyes.
59. Pyoderma gangrenosum is strongly associated with Crohn's disease and ulcerative colitis. Surgical intervention in active pyoderma gangrenosum is contraindicated because it may produce extension of the ulcer.
60. Uremic frost is the presence of white deposits in the head and neck area in patients with severe renal failure. The pruritus of renal failure often responds to ultraviolet light B (UVB) therapy.
61. Small vascular lesions called angiokeratoma corporis diffusum are typically found in a bathing suit distribution in Fabry's disease.
62. Nephrogenic fibrosing dermopathy is a recently described disease characterized by papules, plaques, and thickened skin of the trunk and extremities. It is associated with impaired renal function from many different causes.
63. Papulosquamous eruptions are defined by an inflammatory reaction consisting of red or purple papules or plaques with scale.
64. Oral hairy leukoplakia is a manifestation of Epstein-Barr virus infection.
65. Pellagra (due to deficiency of niacin and/or nicotinic acid) is most common in patients with corn-rich diets, alcoholism, gastrointestinal (GI) disease, carcinoid, and some drugs. The four classic symptoms start with the letter D: diarrhea, dermatitis, dementia, death. Casal's necklace is the distinctive photosensitive eruption that presents around the neck.
66. Malignancy in a small congenital melanocytic nevus does not occur before puberty and overall is minimal.
67. Capillary hemangiomas are the most common vascular tumor of childhood.
68. Pyogenic granulomas are neither pyogenic nor granulomatous; they are neovascularizations, presenting as acute-onset, friable vascular papules that bleed frequently.
69. Direct immunofluorescence of perilesional skin is required in many cases to rule in or exclude the diagnosis of an autoimmune bullous disorder.
70. The majority of nonmelanoma skin cancers are on the face. One half are on the nose.
71. Breslow depth measurement levels are more accurate prognostic indicators than Clark's level in malignant melanomas. The presence of in-transit metastases or satellite lesions indicates a worse prognosis than limited nodal metastases. There is currently no effective single-agent therapy for advanced melanoma.
72. Mycosis fungoides is a low-grade T-cell lymphoma with a median survival of 12 years for patients with patch or plaque stage disease. Management of mycosis fungoides is best accomplished by the involvement of several specialties, such as dermatology, dermatopathology/pathology, hematology/oncology, and radiation oncology.
73. Angiosarcoma, characterized as an erythematous or hemorrhagic macule or plaque, presents in three clinical settings: on the face and scalp of the elderly, in the setting of chronic lymphedema (Stewart-Treves syndrome), and in previously irradiated tissue.
74. Merkel cell carcinoma has a characteristic paranuclear "dot" that stains with cytokeratin but may be confused histologically with oat-cell carcinoma of the lung, malignant lymphoma, sweat gland carcinoma, metastatic carcinoid tumors, and Ewing's sarcoma.
75. Microcystic adnexal carcinoma recurs frequently due to perineural invasion and classically presents on the upper lip (although it may be seen elsewhere on the face and beyond).
76. Dermatofibrosarcoma protuberans stains positively for the human hematopoietic progenitor cell antigen CD-34 and is histologically characterized by intersecting bundles of spindle-shaped cells with a characteristic storiform (cartwheel) arrangement.
77. Approximately 9% of all patients who die from internal malignancy will demonstrate metastatic tumors in the skin. Sister Mary Joseph's nodule is the name applied to metastatic tumor in the umbilicus. It is most commonly seen in intraabdominal malignancies and is a poor prognostic sign.
78. Physicians should teach patients two basic concepts about skin cancer prevention: sun protection and self-examination of skin.
79. Phototoxic reactions clinically and symptomatically resemble sunburn, while photoallergic reactions resemble dermatitis.
80. The safe total maximum dose of 1% lidocaine for adults is 7 mg/kg, if combined with epinephrine, and 4.5 mg/kg, if given without epinephrine. The earliest signs of lidocaine toxicity include talkativeness, tinnitus, metallic taste, lightheadedness, diplopia, and circumoral pallor.
81. Buffering an anesthetic solution with 8.4% sodium bicarbonate in order to diminish the pain of injection will also shorten its duration of action.
82. Suture size does not correspond to a specific diameter, but rather to a specific tensile strength.
83. Pigmentation is determined by the type of melanin synthesized and the amount distributed to the surrounding keratinocytes.

84. Mohs micrographic surgery utilizes frozen sections of fresh tissue. It is indicated for tumor extirpation in zones of the face known to have high recurrence rates (e.g., nasolabial fold, nasal ala, medial canthus, pinna, postauricular sulcus). It offers cure rates of 99% for primary basal cell cancers and 95% for recurrent tumors.

85. Carbon dioxide and erbium:YAG lasers are used for tissue ablation.

86. Erythema nodosum is the most common cause of panniculitis.

87. Black tattoos are removed with the Q-switched 1064-nm Nd:YAG, the Q-switched alexandrite, and the Q-switched ruby lasers. Green tattoo pigment is removed only by the Q-switched alexandrite laser. Red tattoo pigment is removed only with the Q-switched 532-nm Nd:YAG laser.

88. PUVA is the acronym for psoralen plus ultraviolet light, type A.

89. Retinoids are structural analogs of vitamin A (retinol). Their most important functions include tissue differentiation (especially epithelial tissues), general growth, visual function, and reproduction. Systemic retinoids are potent teratogenic drugs.

90. The TORCHES infections are **t**oxoplasmosis; **o**ther (varicella-zoster virus, parvovirus B19); **r**ubella; **c**ytomegalovirus; **h**erpes simplex virus and HIV; **e**nteroviruses and Epstein-Barr virus; and **s**yphilis.

91. The three common causes of acquired circumscribed hair loss are alopecia areata, tinea capitis, and trichotillomania. A circular, scaly, or crusted bald spot on the scalp of a black child should be considered tinea capitis until proven otherwise. When a solitary lesion of alopecia areata is small, no treatment may be needed. The prognosis for such a lesion is excellent, and spontaneous regrowth often occurs.

92. Xerosis (dry skin, asteatosis, dermatitis hiemalis) is the most common geriatric dermatosis and the most common cause of pruritus in elderly patients.

93. Pruritic urticarial papules and plaques of pregnancy are the most common specific dermatosis of pregnancy.

94. Black skin manifests minor physiologic differences, including a stratum corneum with increased layers and cohesiveness and a decreased ability to synthesize vitamin D3.

95. Contact dermatitis is the most common form of occupational skin disease. Irritants cause 75% of occupationally induced contact dermatitis, while allergens are responsible for 25%. Treatment includes allergen and irritant avoidance, protective clothing, moisturizers, and topical steroids.

96. Gottron's papules (erythematous to violaceous papules over the knuckles) are a cutaneous finding that is pathognomic of dermatomyositis.

97. Most viral exanthems are morbilliform.

98. The initial approach to the pruritic patient should focus on identifying and treating a primary skin disorder. If no obvious cause is found, look for evidence of systemic disease.

99. Bullous impetigo is always caused by *Streptococcus aureus* strains, usually phage II, type 71, that produce exfoliative toxins.

100. Syphilis is caused by the spirochete *Treponema pallidum* ssp. *pallidum*.

I

GENERAL

STRUCTURE AND FUNCTION OF THE SKIN

Scott D. Bennion, MS, MD

1. Name the three layers of the skin. What composes them?

The epidermis, dermis, and subcutis (subcutaneous fat). The **epidermis** is the outermost layer and is composed primarily of keratinocytes, or epidermal cells. Beneath the epidermis lies the **dermis**, which is composed primarily of collagen but also contains adnexal structures, including the hair follicles, sebaceous glands, apocrine glands, and eccrine glands. Numerous blood vessels, lymphatics, and nerves also traverse the dermis. Below the dermis lies the **subcutis**, or subcutaneous layer, which consists of adipose tissue, larger blood vessels, and nerves. The subcutis may also contain the base of hair follicles and sweat glands (Fig. 1-1).

2. How many layers are there in the epidermis? How are they organized?

The epidermis has four layers: the basal cell layer, spiny cell layer, granular cell layer, and cornified layer (Fig. 1-2). The basal cell layer (**stratum basalis**) is composed of columnar or cuboidal cells that are in direct contact with the basement membrane, the structure that separates the dermis from the epidermis. The basal cell layer contains the germinative cells, and, for this reason, occasional mitoses may be present.

The three layers above the basal cell layer are histologically distinct and demonstrate differentiation of the keratinocytes as they move toward the skin surface and become "cornified." Just above the basal cell layer is the spiny cell layer (**stratum spinosum**), so called because of a high concentration of desmosomes and keratin filaments that give the cells a characteristic "spiny" appearance (Fig. 1-3A). Above the spiny layer is the granular cell layer (**stratum granulosum**). In this layer, keratohyalin granules are formed and bind to the keratin filaments (tonofilaments) to form large electron-dense masses within the cytoplasm that give this layer its "granular" appearance.

The outermost layer is the cornified layer (**stratum corneum**), where the keratinocytes abruptly lose all of their organelles and nuclei. The keratin filaments and keratohyalin granules form an amorphous mass within the keratinocytes, which become elongated and flattened, forming a lamellar array of "corneocytes." The corneocytes are held together by the remnants of the desmosomes (dense bodies) and a "cementing substance" released into the intracellular space from organelles called Odland bodies.

3. Do other types of cells normally occur in the epidermis?

In addition to keratinocytes, three other cells are normally found in the epidermis. The **melanocyte**, the most common, is a dendritic cell situated in the basal cell layer. There are approximately 36 keratinocytes for each melanocyte. This cell's function is to synthesize and secrete melanin-containing organelles called melanosomes.

The next most common cell is the **Langerhans cell**, which is a bone marrow–derived, antigen-presenting cell that has very important immune surveillance functions. On light microscopy, these dendritic cells are primarily distributed in the stratum spinosum. Langerhans cells were first described by Paul Langerhans in 1868 while he was still a medical student.

Also located in the epidermis in small numbers are **Merkel cells**. The function of these cells is not fully established, but they are frequently in contact with nerve fibrils. Ultrastructurally, Merkel cells contain electron-dense bodies that are also found in APUD (amino acid precursor uptake and decarboxylation) cells of endocrine glands.

4. What is apocopation?

Apocopation is the process by which melanocytes transfer melanosomes to keratinocytes. In this process, the tips of the melanocytic dendritic processes are phagocytized by the keratinocytes.

5. Describe the structure of the basement membrane zone (BMZ).

The BMZ is not normally visible by light microscopy in sections stained with hematoxylin-eosin but can be visualized as a homogeneous band measuring 0.5 to 1.0 mm thick on periodic acid–Schiff staining. Ultrastructural studies and immunologic mapping demonstrate that the BMZ is an extremely complex structure consisting of many components that function to attach the basal cell layer to the dermis (Fig. 1-3B). Uppermost in the BMZ are the cytoplasmic tonofilaments of the basal cells, which attach to the basal plasma membrane of the cells at the hemidesmosome. The hemidesmosome is attached to the lamina lucida and lamina densa of the BMZ via anchoring filaments. The BMZ, in turn, is anchored to the dermis by anchoring fibrils that intercalate among the collagen fibers of the dermis and secure the BMZ to the dermis. The importance of these structures in maintaining skin integrity is demonstrated by diseases such as epidermolysis bullosa, in which they are congenitally missing or damaged.

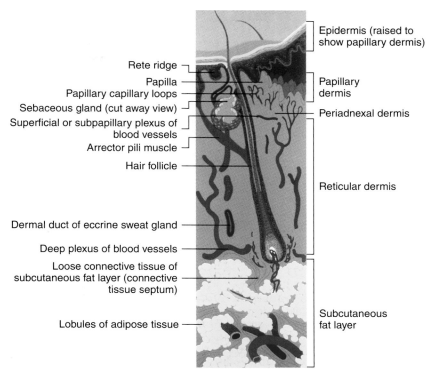

Epidermis (raised to show papillary dermis)

Rete ridge

Papilla

Papillary capillary loops

Sebaceous gland (cut away view)

Superficial or subpapillary plexus of blood vessels

Arrector pili muscle

Hair follicle

Papillary dermis

Periadnexal dermis

Reticular dermis

Dermal duct of eccrine sweat gland

Deep plexus of blood vessels

Loose connective tissue of subcutaneous fat layer (connective tissue septum)

Lobules of adipose tissue

Subcutaneous fat layer

Figure 1-1. Structure of the skin.

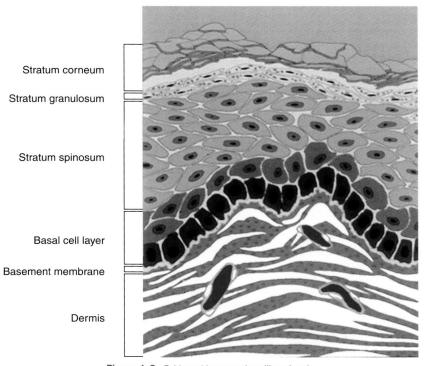

Stratum corneum

Stratum granulosum

Stratum spinosum

Basal cell layer

Basement membrane

Dermis

Figure 1-2. Epidermal layers and papillary dermis.

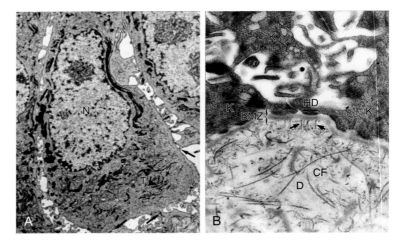

Figure 1-3. A, Keratinocyte. An electron micrograph illustrates the ultrastructural components of a typical keratinocyte in the stratum spinosum, including the nucleus (*N*), tonofilaments (*T*), and desmosomal intercellular connections (*arrow*) that give this layer its "spiny" appearance. **B,** Basement membrane zone (*BMZ*). At the interface of the basal keratinocytes (*K*) of the epidermis and dermis (*D*) is the BMZ. The keratinocytes are attached to the BMZ by hemidesmosomes (*HD*). The BMZ is composed of the lamina lucida, which is the upper clear area, and the lamina densa, which is the dark area just below the lamina lucida. Anchoring fibrils (*arrows*) bind the BMZ to the dermis by intercalating among the collagen fibers (*CF*) of the dermis.

6. How is the structure of the epidermis related to its functions?

The three most important functions of the epidermis are protection from environmental insult (barrier function), prevention of desiccation, and immune surveillance. The stratum corneum is an especially important cutaneous barrier that protects the body from toxins and desiccation. Although many toxins are nonpolar compounds that can move relatively easily through the lipid-rich intracellular spaces of the cornified layer, the tortuous route among cells in this layer and the layers below effectively forms a barrier to environmental toxins. Ultraviolet light, another environmental source of damage to living cells, is effectively blocked in the stratum corneum and the melanosomes. The melanosomes are concentrated above the nucleus of the keratinocytes in an umbrella-like fashion, providing photoprotection for both epidermal nuclear DNA and the dermis.

The prevention of **desiccation** is another extremely important function, as extensive loss of epidermis is often fatal (e.g., toxic epidermal necrolysis). In the normal epidermis, the water content decreases as one moves from the basal layer to the surface, comprising 70% to 75% of weight at the base and decreasing to 10% to 15% at the bottom of the stratum corneum.

Immune surveillance against foreign antigens is a function of the Langerhans cells that are dispersed among the keratinocytes. Langerhans cells internalize external antigens and process these antigens for presentation to T lymphocytes in the lymph nodes. Inflammatory cells (i.e., neutrophils, eosinophils, lymphocytes) are also capable of intercepting and destroying microorganisms in the epidermis.

7. What structural components of the epidermis are involved in blistering diseases?

In the epidermis, the keratinocytes are bound to each other by desmosomal complex. These complexes consist of the desmosome and the tonofilaments of the cytoplasm that are made of cytokeratins. In the upper stratum spinosum, the tonofilaments are composed mainly of keratins 1 and 10. Congenital abnormalities in these keratins produce structural weakness between keratinocytes, producing a disease called **congenital bullous ichthyosiform erythroderma** (epidermolytic hyperkeratosis). Abnormalities in keratin types 5 (KRT5) and 14 (KRT14) in the basal cell layers lead to a mild blistering disease named **epidermolysis bullosa simplex** (EBS) (Fig. 1-4). **Pemphigus** is an acquired group of blistering diseases of the epidermis in which autoantibodies directed against antidesmosomal proteins produce damage to the desmosomes.

The skin diseases associated with antibodies and damage to the desmosomes and their characteristics are listed in Table 1-1.

8. Are there hereditary diseases of the BMZ and dermis that cause blistering and damage to the skin?

Yes. There is a complex group of inherited diseases in which the skin is friable and bullous lesions occur, often with subsequent scarring. The two subgroups within this group are junctional epidermolysis bullosas (JEBs) and dystrophic epidermolysis bullosas (DEBs). Like the EBS diseases, which affect the epidermal layers, these diseases occur because the vital structural elements of the BMZ and dermis are missing, causing the skin to separate easily and blister. In JEBs, the separation occurs within the lamina lucida (LL) of the BMZ. Decreased amounts or abnormalities in the LL components, such as laminins I and V, 19-DEJ-1 protein, XII collagen, plectin, XVII collagen (bullous pemphigoid antigen) and alpha 4 beta 6 integrin have been identified in this group.

In the DEB group, separation occurs below the BMZ in the dermal layer, and a decreased amount or absence of type VII collagen has been noted. As a rule, the deeper in the skin the separation occurs, the more severe the clinical

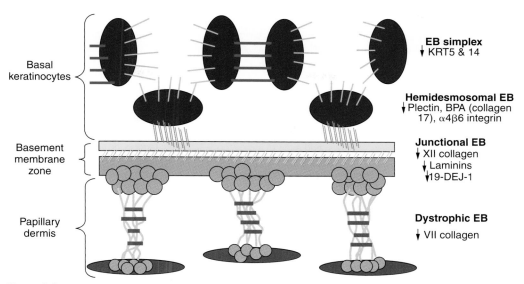

Figure 1-4. This diagram of the dermal epidermal junction illustrates the affected levels in the various types of epidermolysis bullosa (*EB*).

Table 1-1. Diseases Associated with Antibodies and Damage to Desmosomes

DISEASE INVOLVED	CLINICAL APPEARANCE AND LOCATION	MAIN DERMOSOMAL MOLECULES
Pemphigus vulgaris	Oral and diffuse superficial flaccid blisters with ulcers	Desmogleins 1 and 3 (Dsg1 and 3) and plakoglobin
Pemphigus foliaceus	Diffuse superficial blisters and crusting	Desmoglein 1 (Dsg1)
Pemphigus vegetans	Vegetating, weeping lesions in the intertriginous areas	Desmoglein 3 (Dsg3)
Pemphigus erythematosus	Butterfly eruption with blistering in malar areas	Desmoglein 3 (Dsg3)
Paraneoplastic pemphigus	Diffuse erythema multiforme-like painful eruption	Desmoplakins 1 and 2 (Dsg1 and 2), BP antigen 1 (BP230), plectin, desmogleins 1 and 3 (Dsg1 and 3), envoplakin, periplakin
IgA pemphigus	Pustular or vesiculopustular eruption	Desmogleins 1 and 3 (Dsg1 and 3), desmocollin 1

picture with increased scarring and loss of function. DEB patients typically have severe deforming scars and decreased life span (see Fig. 1-4).

9. Are there acquired blistering diseases of the BMZ and dermis?

Yes. There are several diseases in which blistering occurs secondary to disruption of the structures of the BMZ and dermis. As with the epidermal blistering diseases, antibodies to the hemidesmosomes and other structures within the BMZ and dermis cause separation of the skin and blistering. In the uppermost portion of the BMZ, the LL, hemidesmosomes bind the basal keratinocytes to the basement membrane. Bullous pemphigoid (BP) is a classic example of an acquired blistering disease in which antihemidesmosomal antibodies are produced and appear to induce inflammation and subsequent damage of the hemidesmosomes, causing a blister to develop between the cells and the basement membrane.

A partial list of the skin diseases associated with antibodies and damage to the basement membrane structures and dermis are listed in Table 1-2.

10. What abnormalities in structural components of the basement membrane are involved in bullous skin diseases?

Structures within the basement membrane can be congenitally absent or decreased in number, or, as with the epidermal desmosomes, they can be affected by antibodies directed against them. In the uppermost portion of the BMZ, in the lamina lucida, hemidesmosomes bind the basal keratinocytes to the basement membrane.

Table 1-2. Skin Diseases Associated with Antibodies and Damage to Basement Membrane Structures and Dermis

DISEASE	CLINICAL APPEARANCE AND LOCATION	BASEMENT MEMBRANE MOLECULE INVOLVED
Bullous pemphigoid	Tense blisters diffusely	BP antigens 1 (BP230) and 2 (BP180)
Pemphigoid (herpes) gestationis	Urticarial blisters with pruritus in late pregnancy	BP antigen 2 (BP180 or collagen XVII antigen)
Epidermolysis bullosa acquisita	Friable skin and blistering knees, elbows, and sites of increased pressure	Type VII dermal collagen (anchoring fibril antigen)
Bullous lupus erythematosus	Blistering face and trunk with flairs of systemic lupus erythematosus (SLE)	Type VII dermal collagen and lamins 5 and 6
Linear IgA bullous disease (LIBD)	Tense vesicles in annular and target-like patterns on the trunk	BP antigen 2 (BP180 or collagen XVII antigen) and 97 kDa

Bullous pemphigoid is an acquired blistering disease in which antihemidesmosomal antibodies are produced. These antibodies appear to induce inflammation and subsequent damage to the hemidesmosomes, causing a blister to develop between the cells and basement membrane.

11. What is the function of the sebaceous gland?

The sebaceous gland is a holocrine gland that is a part of the pilosebaceous unit. Its function is to produce **sebum**, which is a combination of wax esters, squalene, cholesterol esters, and triglycerides. Sebum is secreted through the sebaceous duct into the hair follicle, where it covers the skin surface, possibly as a protectant. Sebum may also have antifungal properties. Sebaceous glands are located everywhere on the skin except the palms and soles.

Key Points: Anatomy and Function of Skin

1. The skin is composed of an epidermis, dermis, and subcutis (composed mainly of subcutaneous fat).
2. The four primary functions of skin are:
   - Barrier function and prevention of desiccation
   - Immune surveillance
   - Temperature control
   - Cutaneous sensation
3. The main cell types in the epidermis are melanocytes, keratinocytes, Langerhans cells, and Merkel cells.
4. Genetic mutations in critical adhesion molecules cause inherited blistering diseases that are usually evident at birth (e.g., epidermolysis bullosa simplex).
5. Autoimmune diseases characterized by autoantibodies to critical adhesion molecules produce acquired blistering diseases (e.g., pemphigus vulgaris).

---

12. How do the eccrine sweat glands and apocrine sweat glands differ?

Embryologically, eccrine glands derive from the epidermis and are not part of the pilosebaceous unit. The eccrine sweat glands function in temperature regulation via secretion of sweat, a combination of mostly water and electrolytes, which evaporates and cools the skin. Their ducts pass through the dermis and epidermis to empty directly onto the skin surface. Eccrine glands are located everywhere on the skin surface except on modified skin areas, such as the lips, nail beds, and glans penis. Eccrine sweat glands are found only in higher primates and horses.

Apocrine glands originate from the same hair germ that gives rise to the hair follicle and sebaceous gland. The apocrine duct empties into the follicle above the sebaceous gland. Their anachronistic function is to produce scent. They are located primarily in the axillae and perineum, and their activity is sex hormone–dependent. The breast and cerumen glands are both modified apocrine sweat glands.

13. How is the dermis organized?

The dermis is organized into two distinct areas: the papillary dermis and the reticular dermis. The superficial **papillary dermis** is a relatively thin zone beneath the epidermis. On light microscopy, it is composed of thin, delicate collagen fibers and is highly vascularized. The hair follicles are enveloped by a **perifollicular dermis** that is contiguous with, and morphologically resembles, the papillary dermis. Collectively, the papillary dermis and perifollicular dermis are called the **adventitial dermis**, although this term is rarely used in dermatology texts.

The deeper zone is the **reticular dermis**, which comprises the bulk of the dermis. It is less vascular than the papillary dermis and demonstrates thick, well-organized collagen bundles.

14. What are the components of the dermis?

The main cell type in the dermis is the fibroblast. The fibroblast produces the main components of the dermis, including collagen (70% to 80%) for resiliency, elastin (1% to 3%) for elasticity, and proteoglycans to maintain water within the dermis. The bulk of the collagen within the dermis consists of types I and III and is organized into collagen bundles that mostly run horizontally throughout the dermis. The elastic fibers are interspersed among the collagen fibers. Oxytalan fibers are small elastic fibers found primarily in the papillary dermis and are usually oriented perpendicularly to the skin surface. The proteoglycans (primarily hyaluronic acid) comprise the amorphous ground substance around the elastic and collagen fibers.

15. What are the functions of the dermis?

- Temperature regulation through control of cutaneous blood flow and sweating, achieved by the dermal vessels and eccrine sweat glands
- Mechanical protection of underlying structures, achieved primarily by the collagen and hyaluronic acid
- Innervation of the skin that mostly occurs in the dermis and is responsible for cutaneous sensation

16. Which structural component of the dermis is involved in congenital and autoimmune skin diseases?

Collagen. Antibodies against **type VII collagen**, which makes up the anchoring filaments within the dermis, are found in the autoimmune diseases **bullous systemic lupus erythematosus** (SLE) and **acquired epidermolysis bullosa**. Antibodies to laminins 5 and 6, which are also located in the anchoring filaments, are found in bullous SLE patients. The anchoring filaments function to bind the basement membrane to the dermis, and damage to this collagen results in blister formation below the basement membrane. Clinically, blistering damage beneath the basement membrane causes significant scarring in contrast to blisters in the epidermis or above the basement membrane that do not cause scarring. **Congenital epidermolysis bullosa** (EB), in which there is a congenital paucity or absence of type VII collagen and anchoring fibers, can result in severe scarring. The most severe form of this disease, recessive dystrophic EB, is associated with "mitten" deformities of the hands and feet, severe scarring of the upper respiratory and gastrointestinal tracts, and early death (Fig. 1-5A).

Congenital abnormalities in the various collagens in the dermis, especially types I and III, are found in several of the Ehlers-Danlos syndromes. The cutaneous manifestations of these syndromes are hyperextensibility of the skin, easy bruising, and poor healing with resultant wide scar formation (Fig. 1-5B).

17. How does the vasculature of the dermis function in temperature control?

Body temperature is regulated, in part, through control of dermal blood flow. Lowering body temperature is accomplished through increased blood flow in the vascular plexus in the high papillary dermis, allowing heat to be removed through radiation from the skin. The dermal vasculature is composed of a superficial and deep plexus of arterioles and venules that are interconnected by communicating vessels (Fig. 1-6). The incoming blood flow to the superficial capillary plexus in the upper dermis can be decreased by increased smooth muscle tone in the ascending arterioles, or it can be shunted directly from the arterioles to the venous channels in the deeper plexus systems via glomus bodies, which are modified arterioles surrounded by multiple layers of muscle cells. During cold temperatures, decreased papillary blood flow to the papillary dermis, in essence, shunts the blood away from the skin surface and

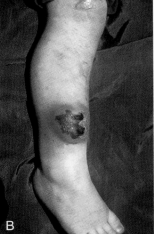

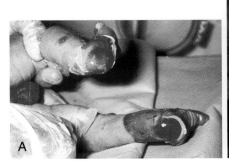

Figure 1-5. A, Epidermolysis bullosa of a newborn. **B,** Ehlers-Danlos syndrome. A large hematoma with poor healing secondary to minor trauma of the lower extremity.

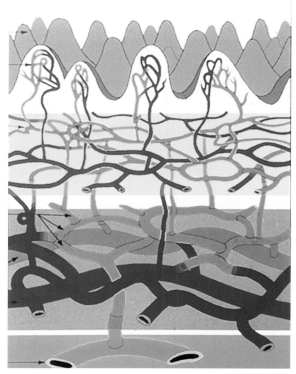

Figure 1-6. Vasculature of the skin.

decreases heat loss from the body. The hot flashes that typically occur in menopausal women are caused by an instability of this system. Periodic dilation of the skin capillaries allows increased blood flow to the skin, which is perceived as heat.

18. How is the skin innervated?

The innervation of the skin recapitulates the blood flow: Large, myelinated, cutaneous branches of the musculocutaneous nerves branch in the subcutaneous tissue to form a deep nerve plexus in the reticular dermis. Nerve fibers from the deep plexus ascend to form a superficial subpapillary plexus. Nerves from these plexuses innervate the skin either as free nerve endings or as corpuscular receptors. The free nerve endings may terminate in the superficial dermis or on Merkel cells in the epidermis. Free nerve endings function as important sensory receptors. They transmit touch, pain, temperature, itch, and mechanical stimuli. These exist in the papillary dermis as individual fibers surrounded by **Schwann's cells**. The other type of receptor in the skin is the **corpuscular receptor**.

19. Name the two main corpuscular (encapsulated) nerve receptors found in the skin.

- **Meissner corpuscle:** Found in highest concentration on the papillary ridge of glabrous skin. It is a touch receptor. Mucocutaneous end organs is the name applied to similar corpuscular nerve receptors found on the areola, labia, glans penis, clitoris, perianal canal, eyelids, and lips.
- **Pacinian corpuscle:** Found in acral areas in the deep dermis and subcutaneous tissue. It has a very distinct capsule associated with multiple lamellated wrapping cells that surround a myelinated axon with an "onion-like" appearance on cross-section. Pacinian corpuscles are mechanoreceptors that respond to vibration.

  Some textbooks list other corpuscular nerve receptors including the Ruffini corpuscle (rare, expanded, myelinated, afferent fibers that connect to collagen in digits), Golgi-Mazzoni corpuscles (laminated like Pacinian corpuscles, found on fingers with simpler organization), and Krause end bulbs (encapsulated myelinated endings found in the papillary dermis).

20. Is loss of cutaneous sensation very serious?

The importance of skin innervation is best illustrated by diseases that destroy cutaneous nerves. The archetypical disease is **Hansen's disease (leprosy)**. This disease attacks and destroys cutaneous nerves, resulting in severe mutilation of the extremities after years of unperceived trauma.

21. How is the subcutis organized?

The subcutis, or subcutaneous fat, is arranged into distinct fat lobules, which are divided by fibrous septae composed primarily of collagen. Blood vessels, nerves, and lymphatics are also found in the fibrous septae. In addition to its role as a caloric reserve, the subcutaneous fat serves as a heat insulator and shock absorber.

BIBLIOGRAPHY

1. Bergstresser PR, Costner MI: Anatomy and physiology. In Bolognia JL, Jorizzo JL, Rapini RP, editors: *Dermatology*, London, 2003, Mosby, pp 25–38.
2. Chan LS: Human skin basement membrane in health and in autoimmune diseases, *Front Biosci* 2:d343–d352, 1997.
3. McGrath JA, Eady RAJ, Pope FM: Anatomy and organization of the human skin. In Burns S, Breathnach SM, Cox N, Griffiths C, editors: *Rook's textbook of dermatology*, ed 7, Malden, MA, 2004, Blackwell, pp 3.1–3.84.

MORPHOLOGY OF PRIMARY AND SECONDARY SKIN LESIONS

Donna M. Corvette, MD

1. Why do dermatologists use words that no one else understands?

The language of dermatology is unique. It encompasses terms that rarely, if ever, are used in other medical specialties. The use of these correct dermatologic terms is important to accurately describe skin lesions to dermatologists during telephone calls and during rounds and teaching. A good description of a skin lesion enables the listener to formulate a series of differential diagnoses, whereas a poor one does not.

2. But why are the descriptions so long?

Use of appropriate terminology and important clues, such as configuration and skin distribution, effectively paints an accurate picture for the listener. Use of vague terms—spot, bump, rash, and lesion—is not helpful. Such vocabulary is counterproductive to formulating an accurate differential diagnoses. "Grouped vesicles on an erythematous base" immediately suggests herpes simplex, and "brown, friable 'stuck-on' papules" accurately describes seborrheic keratoses. "Well-demarcated, erythematous plaques with micaceous, silvery scales located on extensor surfaces" is suggestive of psoriasis. "Violaceous, polygonal papules with Wickham's striae located on flexural surfaces" is consistent with lichen planus. On the other hand, "red, scaly rash on the foot" describes an enormous, nebulous group of disorders.

3. How can I possibly learn the language of dermatology?

First, learn the definitions of the various primary, secondary, and special skin lesions. Each of these groups consists of a short list of terms that specifies basic types. Then, follow this simple template when describing skin lesions:

- Size
- Color or additional descriptive terms (e.g., pigmentation, shape)
- Type of primary, secondary, or special skin lesion (e.g., papule, macule)
- Arrangement (e.g., grouped lesions)
- Distribution (e.g., truncal, generalized)

This template provides a systematic way to add adjectives to the type of lesion. Repetition is key; practice using the template when describing skin lesions.

4. What is a primary skin lesion?

It is the initial lesion that has not been altered by trauma, manipulation (scratching, scrubbing), or natural regression over time. Examples include:

- Macules
- Wheals
- Papules
- Vesicles
- Plaques
- Bullae
- Patches
- Pustules
- Nodules
- Cysts

5. How is each of the primary lesions defined?

See Table 2-1.

6. How do you determine whether a lesion is flat or raised?

Palpation is the most reliable method, but side-lighting also helps. It can be difficult to distinguish a macule from a papule or a patch from a plaque in a photograph.

Table 2-1. Primary Skin Lesions

PRIMARY LESION	DEFINITION	MORPHOLOGY	EXAMPLES
Macule	Flat, circumscribed skin discoloration that lacks surface elevation or depression		Café-au-lait Vitiligo Freckle Junctional nevi Ink tattoo
Papule	Elevated, solid lesion <0.5 cm in diameter		Acrochordon (skin tag) Basal cell carcinoma Molluscum contagiosum
Plaque	Elevated, solid "confluence of papules" (>0.5 cm in diameter) that lacks a deep component		Bowen's disease Mycosis fungoides Psoriasis Eczema Tinea corporis
Patch	Flat, circumscribed skin discoloration; a very large macule		Port wine stain Vitiligo
Nodule	Elevated, solid lesion >0.5 cm in diameter; a larger, deeper papule		Rheumatoid nodule Tendon xanthoma Erythema nodosum Lipoma Metastatic carcinoma

Continued

Table 2-1. Primary Skin Lesions—cont'd

PRIMARY LESION	DEFINITION	MORPHOLOGY	EXAMPLES
Wheal	Firm, edematous plaque that is evanescent and pruritic; a hive		Urticaria Dermographism Urticaria pigmentosa
Vesicle	Papule that contains clear fluid; a blister		Herpes simplex Herpes zoster Dyshidrotic eczema Contact dermatitis
Bulla	Localized fluid collection >0.5 cm in diameter; a large vesicle		Pemphigus vulgaris Bullous pemphigoid Bullous impetigo
Pustule	Papule that contains purulent material		Folliculitis Impetigo Acne Pustular psoriasis
Cyst	Nodule that contains fluid or semisolid material		Acne Epidermal inclusion Trichilemmal cyst

7. How does a primary lesion differ from a secondary lesion?

Secondary skin lesions are created by scratching, scrubbing, or infection. They may also develop normally with time. For example, the primary lesion in a sunburn is a macular erythema (although it could also be a blister), but with resolution, scale and increased pigmentation become prominent. Examples of secondary lesions include:

- Crusts
- Scale
- Ulcers

- Fissures
- Excoriations
- Scars
- Erosions
- Postinflammatory hyperpigmentation

8. How are secondary skin lesions defined?
See Table 2-2.

Table 2-2. Secondary Skin Lesions

SECONDARY LESION	DEFINITION	MORPHOLOGY
Crust	A collection of cellular debris, dried serum, and blood; a scab Antecedent primary lesion is usually a vesicle, bulla, or pustule	
Erosion	A partial focal loss of epidermis; heals without scarring	
Ulcer	A full-thickness, focal loss of epidermis and dermis; heals with scarring	
Fissure	Vertical loss of epidermis and dermis with sharply defined walls; crack in skin	

Continued

Table 2-2. Secondary Skin Lesions—cont'd

SECONDARY LESION	DEFINITION	MORPHOLOGY
Excoriation	Linear erosion induced by scratching	
Scar	A collection of new connective tissue; may be hypertrophic or atrophic Scar implies dermoepidermal damage	
Scale	Thick stratum corneum that results from hyperproliferation or increased cohesion of keratinocytes	

9. What is a maculopapular eruption?

A dermatitic lesion that is composed of both macules and papules. Maculopapular eruptions are commonly seen with viral exanthems and drug-induced reactions. The cutaneous eruption of measles is an example of a maculopapular eruption.

10. Give some examples of special skin lesions.

- Telangiectasias
- Purpura
- Petechiae
- Comedones
- Burrows
- Target lesions

11. What are telangiectasias?

Telangiectasias (Fig. 2-1) are small, dilated, superficial blood vessels (capillaries, arterioles, or venules) that blanch (disappear) with pressure.

12. Are telangiectasias pathognomonic for a certain disease?

No. Telangiectasias may occur in many cutaneous disorders, including collagen vascular diseases such as dermatomyositis, systemic lupus erythematosus, and progressive systemic sclerosis. They are also

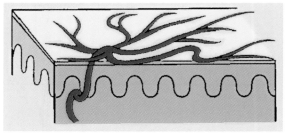

Figure 2-1. Telangiectasia.

commonly seen as a consequence of chronic ultraviolet radiation and topical steroid usage. Telangiectasias may also be seen in tumors such as a noduloulcerative basal cell carcinoma, which is classically described as a pearly colored papule with telangiectasias and central ulceration.

13. What is a burrow?

A burrow (Fig. 2-2) is an elevated channel in the superficial epidermis produced by a parasite, such as the mite *Sarcoptes scabiei*. Scabies burrows characteristically are located on the wrists and in fingerwebs; the diagnosis is confirmed by demonstrating the mite microscopically in skin scrapings. The human hookworm may also produce a serpiginous burrow; however, demonstrating this organism is much more difficult.

14. What is a comedo?

A comedo (Fig. 2-3) is a folliculocentric collection of sebum and keratin. Comedonal acne characteristically consists of both open (blackheads) and closed comedones (whiteheads). When the contents of a closed comedo are exposed to air, a chemical reaction occurs, imparting the black color of an open comedo.

15. What is the difference between petechiae and purpura?

The size of the lesion is the major difference. Both petechiae and purpura result from extravasation of red blood cells into the dermis; hence, they do not blanch with pressure. Petechiae, however, are much smaller than purpura; they are <5 mm in diameter.

16. What are targetoid (target) lesions?

Targetoid lesions typically consist of three zones. The first zone consists of a dark or blistered center (bull's-eye) that is surrounded by a second, pale zone. The third zone consists of a rim of erythema. Target lesions classically are found in patients with erythema multiforme (Fig. 2-4).

17. List some of the additional descriptive adjectives used in dermatology that refer to color or pigmentation.

- **Depigmented:** Absence of melanin, a lack of color. Depigmented macules and patches are commonly found in vitiligo.
- **Hypopigmented:** Lighter than normal skin color; normal number of melanocytes but decreased production of melanin by the melanocytes. The ash-leaf macule of tuberous sclerosis is an example of a hypopigmented macule.
- **Hyperpigmented:** Darker than normal skin color. Junctional nevi and café-au-lait macules (neurofibromatosis) are hyperpigmented macules.
- **Erythematous:** Showing redness of the skin.

18. How do atrophy and lichenification differ?

Atrophy (Fig. 2-5) is thinning of the epidermis, dermis, or subcutis (fat). Epidermal atrophy leads to a fine, cigarette-paper wrinkling of the skin surface,

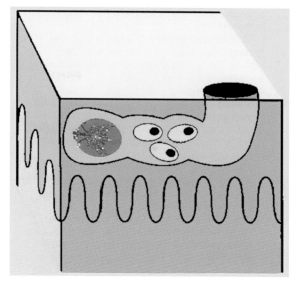

Figure 2-2. Scabies.

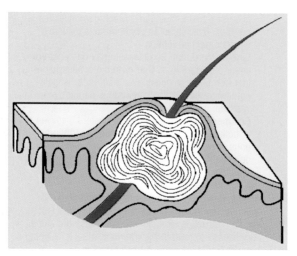

Figure 2-3. Comedo.

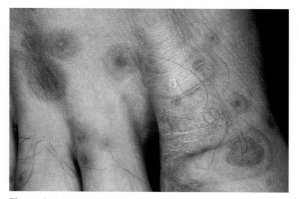

Figure 2-4. Targetoid lesions. Patient with classic erythema multiforme demonstrating lesions resembling a "bull's-eye" Note that some lesions demonstrate a small, centrally placed blister. (Courtesy of the Fitzsimons Army Medical Center teaching files.)

whereas dermal and fat atrophy cause a depression in the skin surface.

A **lichenified lesion** (Fig. 2-6) is a focal area of thickened skin produced by chronic scratching or rubbing. The skin lines are accentuated, resembling a washboard (Fig. 2-7).

19. Do skin diseases have characteristic arrangements or configurations?

Some, but not all, cutaneous diseases demonstrate characteristic arrangements or configurations of lesions. Commonly used adjectives include:

- **Annular:** Used to describe lesions that are ring shaped. Annular plaques are typical findings in granuloma annulare, tinea corporis (ringworm), and erythema marginatum.
- **Gyrate:** From the Latin *gyratus*, which means "to turn around in a circle," gyrate skin lesions are rare presentations. Gyrate erythema that resembles wood grain or topographic maps is seen in erythema gyratum repens, which usually heralds the presence of an internal malignancy.
- **Dermatomal:** Used to describe lesions that follow neurocutaneous dermatomes. The classic example is herpes zoster (shingles), which demonstrates grouped vesicles on an erythematous base in a dermatomal distribution.
- **Linear:** More than 20 diseases may demonstrate linear configurations. One example is allergic contact dermatitis to poison ivy; it characteristically demonstrates linear erythematous papules or vesicles.
- **Grouped:** Papules, pustules, or blisters (vesicles or bullae) may demonstrate grouped configurations. A typical example is herpes simplex, which demonstrates grouped vesicles on an erythematous base.

20. What is the Koebner phenomenon?

Traumatizing the epidermis of a patient with a certain preexisting skin disease will cause the same skin disease to form in the traumatized skin. Noticing this skin finding is helpful when creating a differential diagnosis. Only certain diseases are associated with a Koebner phenomenon; lichen planus, lichen nitidus, and psoriasis (Fig. 2-8) are examples.

21. Do skin diseases characteristically occur in certain locations?

Yes. This is the reason that a complete skin examination should be performed on all patients. Seborrheic dermatitis characteristically occurs on the scalp, nasolabial folds, retroauricular areas, eyelids, eyebrows, and presternal areas; it tends to spare the extremities. Psoriasis may resemble seborrheic dermatitis, but it characteristically demonstrates a different distribution, usually involving the extremities (elbows, knees), intergluteal fold, scalp, and nails.

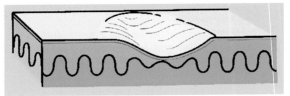

Figure 2-5. Atrophy.

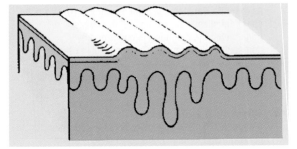

Figure 2-6. Lichenification.

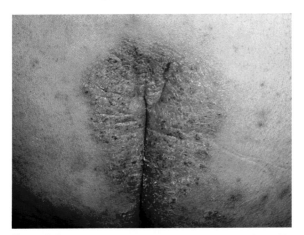

Figure 2-7. Lichen simplex chronicus. Patient with atopic dermatitis and secondary lichenification manifesting as thickened skin with accentuation of skin markings. Secondary excoriations are also present. (Courtesy of the Fitzsimons Army Medical Center teaching files.)

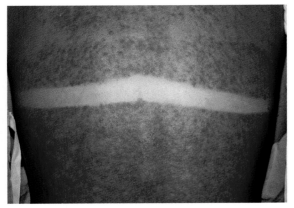

Figure 2-8. Koebner (isomorphic) phenomenon. Patient with acute explosive psoriasis demonstrating restriction of lesions to the site of minor trauma in the form of a sunburn. (Courtesy of the William L. Weston, M.D. collection.)

Key Points: Primary and Secondary Lesions

1. The clinical diagnosis of skin disease is accomplished by a complex appreciation of the primary and secondary skin lesions, distribution, color, arrangement, and body site.
2. Palpation of skin lesions is an underappreciated physical skill that augments the visual clues.
3. Not all lesions can be diagnosed by the initial physical examination and the presence or absence of symptoms (e.g., pruritus, burning); history and clinical course are often required to establish a diagnosis.
4. Not all skin diseases can be diagnosed in a single or even multiple visits.

BIBLIOGRAPHY

1. Cox NH, Coulson IH: Diagnosis of skin disease. In Burns S, Breathnach SM, Cox N, Griffiths C, editors: *Rook's textbook of dermatology*, ed 7, Malden, MA, 2004, Blackwell, pp 5.1–5.10.
2. Rapini R: Clinical and pathologic differential diagnosis. In Bolognia JL, Jorizzo JL, Rapini R, editors: *Dermatology*, London, 2003, Mosby, pp 3–12.

DIAGNOSTIC TECHNIQUES

Stephen Thomas Spates, MD

1. What is the most sensitive office laboratory test for diagnosing dermatophyte infections of the skin?

Microscopic examination of a potassium hydroxide (KOH) preparation of scrapings taken from the affected area is the most sensitive office laboratory test. A study of 220 specimens examined by both KOH and culture demonstrated positive KOH preparations and positive cultures in 45% of samples, a positive KOH preparation and negative culture in 52% of samples, and a negative KOH preparation and a positive culture in only 3% of samples. However, cultures can be useful because other studies have shown a 5% to 15% increase in positive specimens by culturing KOH-negative materials. Moreover, it is important to realize that the diagnostic accuracy of the KOH preparation depends on the skill of the individual performing the test.

Lefler E, Haim S, Merzbach D: Evaluation of direct microscopic examination versus culture in the diagnosis of superficial fungal infections, *Mykosen* 24:102–106, 1981.

2. How is a KOH examination performed?

The highest rate of recovery of organisms occurs in specimens taken from the tops of vesicles, the leading edges of annular lesions, or deep scrapings from the nails suspected to be infected with fungi. The site should be swabbed with an alcohol pad or water and scraped with a no. 15 blade. In some instances, such as the scalp or nail, a curette may be more effective. The moist corneocytes are then easily transferred from the blade to a glass slide. One or two drops of KOH (10% to 20%) are added, and a coverslip is applied to the specimen. The KOH preparation is gently warmed, but not boiled, and then examined under the microscope. It is important to focus back and forth through the material so that the refractile hyphae can be visualized. Fungal hyphae can be recognized by their regular cylindrical shapes with branching and the presence of septae that may demonstrate a subtle greenish hue (Fig. 3-1). A pencil eraser or pen cap gently applied to the surface of the coverslip may enhance keratinocyte breakdown, especially for clumped specimens. If no organisms are observed initially, waiting 10 to 15 minutes may aid visualization.

3. What laboratory tests are useful for diagnosing tinea capitis?

Testing for fluorescence in the affected area using a Wood's light is the quickest technique. If the hair fluoresces yellow-green, then a fungal infection is likely. However, lack of fluorescence does not exclude tinea capitis, because *Trichophyton tonsurans* accounts for 80% to 95% of scalp ringworm infections in the United States, and it does not fluoresce. Therefore, examination of KOH-treated infected hair is more sensitive and can also be rapidly performed. The best results are obtained when broken-off hairs are examined, because these are the ones infected by hyphae and arthrospores. Most dermatophytes, such as *T. tonsurans*, grow within the hair shaft (endothrix), and a few minutes are required to let KOH break down the hair shaft and visualize the infection. Finally, the diagnosis can also be proved by fungal cultures. The easily broken, infected hairs are embedded in the media. The specimen can be obtained using a no. 15 blade, curette, or hemostat.

Lucky AW: Epidemiology, diagnosis, and management of tinea capitis in the 1980s, *Pediatr Dermatol* 2:226–228, 1985.

4. What is a Wood's light or lamp? How is it useful in skin diseases?

A Wood's light produces invisible long-wave ultraviolet radiation, or "black light," at a wavelength of 360 nm. When this light strikes the surface of the skin or urine, fluorescence is produced in some disorders. This fluorescence is best observed in a completely dark room. The Wood's lamp is useful in diagnosing cases of several skin conditions: tinea capitis (see preceding text), tinea versicolor (dull yellow fluorescence), erythrasma (coral red fluorescence; Fig. 3-2), and *Pseudomonas* infections of the skin (green fluorescence). It is also useful as a screening test in porphyria cutanea tarda as the urine fluoresces a coral red color (Fig. 3-3). The Wood's light may also be used in certain disorders of pigmentation. In patients with hyperpigmentation, it is used to localize the site of the pigment because it accentuates superficial epidermal pigment, whereas deeper dermal pigment is unchanged. It is also used in patients with vitiligo because it demonstrates complete depigmentation. Finally, it can be used to delineate the borders of melanocytic lesions, such as lentigo maligna, prior to surgery.

5. Name common culture media used for isolating dermatophytes.

Dermatophyte test media (DTM) and Sabouraud's dextrose agar, with or without antibiotics (e.g., Mycosel agar, Mycobiotic agar), are the two most common types of culture media used. Many dermatologists prefer DTM because it has the advantage of a color indicator that changes the media from yellow to red when a dermatophyte is present. DTM is 95% to

97% accurate in differentiating dermatophytes from nondermatophytes. Sabouraud's dextrose agar is a standard in mycology laboratories and also in many dermatologists' offices. It consists of dextrose (energy source), peptone (protein source), and agar (for a firm surface). Antibiotics can be added to suppress bacterial contaminants, and cycloheximide is added to suppress yeasts and nondermatophytes. Plain Sabouraud's agar is an especially good culture medium for *Candida albicans*.

Taplin D, Zaias N, Rebell G, Blank H: Isolation and recognition of dermatophytes on a new medium (DTM), *Arch Dermatol* 99:203–209, 1969.

Head E: Laboratory diagnosis of the superficial fungal infections, *Dermatol Clin* 2:93–108, 1984.

6. Describe a simple test for tinea versicolor other than a KOH preparation.

Clear cellophane tape preparations are an excellent diagnostic testing material because the organism is found in the upper stratum corneum. First, the skin is scraped to ensure there is adequate scale. The tape is applied over the scale and then mounted on a glass slide and examined under the microscope. Clusters of short hyphae and yeasts are seen producing a "spaghetti and meatballs" pattern. Methylene blue may also be added to the slide, selectively staining the organism and thus enhancing visualization (Fig. 3-4). It is important to note that *Malassezia globosa* and *M. furfur*, the most common etiologic agents of tinea versicolor, cannot be cultured on any of the routine fungal media kept in most laboratories.

Martin AG, Kobayashi GS: Yeast infections: candidiasis, pityriasis (tinea) versicolor. In Fitzpatrick TB, Eisen AZ, Wolff K, et al, editors: *Dermatology in general medicine*, ed 4, New York, 1993, McGraw-Hill, pp 2462–2467.

7. What is a Tzanck preparation or smear?

A Tzanck smear is a standard technique for the rapid diagnosis of herpes simplex virus (HSV) or varicella-zoster virus (VZV) infections. It cannot distinguish between these two agents, nor can it distinguish between HSV subtypes (HSV type 1 or 2). It is performed by scraping the base of a fresh blister with a scalpel blade and then spreading the adhering cells and material onto a glass slide. The slide is then stained with a Giemsa, Wright, or Sedi stain. The typical multinucleated giant cells or atypical keratinocytes with large nuclei are then easily visualized (Fig. 3-5).

Nahass GT, Goldstein BA, Zu WY, et al: Comparison of Tzanck smear, viral culture, and DNA diagnostic methods in detection of herpes simplex virus and varicella-zoster infection, *JAMA* 268:2541–2544, 1992.

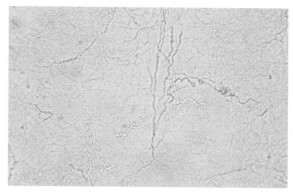

Figure 3-1. Refractile and cylindrical hyphae traversing KOH preparation of skin scraping.

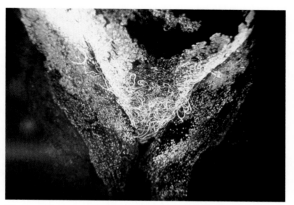

Figure 3-2. Wood's light examination of the groin area demonstrating classic coral red fluorescence associated with erythrasma. (Courtesy of John L. Aeling, MD.)

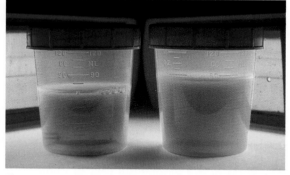

Figure 3-3. Wood's light examination of the urine in a patient with porphyria cutanea tarda demonstrating classic coral red fluorescence with normal urine specimen exhibited for comparison. (Courtesy of James E. Fitzpatrick, MD.)

8. What is the best method of diagnosing scabies?

The best method is to scrape a burrow and demonstrate the parasite inside it. A classic burrow appears as an irregular, linear, slightly elevated lesion, best found on the flexor wrists, fingerwebs, and genitalia. Eighty-five percent of adult male patients with scabies will have mites on the hands or wrists. Occasionally, the mite can be seen with the naked eye as a small dot at one end of the burrow. Following the application of mineral oil, on either the blade or skin, the burrow is scraped vigorously with a no. 15 scalpel blade, but not so vigorously as to draw blood. The mineral oil is collected from the skin and blade and transferred to a glass slide, which is then examined under the microscope. The diagnosis is established by identifying either the fecal pellets (scybala), eggs, or the mite itself (Fig. 3-6).

Hay RJ: Scabies and pyodermas—diagnosis and treatment, *Dermatol Ther* 22:466–464, 2009.

9. How do you diagnose mite bites acquired from an animal?

Clinically, patients present with pruritic red bumps, most commonly on the arms, breasts, and abdomen. The most common sources of these animal mites are cats infested with *Cheyletiella* species. This nonburrowing mite exhibits "bite and run" tactics, so it is not likely to be found on the patient's body. The key to making the diagnosis is to have the animal examined by a veterinarian who is familiar with these parasites. The diagnosis is established by a cellophane tape preparation taken from the cat, dog, or rabbit, demonstrating either the six-legged larval form or the eight-legged adult. Unlike the scabies mite, *Cheyletiella* has well-developed, clawlike mouth parts.

10. How do you diagnose lice infestation?

Lice infestation is caused by *Pediculus humanus capitis* (head louse), *P. humanus corporis* (body louse), or *Phthirus pubis* (pubic louse). Lice can be identified by eye or by using a hand lens, but they can be very difficult to locate. If body lice infestation is suspected, examination of the seams of clothing is more likely to be diagnostic than is examining the skin. Lice will appear as brownish-gray specks. Head and pubic lice are more often seen in hairy areas and are often found with their mouth parts embedded in the skin with outstretched claws grasping hairs on either side. Usually more numerous are nits (eggs), which are white-gray oval structures smaller than 1 mm in size and are firmly attached to the hair shaft. Eggs that are near the junction of the hair shaft and the skin are indicative of active or recent infection. Since hair casts are white and may resemble nits, it is sometimes necessary to examine possible nits under the microscope to prove their identity (Fig. 3-7).

11. What is the diagnostic test of choice for a patient presenting with a suspected syphilitic chancre on his penis?

Dark-field examination of the chancre is the most specific test for the diagnosis of syphilis. This test is typically positive unless the patient has applied or ingested antibiotics. In addition to primary syphilis, dark-field microscopy can also be used to diagnose all of the mucocutaneous lesions of secondary syphilis. However, it is less reliable for examining specimens from the mouth or rectum because of the high prevalence of commensal, nonpathogenic treponemes in these locations that may be mistaken for *Treponema pallidum*, the agent of syphilis. The best specimens for dark-field examination are serous fluid expressed from the bases of the chancre

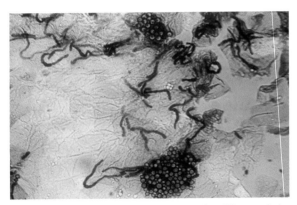

Figure 3-4. A positive cellophane tape preparation of tinea versicolor that has been stained with methylene blue. The characteristic clusters of spores and short hyphae are demonstrated. (Courtesy of James E. Fitzpatrick, MD.)

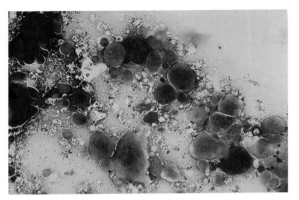

Figure 3-5. A positive Tzanck preparation demonstrating large multinucleated keratinocytes. The nuclei of normal keratinocytes are the size of neutrophils, which are the other cells present in this preparation. (Courtesy of James E. Fitzpatrick, MD.)

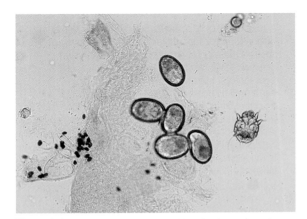

Figure 3-6. A positive scraping for scabies showing an immature mite, eggs, and numerous fecal pellets. (Courtesy of James E. Fitzpatrick, MD.)

following cleaning with sterile saline and clean gauze. The specimen then should be immediately evaluated for the organism's characteristic corkscrew morphology and flexing, hairpin motility. If a patient is suspected of having a syphilitic chancre and a dark-field evaluation is negative, it should be repeated at least once before the diagnosis is excluded. Fluorescent antibody microscopy, although not widely available, offers a sensitive alternative and has the advantage that it does not require live organisms and it can be done on fixed slides. This technique utilizes antibodies to *T. pallidum*.

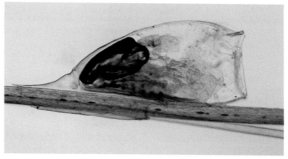

Figure 3-7. Microscopic examination of a hair shaft demonstrates an empty hair louse egg that is glued to the hair shaft. (Courtesy of James E. Fitzpatrick, MD.)

12. How is secondary syphilis diagnosed?

As with primary syphilis, the most specific test is dark-field microscopy. Special stains on skin biopsies are diagnostic as well. More often, screening tests for syphilis such as nontreponemal serologic tests are utilized, usually a rapid plasma reagin (RPR) or a Venereal Disease Research Laboratory (VDRL) test is ordered. Nontreponemal serologic tests for syphilis detect antibodies to reagin, a cholesterol-lecithin-cardiolipin antigen that cross-reacts with antibodies present in the sera of patients with syphilis. These antibodies are not specific for syphilis and should always be confirmed by a specific test for syphilis, usually a fluorescent treponemal antibody–absorption (FTA-ABS) or the microhemagglutination–*T. pallidum* (MHA-TP) test. Nontreponemal serologic tests for syphilis are positive in almost all cases of secondary syphilis. Adequate treatment causes the titer to decline to low titers or nonreactivity.

Domantay-Apostol GP, Handog EB, Gabriel MT: Syphilis: the international challenge of the great imitator, *Dermatol Clin* 26:191–202, 2008.

13. How long do serologic tests for syphilis remain positive?

Nontreponemal test antibody titers (e.g., VDRL) are reported quantitatively in the form of the highest positive titer. This titer correlates with disease activity and treated patients may demonstrate negative results or very low titers. More than 50% of patients will be seronegative 1 year after treatment. A patient with a positive treponemal test (e.g., FTA-ABS) is less likely to revert to negative and only 24% of patients will be seronegative 1 year after treatment; both treated and untreated patients may demonstrate positive serologic tests for the rest of their lives.

14. In patients with symptomatic gonococcal urethritis, how efficacious is a Gram stain of the exudate in comparison to a culture utilizing selective media for gonococcus?

A Gram stain of a urethral discharge in symptomatic males is an excellent method of diagnosing gonorrhea. A positive Gram stain showing multiple neutrophils, some containing clusters of gram-negative diplococci with the sides flattened toward one another, is cited as having a sensitivity of 98%. With such a Gram stain, a culture is expensive and adds little diagnostic yield (about 2%). Cultures are usually done in males with a urethritis and a negative or nondiagnostic Gram stain of the urethral exudates. In women suspected of having gonorrhea, the site of choice for obtaining specimens is the endocervix. However, gram-stained smears are relatively insensitive (30% to 60%), and their interpretation is difficult. A culture on selective media is essential to diagnose gonorrhea in women.

Holder NA: Gonococcal infections, *Pediatr Rev* 29:228–234, 2008.

15. What is the best way to diagnose allergic contact dermatitis?

The diagnostic test of choice is a properly applied and correctly interpreted patch test. Contact dermatitis is divided into irritant or allergic subtypes. Allergic contact dermatitis is immunologically mediated and is an acquired sensitivity that affects only certain individuals. Irritant contact dermatitis is not immunologically mediated and is due to chemical damage of the skin. For example, excessive hand washing or exposure to battery acid will involve almost everyone exposed in such fashion.

Goossens A: Recognizing and testing allergens, *Dermatol Clin* 27:219–226, 2009.

Key Points: Diagnosis of Fungal Infections

1. Microscopic examination of KOH-treated clinical material (epidermal scale, hair, nails) is more sensitive in experienced hands than are cultures for establishing the diagnosis of dermatophyte infections.
2. The Wood's light is very specific but not sensitive for establishing the diagnosis of tinea capitis because the majority of cases are produced by *Trichophyton tonsurans*, a species that does not fluoresce.
3. Dermatophyte test medium is excellent for establishing the diagnosis of a dermatophyte infection but will miss most infections by yeast such as *Candida* species.
4. When examining or culturing hairs in suspected cases of tinea capitis, pluck or remove the broken hairs, which are infected, and not the intact hairs.

> ### Key Points: Biopsy Techniques
> 1. Shave biopsies are often poor choices for melanocytic lesions such as dysplastic nevi or melanoma, as they may fail to allow full and complete microscopic assessment of the lesion.
> 2. An incisional biopsy is used to remove the thickest or clinically most worrisome portion of a larger lesion not amenable to complete removal for diagnostic pathologic examination.
> 3. When splitting a punch biopsy, the specimen is cut through the dermal rather than the epidermal side to reduce crush artifact.

16. How are patch tests applied?

The suspected allergen is usually placed in an appropriate vehicle at an appropriate concentration. The patch test allergens are usually purchased in prepared forms, but less common allergens can be prepared individually. The allergens are placed in special wells that are taped against the skin of the back for 48 hours and then removed. It is important to instruct patients to keep the testing area completely dry. This skin area is then examined 24 to 72 hours after the patch is removed for a reading. A strong positive reaction has erythema, infiltration, papules, and vesicles. A bullous reaction is extremely positive. Interpretation of patch tests and correlation with the clinical disease are complex and usually performed by dermatologists.

17. In what diseases is a skin biopsy helpful?

A skin biopsy with routine hematoxylin-eosin staining is the best diagnostic technique for many cutaneous neoplasms that cannot be diagnosed visually. It is also helpful in many inflammatory skin disorders, especially those in which a specific diagnosis cannot be made from clinical examination, blood tests, or scrapings of the skin. The skin biopsy is a common office procedure, and specimens may also be submitted for more advanced studies such as immunofluorescence, electron microscopy, special stains, cultures, or polymerase chain reaction studies.

18. When are shave biopsies indicated?

The choice of the biopsy technique requires knowledge of basic dermatology, most specifically, where in the skin the pathology is likely to be located. A shave biopsy is usually the most superficial of the skin biopsies and particularly useful when the lesion is in or close to the epidermis. A shave biopsy is best for pedunculated, papular, or otherwise exophytic lesions. It is particularly useful for diagnosis of basal cell and squamous cell carcinomas, seborrheic keratoses, warts, intradermal nevi, and pyogenic granulomas. Shave biopsies are often poor choices for biopsies of melanocytic lesions such as dysplastic nevi or melanoma. Unlike punch biopsies, shave biopsies only require a clean, nonsterile field and do not require sutures.

19. What are the indications for punch biopsies?

A punch biopsy utilizes a round knife that takes a cylinder of tissue including the epidermis, dermis, and often the subcutaneous fat. Although punch biopsies from 2 to 10 mm in diameter can be used, the most common diameter is 4 mm. A larger punch biopsy may be useful if the specimen is to be divided for culture or other procedures. When splitting the biopsy, the specimen is cut through the dermal rather than the epidermal side to reduce crush artifact. A larger punch biopsy of the skin is also helpful in the diagnosis of cutaneous T-cell lymphoma and for scalp biopsies, where a generous specimen is often necessary to establish the diagnosis. The surgical defect left by punch biopsies may be allowed to heal-in secondarily, but most dermatologists close the defect with a single suture.

20. Describe the indications for an excisional or incisional biopsy.

Excisional or incisional biopsies are usually elliptical in shape and typically deeper than punch biopsies. An excisional biopsy is the complete removal of a lesion into the fat, followed by layered closure of the skin. It is particularly helpful in the complete removal of malignancies, such as malignant melanoma, basal cell carcinoma, and squamous cell carcinoma. Excisional biopsies can also be performed when the cosmetic result is felt to be superior to that of a punch biopsy. An incisional biopsy is the incomplete or partial removal of a lesion. If a suspected malignancy is felt to be too large to remove with simple surgery, an incisional biopsy is used to remove the thickest or clinically most worrisome portion for diagnostic pathologic examination. It is also useful for diagnosing panniculitis, sclerotic, or atrophic lesions in which it is important to compare normal adjacent skin to that of the lesion, and to lesions with active expanding borders, such as pyoderma gangrenosum.

Arndt KA: Operative procedures. In Arndt KA, editor: *Manual of dermatologic therapeutics with essentials of diagnosis*, ed 4, Boston, 1989, Little, Brown and Co, pp 171–180.

21. Define and describe direct immunofluorescence of the skin.

Direct immunofluorescence (DIF) of the skin is a histologic stain for antibodies or other tissue proteins in skin biopsy specimens. A skin sample obtained from the patient is immediately frozen in liquid nitrogen or placed in special media to preserve the immunoreactants. Arrangements should be made to ensure proper and timely transport to the immunofluorescence laboratory. Once received, the tissue is sectioned and then incubated with antibodies to human immunoglobulins or complement components that have been tagged with a fluorescent molecule to allow their visualization. The samples are then examined with a fluorescence microscope, where fluorescence indicates that immunoreactants were deposited in the patient's tissue. The specific immunoreactants present, and the pattern and intensity of staining, are used to determine the diseases most likely to be associated with the DIF findings.

Zillikens D: Diagnosis of autoimmune bullous skin disease, *Clin Lab* 54:491–503, 2008.

22. Name some skin diseases in which DIF is helpful in making a diagnosis.

Many of the immunobullous diseases are associated with specific DIF findings: bullous pemphigoid, herpes gestationis, cicatricial pemphigoid, epidermolysis bullosa acquisita, dermatitis herpetiformis, linear IgA bullous dermatosis, and the various types of pemphigus. In addition, DIF may be helpful in evaluating cutaneous and systemic lupus erythematosus, other collagen vascular diseases, vasculitis such as Henoch-Schönlein purpura (Fig. 3-8), and certain types of porphyria.

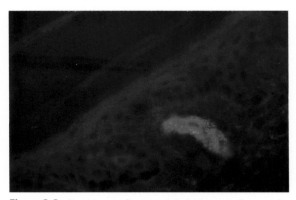

Figure 3-8. Direct immunofluorescent study demonstrating granular deposits of IgA within a blood vessel of a patient with Henoch-Schönlein purpura. (Courtesy of James E. Fitzpatrick, MD.)

23. How does indirect immunofluorescence of the skin differ from direct immunofluorescence of the skin?

Indirect immunofluorescence studies test for the presence of circulating autoantibodies in the serum, in contrast to direct immunofluorescence studies, which test for the presence of autoantibodies deposited in the skin. The serum from the patient is incubated with an appropriate normal substrate such as monkey esophagus, rat bladder, or human skin. The substrate is incubated with fluorescein-labeled antibodies directed against the antibody in the tissue. The specimen is then examined under a fluorescence microscope. By running this test at various dilutions, the amount of circulating antibody can be determined and reported as a titer. Titers are useful in some diseases, such as pemphigus vulgaris, in determining disease activity and treatment.

24. Is ELISA ever used for the diagnosis of immunobullous disease?

Yes. In recent years the enzyme-linked immunosorbent assay (ELISA) has been increasingly used for the diagnosis and differentiation of various forms of pemphigus, based on the presence of IgG autoantibodies directed against desmoglein-1 (dsg-1) and desmoglein-3 (dsg-3), which are proteins found in the intercellular junctions between keratinocytes. The ELISA is also, but less commonly, used to detect IgG autoantibodies against BP180 and BP230, which are the major antigens associated with bullous pemphigoid. The ELISA is both more specific and sensitive when compared to indirect immunofluorescence testing.

Mihai S, Sitaru G: Immunopathology and molecular diagnosis of autoimmune bullous disease, *J Cell Mol Med* 11:462–481, 2007.

25. How are bacterial skin cultures performed, and when are they useful?

Bacterial cultures are useful when active infection of the skin is suspected. Bacterial cultures demonstrate high yields in superficial infections such as impetigo, ecthyma, and infected ulcers, and lower yields in cellulitis. When culturing superficial infections, the involved area should first be cleaned with an alcohol pad and then thoroughly swabbed. A higher concentration of bacteria may be found at the point of maximal inflammation. The best results in cellulitis are obtained when the leading edge is injected with nonbacteriostatic saline using a 20-gauge needle mounted on a tuberculin syringe. The aspirate may be sent for culture while still in the syringe if it can be taken to the laboratory immediately, or the aspirated material may be submitted in a bacterial culturette.

DISORDERS OF KERATINIZATION

H. Alan Arbuckle, MD, FAAP, FAAD, and Lori D. Prok, MD

1. What are the ichthyosiform dermatoses?

The ichthyosiform dermatoses are a heterogeneous group of disorders presenting with excessive scaling of the skin. The inherited forms of the ichthyoses are most common, although the condition can occur secondary to other diseases.

2. What does "ichthyosis" mean?

The term *ichthyosis* is derived from the Greek root *ichthy*, meaning fish, indicative of the scales on the skin of affected individuals.

3. How common are the congenital ichthyoses? How are they inherited?

- **Ichthyosis vulgaris:** Incidence of 1:250; autosomal dominant
- **X-linked ichthyosis:** Incidence of 1:6000; X-linked recessive
- **Epidermolytic hyperkeratosis:** Incidence of 1:300,000; autosomal dominant
- **Congenital ichthyosiform erythroderma (CIE):** Incidence of 1:100,000; autosomal recessive
- **Lamellar ichthyosis:** Incidence of 1:300,000; autosomal recessive
- **Harlequin fetus:** Rare; autosomal recessive

Akiyama M: The clinical spectrum of nonbullous congenital ichthyosiform erythroderma and lamellar ichthyosis, *Clin Exp Dermatol* 28(3):235–240, 2003.

DiGiovanna J: Ichthyosis: etiology, diagnosis, and management, *Am J Clin Dermatol* 4(2):81–95, 2003.

Shwayder T: Disorders of keratinization: diagnosis and management, *Am J Clin Dermatol* 5(1):17–29, 2004.

4. What features help differentiate the most common inherited ichthyoses?

Both clinical and histologic features are helpful in the diagnosis of ichthyoses (Table 4-1). Onset of symptoms, anatomic location of skin changes, birth history, and the condition of the infant's skin at birth are helpful clues. In some instances, a skin biopsy can be diagnostic.

Ichthyosis vulgaris (Fig. 4-1A,B) usually develops around school age, and is characterized by generalized xerosis and scale, with characteristic sparing of the flexural skin. Additional findings include follicular accentuation (keratosis pilaris), hyperlinearity of palms and soles, and a personal or family history of atopy. Rare patients may have an associated palmar-plantar keratoderma. Skin biopsy demonstrates a decreased granular cell layer associated with moderate hyperkeratosis.

X-linked ichthyosis, in contrast, is usually present by one year of age, affects the posterior neck with "dirty"-appearing scales, and spares the palms and soles (Fig. 4-1C). The skin changes—gradually worsening with age—with the neck, face, and trunk ultimately developing thick, brown scales. The disease is caused by a defect in steroid sulfatase, an enzyme important in cholesterol synthesis and vital for normal development and function of the stratum corneum. Accumulation of cholesterol sulfate and a lack of tissue cholesterol ensue, leading to a disturbance in steroid hormone metabolism. Skin biopsy of X-linked ichthyosis is rarely diagnostic, and demonstrates a normal granular layer with hyperkeratosis.

5. What genetic defect is responsible for X-linked ichthyosis (XLI)?

Ninety percent of patients with XLI have deletions in the *STS* gene on chromosome Xp22.3, leading to steroid sulfatase deficiency and the classic phenotype of XLI. However, some patients have larger deletions at this site, encompassing neighboring genes. These patients present with more complicated forms of XLI representing contiguous gene deletion syndromes (OMIM [Online Mendelian Inheritance in Man] #308100).

6. What additional phenotypes may patients with XLI contiguous gene syndromes exhibit?

Hypogonadotropic hypogonadism and anosmia (Kallman's syndrome), chondrodysplasia punctata, short stature, and/or ocular albinism may be present in these patients in addition to X-linked ichthyosis.

7. What important birth history may be obtained in patients with XLI?

Labor may be protracted or fail to progress when the fetus is affected with XLI. This is directly related to the defect in steroid sulfatase, which leads to abnormal steroid hormone metabolism. Female carriers may also exhibit asymptomatic corneal opacities.

Table 4-1. Clinical Features of the Major Inherited Ichthyoses

DISORDER	ONSET	TYPE OF SCALE	SITES	HISTOLOGY	OTHER FINDINGS	DEFECT
Ichthyosis vulgaris	Childhood	Fine	Palms, soles, extensors	Diminished granular layer	Atopy, keratosis pilaris	Filaggrin
X-linked ichthyosis	Birth or infancy	Coarse, brown	Neck, face, trunk, flexors	Normal granular layer	Corneal opacities	Steroid sulfatase
Epidermolytic hyperkeratosis	Birth	Erosions/bullae, coarse, verrucous	Generalized, especially flexors	Epidermolytic hyperkeratosis	Foul odor, pyogenic infections	Keratin
Congenital ichthyosiform erythroderma (CIE)	Birth	Fine, white, with erythroderma	Generalized with flexors, palms, soles	Increased granular layer, focal parakeratosis	Ectropion, nail dystrophy, poor growth, alopecia	ALOXE3/ ALOX12B
Lamellar ichthyosis	Birth	Platelike, dark, erythroderma	Generalized with flexors, palms, soles	Increased granular layer, hyperkeratosis	Same as CIE	Transglutaminase
Harlequin fetus	Birth	Massive thick plates	Generalized	Massive compact hyperkeratosis	Ectropion, eclabium, ear and limb deformities	ACBA12

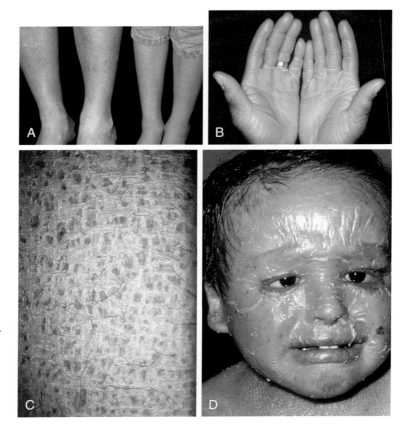

Figure 4-1. A, Grandfather and grand-daughter with ichthyosis vulgaris. **B,** Palmar hyperkeratosis, a finding often associated with ichthyosis vulgaris. **C,** X-linked ichthyosis, showing characteristic coarse, brown scales. **D,** Young child with congenital ichthyosiform erythroderma demonstrating diffuse erythema and scale. (A, B, and D, courtesy of James E. Fitzpatrick, MD.)

8. Name the hereditary syndromes presenting with ichthyosis as a component.
See Table 4-2.

9. What is a collodion baby?
A collodion baby is a newborn infant whose skin looks like a "baked apple," with a shiny, tough, membrane-like covering. This term describes a phenotype that occurs in several types of ichthyosis. Although congenital ichthyosiform erythroderma is the most common underlying condition (Fig. 4-1D), lamellar ichthyosis, Netherton's syndrome, Conradi's syndrome and others may also present as a collodion baby. Collodion babies may also go on to have normal skin. These infants are at increased risk for infections and fluid and electrolyte imbalances due to cutaneous fissures and impaired barrier function of the skin. Treatment in a high-humidity environment with frequent application of petrolatum allows gradual sloughing of the collodion membrane. Manual debridement and keratolytics are not recommended.

10. What is a harlequin fetus?
The most severe manifestation of congenital ichthyosis, the harlequin fetus, is born with massive hyperkeratotic plates associated with limb deformities, rudimentary ears, ectropion, and eclabium (Fig. 4-2). These infants rarely survive beyond the first week of life. The use of acitretin in harlequin ichthyosis may be lifesaving, although side effects are numerous and may be severe.

11. Name several conditions associated with acquired ichthyosis.
See Table 4-3.
- **Malignancy:** The pathogenesis of the skin changes associated with malignancies is unknown, although reduced dermal lipid synthesis, malabsorption, and immunologic abnormalities have been identified.
- **Nutritional and metabolic disorders:** Many of nutritional problems involve abnormal vitamin A metabolism. Chronic renal failure may result in hypervitaminosis A, which produces rough, scaly skin. Hypovitaminosis A produces follicular hyperkeratosis and dry skin.
- **Drugs and other therapies:** Medications produce ichthyosis by various mechanisms. Niacin, triparanol, butyrophenones, dixyrazine, and nafoxidine alter cholesterol synthesis. Cimetidine and retinoids are antiandrogenic and reduce sebum secretion (Fig. 4-3).

Homayoun A: Acquired ichthyosis and related conditions, *Int J Dermatol* 23:458–461, 1984.

Table 4-2. Hereditary Syndromes with Ichthyosis

SYNDROME	CLINICAL FEATURES	SKIN FINDINGS	DEFECT
Conradi-Hünermann disease (chondrodysplasia punctata)	Chondrodysplasia punctata, limb defects, cataracts, cardiovascular and renal abnormalities, mental retardation	Congenital ichthyosiform erythroderma (CIE), whorled hyperpigmentation, palmoplantar keratoderma	Sterol isomerase emopamil–binding protein
CHILD (congenital hemidysplasia with ichthyosiform erythroderma and limb defects) syndrome	Hemidysplasia and limb defects with sharp midline demarcation	CIE	NAD(P)H steroid dehydrogenase–like protein
Sjögren-Larsson syndrome	Spasticity, mental retardation, retinal degeneration	Lamellar scales	Fatty aldehyde dehydrogenase
Chanarin-Dorfman syndrome (neutral lipid storage disease)	Fatty liver, myopathy, cataracts, deafness, CNS defects	CIE	Impaired long-chain fatty acid oxidation
Netherton's syndrome	Trichorrhexis invaginata (bamboo hairs), atopy, aminoaciduria	Ichthyosis linearis circumflexa	*SPINK5* gene
Refsum's disease	Cerebellar ataxia, peripheral neuropathy, retinitis pigmentosa	Like ichthyosis vulgaris	Phytanoyl-CoA hydroxylase
Multiple sulfatase deficiency	Metachromatic leukodystrophy, hepatosplenomegaly	Like X-linked ichthyosis	Sulfatase modifying factor-1 gene
Trichothiodystrophy (PIBIDS)	Photosensitivity, ichthyosis, brittle hair, intellectual impairment, decreased fertility, short stature	CIE	Xeroderma pigmentosa D or B gene
KID (keratitis-ichthyosis-deafness) syndrome	Keratitis, neurosensory deafness, alopecia	Grainy, spiculated scaling	Connexin 26 gene

12. Are laboratory tests helpful in the diagnosis of ichthyoses?

In general, no. However, with recent advancements in genetic testing and microarray analysis, genetic testing is becoming easier and more readily available for this group of disorders. In ichthyosis vulgaris, cultured keratinocytes demonstrate absent or reduced filaggrin keratohyalin granules, and fail to react to antifilaggrin monoclonal antibodies. The defective enzyme in X-linked ichthyosis, steroid sulfatase, can be assayed in cultured keratinocytes, fibroblasts, leukocytes, or skin scales. Low levels of cholesterol sulfate in blood can be detected by the increased mobility of low-density lipoproteins on serum protein electrophoresis. Female heterozygotes can be detected by Southern blot hybridization from peripheral blood leukocytes. The gene has been mapped to the short arm of the X chromosome (Xp22.3). Several of the rarer ichthyosiform syndromes are also associated with enzyme deficiencies detectable in cell cultures.

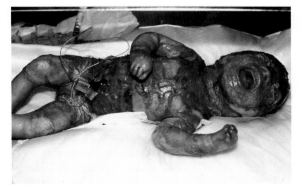

Figure 4-2. Fatal case of harlequin fetus demonstrating large, fissured, keratotic platess. (Courtesy of the Fitzsimons Army Medical Center teaching files.)

Oji V, Traupe H: Ichthyoses: differential diagnosis and molecular genetics, *Eur J Dermatol* 16(4):349–359, 2006.

Scharschmidt TC, Man MQ, Hatano Y, et al: Filaggrin deficiency confers a paracellular barrier abnormality that reduces inflammatory thresholds to irritants and haptens, *J Allergy Clin Immunol* 124(3):496–506, 2009.

13. Is prenatal diagnosis of congenital ichthyosis possible?

Prenatal diagnosis is available for many of the congenital ichthyoses, if one is suspected, based on family history. Fetal skin biopsy performed at 19 to 21 weeks will demonstrate early development of a thickened stratum corneum,

Table 4-3. Conditions Associated with Acquired Ichthyosis

MEDICATIONS	MALIGNANCIES	NUTRITIONAL DISORDERS	METABOLIC DISORDERS	MISCELLANEOUS DISORDERS
Butyrophenone	Non–Hodgkin's lymphoma	Essential fatty acid deficiencies	Chronic renal failure	Systemic lupus erythematosus
Cimetidine	Hodgkin's lymphoma	Hypervitaminosis A	Hypothyroidism	Sarcoidosis
Clofazimine	Carcinoma of solid organs	Hypovitaminosis A	Panhypopituitarism	Leprosy
Dixyrazine	Mycosis fungoides	Kwashiorkor		Dermatomyositis
Isoniazid	Leukemia	Pellagra		HIV infection
Nafoxidine	Lymphosarcoma			Polycythemia
Niacin	Rhabdomyosarcoma			Haber's syndrome
Triparanol	Kaposi's sarcoma			
Allopurinol	Leiomyosarcoma			
Retinoids	Multiple myeloma			

normally not present until 24 weeks. This is useful in lamellar ichthyosis, epidermolytic hyperkeratosis, Sjögren-Larsson syndrome, and harlequin fetus. Lamellar ichthyosis may also be detected via a transglutaminase activity assay from a fetal skin sample. Epidermolytic hyperkeratosis, known to result from mutations in keratins 1 and 10, can be detected by direct gene sequencing done on chorionic villus sampling in the second trimester. Cultured chorionic villi cells or amniocytes will demonstrate the enzyme deficiency in XLI, Sjögren-Larsson syndrome, and Refsum's disease. A high ratio of maternal urinary estrogen precursors in a male fetus also suggests the diagnosis of XLI. Trichothiodystrophy can be identified by unscheduled DNA synthesis in cultured amniocytes exposed to ultraviolet light.

Rothnagel JA: Prenatal diagnosis of epidermolytic hyperkeratosis by direct gene sequencing, *J Invest Dermatol* 102:13–16, 1994.

14. How is ichthyosis treated?

Acquired ichthyosis usually improves with treatment of the underlying condition. Congenital ichthyosis is difficult to treat, especially in its severe forms.

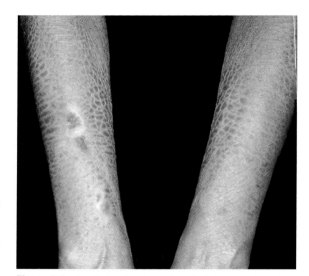

Figure 4-3. Acquired ichthyosis due to clofazimine. (Courtesy of the Fitzsimons Army Medical Center teaching files.)

Topical emollients containing glycolic acid, lactic acid, urea, or glycerin may partially improve dryness and scaling. Topical tretinoin (Retin-A) is effective but poorly tolerated due to irritation. Oral retinoids, including isotretinoin, etretinate, and acitretin, are very effective, but relapses after treatment cessation are common. The use of oral retinoids is limited by major side effects (including teratogenic effects), and chronic use, which is often required in congenital disorders, is associated with hyperostoses. Blistering may indicate bacterial infection and should be cultured and managed with oral antibiotics. The foul odor present in epidermolytic hyperkeratosis may be due to bacterial colonization and can be improved by the use of an antibacterial soap.

Oji V, Traupe H: Ichthyosis: clinical manifestations and practical treatment options, *Am J Clin Dermatol* 10(6):351–364, 2009.

15. What is Hailey-Hailey disease?

Hailey-Hailey disease, also known as benign familial pemphigus, is an autosomal dominant condition in which mutations in the *ATP2C1* gene result in abnormal intracellular calcium signaling. It is characterized histologically by acantholysis (loss of cohesion between keratinocytes) and clinically by patches of minute vesicles that break and form crusted erosions.

16. How does Hailey-Hailey disease present?

Skin changes consisting of localized patches of minute vesicles and erosions start in areas of friction, usually the neck, groin, and axilla (Figs. 4-4 and 4-5). Patches spread peripherally with serpiginous borders and show central healing with hyperpigmentation or granular vegetations. Onset of lesions is often delayed until the second or third decade. Associated symptoms include itching, pain, and foul odor.

17. Do any factors exacerbate the skin changes of Hailey-Hailey?

Physical trauma, heat, or sweating worsen skin lesions. Patients have reported the onset of new lesions within hours of wearing restrictive shirt collars, tight bra straps, and electrocardiogram electrodes. Most patients report a worsening of lesions in the summer.

18. Which diseases may be confused with Hailey-Hailey disease?

Eczema, impetigo, fungal or viral infections, pemphigus vulgaris, pemphigus vegetans, or Darier's disease. The recurring, chronic nature of Hailey-Hailey disease, lack of oral and ocular involvement, and intertriginous predilection help to differentiate these conditions.

19. How is Hailey-Hailey disease treated?

Topical steroids are generally helpful in relieving burning and itching. Both *Staphylococcus aureus* and *Candida albicans* infections may exacerbate lesions, requiring treatment with appropriate antibacterial and antifungal agents. Recalcitrant cases have been treated with localized steroid injections, carbon dioxide laser, dermabrasion, topical cyclosporine, dapsone, vitamin E, psoralen plus ultraviolet A (PUVA), methotrexate, thalidomide, and vitamin D analogs, with variable results.

Aoki T: 1-Alpha,24-dihydroxyvitamin D3 (tacalcitol) is effective against Hailey-Hailey disease both in vivo and in vitro, *Br J Dermatol* 139:897–901, 1998.

Kartamaa M: Familial benign chronic pemphigus (Hailey-Hailey disease): treatment with carbon dioxide laser vaporization, *Arch Dermatol* 128:646–648, 1992.

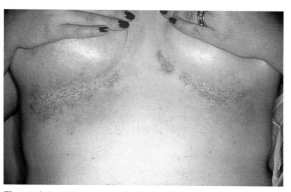

Figure 4-4. Patient with Hailey-Hailey disease demonstrating characteristic involvement of flexural areas of inflammatory crease.

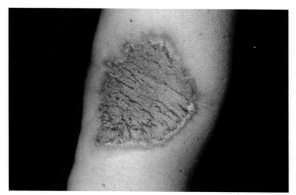

Figure 4-5. Hailey-Hailey disease showing a patch of minute vesicles, erosions, and crusting in the antecubital fossa.

Key Points: Disorders of Keratinization

1. Ichthyosis vulgaris, with an incidence of 1:250, is by far the most common ichthyosis.
2. Congenital ichthyosiform erythroderma and lamellar ichthyosis are the two disorders of keratinization that are most likely to present as a collodion baby.
3. Topical emollients containing glycolic acid, lactic acid, urea, and glycerin are the mainstay of therapy in mild disorders of keratinization.
4. Oral retinoids are the most effective therapy for severe ichthyoses, but their use is limited by side effects of chronic use.

---

20. What is Darier's disease?

Darier's disease, also known as keratosis follicularis and Darier-White disease, is a dominantly inherited disorder of keratinization caused by mutations in the *ATP2A2* gene, resulting in dysfunction of intracellular calcium signaling. Typically, the disease presents in the first or second decade of life. Microscopically, it is characterized by distinctive changes of both premature keratinization and acantholysis.

21. How is Darier's disease diagnosed?

The diagnosis is based on clinical manifestations and histologic features. The primary lesions are flesh-colored papules that may coalesce into plaques and develop tan, scaly crusts (Fig. 4-6). These keratotic papules are located in "seborrheic areas," such as the chest, back, ears, nasolabial folds, scalp, and groin. Thick, foul-smelling, warty masses can develop. Flat, wartlike papules may be seen on the dorsa of distal extremities, and 1- to 2-mm punctate keratoses may be present on the palms and soles. Oral and rectal mucosal surfaces often demonstrate small, cobblestone-like papules. The diagnosis can be confirmed by skin biopsies that reveal acantholytic dyskeratosis.

22. Are there any nail or hair changes in Darier's disease?

Nails demonstrate longitudinal ridging, as well as red and white longitudinal streaks. Distal nail edges show V-shaped notching and subungual thickening. Rarely, alopecia results from extensive scalp involvement.

23. Is Darier's disease difficult to treat?

Complete clearing of Darier's disease is rare. Soothing moisturizers containing urea or lactic acid reduce scaling and irritation. Salicylic acid in a propylene glycol gel and topical retinoids are also effective in reducing crusts and scale, although retinoids may need to be initiated on an alternate-day schedule in combination with midpotency topical steroids to minimize irritation. Aggravating factors such as heat, humidity, sunlight, and lithium should be avoided. Infection should be prevented with antibacterial soaps and treated with antibiotics. Oral retinoids are effective, but toxicity limits their use; intermittent use may be preferable, such as starting the medication before a summer holiday to prevent sun-induced exacerbations. Recalcitrant verrucous lesions have been treated with dermabrasion, carbon dioxide laser vaporization, and surgery.

Burge SM: Darier-White disease: a review of the clinical features in 163 patients, *J Am Acad Dermatol* 27:40–50, 1992.

Burge SM: Management of Darier's disease, *Clin Exp Dermatol* 24:53–56, 1999.

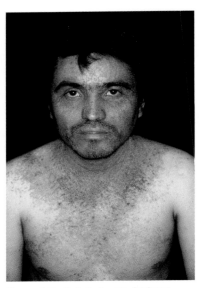

Figure 4-6. Darier's disease. Confluent, crusted papules involving the face, scalp, and chest.

CHAPTER 5

NEUROCUTANEOUS DISORDERS

Anne R. Halbert, MB BS (Hons), FACD

NEUROFIBROMATOSIS

1. What are the two main forms of neurofibromatosis?
Neurofibromatosis type 1 (NF-1 or von Recklinghausen's disease) and neurofibromatosis type 2 (NF-2). NF-1 accounts for 90% of all cases of neurofibromatosis and affects approximately 1 in 3500 individuals. NF-2 is a genetically distinct entity with a prevalence of 1 in 25,000. Both conditions have autosomal dominant inheritance with 50% of cases representing new mutations.

2. Outline the diagnostic criteria for NF-1.
The diagnosis can be made if two or more of the following criteria are present:
- Six or more café-au-lait macules >5 mm in greatest diameter in prepubertal children and >15 mm diameter in postpubertal individuals
- Two or more neurofibromas of any type or one plexiform neurofibroma
- Freckling in axillary or inguinal regions
- Two or more Lisch nodules
- Optic glioma
- Distinctive osseous lesion, such as sphenoid dysplasia or thinning of long bone cortex, with or without pseudoarthrosis
- First-degree relative with NF-1

National Institutes of Health Consensus Development Conference: Conference statement: neurofibromatosis, *Arch Neurol* 45, 575–578, 1988.

3. Where is the gene for NF-1 located? What protein does it encode?
The NF-1 gene is a large gene mapping to chromosome 17q11.2. It encodes a protein called neurofibromin, which has a role in tumor suppression.

4. What is the earliest skin sign of NF-1?
Café-au-lait macules. These sharply defined, light brown patches may be present at birth but more commonly start appearing in the first year of life (Fig. 5-1). They are noted initially by 4 years or less in all affected children and within the first year in 82% of cases.

Huson SM, Compston DAS, Harper PS: A genetic study of von Recklinghausen neurofibromatosis in southeast Wales. II. Guidelines for genetic counselling, *J Med Genet* 26:712–721, 1989.
Boyd KP, Korf BR, Theos A: Neurofibromatosis type 1, *J Am Acad Dermatol* 61:1–14, 2009.

5. What is Crowe's sign? When does it develop?
Crowe's sign is freckling of the axillae or other body folds. It develops in 90% of NF-1 patients, usually in middle childhood. These lesions are not really freckles, but multiple small café-au-lait macules.

Key Points: Neurocutaneous Disorders

1. Multiple Lisch nodules are pathognomonic of NF-1.
2. Multiple café-au-lait macules are the earliest skin sign of NF-1, occurring in approximately 80% of affected babies by the end of the first year of life.
3. NF-2 most commonly presents with deafness or tinnitus related to underlying vestibular schwannomas.
4. There are two genetic loci for tuberous sclerosis on chromosomes 9 and 16.
5. In virtually all cases of Sturge-Weber syndrome, the facial port wine stain involves some of the V1 distribution.
6. Hypomelanotic macules are a useful diagnostic skin sign for tuberous sclerosis in infants with seizures.

---

6. When do peripheral neurofibromas appear in NF-1?
Peripheral neurofibromas usually start to develop during puberty but increase in size and number in early adult life. They are soft, pink, or flesh-colored papules, nodules, or tumors distributed mainly over the trunk and limbs (Fig. 5-2). Multiple neurofibromas can develop or existing neurofibromas may enlarge during pregnancy.

7. What is a plexiform neurofibroma?

It is a diffuse, elongated neurofibroma occurring along the course of a nerve, usually the trigeminal or upper cervical nerves. Present in 30% of patients with NF-1, these lesions are mostly congenital. They are often disfiguring, associated with overlying skin hypertrophy, hyperpigmentation, and increased hair (Fig. 5-3).

8. What are Lisch nodules?

Melanocytic hamartomas of the iris. When multiple, these lesions are pathognomonic of NF-1, occurring in more than 90% of patients by the second decade of life. They are best seen on slit lamp examination.

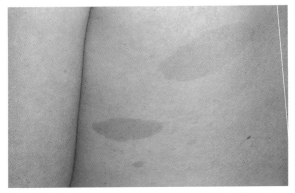

Figure 5-1. Multiple café-au-lait macules >5 mm in diameter.

9. What is the most common central nervous system (CNS) tumor occurring in NF-1?

Optic glioma occurs in 15% of patients, usually before 6 years of age. Two percent of affected individuals develop other CNS neoplasms including astrocytomas, schwannomas, and hamartomas. Epilepsy occurs in 6% of patients, often due to these underlying focal lesions.

Friedman JM, Birch PH: Type 1 neurofibromatosis: a descriptive analysis of the disorder in 1728 patients, *Am J Med Genet* 70:138–143, 1997.

10. How common is intellectual impairment in NF-1?

Nearly 50% of patients have mild intellectual impairment or learning difficulties; 5% have moderate to severe retardation.

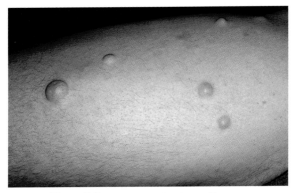

Figure 5-2. Multiple peripheral neurofibromas.

11. What are the most common skeletal abnormalities in NF-1?

- Macrocephaly: 45%
- Short stature: 34%
- Dysplasia of a long bone, most commonly tibia: 14%
- Kyphoscoliosis: 11.5%

12. How frequently should patients with NF-1 be assessed? What should this assessment include?

An annual assessment is usually sufficient. The clinical examination should include a blood pressure measurement (hypertension occurs in 6% due to renovascular stenosis or pheochromocytoma) and a full neurologic examination. Children also require a regular eye examination; surveillance for kyphoscoliosis, precocious puberty, and hypogonadism; and regular developmental assessments. Investigations should be guided by symptoms or physical signs.

Drappier J-C, Khosrotehrani K, Zeller J, et al: Medical management of neurofibromatosis 1: a cross sectional study of 383 patients, *J Am Acad Dermatol* 49: 440–444, 2003.

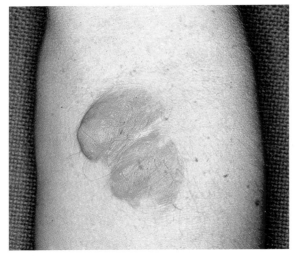

Figure 5-3. Soft baglike lesion of a plexiform neurofibroma.

13. What are the diagnostic criteria for NF-2?

The diagnostic criteria are met by an individual who has

- Bilateral vestibular schwannomas **or**
- First-degree relative with NF-2 **and** unilateral eighth nerve mass **or** two of the following: neurofibroma, meningioma, glioma, schwannoma, or juvenile posterior subcapsular lenticular opacity

14. Where is the gene for NF-2? What is the gene product?

The *NF-2* gene is located on chromosome 22q12.1. It encodes a cytoskeletal protein, merlin (also called schwannomin), which acts as a tumor suppressor.

15. What are the most common presenting symptoms of NF-2?

Hearing loss or tinnitus related to underlying vestibular schwannomas is the presenting symptom in the majority of patients, developing at a mean age of 20 years. Other presenting symptoms relate to underlying CNS tumors (20% to 30%), skin tumors (12.7%), and ocular abnormalities (12.7%).

Evans DGR, Sainio M, Baser ME: Neurofibromatosis type 2, *J Med Genet* 37:897–904, 2000.
Asthagiri AR, Parry DM, Butman JA, et al: Neurofibromatosis type 2, *Lancet* 373:1974–1986, 2009.

16. What are the skin signs of NF-2?

Café-au-lait macules (usually fewer than six) occur in approximately half the affected individuals. Cutaneous schwannomas (mean number seven) occur in two thirds, presenting as soft, raised, hypertrichotic areas or subcutaneous spherical tumors along peripheral nerves.

17. What is the ocular sign of NF-2?

Posterior subcapsular cataracts (60% to 80%). Unlike in NF-1, Lisch nodules or optic gliomas do not occur.

TUBEROUS SCLEROSIS

18. Tuberous sclerosis is also known as epiloia. What does this term mean?

Epiloia was a term coined from the diagnostic triad of epilepsy, low intelligence, and adenoma sebaceum:
- Epilepsy: 60%
- Mental retardation: 40% to 60%
- Skin signs: 60% to 70%

19. What is the inheritance of tuberous sclerosis?

Inheritance is autosomal dominant, with high penetrance but variable expression. Up to 60% of cases are said to represent new mutations, but "normal" parents must undergo thorough clinical and radiologic evaluation to exclude subclinical disease.

20. Where are the genetic defects for tuberous sclerosis?

Genetic linkage studies of familial cases have demonstrated two separate genes linked to tuberous sclerosis: *TSC 1,* located at chromosome 9q34, encoding a protein called hamartin, and *TSC 2,* located at chromosome 16p13.3, encoding a protein called tuberin.

Narayanan V: Tuberous sclerosis complex: genetics to pathogenesis, *Pediatr Neurol* 29:404–409, 2003.
Curatolo P, Bombardieri R, Jozwiak S: Tuberous sclerosis, *Lancet* 372:657–668, 2008.

21. What is the earliest skin sign of tuberous sclerosis?

Hypomelanotic macules (Fig. 5-4). Frequently present at birth or in early infancy, these lesions are a helpful sign in infants with convulsions. Best seen with Wood's lamp examination, they are polygonal or ash-leaf in shape, ranging in size from 1 to 3 cm and numbering 1 to 100. Occasionally, they are accompanied by 1- to 3-mm confetti-like white spots scattered over the trunk and limbs. Common skin signs of tuberous sclerosis include the following:
- Ash-leaf hypomelanotic macules
- Facial angiofibromas
- Periungual fibromas (Koenen's tumors)
- Shagreen patch
- Forehead fibromatous plaque

22. Adenoma sebaceum is a misnomer. What is the correct term for the facial lesions seen in tuberous sclerosis?

Angiofibromas (Fig. 5-5). These lesions consist of hyperplastic blood vessels and collagen and are not tumors of sebaceous glands. Facial angiofibromas appear at 4 to 9 years of age and increase in size and number during puberty. They are firm, discrete, reddish papules of 1 to 10 mm, developing initially in the nasolabial folds and frequently progressing over the malar region, forehead, and chin.

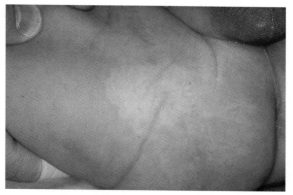

Figure 5-4. Ash-leaf macule in an infant.

23. What are Koenen's tumors?

Subungual and periungual fibromas (Fig. 5-6). These develop at or after puberty and present as firm, flesh-colored growths of 5 to 10 mm in length, projecting from the nail folds and beneath the nail plate.

24. What is a shagreen patch?

An irregularly thickened, slightly elevated, flesh-colored plaque consisting of collagen. It is most commonly located over the lumbosacral area. Fibromatous plaques are also frequently found on the forehead (Fig. 5-7).

25. What are tubers, and where do they occur?

Tubers are potato-like nodules of glial proliferation and are the characteristic CNS lesion of tuberous sclerosis. They may occur anywhere in the cerebral cortex, basal ganglia, and ventricular walls (subependymal nodules), and their number and size correlate with clinical features of seizures and mental retardation. Cortical tubers are often isodense with normal brain tissue and are best detected with magnetic resonance imaging (MRI). Subependymal nodules may calcify and are readily detectable with computed tomography (CT) scanning. Fifty percent of plain skull x-rays taken in later childhood also reveal bilateral areas of calcification in the brain.

26. What signs of tuberous sclerosis may be revealed on funduscopic examination?

Retinal hamartomas (phacomata) may occur in 50% of patients. They may be seen as white streaks along the retina or elevated multinodular lesions near the optic disc.

27. Which cardiac abnormality is characteristic of tuberous sclerosis?

Congenital rhabdomyomas (50%). These tumors are due to abnormal differentiation of embryonic myocardium into atypical Purkinje cells. They are usually multiple and often clinically silent, although ventricular outflow obstruction may occur. They may regress later in childhood.

28. Can renal involvement occur in tuberous sclerosis?

Yes. Angiomyolipomas are common hamartomatous tumors in the kidney. They may be multiple and bilateral and are usually asymptomatic. Renal cysts are common.

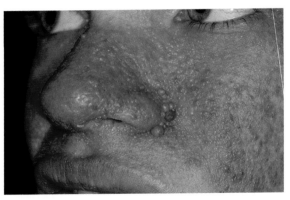

Figure 5-5. Facial angiofibromas in tuberous sclerosis (adenoma sebaceum).

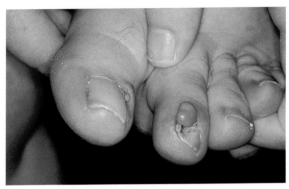

Figure 5-6. Koenen's tumor (periungual fibroma).

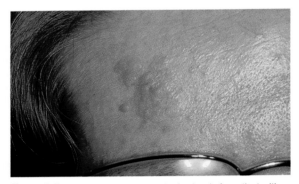

Figure 5-7. Fibromatous plaque on the forehead of a patient with tuberous sclerosis.

29. What is the prognosis for patients with tuberous sclerosis?

The prognosis is extremely variable and depends on the severity of the clinical manifestations. In severe cases, death may occur from epilepsy, infection, cardiac failure, or, rarely, pulmonary fibrosis.

STURGE-WEBER SYNDROME

30. Name the two essential components of the Sturge-Weber syndrome.

A facial port wine stain and homolateral leptomeningeal angiomatosis.

31. What is the inheritance of the Sturge-Weber syndrome?

It is not inherited. It is a sporadic developmental malformation.

32. Where does the port wine stain most commonly occur in Sturge-Weber syndrome?

The port wine stain most commonly involves the areas innervated by the ophthalmic (V1) and maxillary (V2) divisions of the trigeminal nerve. In virtually all cases, some portion of the forehead, upper eyelid, and nasal root (V1) is involved. The port wine stain may be bilateral (Fig. 5-8) and may involve nasal or oral mucosa. Port wine stains are present on the extremities or trunk in addition to the face in 40% of cases.

Tallman B, Tan OT, Morelli JG, et al: Location of port wine stains and the likelihood of ophthalmic and/or central nervous system complications, *Pediatrics* 87:323–327, 1991.

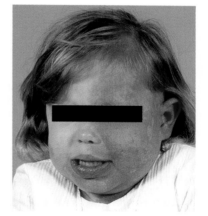

Figure 5-8. Sturge-Weber syndrome. The bilateral port wine stain involves the left V1, V2, and V3 regions and right V3 region.

33. What are the complications of leptomeningeal angiomatosis?

The vascular malformation of the cerebral meninges becomes complicated by meningeal artery calcification, calcification of the subjacent cortex, and cerebral atrophy. This results in epilepsy in 75% to 90% of cases, mental retardation (particularly in those with severe epilepsy), and, occasionally, contralateral hemiplegia.

Paller AS: The Sturge-Weber syndrome, *Pediatr Dermatol* 4:300–304, 1987.
Thomas-Sohl KA, Vaslow DF, Maria BL: Sturge-Weber syndrome: a review, *Pediatr Neurol* 30:303–310, 2004.

34. When does epilepsy usually begin in the Sturge-Weber syndrome?

The onset is usually between the second and seventh months of life, although this is occasionally delayed until later childhood.

35. Can the extent of neurologic involvement be predicted from the size of the facial port wine stain?

No. There is no correlation between extent of facial port wine stain, leptomeningeal angiomatosis, and degree of neurologic impairment.

36. What investigations confirm leptomeningeal angiomatosis?

MRI or CT scanning with contrast localizes the pial vascular anomalies and reveals intracranial calcification early in life. In later childhood (mean age, 7 years), a plain skull x-ray may reveal the typical double-contoured, curvilinear, "tram tracks" of calcification.

37. Do ocular complications occur in the Sturge-Weber syndrome?

Ocular complications occur in 30% to 60% of cases and include capillary malformations of the conjunctiva, iris, and choroid (ipsilateral to the facial port wine stain), glaucoma, and megalocornea. These complications may be associated only with a facial port wine stain involving the V1 distribution and do not necessarily imply CNS involvement. Glaucoma most commonly begins in the first 2 years of life; hence, regular ophthalmologic review from birth is vital in patients with V1 port wine stains.

38. How can the facial port wine stain be treated?

The pulsed dye laser (wavelength = 585/595 nm) is the most effective treatment modality. Regular laser treatments may result in significant fading and may also help prevent the soft tissue hypertrophy that gradually develops with many port wine stains.

39. In what other neurocutaneous disorders do facial or occipitocervical port wine stains occur?

Von Hippel-Lindau disease. Other features of this autosomal dominant disorder may include bilateral retinal angiomatosis (50%); cerebellar, medullary, or spinal hemangioblastoma (40%); renal cell carcinoma (25%); and, occasionally, pheochromocytoma.

ATAXIA-TELANGIECTASIA

40. What is the inheritance of ataxia-telangiectasia?

An autosomal recessive gene with the defective gene located on chromosome 11q22.3; it encodes an ataxia-telangiectasia mutated gene (*ATM*) that is a member of the phosphotidylinositol 3–kinase family.

41. What is the earliest clinical sign of ataxia-telangiectasia?

Progressive cerebellar ataxia due to degeneration of Purkinje cells, beginning at age 12 to 18 months. Choreoathetoid movements, hypotonia, dysarthria, and abnormal eye movements gradually develop, and intelligence frequently declines.

Smith SL, Conerly SL: Ataxia-telangiectasia or Louis-Bar syndrome, *J Am Acad Dermatol* 12:681–696, 1985.

42. Name the typical skin sign of ataxia-telangiectasia.

Mucocutaneous telangiectases. These begin on the bulbar conjunctiva and ears between 2 and 6 years of age and may progress to involve the periorbital skin, trunk, extremities, body folds, and other mucosal surfaces.

43. What are the two most common causes of death in ataxia-telangiectasia?

Severe respiratory infections and lymphoreticular malignancies.

NEUROCUTANEOUS MELANOCYTOSIS

44. What are the essential features of neurocutaneous melanocytosis (NCM)?

The presence of a congenital melanocytic nevus with melanotic rests in the brain or meninges.

45. What type of congenital nevus is usually present?

NCM occurs in 7.5% of patients with giant truncal nevi and approximately 70% of patients with medium-sized congenital nevi and multiple progressive satellite lesions.

Bett BJ: Large or multiple congenital melanocytic nevi: occurrence of neurocutaneous melanocytosis, *J Am Acad Dermatol* 54:767–777, 2006.

46. Is it always symptomatic?

No. One third of cases are asymptomatic. Those with symptoms present with seizures, hydrocephalus, spinal cord compression, and developmental delay.

47. How is it diagnosed?

MRI scanning done before 4 months of age is the most appropriate investigation in high-risk babies.

ACKNOWLEDGMENT

Some of the clinical photographs were kindly provided by Drs. William Weston and Joseph Morelli.

MECHANOBULLOUS DISORDERS

H. Alan Arbuckle, MD, FAAP, FAAD, and Ronald E. Grimwood, MD

CHAPTER 6

1. What are the mechanobullous disorders?

This is a group of disorders, either inherited or acquired, that result in small blisters (vesicle) or large blisters (bulla) that form after trauma to the skin. The most common acquired lesion would be a typical blister that one can develop on a foot after the skin rubs on a shoe or boot. The most common inherited mechanobullous disorders are those that fall into the category of epidermolysis bullosa (EB). Vesicles and bullae develop in these individuals with very minor trauma. The remaining portion of this chapter will deal with EB and its complications.

2. Do all of the blisters that form in EB develop in the same layer of the skin?

No. Depending on the type of EB there are three basic levels of separation within the skin. The two basic layers of skin are the epidermis and dermis. The junction between these two layers contains important structural proteins and is called the dermal–epidermal junction (DEJ) (Fig. 6-1). Separation due to trauma may occur in any one of these three anatomic sites.

Key Points: Heritable Blistering Disorders

1. Epidermolysis bullosa is an inherited group of disorders characterized by genetic defects of structural proteins needed for the normal attachment and integrity of the epidermis.
2. There are four major subtypes with different ultrastructural localization of the blister: EB simplex (epidermal cleavage plane), junctional EB (cleavage plane between epidermis and dermis), dystrophic EB (cleavage plane in superficial dermis), and Kindler's syndrome (with a mixed split of both epidermis and dermis).
3. Fetoscopy with a skin biopsy can be used to provide a prenatal diagnosis.
4. At the present time, there is no specific therapy for the treatment of any of the forms of EB.
5. The management of EB consists of genetic counseling, prevention of mechanical forces that produce new blisters, wound care, nutritional support, and infection control.

3. How is EB classified, and what are the major modes of inheritance?

In the past, there were three major categories of EB, depending on the level of the blister, and numerous subtypes within each category. In 2008, the Third International Consensus Meeting on Diagnosis and Classification of EB was published. In this manuscript, there was an attempt to simplify classification and eliminate misleading terms and acronyms. EB is now divided into four major categories:

1. Epidermolysis bullosa simplex
   - **Localized:** Epidermis (basal layer); autosomal dominant
   - **Generalized:** Epidermis (basal layer); autosomal dominant
2. Junctional epidermolysis bullosa
   - **Lethal:** DEJ; autosomal recessive
   - **Nonlethal:** DEJ; autosomal recessive
3. Dystrophic epidermolysis bullosa
   - **Dominant DEB:** Dermis; autosomal dominant
   - **Recessive DEB:** Dermis; autosomal recessive
4. Kindler's syndrome: Mixed; autosomal recessive

Fine JD, Eady RA, Bauer EA, et al: The classification of inherited epidermolysis bullosa (EB): report of the Third International Consensus Meeting on Diagnosis and Classification of EB, *JAAD* 58(6):931–950, 2008.

4. Describe the clinical findings in EB simplex.

In the common **localized** variety, the presentation is that of easy blistering noted on the hands and feet. These individuals may go undiagnosed until they are placed in a situation that generates increased pressure to these surfaces, such as marching in the military (Fig. 6-2). The **generalized** form is also usually present at birth, but, on rare occasions, it may not appear until 6 to 12 months of age in areas of trauma. The affected areas generally heal without scarring. In the simplex forms, generally the skin is the only thing affected; however, in the more severe forms of generalized simplex, they can have oral mucosa involvement and, on rare occasions, have esophageal strictures. The good news is that in some of the severe forms of generalized simplex EB the blistering tends to improve as the child ages. This is true for both the intraoral and cutaneous lesions.

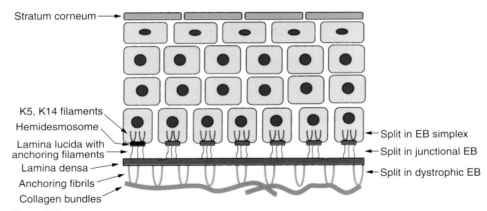

Figure 6-1. Layers of the skin with major sites of splitting in epidermolysis bullosa (EB). (Courtesy of James E. Fitzpatrick, MD.)

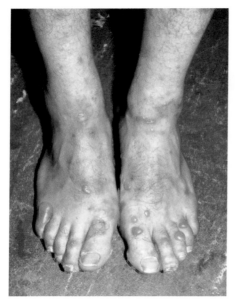

Figure 6-2. Localized junctional EB confined to the feet occurring in an infantry soldier. This exacerbation was produced by a long forced march. (Courtesy of the Fitzsimons Army Medical Center teaching files.)

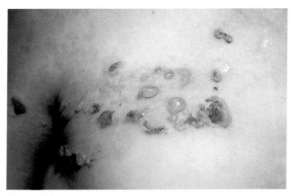

Figure 6-3. Generalized EB simplex demonstrating generalized truncal blistering.

5. Is the cause of EB simplex known?

Yes. In the vast majority of cases simplex EB is due to a mutation in either keratin 5 or 14 (Fig. 6-3). Keratins are structural proteins within keratinocytes that give the keratinocytes their shape and size, similar to the frame in a house. Keratins 5 and 14 are expressed in the basal layer of the epidermis, which is why the split is in the epidermis in EB simplex. There are rare forms of EB simplex that involve other structural proteins within the epidermis, such as plakophilin, desmoplakin, plectin, and integrins. Of interest is the simplex form of EB involving the protein plectin. Plectin is also important in skeletal muscle and individuals affected by the plectin form of EB simplex develop muscular dystrophy, usually after puberty.

Charlesworth A, Gagnous-Palacios L, Bonduelle M, et al: Identification of a lethal form of epidermolysis bullosa simplex associated with a homozygous mutation in plectin, *J Invest Dermatol* 121:1344–1348, 2003.

6. What are the clinical findings in junctional EB?

At birth, a few blisters may be present over areas of trauma, and it may be impossible to tell this type from EB simplex or the dystrophic type. However, infants may have oral erosions that are not found in EB simplex. Junctional EB includes

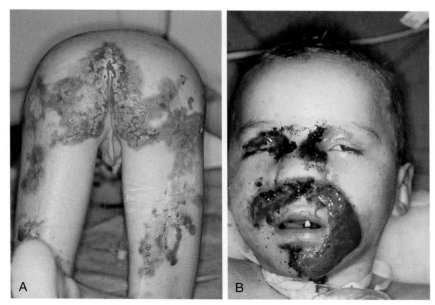

Figure 6-4. A and **B,** Junctional epidermolysis bullosa, lethal type. Chronic central erosions are characteristic.

localized variants that are not as involved and a severe generalized form (lethal) that typically results in death prior to the age of two (Fig. 6-4). As with EB simplex, blisters and erosions over areas of trauma are common. In contrast to those with EB simplex, children with the lethal form of JEB have prominent central facial erosions with hypergranulation tissue that is difficult to treat. They also have dental defects, nail dystrophy, and tracheal and bronchiolar involvement producing respiratory distress, which is often the cause of death. The other common cause of death in infants with the lethal JEB is sepsis.

7. Is the cause of junctional EB known?

Yes. The most common cause of JEB is a defect in a protein at the DEJ called laminin 5. Laminin 5 is very important in keeping the epidermis attached to the dermis; therefore the split in JEB is at the lamina lucida within the DEJ. Many of the mutations in the laminin 5 gene that result in the lethal form of JEB cause a stop codon, which results in early termination of transcription; so, very little laminin 5 is made. In the milder forms of JEB, having a laminin 5 mutation, the result is just an abnormal or truncated protein that still maintains some function. There are other rarer forms of JEB that can result from mutations to the genes that encode for either bullous pemphigoid antigen-2 (also referred to as type XVII collagen) or α6β4 integrin. Both proteins are found in the anchoring filaments at the DEJ. Of note, the form of JEB involving α6β4 integrin results in pyloric atresia in addition to blistering.

Bauer JW, Lanschuetzer C: Type XVII collagen gene mutations in junctional epidermolysis bullosa and prospects for gene therapy, *Clin Exp Dermatol* 28:53–60, 2003.

Iacovacci S, Cicuzza S, Odorisio T, et al: Novel and recurrent mutations in the integrin beta 4 subunit gene causing lethal junctional epidermolysis bullosa with pyloric atresia, *Exp Dermatol* 12:925, 2003.

8. What are the clinical findings in dystrophic EB?

In the recessive form of this condition, hemorrhagic blisters are typically present at birth. The blistered areas heal with scarring that can lead to the loss of functional digits in the hands (Fig. 6-5). Oral and esophageal involvement causes feeding problems with resultant esophageal stricture. The teeth are malformed, and multifactorial anemia is common. The dominant form of the disease is less severe and tends to be more localized. Atrophic scarring is still the rule over affected areas. A unique dominant dystrophic form exists (transient bullous dermolysis in the newborn) that is only transient. The blistering tendency decreases with age.

Christiano AM, Fine JD, Uitto J: Genetic basis of dominantly inherited transient bullous dermolysis of the newborn: a splice site mutation in the type VII collagen gene, *J Invest Dermatol* 109:811–814, 1997.

Das BB, Sahoo S: Dystrophic epidermolysis bullosa, *J Perinatol* 24:41–47, 2004.

9. Is the cause of dystrophic EB known?

The primary defect in dystrophic EB is an absent or structurally altered protein found in the dermis. This protein is type VII collagen, which makes up the anchoring fibrils that connect the basement membrane with the dermal collagen. Recently, mutations in the type VII collagen gene (*COL7A1*) located on the short arm of chromosome 3 have been found in families with both the autosomal dominant and autosomal recessive form of dystrophic EB.

Individuals with both the recessive and dominant forms are at increased risk of squamous cell carcinomas as they age. In the severe recessive form, the cumulative risks are 38.7% by age 35, 70% by age 45, and 78.7% by age 55.

Fine JD, Johnson LB, Weiner M, et al: Epidermolysis bullosa and the risk of life-threatening cancers: the National EB Registry experience, *JAAD* 60(2):203–211, 2009.

Masse M, Cserhalmi-Friedman PB, Falanga V, et al: Identification of a novel type VII collagen gene mutations resulting in severe recessive dystrophic epidermolysis bullosa, *Clin Exp Dermatol* 30:289–293, 2005.

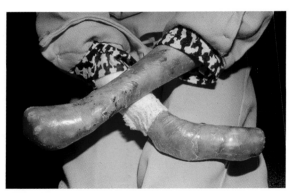

Figure 6-5. Recessive dystrophic epidermolysis bullosa. Severe scarring resulting in loss of functional digits.

10. What is Kindler's syndrome?

Kindler's syndrome was added as a subtype of EB, in 2008, with the release of the Third International Consensus Meeting on EB. Prior to this, it was considered a separate mechanobullous disease. Kindler's syndrome is an autosomal recessive form of EB that is characterized by poikiloderma, blistering in areas of trauma, mucosal inflammation, and photosensitivity. Like some forms of EB simplex, the blistering in Kindler's syndrome tends to improve with age. The cause of Kindler's syndrome is a loss of function mutation in the *FERMT1* gene. This mutation causes an alteration in the actin cytoskeleton-extracellular matrix and results in a variable plane of blister formation at or close to the DEJ. Because of the severe mucosal inflammation, patients with Kindler's syndrome have significant dental issues as well as anal stenosis and phimosis.

Burch JM, Fassihi H, Jones CA, et al: Kindler syndrome: a new mutation and new diagnostic possibilities, *Arch Dermatol* 142:620–624, 2006.

Lai-Cheong JE, McGrath JA: Kindler syndrome, *Dermatol Clin* 28(1):119–124, 2010.

11. Can a definitive diagnosis of the various EB types be made on clinical presentation?

No. In newborns and infants, it is virtually impossible to tell these disorders apart. Several techniques can aid in establishing the correct diagnosis. One such technique is immunomapping, which involves the use of antibodies directed against known proteins located at specific sites in the skin. The patient's skin is subjected to minor trauma followed by a biopsy. The specimen is then "mapped" with the locating antibodies (Fig. 6-6). This technique locates the actual level of the blister formation in the skin specimen and determines the major category of mechanobullous disorder (i.e., epidermal, junctional, or dystrophic). The diagnosis can be further refined by using monoclonal antibodies that are specific for the

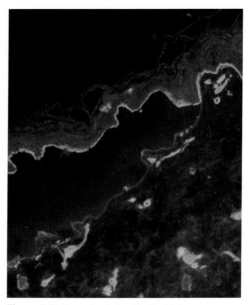

Figure 6-6. Recessive dystrophic EB with immunomapping with fluorescent marker for laminin. Note that the laminin that is found on the dermal side of the basement membrane zone is on the roof of an induced blister. (Courtesy of James E. Fitzpatrick, MD.)

missing or altered proteins. At many institutions, where electron microscopy (EM) is available, the tissue is also examined under EM, which can add additional information in making the diagnosis of EB (Fig. 6-7).

12. Are there any treatments for the mechanobullous disorders?

There are no specific treatments for this group of disorders. The current standard of care for these infants is strict wound care and infection control. Nonadherent dressings and padding are used to help blister heal and decrease trauma to the skin. Bathing can be quite painful for these children, especially for those that have the more severe forms of EB. Adding one pound of pool salt to a full tub of water has been found to help alleviate the pain with bathing.

In variants with oral manifestations, such as junctional EB and recessive dystrophic EB, meticulous oral hygiene with close dental follow-up is essential. Capping, crowns, and restorations can be helpful. Blenderized food is necessary early on for patients with recessive dystrophic EB to help minimize trauma to the esophagus and prevent esophageal webbing. Hand deformities in dystrophic EB can be surgically corrected, but the recurrence rate is high. There is extensive research in the area of gene therapy for the various forms of epidermolysis bullosa.

When dealing with a newborn with suspected EB it is best to contact one of the national organizations that deals with EB, such as the Dystrophic EB Research Association (www.DebRA.org), which can provide both clinical as well as family support. In addition, one can contact one of the five large multidisciplinary EB clinics in North America (Stanford University, Stanford, CA; Children's Hospital, Aurora, CO; Cincinatti Children's Hospital, OH; Hospital for Sick Children, Toronto, Canada; and Columbia University, New York).

13. Are prenatal diagnostic techniques useful for this group of disorders?

Fetoscopy with fetal skin biopsy has been the primary method of prenatal diagnosis for EB and other inherited skin diseases. More recently, it has been found that fetal DNA can be obtained as early as 10 weeks estimated gestational age (EGA) from chorionic villi or 12 weeks EGA from amniotic fluid.

Fassihi H, Ashton GH, Denyer J, et al: Prenatal diagnosis of Herlitz junctional epidermolysis bullosa in nonidentical twins, *Clin Exp Dermatol* 30:180–182, 2005.

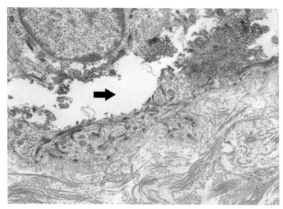

Figure 6-7. Electron microscopic study of an induced blister in EB simplex demonstrating a split (*arrow*) in the cytoplasm of the basilar keratinocyte. (Courtesy of James E. Fitzpatrick, MD.)

PAPULOSQUAMOUS SKIN ERUPTIONS

Alison S. Klenk, MD, and Jeffrey B. Travers, MD, PhD

1. Name the papulosquamous skin eruptions.

Papulosquamous skin disorders are inflammatory reactions characterized by red or purple papules and plaques with scale. These diseases include psoriasis, pityriasis rubra pilaris, seborrheic dermatitis, pityriasis rosea, pityriasis lichenoides et varioliformis acuta, and parapsoriasis. Lichen planus and lichen nitidus are also considered papulosquamous disorders (see Chapter 12).

Habif TP: *Clinical dermatology: a color guide to diagnosis and therapy*, ed 4, St Louis, 2004, Mosby.

2. What is psoriasis?

Psoriasis is a common, genetically determined, inflammatory, and hyperproliferative skin disease. Although there are morphologic variations, the most characteristic lesions consist of chronic, well-demarcated, dull-red plaques (Fig. 7-1A) with silvery scale found commonly on extensor surfaces and the scalp (Fig. 7-1B).

3. What is its incidence of psoriasis?

Psoriasis occurs in about 1% to 2% of the population worldwide. Its incidence varies among population groups, being highest in those of Western Europe and Scandinavia. It is less common in blacks and Chinese and rare in pure Native Americans.

4. List the different types of psoriasis.

The different clinical presentations of psoriasis can be separated by morphology or location.

Morphologic variants	Locational variants
Chronic plaque psoriasis	Scalp psoriasis
Guttate psoriasis	Palmoplantar psoriasis
Pustular psoriasis	Inverse psoriasis
Erythrodermic psoriasis	Nail psoriasis
Psoriatic arthritis	

5. What is guttate psoriasis?

Guttate psoriasis is a variant of psoriasis usually seen in adolescents and young adults. It is characterized by crops of small, droplike, psoriatic papules and plaques (Fig. 7-2A). The word guttate is derived from the Latin *gutta*, which means "drop." This type of psoriasis is often found in association with streptococcal pharyngitis, and treatment of the pharyngitis with oral antibiotics may improve or even clear the psoriasis.

6. Does pustular psoriasis refer to psoriasis that is secondarily infected?

No. The pustular forms are uncommon, less stable variants of psoriasis. Instead of erythematous plaques with silvery scale as seen in typical psoriasis, pustular psoriasis is characterized by superficial pustules, often with fine desquamation. Although triggers such as infection can precipitate a flare of pustular psoriasis, the pustules are sterile. Patients often need systemic treatments, such as retinoids, immunosuppressives, or phototherapy, to keep their disease under control.

7. What is inverse psoriasis?

Inverse psoriasis refers to psoriasis that involves intertriginous areas (axillae, groin, umbilicus). This distribution is opposite to the usual extensor distribution of psoriasis vulgaris. Psoriatic lesions with both distributions sometimes can be found in the same patients. Clinically, psoriatic lesions found in these "inverse" distributions often do not have scale, but consist of sharply demarcated red plaques that may become macerated and eroded (Fig. 7-2B). Treatment of inverse psoriasis usually involves low-potency (nonfluorinated) topical corticosteroids.

8. Is there a genetic basis for psoriasis?

Although a specific genetic abnormality has not been identified, psoriasis is generally considered to be a genetically determined disease. There are reports of striking family pedigrees that suggest an autosomal dominant inheritance, but with only partial penetrance. Keep in mind that psoriasis is probably not a single disease, but a family of diseases involving epidermal hyperproliferation. The external environment presumably plays a role in the clinical expression.

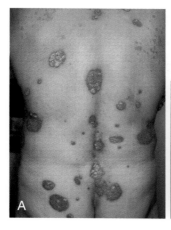

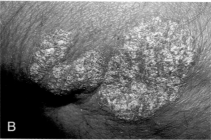

Figure 7-1. Psoriasis vulgaris. **A,** Numerous well-demarcated scaly plaques on the trunk. **B,** Close-up of elbow involvement demonstrating typical, well-demarcated, red plaques with silvery scale. (Panel A courtesy of the Fitzsimons Army Medical Center teaching files).

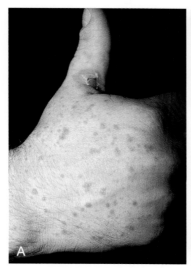

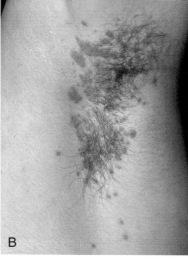

Figure 7-2. **A,** Guttate, or the acute type of psoriasis, showing widespread droplike lesions. This type of psoriasis is associated with streptococcal infections, probably through the immune-stimulating effects of exotoxins secreted by the bacteria. **B,** Inverse psoriasis involves intertriginous areas such as the axilla, as shown here. Note the lack of silvery scale seen in psoriasis vulgaris.

The strongest evidence for the importance of external factors in the expression of psoriasis is seen in acute guttate psoriasis, which often occurs in association with streptococcal pharyngitis.

Travers JB, Hamid QA, Norris DA, et al: The environment of psoriasis allows enhanced reactivity to epicutaneously applied bacterial exotoxins, *J Clin Invest* 104:1181–1189, 1999.

9. If one of my relatives has psoriasis, what is the chance that I will get psoriasis?

Questionnaire-based studies reveal that almost 5% of first-degree relatives of psoriasis patients also have psoriasis, compared to 1.2% of relatives of nonpsoriatic spouses of probands. If a sibling has psoriasis, other siblings have a 16% incidence if one parent has psoriasis and a 50% chance if both parents are affected. Twin studies indicate that if one twin has psoriasis, the other twin is similarly affected in 20% of dizygotic pairs and in 73% of monozygotic pairs. The absence of 100% concordance in monozygotic twins (who have identical genetic material) indicates that environmental factors also contribute to the expression of psoriasis.

10. Name the types of psoriatic arthritis.

Although the exact incidence of psoriatic arthritis is unknown, an estimated 5% to 10% of patients with psoriasis suffer from psoriatic arthritis. The arthritis may precede, accompany, or, more commonly, follow the development of the skin disease. The five types of psoriatic arthritis are

- Asymmetric oligoarthritis, monoarthritis (60% to 70%)
- Symmetric polyarthritis (15%)
- Distal interphalangeal joint (DIP) disease (5%)
- Destructive arthritis (5%)
- Axial arthritis (5%)

11. Describe the clinical features of the psoriatic arthritides.

Asymmetrical arthritis, the most common form of psoriatic arthritis, usually involves one or several joints of the fingers or toes. The appearance of this type of arthritis can be similar to subacute gout and include "sausage-like" swelling of a digit due to involvement of the proximal and DIP joints and the flexor sheath (Fig. 7-3). Symmetrical polyarthritis resembles rheumatoid arthritis, but tests for rheumatoid factor are negative, and the condition is clinically less severe than rheumatoid arthritis. Although not common, DIP joint disease of hands and feet is the most classic presentation of arthritis with psoriasis. Destructive arthritis (arthritis mutilans) is a rare, severely deforming arthritis involving predominantly fingers and toes. Gross osteolysis of the small bones of the hands and feet can result in shortening, subluxations, and, in severe cases, telescoping of the digits, resulting in an "opera glass" deformity. Axial arthritis of the spine, which resembles idiopathic ankylosing spondylitis, manifests by itself or with peripheral joint disease.

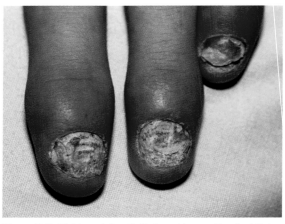

Figure 7-3. Distal psoriatic arthritis in an 11-year-old patient. Note the extensive nail changes. (Courtesy of the William L. Weston, M.D. collection.)

12. What are the abnormal nail findings seen in psoriasis? Which is most common?

A careful examination of the nails should be part of the skin exam, especially when evaluating a rash that might be psoriasis. Characteristic nail changes are found in 25% to 50% of psoriatics. These changes include nail pitting, discoloration, onycholysis, subungual hyperkeratosis, and nail deformity. Nail pitting, the most common nail finding in psoriasis, consists of small, discrete, punched-out depressions on the nail surface (Fig. 7-4). Circular areas of nail bed discoloration that resemble oil drops are often seen under the nail plate (hyponychium). The nail can become thin and brittle at the distal edge with separation from the nail bed (onycholysis) or thickened with subungual debris.

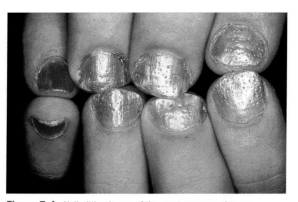

Figure 7-4. Nail pitting is one of the most common changes associated with psoriasis. As demonstrated here, even nail polish cannot hide these discrete pits.

Ridges, grooves, or even frank deformity of the nail plate can also be seen.

13. Are there other nonskin manifestations of psoriasis?

Recent studies have confirmed that psoriasis is associated with medical and psychiatric co-morbidities. Patients with psoriasis have a higher incidence of obesity, diabetes mellitus, hypertension, hypercholesterolemia, and myocardial infarction. Rates of Crohn's disease and ulcerative colitis are also increased in patients with psoriasis. In addition, the emotional distress of having a severe skin disease may have a profoundly negative psychological impact. Depressed mood, anxiety, suicidal ideation, and clinical depression are found at a higher incidence in psoriatic patients. Care of the psoriatic patient does not stop at the skin and joints.

14. You are working in a dermatology clinic, seeing a patient with a rash that is possibly psoriasis. Outside the room, the attending asks if you noticed any evidence of the "Koebner phenomenon" or an "Auspitz sign" when you examined the patient. What are these?

The isomorphic or Koebner phenomenon is the development of a cutaneous eruption at the site of physical trauma (scratch, surgical wound, or sunburn). Other skin conditions that exhibit the Koebner phenomenon include lichen planus, lichen nitidus, and vitiligo. Patients with psoriasis should be warned of this tendency before subjecting themselves to cosmetic procedures involving physical trauma (such as having a tattoo).

The Auspitz sign is the presence of small bleeding points seen on a psoriatic lesion when the scales are removed. This bleeding is due to thinning of the epidermis between the elongated rete ridges. Note that it is not a good idea to attempt to elicit these two signs on your psoriatic patients.

15. Name three types of drugs that precipitate or exacerbate psoriasis.

Beta-blocking agents, antimalarials (i.e., hydroxychloroquine), and lithium. All three can precipitate or exacerbate psoriasis. These medications should be used with caution in psoriatics.

16. What other factors can provoke or exacerbate psoriasis?

Any evidence of skin or other systemic infection (especially streptococcal pharyngitis) should warrant appropriate oral antibiotics.

17. Do systemic corticosteroids help psoriasis?

Although treatment with systemic corticosteroids rapidly clears psoriasis, the disease usually "breaks through," requiring higher doses of corticosteroids. If systemic corticosteroid treatment is withdrawn, the psoriasis usually relapses and may worsen. This "rebound" worsening of psoriasis may even result in a severe flare of erythrodermic (total body) or generalized pustular psoriasis.

18. What topical medications are used to treat psoriasis?

Patients with limited disease (usually <20% of their body surface) can often be managed on topical agents alone. Although systemic corticosteroids generally should not be used, topical and intralesional corticosteroids are a first-line treatment. For plaques, medium- to high-potency corticosteroids used daily can result in a rapid response, often controlling the inflammation and itching. Unfortunately, the relief is often temporary, and tolerance can occur. Side effects include atrophy and telangiectasias, especially if high-potency topical preparations are used on the face or intertriginous areas (see also Chapter 54).

Coal tar preparations can also be effective, especially if used with topical corticosteroids. Anthralin, a synthetic derivative of chrysarobin, a tree bark extract, is effective in daily, short applications for chronic plaque psoriasis, but its irritant qualities often worsen inflammatory psoriasis. Calcipotriene (Dovonex), a vitamin D3 analog, is an effective treatment for localized psoriasis, but its cost and the possibility of systemic absorption resulting in changes in calcium homeostasis preclude its use in extensive disease. Calcipotriene should be limited to a maximum dosage of 100 gm/wk. A newer and potentially more effective treatment is the combination of calcipotriene and the corticosteroid, betamethasone diproprionate (Taclonex).

Menter A, Gottlieb A, Feldman SR, et al: Guidelines of care for the management of psoriasis and psoriatic arthritis. Section 1. Overview of psoriasis and guidelines of care for the treatment of psoriasis with biologics, *J Am Acad Dermatol* 58:826–850, 2008.

19. How is ultraviolet radiation used to treat psoriasis?

It has been known for centuries that sunlight exposure can improve psoriasis. Two forms of ultraviolet radiation are used clinically: ultraviolet B (UVB, 290 to 320 nm) and ultraviolet A (UVA, 320 to 400 nm) combined with an oral photosensitizer, psoralen plus UVA (PUVA). Although not as effective as PUVA, use of UVB results in less incidence of side effects and is often used first in the treatment of light-sensitive psoriasis (see also Chapter 54).

20. What systemic drugs are used to treat psoriasis?

Methotrexate, cyclosporine, and retinoids (i.e., acitretin). Because of the potential side effects of these agents, their use should be carefully considered by the physician and patient. Methotrexate suppresses DNA synthesis by inhibiting the enzyme dihydrofolate reductase. In addition to its antimitotic effects, methotrexate inhibits neutrophil function. Side effects include bone marrow suppression, stomach upset, and hepatotoxicity. Although the incidence of hepatic fibrosis and cirrhosis is low with cumulative doses <1.5 gm, liver function tests are not a reliable indicator of methotrexate-induced hepatotoxicity, and a liver biopsy is recommended after 1.5 gm and every 1.0 to 1.5 gm thereafter. Methotrexate should be avoided in psoriatic patients who have underlying liver disease, renal disease, or are heavy drinkers. Patients who take methotrexate should be aware of its interactions with many other medications.

The antilymphocytic drug cyclosporine can be used for severe psoriasis. It has a relatively rapid onset of action, but side effects such as hypertension and nephrotoxicity limit its use as a long-term agent. The doses used, 3 to 5 mg/kg/day, are usually lower than the dosages used to inhibit organ transplant rejection.

Systemic retinoids such as acitretin are first-line agents in pustular psoriasis and also may be used to treat chronic plaque psoriasis. Unlike methotrexate and cyclosporine, retinoids do not suppress the immune system. Rather, retinoids likely mitigate the epidermal hyperproliferation seen in psoriasis. Acitretin is a potent teratogen and must be avoided in women of child-bearing age. Other systemic treatments include the "biologicals," which will be covered in the next question.

21. What biologic agents may be used in the treatment of psoriasis?

Biologic agents are proteins derived from living cells that are used to modulate specific portions of the aberrant immune response that leads to psoriasis. They are administered by subcutaneous, intramuscular, or intravenous injection. Tumor necrosis factor (TNF) alpha inhibitors (etanercept, adalimumab, and infliximab), as well as alefacept, are used in the treatment of refractory or extensive psoriasis. The TNF-α inhibitors block the proinflammatory action of TNF-α, a potent cytokine that mediates the formation of psoriatic plaques. Risks of TNF-α inhibitors include increased susceptibility to infections, such as reactivation of tuberculosis or hepatitis B, and higher rates of malignancy such as lymphoma.

Alefacept binds to and inhibits memory T lymphocytes that express CD2, which reduces the number of these pathogenic T cells. Patients undergoing alefacept therapy must be monitored for lymphopenia. Alefacept is less effective than the TNF-α inhibitors and is rarely used in clinical practice.

The newest biologic agent (FDA-approved in September, 2009) is ustekinumab, a humanized antibody against the p40 subunit found in the cytokines interleukin (IL)-12 and IL-23. In particular, the inhibition of IL-23 blocks the T-cell pathway (TH17) recently implicated in the pathogenesis of psoriasis.

Although these systemic psoriasis therapies may be more effective, care must be exercised in their use, especially because the long-term side effects of biological agents are not completely clear.

22. Describe the rash of pityriasis rubra pilaris.

Pityriasis rubra pilaris (PRP) is a rare disease in which the primary abnormality appears to be hyperproliferation of the epidermis (Fig. 7-5). Five variants have been described, the most common being type I, the classic adult-onset form. In this type, the eruption commonly begins on the head and neck as reddish-orange, slightly scaly macules and thin plaques. The rash extends in a cephalocaudal fashion, and within several weeks, red, perifollicular papules with central plugs develop in the lesions. The scalp often develops extensive yellowish scale. The palms and soles become thickened and yellow, which is called keratoderma. This results in a well-demarcated, very characteristic "PRP sandal." Although total body involvement (erythroderma) is not uncommon, the rash of PRP often has characteristic skip areas of normal skin ("islands of sparing"). Considering that the rash usually looks very impressive, it is surprising that patients often complain of only mild irritation and pruritus.

23. Although pityriasis rubra pilaris can occur at any age, in what decades is it most often seen? What is the prognosis?

PRP has a bimodal age distribution, with the highest incidence in the fifth and sixth decades and a smaller peak in childhood. The prognosis is variable, but usually 80% of patients clear spontaneously in several years.

24. How is pityriasis rubra pilaris treated?

Treatment strategies for PRP depend on the extent of involvement and how much the patient is bothered. Lubrication with emollients and topical corticosteroids are rarely helpful. The treatment of choice is oral retinoids, with methotrexate being reserved for retinoid-resistant cases.

Key Points: Papulosquamous Disorders

1. Psoriasis classically has symmetrical red plaques with silver-white scale on elbows, knees, and scalp.
2. Nail changes in psoriasis can mimic those seen with a dermatophyte fungal infection.
3. Pityriasis rubra pilaris has large areas of orange-colored plaques with islands of sparing, and hand/foot thickened skin.
4. Seborrheic dermatitis can be found not only on scalp, but also on the face around the nares, central chest, axillae, and even on the penis.
5. Pityriasis rosea has oval papules and plaques that tend to line up along skin lines ("Christmas tree" pattern) with trailing scale (scale does not reach the end of the lesion).

25. Describe the distribution of the "seborrheic areas."

Seborrheic areas have a rich supply of sebaceous glands and include the scalp, face, central chest, and intertriginous areas. Skin diseases that can have a "seborrheic distribution" include seborrheic dermatitis, psoriasis, Darier's disease, and pemphigus foliaceus.

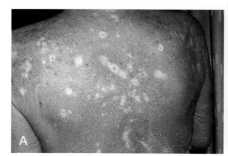
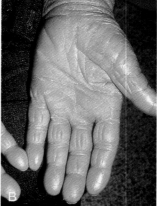

Figure 7-5. Pityriasis rubra pilaris. **A,** Extensive involvement in adult showing characteristic salmon color and "islands of sparing." **B,** Characteristic thickened yellow palmar changes.

26. What does seborrheic dermatitis look like?

Seborrheic dermatitis is a chronic dermatitis with a typical morphologic appearance of red plaques with greasy yellow scales, distributed in the seborrheic areas. Scalp involvement is almost universal. Facial involvement is common and manifests itself as erythema and scaling on the medial sides of the eyebrows, glabella, and nasolabial folds. Ocular involvement (blepharitis and conjunctivitis) and ear involvement (external auditory canal and posterior auricular scalp) are also frequently seen. Visible scalp desquamation, commonly known as dandruff, is probably the precursor and/or a mild form of seborrheic dermatitis.

Naldi L, Rebora A: Clinical practice. Seborrheic dermatitis, *N Engl J Med* 360:387–396, 2009.

27. What causes seborrheic dermatitis?

Seborrheic dermatitis is probably a hypersensitivity response to common skin yeasts, of the genus *Malassezia* (*Pityrosporum*). Seborrheic dermatitis may be more severe when associated with HIV infection, the use of dopamine antagonist antipsychotics, and Parkinson's disease.

28. How can you differentiate between seborrheic dermatitis and psoriasis of the scalp?

The differentiation between these two disorders can be difficult. However, in contrast to seborrheic dermatitis, scalp psoriasis is often patchy, consisting of thicker plaques with silvery scale. The rest of the skin should be examined, including the nails, to look for other evidence of psoriasis. The patient should also be questioned about a possible family history of psoriasis.

29. How is seborrheic dermatitis treated?

Although treatment of seborrheic dermatitis is suppressive, it is not curative. The scalp is best treated with medicated shampoos (selenium sulfide, zinc pyrithione, and tar). Patients should be instructed to leave the shampoo on their scalp for at least 5 minutes before rinsing (or two or three songs for patients who are inclined to sing in the shower). Use of a medium- or high-potency topical steroid solution on the scalp is often helpful for patients who experience burning or pruritus or have resistant areas. Facial seborrheic dermatitis is very responsive to low-potency topical corticosteroids (hydrocortisone) or topical antifungal creams. Oral antibiotics should be given if there is evidence of secondary infection.

30. What is pityriasis rosea? Describe the characteristic rash.

Pityriasis rosea is an acute, benign, self-limiting disorder that affects teenagers and young adults. The eruption has a characteristic pattern, and three fourths of cases start with a single 2- to 4-cm, sharply defined, thin, oval plaque. Within a few days to weeks, crops of similar-appearing, though usually smaller, papules follow the initial "herald patch" (Fig. 7-6). The eruption characteristically involves the trunk and proximal extremities, usually sparing the face, palms, and soles. Lesions on the trunk tend to run parallel to the lines of skin cleavage, resulting in a "Christmas tree" pattern. The lesions usually resolve within several weeks to a month but may persist longer. Except for a mild prodrome, affected patients are usually asymptomatic. The lesions of pityriasis rosea often have "trailing scale" (e.g., collarette of scale that does not extend to the border of the lesion), and papular variants can be seen, especially in children.

Drago F, Broccolo F, Rebora, A : Pityriasis rosea: an update with a critical appraisal of its possible herpesviral etiology, *J Am Acad Dermatol* 61:303–318, 2009.

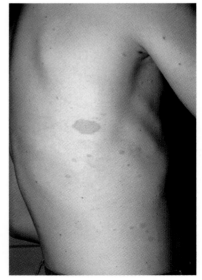

31. What is the cause of pityriasis rosea?

Although the etiology of pityriasis rosea is unknown, the occasional prodromal symptoms, characteristic disease course, tendency for lifelong immunity, seasonal variance, and reports of epidemics all point to an infectious (viral) agent. Treatment consists of reassurance, emollients, and antipruritic agents for symptomatic patients. Ultraviolet radiation treatment (sunshine or UVB) hastens the disappearance of the eruption. Some studies suggest that human herpesvirus 7 is the causative agent.

32. In the dermatology clinic, a 20-year-old man presents who has been referred from the primary care clinic with a diagnosis of pityriasis rosea. He has a rash that looks like pityriasis rosea, but he complains of fevers, myalgias, and swollen lymph glands. He remembers having an ulcer on his penis several months ago. What test do you recommend?

The eruption of secondary syphilis can mimic pityriasis rosea, though patients often have systemic manifestations such as fever, lymphadenopathy, headache, or bone pain. Unlike pityriasis rosea, secondary syphilis often involves the palms, soles, and mucous membranes. A sexual history should be elicited in such patients, and a rapid plasma reagin (RPR) or Venereal Disease Research Laboratory

Figure 7-6. Pityiasis rosea. A young adult demonstrates a characteristic large herald patch near the axilla associated with numerous oval secondary lesions that follow skin lines.

(VDRL) test should be obtained. Because syphilis is readily treated, and because untreated syphilis can result in life-threatening cardiovascular and neurologic sequelae, many dermatologists customarily obtain an RPR or VDRL test on every sexually active patient who presents with a pityriasis rosea–like eruption.

33. What are the two major types of parapsoriasis? Why is it important to differentiate between them?

Parapsoriasis is a term often used to describe slowly evolving, asymptomatic, scaly plaques, often found on the trunk and proximal extremities. Parapsoriasis is divided into small plaque (1- to 5-cm diameter) and large plaque (5- to 15-cm diameter) forms. The prognosis of the two types differs, and approximately 10% of cases of large-plaque parapsoriasis eventuate in T-cell lymphoma. Parapsoriasis is resistant to most topical treatments but often responds to phototherapy.

34. What is pityriasis lichenoides et varioliformis acuta?

Pityriasis lichenoides et varioliformis acuta (PLEVA or Mucha-Habermann disease) is a rare disease characterized by crops of polymorphous lesions on the trunk, thighs, and upper arms. The eruption consists of red-brown papules that can become purpuric, scaly, and even necrotic (Fig. 7-7). The patients usually are asymptomatic, although itching and low-grade fevers and malaise are not uncommon. Individual lesions resolve in several weeks leaving postinflammatory hyper- or hypopigmentation and occasionally scars. The clinical course of PLEVA often waxes and wanes and can last months to years.

Khachemoune A, Blyumin ML: Pityriasis lichenoides: pathophysiology, classification, and treatment, *Am J Clin Dermatol* 8:29–36, 2007.

35. How is PLEVA treated?

Oral antibiotics (erythromycin or tetracycline) have been suggested, but no controlled studies exist. Phototherapy and immunosuppressive agents, such as methotrexate, have been used for recalcitrant or severe cases.

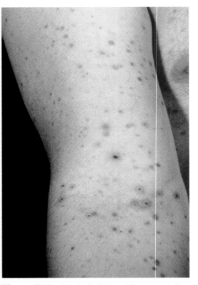

Figure 7-7. Pityriasis lichenoides et varioliformis acuta. Characteristic polymorphic appearance with red scaly papules, hemorrhagic papules, and necrotic papules.

CHAPTER 8

DERMATITIS (ECZEMA)

Thomas W. McGovern, MD

1. What is dermatitis and why is it so important?

Dermatologists use the interchangeable terms "dermatitis" or "eczema" to refer to a specific group of inflammatory skin diseases. Dermatitis presents with pruritic, erythematous macules, papules, vesicles, or plaques with or without distinct margins. Lesions pass through acute (vesicular), subacute (scaling and crusting), and chronic (acanthotic with thick epidermis) phases. Oozing, crusting, scaling, fissuring, and lichenification frequently accompany the primary lesions. Up to 25% of all patients presenting with a new skin disease have a form of dermatitis. Patients typically suffer from intense pruritus that distracts them from their daily activities, including sleep, and they are desperate for relief.

2. What is atopy?

Atopy is derived from the Greek word *atopos,* meaning "out-of-place," and refers to the predisposition to develop dermatitis, asthma, and allergic rhinitis. The surfaces where the body contacts the external environment are "overreactive" (the lower airways in asthma, the upper airways and conjunctiva in allergic rhinoconjunctivitis, and the skin in atopic dermatitis).

"Atopic dermatitis is not an allergic disease, but a skin disease with allergies" (Jon Hanifin, Dermatology Foundation Clinical Symposia, 2007): upper airway (allergic rhinitis) or lower airway (allergic asthma). For example, atopic dermatitis typically improves in the spring when allergic rhinitis is at its peak.

3. Why is atopic dermatitis becoming more common?

The prevalence of atopic dermatitis in six- and seven-year-old children varies from less than 2% in Iran and China to 10% to 20% in the United States, United Kingdom, Australia, and Scandinavia. The incidence was only 2% in those born before 1960. The increase over time and difference between more- and less-developed nations has been explained by the "hygiene hypothesis." This postulates that a reduction in the frequency of childhood infections results in an increased incidence of various allergic and autoimmune diseases including atopic dermatitis, asthma, allergic rhinitis, childhood insulin-dependent diabetes mellitus, and Crohn's disease.

4. What are the diagnostic criteria for atopic dermatitis?

Three of the four following features must be present:
- Pruritus—the primary symptom, and even referred to as the "primary lesion" by some
- Typical morphology and distribution of lesions for age
- Chronic or chronically relapsing course
- Personal or family history of asthma, allergic rhinitis, or atopic dermatitis

5. What is the underlying defect in patients with atopic dermatitis?

At least 50% of patients with moderate to severe atopic dermatitis have a defect in the gene coding for filaggrin, a protein essential to maintaining the barrier function of the stratum corneum. The stratum corneum then allows various irritants, microbes, or allergens to penetrate the skin surface, elicit cytokine release from keratinocytes, and initiate a Th2 immune response acutely that leads to the clinical manifestations of disease and increased IgE levels. In chronic cases of atopic dermatitis, the Th2 response is replaced by a Th1 response. A primary immune defect, at least in some atopic patients, cannot yet be ruled out because bone marrow stem cell transplants from atopic patients have transferred atopic dermatitis to recipients.

Terui T: Analysis of the mechanism for the development of allergic skin inflammation and the application for its treatment: overview of the pathophysiology of atopic dermatitis, *J Pharmacol Sci* 110:232–236, 2009.

6. In atopic dermatitis, which comes first—the itch or the rash?

The itch. Atopic dermatitis is "an itch, which, when scratched, erupts." Atopic dermatitis is pruritus enfleshed.

7. Why does atopic dermatitis itch?

Neural and chemical mechanisms are involved. When the epidermis and its nerve fibers are stripped from skin, pruritus is abolished. Keratinocytes and mast cells release high levels of nerve growth factor (NGF), which increases the sensitivity of cutaneous pruritus receptors. These sensitized nerve endings demonstrate an increased capacity to transmit signals that are perceived as pruritus (allokinesis). Chemical mediators associated with itch include serine proteases, interleukins 2 and 31, opioids, acetylcholine, prostanoids, and substance P. Histamine may play a limited role in the pruritus of atopic dermatitis. These mediators act either on nerve endings or directly on keratinocytes. They are produced by mast cells, keratinocytes, T cells, and nerve fibers.

Yosipovitch G, Papoiu ADP: What causes itch in atopic dermatitis? *Curr Allergy Asthma Rep* 8:306–311, 2008.

8. Why do people like to scratch an itch?

Scratching suppresses areas of the brain associated with negative experiences of pruritus and activates pleasure centers of the brain. In other words, there is an emotional reward for scratching. Unfortunately, scratching damages the skin and worsens dermatitis so that it itches even more. Therefore, people scratch even more and get caught in an "itch-scratch cycle" that they cannot exit without medical help or supreme levels of self-restraint.

Yosipovitch G, Ishiuji Y, Patel TS, et al: The brain processing of scratching, *J Invest Dermatol* 128:1806–1811, 2008.

9. Does psychological stress worsen atopic dermatitis?

Probably. In mice, various stressors can produce atopic dermatitis skin lesions, possibly due to an upregulation of substance P–sensitive nerve fibers. Transepidermal water loss increases in humans who are under mental stress compared to control subjects. Such water loss is an indicator of a defective epidermal barrier.

10. Did John Phillip Sousa write the "Atopic March?"

No, but if he did, it would have a lot of scratching, sneezing, and wheezing coming from the percussion section! The atopic march is not music but the subsequent development of allergic rhinitis (70%) and/or asthma (50%) in patients with atopic dermatitis. Filaggrin mutations predispose to airway disease in atopic dermatitis patients. Evidence points to the necessity of *epicutaneous* exposure to allergens (e.g., dust mites) that cause allergic *airway* disease in these patients. If infants with atopic dermatitis have good barrier protection, it is likely that the airway disease of the atopic march can be prevented!

Marenholz I: Filaggrin loss-of-function mutations predispose to phenotypes involved in the atopic march, *J Allergy Clin Immunol* 118(4):866–871, 2006.

11. How does atopic dermatitis present at different ages?

Atopic dermatitis may present at any age, but 60% of patients experience their first outbreak by their first birthday, and 90% by their fifth. Four clinical phases are recognized:

1. Infantile (2 months to 2 years)
   - Distribution: Cheeks (Fig. 8-1A), face and scalp, extensor surfaces of extremities and trunk (due to friction from crawling)
   - Morphology: Erythema, papules, vesicles, oozing, and crusting
   - Clearing: Dermatitis clears in half of the patients by 3 years of age
2. Childhood (3 to 11 years)
   - Distribution: Wrists, ankles, backs of the thighs, buttocks, and antecubital and popliteal fossae (Fig. 8-1B)
   - Morphology: Chronic, lichenified scaly patches and plaques that may have crusting and oozing (see Fig. 8-1B)
   - Clearing: Two thirds of patients clear by age 6
3. Adolescent/young adult (12 to 20 years)
   - Distribution: Face, neck, arms, back, and flexures (Fig. 8-1C)

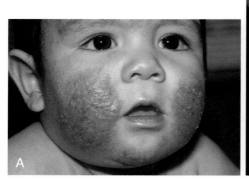
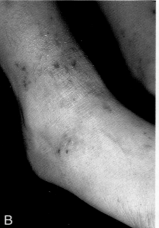
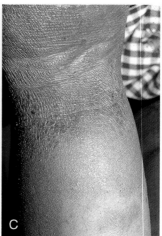

Figure 8-1. Phases of atopic dermatitis. **A,** Infantile phase. Typical erythematous, oozing, and crusted plaques seen on the cheek of an infant with atopic dermatitis. **B,** Childhood phase. A 5-year-old child with oozing, crusted lesions with secondary excoriations on the thigh and calf. **C,** Adolescent/young adult phase. Characteristic chronic flexural dermatitis in an adolescent. (Panel A courtesy of the William L. Weston, M.D. collection; panel C courtesy of James E. Fitzpatrick, MD.)

- Morphology: Thick, dry, lichenified plaques without weeping, crusting, or oozing
- Clearing: 90% or patients clear by age 18
4. Adult (>20 years)—50% of all patients will have recurrences as adults
    - Distribution: Most commonly involves the hands, sometimes the face and neck, and rarely diffuse areas
    - Morphology: Lichenified plaques, fissures on the hands, occasional vesicular outbreaks, one subset of "sensitive skin" patients

Key Points: Dermatitis

1. Dermatitis and eczema are two interchangeable terms.
2. Moisturization (especially with ceramide- or glycerin-containing products) and topical corticosteroids remain the mainstay of atopic dermatitis treatment.
3. Wet-to-dry dressings with topical corticosteroids are rapid, effective therapy for moderate-to-severe forms of dermatitis.
4. Exfoliative dermatitis can be a life-threatening disorder that requires urgent evaluation and treatment by a dermatologist.

12. What physical findings are associated with atopic dermatitis?

- Dry skin due to decreased ability of the skin to hold onto water
- Keratosis pilaris: Horny plugs in follicular orifices, especially on dorsal arms, anterior thighs, buttocks, and upper back
- Pityriasis alba: Hypopigmented patches with fine scale, particularly on the face of darker-skinned children
- Hyperlinear palm and sole creases
- Vascular abnormalities: Skin pallor, low finger and toe temperatures, pronounced vasoconstriction on exposure to cold

13. What factors provoke or exacerbate atopic dermatitis?

- Wool clothing: The size of wool fibers stimulates intense itching via allokinesis
- Clothing made of blended or synthetic fabrics and shirt collar tags
- Prolonged bathing/hot water bathing: Both promote transepidermal water loss
- Soaps, especially soaps with a high (basic) pH
- Infection: *Staphylococcus aureus* colonizing skin releases superantigens that trigger dermatitis flares
- Climate extremes: Heat, cold, low humidity, and high humidity
- Food: Food antigens appear to play a minor role in the cause of atopic dermatitis

14. How can your atopic patients relieve their pruritic agony and discomfort?

- Avoid provoking factors (scrubbing, bathing >10 minutes, hot water bathing, scented soaps, irritating clothing, low humidity, temperature extremes, copious sweating, etc.).
- Moisturize by hydrating the skin and then applying moisturizers within 3 minutes of bathing to prevent evaporation. Moisturizers containing ceramide, such as CeraVe, or glycerin, such as Vaseline Intensive Rescue products, are especially beneficial in atopic patients. Alpha-hydroxy acid products often sting and burn in dermatitis patients.
- Limit soap use to mild, unscented soaps on hairy or oily areas.
- Wear 100% cotton clothing as much as possible, and if the arms and forearms are affected during dry seasons, wear long-sleeved shirts to reduce evaporation from the skin.
- During dry times of the year, use a humidifier to keep the humidity between 35% to 40%.
- Topical corticosteroids are the treatment of choice for subacute or chronic lesions.
- Twice-daily use or corticosteroids is only minimally more effective than once-daily use, but application in the evening is more effective than application in the morning!
- Corticosteroids can be safely used on skin colonized by bacteria.
- Younger patients require less potent steroids than older patients. Use occlusive vehicles (ointments, emollient creams) on dry and/or exposed lesions; use nonocclusive vehicles (creams, lotions, foams, liquids) on moist or occluded areas. Foams have the highest level of patient compliance among all vehicles.
- For acutely inflamed and weeping skin, use wet-to-dry compresses (see "Two-Pajama Treatment") because they are soothing, antipruritic, cleansing, hydrating, and cooling. Use a topical corticosteroid with this for improved effectiveness.
- A new class of topical agents, calcineurin inhibitors, includes tacrolimus and pimecrolimus and can be safely used by following the Food and Drug Administration (FDA) guidelines.
- If lesions are secondarily infected, antibiotic therapy for 2 weeks should be prescribed. Antibiotics should not be used if clinical infection is not present.
- Severe atopic dermatitis may require systemic treatment with cyclosporine, azathioprine, methotrexate, or mycophenolate mofetil.
- Ultraviolet A-1 (UVA-1), ultraviolet B (UVB), and psoralen plus ultraviolet A (PUVA) phototherapy are also effective for more severe cases of atopic dermatitis.

15. What is the role of antihistamines in atopic dermatitis?

Minimal, if any. Certain antihistamines may help patients sleep better due to soporific side effects. However, no benefit has been demonstrated in reducing pruritus, because histamine either has no role or a minor role in causing pruritus in atopic dermatitis.

16. Describe the "two-pajamas treatment."

One especially effective method for applying topical antiinflammatory medications under occlusion to areas of widespread dermatitis is known as the "two-pajamas treatment" (a type of wet-to-dry dressing especially suited for young children).

- At bedtime, take two pairs of cotton pajamas and soak one pair in warm water.
- Apply a mild- or moderate-strength corticosteroid to involved skin immediately after bathing.
- Don the wet (wrung-out) pajamas.
- Put the dry pair on top of the wet pair and wear while sleeping.
- Upon waking, remove pajamas, bathe, apply moisturizers, and get dressed.
- Modify this therapy as the "two-socks," "two-gloves," "two-caps," "two-shirts," or "two-pants" treatment as the distribution of lesions dictates.

17. Is "hand dermatitis" a specific entity?

No. This "lumping" term includes any dermatitis confined mostly to the hands. Irritants, allergens, infection, id reactions, atopic dermatitis, and many other causes may be responsible.

18. What is pompholyx?

Pompholyx, from the Greek word for "bubble," accounts for up to 20% of hand dermatitis cases. It also has been called dyshidrotic eczema, even though no definite relationship to sweating has been demonstrated. Patients develop crops of clear, deep-seated, tapioca-like vesicles on the palms and sides of the fingers in 80% of cases (Fig. 8-2). Another 10% also have sole involvement, whereas the remaining 10% have only sole involvement. Erythema is often absent, and heat and prickling sensations may precede attacks. Nails may become dystrophic. The cause is unknown, but it may be a manifestation of atopic dermatitis and is exacerbated by stress in many patients.

19. How can pompholyx be managed?

Most attacks resolve spontaneously within 1 to 3 weeks. However, because pompholyx is generally symptomatic, certain measures should be tried. Hand protection, aluminum subacetate (Burow's solution) soaks for debridement when oozing, and bland emollients help. Large blisters can be drained (and this rapidly relieves itching). Potent topical corticosteroids can be used with or without occlusion for moderate or severe acute disease. Soaking hands in warm water for 15 minutes before applying superpotent steroids and then applying white, cotton gloves overnight is especially helpful. Occasionally, oral or intramuscular corticosteroids are required to bring relief to patients. Oral methotrexate can be used in severe cases as a steroid-sparing agent. Keratolytics, tar, UVB light, or even PUVA can help chronic and/or hyperkeratotic disease.

20. Describe the typical presentation of nummular eczema.

Typically, patients are men 55 to 65 years old who report the rapid onset of tiny papules and juicy vesicles that form erythematous, 1- to 10-cm diameter, coin-shaped (i.e., nummular) plaques studded by pinpoint vesicles and erosions on a background of dry skin (Fig. 8-3). Plaques sometimes clear centrally and resemble tinea corporis. They are found most commonly on the extensor surfaces of the lower extremities, are often bilaterally symmetrical, may recur at sites of previous involvement, and are intensely pruritic. The upper extremities and trunk are involved less frequently. When the trunk is involved, only the back is usually affected.

21. What causes nummular eczema?

Nobody knows for sure, but it is probably a form of irritant dermatitis combined with very dry skin. It is rarely seen in humid environments. Up to 95% of patients have *S. aureus*–colonizing or -infecting lesions, which supports the idea that nummular eczema may be a hypersensitivity reaction to bacteria.

22. Is there a cure for nummular eczema?

No, but the disease can be controlled. Limiting baths and soap exposure, avoiding irritants, frequent use of moisturizers, topical corticosteroids, and avoiding dry environments all have a role in treatment. Topical corticosteroids are the mainstay of therapy. With the high rate of staphylococcal colonization, many dermatologists routinely prescribe a 2-week course of oral antibiotics such as trimethoprim-sulfamethoxazole, dicloxacillin, or cephalexin. I find 1 mg/kg triamcinolone acetonide mixed with 0.1 mg/kg Celestone intramuscularly particularly helpful, and it causes far fewer side effects than oral steroids that may also be used in severe cases, limited to a tapered 2 to 3 week course. Severe chronic cases may also benefit from PUVA.

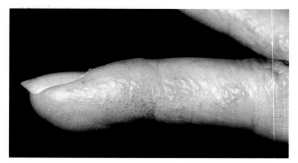

Figure 8-2. Pompholyx. Characteristic "tapioca" or "sago-grain" vesicles on the sides of the fingers. (Courtesy of Fitzsimons Army Medical Center.)

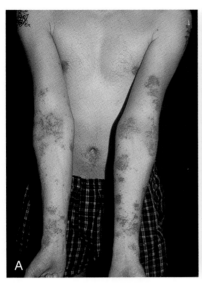
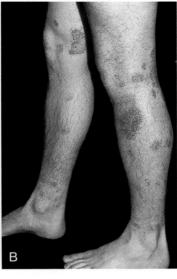

Figure 8-3. Nummular dermatitis. **A,** Typical upper-extremity distribution of coin-shaped lesions in an adult man. **B,** Close-up of coin-shaped lesions of nummular dermatitis, also known as discoid eczema. Note the peripheral margin studded with vesicles and erosions.

23. How does seborrheic dermatitis present in children?

Retention hyperkeratosis of the scalp known as "cradle cap" (Fig. 8-4A) is the most common presentation, while "napkin dermatitis" in the diaper area is the next most frequent. The primary lesions are round to oval patches of dry scales or yellowish-brown, greasy crusts with variable erythema. Seborrheic dermatitis presents in infants 2 to 10 weeks of age and generally clears by 8 to 12 months of age before reappearing at puberty. However, there are exceptions, and children of all ages may have this condition, even though they do not produce sebum as much as adults do.

24. How does seborrheic dermatitis present in adults?

Dandruff—visible scalp desquamation—is the precursor lesion. The scalp may become inflamed and covered with greasy scale (Fig. 8-4B). Dull or yellowish-red, sharply marginated, nonpruritic lesions, covered with greasy scales are seen in areas with a rich supply of sebaceous glands. Characteristically, the medial eyebrows, glabella, melolabial folds, nasofacial sulci, and eyelid margins (blepharitis) are involved. Preauricular cheeks, postauricular sulci, and external auditory canal lesions are also commonly affected sites. The trunk may demonstrate presternal or interscapular involvement. Intertriginous areas, such the inframammary creases, umbilicus, and genitocrural folds, are occasionally involved. Seborrheic dermatitis is one of the most common causes of chronic dermatitis of the anogenital area.

25. What causes seborrheic dermatitis, and with what disease states is it commonly found?

Current theories suggest that immune hyperreaction to the commensal lipophilic yeast *Malassezia* (that lives in our sebaceous glands) and/or sebum causes the dermatitis. An increased incidence and severity of seborrheic dermatitis are seen in persons with central nervous system (CNS) diseases such as Parkinson's disease, facial paralysis, poliomyelitis, syringomyelia, and quadriplegia. The CNS may stimulate increased rates of sebum production. HIV-infected individuals also frequently demonstrate severe seborrheic dermatitis.

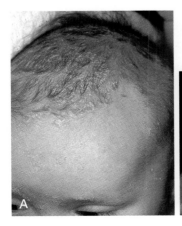
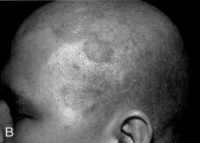

Figure 8-4. Seborrheic dermatitis. **A,** Infant demonstrating characteristic scalp seborrheic dermatitis commonly known as "cradle cap." **B,** Adult demonstrating yellowish-red, sharply demarcated lesions with greasy scale. (Courtesy of James E. Fitzpatrick, MD.)

26. Discuss the treatment approaches to seborrheic dermatitis.

- Like all forms of dermatitis, seborrheic dermatitis can be controlled, not cured.
- Wash hair and scalp daily with anti-*Malassezia* shampoos containing ketoconazole (best combination of price and effectiveness), selenium sulfide, or zinc pyrithione.
- For scalp with moderate scale, use shampoos containing keratolytics, such as tar, salicylic acid, or sulfur to debride scale.
- For extremely thick scalp scale, massage Baker's P&S Liquid or Derma-Smoothe F/S oil into the scalp at bedtime and remove by shampooing in the morning.
- Apply a corticosteroid scalp solution or foams, after shampooing, to reduce inflammation.
- For blepharitis, use warm water compresses, gentle cleansing with diluted nonirritating shampoo (such as baby shampoo), and topical sodium sulfacetamide ointment.
- Treat the face and trunk with mild steroid lotions or creams such as 1% hydrocortisone or desonide 0.05%, pimecrolimus, or antiyeast products such as ketoconazole or ciclopirox.

27. What is an "id" reaction, and what does it have to do with Sigmund Freud?

An id reaction, also known as autosensitization dermatitis, is an immunologically mediated cutaneous inflammation in the absence of locally viable organisms or other locally inciting cause. It presents suddenly as an acute, monomorphous, papulovesicular dermatitis distant to an area of primary dermatitis. It usually erupts symmetrically on the hands, forearms, flexor aspects of the arms, extensor aspects of the arms and thighs, and, less commonly, on the face and trunk. Juicy papules often coalesce into small plaques with associated red macules or wheals. Sigmund Freud did not discover id reactions. In dermatologic usage, "id" derives from a Greek suffix for a father–son relationship or resemblance. Freud's id derives from a third-person Latin pronoun.

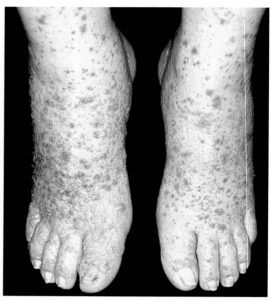

Figure 8-5. Severe papulosquamous id reaction of the lower legs secondary to a severe dermatophyte infection. (Courtesy of James E. Fitzpatrick, MD.)

28. What are the most common settings for an id reaction and how should you treat it?

Stasis dermatitis, scabies, and dermatophyte infections (Fig. 8-5) are the most common settings. The distant lesions often take on the characteristics of the primary cutaneous lesions. The cure lies in treating the primary lesion because, by definition, an id reaction resolves when the primary dermatitis departs. Many id reactions require symptomatic treatment with antipruritics, wet-to-dry soaks, and topical corticosteroids. Often, systemic corticosteroids are necessary to bring relief.

29. What do you call dermatitis that covers virtually the whole cutaneous surface?

Bad news! This extreme condition is called exfoliative dermatitis in the United States and erythroderma in the United Kingdom. Often, over 90% of the body surface is red and scaly, and about 20 to 30 g of scale are shed daily (Fig. 8-6).

30. How can you determine the cause of a patient's exfoliative dermatitis?

History and skin biopsy are the two most helpful aids. Lymph node biopsy helps rule out lymphoma. In many cases, the underlying cause is never established. Of a total of 746 patients, dermatitis was due to

- Idiopathic (causes not determined) (25%)
- Dermatitis (24%)

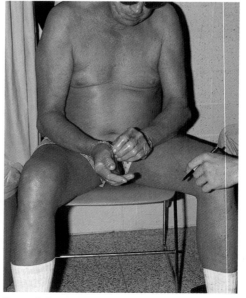

Figure 8-6. Exfoliative dermatitis. Patient with full-body erythroderma of unknown cause. Note the normal hand for comparison. (Courtesy of Fitzsimons Army Medical Center.)

- Atopic (9%)
- Contact (6%)
- Seborrheic (4%)
- Chronic actinic dermatitis (3%)
- Other (2%)
- Psoriasis (20%)
- Drug reactions (19%)
- Cutaneous T-cell lymphoma (8%)
- Other rare causes (4%)

31. What general treatment measures are used to treat patients with exfoliative dermatitis?

- Treat the underlying disorder, if known.
- Wet-to-dry dressings with desonide 0.05% ointment, a mild topical corticosteroid, reliably, significantly, and rapidly improves almost any case of exfoliative dermatitis.
- Problems arising from the erythema and exfoliation such as dehydration, high-output heart failure, and hypothermia must be treated empirically.
- Stop all nonessential drugs.
- Systemic corticosteroids can exacerbate psoriasis and should not be used unless the underlying disease is clearly steroid responsive.
- Phototherapy may be helpful in selected patients, particularly if psoriasis is suspected.
- Oral antibiotics should be used for secondary infections.

CONTACT DERMATITIS

Leslie A. Stewart, MD

1. Name the two pathogenic types of contact dermatitis.

Contact dermatitis refers to cutaneous inflammation resulting from the interaction of an external agent and the skin. These reactions occur through one of two mechanisms: a nonimmunologic irritant contact dermatitis (ICD) or an immunologic allergic contact dermatitis (ACD). ICD accounts for 80% of all reactions, while ACD is responsible for approximately 20%. Although over 3700 substances have been identified as contact allergens, almost any substance, under the right circumstances, can act as an irritant. It is important to note that irritating compounds can be allergenic, and allergenic compounds can be irritating.

Marks JG, Elsner P, DeLeo VA: *Contact and occupational dermatology*, ed 3, St Louis, 2002, Mosby.

2. Name the two subtypes of irritant contact dermatitis, and describe them.

ICD can be divided into acute toxic and cumulative insult subtypes. Acute toxic eruptions occur from a single exposure to a strong toxic chemical, such as an acid or alkali, inducing erythema, vesicles, bullae, or skin sloughing. Reactions occur within minutes to hours after exposure, localize to the areas of maximal contact, and have sharp borders. In most cases, healing occurs soon after exposure. Chronic cumulative insult reactions are the more common type of ICD. These are due to multiple exposures of many low-level irritants, such as soaps and shampoos, over time. This dermatitis may take weeks, months, or even years to appear. It is characterized by erythema, scaling, fissuring, pruritus, lichenification, and poor demarcation from the surrounding skin.

Przybilla B, Rueff F: Contact dermatitis. In Burgdorf WH, Plewig G, editors: *Braun-Falco's dermatology*, ed 3, Heidelberg, 2009, Springer, pp 377–401.

3. Explain the pathogenesis of allergic contact dermatitis (ACD).

ACD is a type IV, delayed, cell-mediated, hypersensitivity reaction. Initially, a low-molecular-weight antigen hapten (<500 Daltons) contacts the skin and forms a hapten–carrier protein complex. This complex then associates itself with an epidermal Langerhans' cell, which presents the complete antigen to a T-helper cell, causing the release of various mediators. Subsequently, T-cell expansion occurs in regional lymph nodes, producing specific memory and T-effector lymphocytes, which circulate in the general bloodstream. This whole process of sensitization occurs in approximately 5 to 21 days. Upon reexposure to the specific antigen, there is proliferation of activated T cells, mediator release, and migration of cytotoxic T cells, resulting in cutaneous eczematous inflammation at the site of contact. This phase occurs within 48 to 72 hours after exposure. Because many allergens are irritants, preceding irritation is common and may enhance allergen absorption. In contrast to irritant reactions, relatively small concentrations of an allergen can be enough to elicit an inflammatory reaction. Acute ACD may have erythema, edema, and vesicle formation. Chronic ACD reactions are scaly, erythematous, possibly lichenified, and can mimic chronic ICD. Table 9-1 compares ACD and ICD.

Li L, Cruz P: Allergic contact dermatitis: pathophysiology applied to future therapy, *Dermatol Thera* 17:219–223, 2004.

Table 9-1. Comparison of Irritant and Allergic Contact Dermatitis

	IRRITANT	ALLERGIC
Examples	Water, soap	Nickel, fragrance, hair dye
Number of compounds	Many	Fewer
Distribution of reaction	Localized	May spread beyond area of maximal contact and become generalized
Concentration of agent needed to elicit reaction	High	Can be minute
Time course	Immediate to late	Sensitization in 2 weeks; elicitation takes 24–72 hrs
Immunology	Nonspecific	Specific type IV delayed hypersensitivity reaction
Diagnostic test	None	Patch test

4. Can urticarial reactions occur from contact with a substance?

Occasionally, urticarial reactions may occur with certain exposures, instead of the eczematous changes seen with ACD and ICD (Fig. 9-1). Allergic contact urticaria involves a specific IgE–mast cell interaction, resulting in the release of vasoactive compounds. While urticaria occurs at the site of contact, more generalized symptoms can appear, including angioedema, anaphylaxis, rhinoconjunctivitis, and widespread urticaria. A good example is the latex glove immediate reaction reported in health care professionals. Nonimmunologic contact urticaria occurs secondary to a non–antibody-mediated release of vasoactive mediators or due to a direct effect on the cutaneous vasculature. Many agents found in cosmetic products can cause a nonimmunologic contact urticaria. These include sorbic acid, benzoic acid, and cinnamic acid. This may explain the facial burning and stinging that some patients experience using cosmetics. To diagnose contact urticaria, a prick test is usually performed. In this test, a small amount of the allergen is placed on the skin, and a needle is used to prick the skin. An urticarial wheal of appropriate size constitutes a positive test, usually developing within 15 to 20 minutes after allergen administration (Fig. 9-2).

Rietschel RL, Fowler JF: Contact urticaria. In Rietschel RL, Fowler JF, editors: *Fisher's contact dermatitis*, Hamilton, Ontario, 2008, BC Decker, pp 615–634.

5. Why is the distribution of a contact dermatitis rash important?

The location and distribution of the dermatitis are vital clues to the underlying culprit (Table 9-2). For example, an eczematous dermatitis on the dorsal feet should alert the clinician to the possibility of shoe dermatitis.

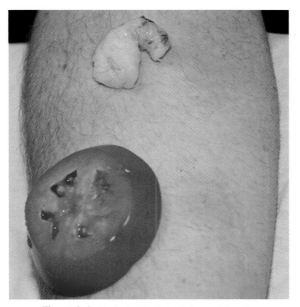

Figure 9-1. Contact urticaria to shrimp and tomato.

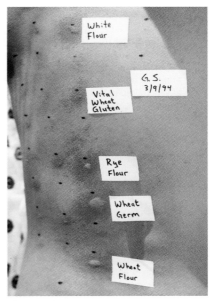

Figure 9-2. Prick test for the diagnosis of contact urticaria. The patient was a baker allergic to flours and wheat.

Table 9-2. Location of Contact Dermatitis and Suspicious Agents

LOCATION	SUSPICIOUS AGENT
Eyelids	Nail polish, eye makeup, airborne allergens
Earlobes or neck	Metal jewelry
Forehead, scalp margins	Hair dyes
Face	Cosmetic fragrances and preservatives, airborne allergens
Axilla	Deodorants
Hands	Gloves, occupational contacts
Waistband	Elastic
Dorsal feet	Shoes

6. List three common misperceptions regarding the location of a contact dermatitis.

1. Dermatitis has to be bilateral if the exposure is bilateral, that is, with a shoe or glove allergy. In most cases, contact reactions tend to be patchy and do not have the same intensity at all sites of exposure.
2. The rash of contact dermatitis occurs only at the site of maximal contact. Allergens can frequently be spread to distant sites of contact (Fig. 9-3), as when nail polish is transferred to the eyelid, inducing dermatitis when a sensitized patient rubs her eyelids with her fingernails.
3. Contact dermatitis does not affect the palms and soles because of their thick stratum corneum. Although it is true that other more sensitive areas such as the eyelids, face, and genitalia are more likely to be reactive, contact dermatitis definitely should be considered when dealing with an eczematous dermatitis of the palms or soles.

7. How is patch testing done?

Because ICD and ACD can be indistinguishable both clinically and histologically, patch testing is the only method available to diagnose ACD and differentiate it from ICD. Two patch test methods are currently in widespread use: the Finn chamber (Fig. 9-4A) and True Test systems (Fig. 9-4B). With the Finn chamber method, a small amount of the allergen, usually in a petrolatum vehicle, is placed into individual aluminum wells affixed to a strip of paper tape. With the True Test method, no

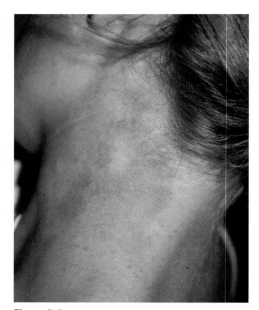

Figure 9-3. Allergic contact dermatitis of the neck due to a nail polish transfer reaction.

advance preparation is necessary, as the allergens have already been commercially incorporated into the back of the paper tape strips. Only 28 "screening" allergens are currently available with the True Test, while hundreds are available with the Finn chamber method. These strips are applied to the patient's upper back, which is the preferred testing site. After 48 hours, the patches are removed and the initial reading is recorded. Because these allergic reactions are delayed, a second interpretation must be performed at 72 hours, 96 hours, or even at 1 week after the initial test application. Additional readings beyond 48 hours increase the positive patch test yield by 34%. The classic positive allergic patch test reaction shows spreading erythema, edema, and closely set vesicles that persist after removal of the patch or that appear after 2 to 7 days. Irritant reactions may have a glazed, scalded, follicular, or pustular appearance that usually fades after the patch is removed.

Davis MD, Bhate K, Rholinger AI, et al: Delayed patch test reading after 5 days: the Mayo Clinic experience, *J Am Acad Dermatol* 59:225–233, 2008.

Rietschel RL, Adams RM, Mailbach HI, et al: The case for patch test readings beyond day 2, *J Am Acad Dermatol* 18:42–45, 1988.

8. What substances are tested in the standard "screening" patch test?

Because of its convenience, most patients with a suspected allergic contact dermatitis are patch tested with the True Test "standard" panel of 28 allergens, which can detect many common sensitivities (Table 9-3). However, this panel only detects 62% to 75% of the most common allergens. The North American Contact Dermatitis Group's Standard 65-allergen tray, which utilizes the Finn Chamber method, is a more efficacious screening series than more limited patch

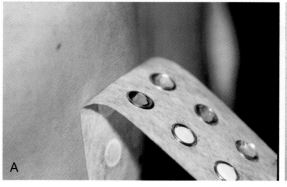
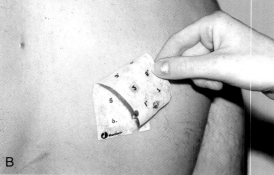

Figure 9-4. A, Finn chamber method. **B,** True Test method.

Table 9-3. Allergens Evaluated by the True Test and the Finn Chamber Test

ALLERGEN	SOURCES
Benzocaine 5%	Topical anesthetic
Caine mix	Topical anesthetic
Nickel sulfate 2.5%	Metal jewelry
Potassium dichromate 0.25%	Leather, cement
Cobalt	Metal jewelry, paint
Neomycin sulfate 20%	Topical antibiotics
p-Phenylenediamine 1%	Hair dye
Ethylenediamine 1%	Topical medications
Cinnamaldehyde 1%	Perfume, flavors
Balsam of Peru 25%	Perfume, medications
Fragrance mix	Perfume, flavors
Formaldehyde 1%	Preservative, fabric finishes
Quaternium-15 2%	Cosmetic and industrial preservative
Imidazolidinyl urea 2%	Cosmetic preservative
Paraben mix	Cosmetic preservative
Thimerosal	Cosmetic and medicament preservative
Cl^+Me^- Isothiazoline (MCI/MI)	Cosmetic and industrial preservative
Lanolin alcohol 30%	Topical skin care products
Epoxy resin 1%	Glues, plastics
p-tert-butylphenol formaldehyde resin 1%	Glues
Colophony (resin) 2%	Adhesives, solder flux
Mercaptobenzothiazole 1%	Rubber, fungicide
Carba mix 3%	Rubber, fungicide
Thiuram mix 1%	Rubber, fungicide
Mercapto mix 1%	Rubber, fungicide
Black rubber mix 0.6%	Black rubber
Budesonide	Topical corticosteroid
Tixocortol 21-pivalate	Topical corticosteroid

test series. Additional testing with more specialized allergen panels is frequently warranted to enhance allergen detection. Testing should only be done with known materials in accepted concentrations.

Cohen DE, Rao S, Brancaccio RR: Use of the North American Contact Dermatitis Group standard 65-allergen series alone in the evaluation of allergic contact dermatitis: a series of 794 patients, *Dermatitis* 19:137–141, 2008.

James WD, Rosenthal LE, Brancaccio RR, Marks JG Jr: American Academy of Dermatology Patch Test Survey: use and effectiveness of this procedure, *J Am Acad Dermatol* 26:991–994, 1992.

Key Points: Contact Dermatitis

1. Eighty percent of contact dermatitis reactions are due to irritation and 20% are due to allergic causes.
2. Location of the dermatitis can help identify the causative agent.
3. Patch testing is the only way to distinguish between allergic and irritant contact dermatitis.
4. Allergic contact dermatitis is frequently patchy and can spread beyond the site of maximal contact.
5. Allergen and irritant avoidance, moisturization, and topical therapy are the keys to therapy.

---

9. An astute physician should not need to patch test. Right?

Many clinicians believe that a thorough history and physical exam are sufficient for an accurate diagnosis of ACD. They believe that patch testing is unnecessary because they can tell whether a reaction is ICD or ACD simply by evaluating the dermatitis. Results of several studies, however, show that clinicians are often wrong when guessing whether contact dermatitis is irritant or allergic. In fact, experienced dermatologists may only suspect the true allergen in 50% of cases. Patch testing is the only way to differentiate between the two conditions because clinically and histologically ICD and ACD cannot be reliably differentiated.

Podmore P, Burrows D, Bingham EA: Prediction of patch test results, *Contact Dermatitis* 11:283–284, 1984.

10. What is a repeated open application test (ROAT)?

The ROAT, or usage test, is used when patch testing is negative, and yet there remains a strong clinical suspicion for ACD. Remember, patch testing is a one-time occlusive test that does not always duplicate low-level chronic daily exposure. With the ROAT, patients apply the suspected product to a quarter-sized area on the forearm twice a day for 1 week. If the patient is allergic, a localized dermatitis will occur, confirming the suspected allergy (Fig. 9-5).

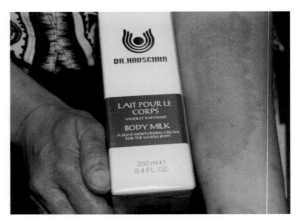

Figure 9-5. Positive ROAT test from a moisturizing cream.

11. What is the differential diagnosis of contact dermatitis?

Contact dermatitis, with its scaling, erythema, lichenification, and/or vesicles, belongs in the group of eczematous disorders. Other such conditions—atopic dermatitis, nummular eczema, neurodermatitis, stasis dermatitis, seborrheic dermatitis, photodermatoses, dermatophyte infections, drug eruptions, and dyshidrotic eczema (pompholyx)—should always be considered when evaluating a prospective patient for contact dermatitis. A complete history including previous skin diseases, drug and exposure histories, location and course of the eruption, patch testing, and potassium hydroxide tests should help point to the diagnosis of contact dermatitis.

Marks JG, Elsner P, DeLeo VA: *Contact and occupational dermatology*, ed 3, St Louis, 2002, Mosby, pp 20–25.

12. Which is the most common allergen on the standard tray?

The metal nickel, found commonly in costume jewelry, is the most common allergen on the standard tray. Approximately 5.8% of the general population in the United States is sensitized, while patch test clinics around the country note a prevalence rate of 19% in their dermatitis populations (Fig. 9-6). The high rate of sensitization is felt to be secondary to ear piercing, which is why this allergy is more common in females. In men, nickel dermatitis is predominantly of occupational origin.

Zug KA, Warshaw EM, Fowler JF, et al: Patch test results of the North American Contact Dermatitis Group 2005-2006, *Dermatitis* 20:149–160, 2009.

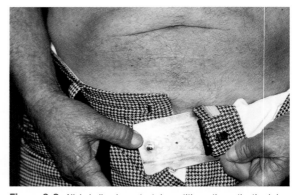

Figure 9-6. Nickel allergic contact dermatitis on the patient's abdomen due to the presence of nickel in the metal buckle on his pants. The rash had been previously misdiagnosed as a nummular eczema.

13. Is nickel the most common allergen overall?

Poison ivy is actually the most common type IV allergen, with approximately 50% to 70% of the general population being sensitized.

14. If a change in a skin care product does not lead to clearing of a patient's rash, does this mean that the original product was not the culprit?

Not necessarily. Many consumer cosmetic and toiletry products contain the same allergens (usually fragrances and preservatives). Moreover, many products contain cross-reacting agents that can exacerbate the original problem. For example, patients who are allergic to the hair dye allergen paraphenylenediamine will need to avoid the over-the-counter topical anesthetic benzocaine. Both compounds belong to the para-amino group and can cross-react with one another.

15. How is contact dermatitis managed?

If the patient has ACD, the allergen should be detected by patch testing, and subsequently it should be thoroughly avoided. Sources of the allergen as well as cross-reacting agents should be explained to the patient. An acceptable nonsensitizing substitute should be offered. For ICD, avoidance of as many irritants as possible is crucial. Frequent water exposure, which desiccates and chaps the skin, should be kept to a minimum. Frequent moisturization and hand protection with gloves, if indicated, are important. With contact dermatitis, systemic steroids should be used only in acute situations. Compresses may be helpful if vesicles are present. When the condition is chronic, topical steroids of appropriate strength and moisturizers are the mainstay of therapy. Recently, the newer nonsteroidal macrolide immunosuppressive agents, tacrolimus and pimecrolimus, have been used increasingly with good results. Lastly, phototherapy and Grenz ray therapy has also been used in difficult cases.

Rietschel RL, Fowler JF: Treatment of contact dermatitis. In Rietschel RL, Fowler JF, editors: *Fisher's contact dermatitis*, ed 6, Hamilton, Ontario, BC Decker, 2008, pp 722–729.

CHAPTER 10

VESICULOBULLOUS DISORDERS

Todd T. Kobayashi, MD, Lt Col, USAF, MC, and
Kathleen M. David-Bajar, MD

1. What is the difference between a vesicle and a bulla?

If the blister is less than 5 mm in diameter, it is referred to as a vesicle; if it is 5 mm or larger, it is called a bulla. Some dermatologists require that blisters be 1 cm before using the term bulla. The term vesiculobullous disorder is often used clinically since some patients may have both vesicles and bullae.

2. How are the bullous diseases defined?

Bullous diseases are characterized by blisters. Blisters are defined as circumscribed skin lesions containing fluid. They may arise at various depths in the epidermis and dermis and are sometimes classified on the basis of the depth of skin involved. One broad classification divides blisters into those that develop within the epidermis (intraepidermal) versus those that develop below the epidermis (subepidermal) (Table 10-1). Some blistering disorders develop because of autoantibodies directed against a component of the epidermis or basement membrane zone, or they develop because of structural defects of these components. Refer to Fig. 10-1 for the location of these components in normal skin as they are discussed during questions.

3. What things cause vesicles and bullae?

Blisters of the skin may be induced by a wide variety of external agents and diseases, including trauma, infections, metabolic disorders, genetic deficiencies, and inflammatory diseases. Infectious causes of blisters are discussed in Chapters 25 (viral) and 27 (bacterial).

4. How do you approach a patient who presents with an acute onset of a vesiculobullous eruption?

The patient history is very important in the initial evaluation of blisters. If the onset of lesions was acute, exposure to contact allergens, arthropods, phototoxic and other drugs or chemicals, trauma, and infectious agents should be queried. Certain chronic vesiculobullous diseases may have an acute onset but may then persist or recur and become chronic (Table 10-2).

5. Which skin findings are helpful in evaluating a patient with blisters?

Several features of vesiculobullous lesions are important to note, including the distribution, symmetry, involvement of mucosal surfaces, and associated lesions (such as erosions, ulcers, and crusts). Additional types of skin lesions, such as urticarial lesions, should be noted. In bullous pemphigoid, urticarial lesions often precede the development of blisters. In some vesiculobullous diseases such as dermatitis herpetiformis, secondary excoriations may be the only lesions visible, with no intact blisters.

The character of the blisters also may provide useful information. Flaccid blisters may indicate a more superficial blistering process than is seen with tense blisters. However, factors other than the depth of the blister are important, including site (blisters on acral skin, which has a thick stratum corneum, are often tense even when superficial) and

---

Table 10-1. Intraepidermal versus Subepidermal Blisters

INTRAEPIDERMAL BLISTERS	SUBEPIDERMAL BLISTERS
Allergic contact dermatitis (spongiotic)	Porphyria cutanea tarda
Bullous dermatophyte infection (spongiotic)	Bullous pemphigoid
Herpes simplex (acantholytic)	Cicatricial pemphigoid
Herpes zoster/varicella (intraepidermal acantholytic)	Dermatitis herpetiformis
Bullous impetigo (subcorneal)	Linear IgA bullous dermatosis
Miliaria crystallina (subcorneal)	Bullous systemic lupus erythematosus (SLE)
Epidermolysis bullosa simplex (mechanobullous)	Epidermolysis bullosa acquisita
Pemphigus vulgaris (suprabasilar acantholytic)	Dystrophic epidermolysis bullosa
Pemphigus foliaceus (subcorneal acantholytic)	Junctional epidermolysis bullosa
Paraneoplastic pemphigus	Anti–p200 pemphigoid
Hailey-Hailey disease (intraepidermal acantholytic)	Anti–p105 pemphigoid
Incontinentia pigmenti (spongiotic)	
Bullous congenital erythroderma (mechanobullous)	

STRUCTURAL COMPONENTS OF THE BASEMENT MEMBRANE ZONE

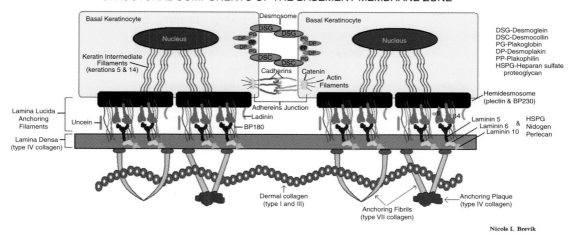

Figure 10-1. Structural components of the basement membrane zone. (Courtesy of Nicole L. Brevik.)

Table 10-2. Acute versus Chronic Onset of Vesiculobullous Eruption

ACUTE	CHRONIC
Allergic contact dermatitis	Bullous pemphigoid
Arthropod bites	Bullous SLE
Drug eruptions (may become chronic if drug is not withdrawn)	Cicatricial pemphigoid
Erythema multiforme (may recur, especially with herpes simplex)	Dermatitis herpetiformis
Hand, foot, and mouth disease	Epidermolysis bullosa acquisita
Herpes simplex	Linear IgA bullous dermatosis
Varicella zoster virus infections	Pemphigus foliaceus
Impetigo	Pemphigus vulgaris
Miliaria crystallina	Genetic blistering diseases
Physical, thermal, or chemical-induced blisters	
Toxic epidermal necrolysis/Stevens-Johnson syndrome	

the specific disease process (in toxic epidermal necrolysis, the blistering is subepidermal, but vesicles and bullae are usually flaccid with large sheets of skin sloughing).

6. **Do particular vesiculobullous diseases occur in characteristic distributions?**
   See Table 10-3.

7. **Which tests are most useful in evaluating vesiculobullous diseases?**
   Most of the tests helpful in determining the cause of vesiculobullous eruptions are performed on the blister itself. When infectious causes are being considered, appropriate cultures (aerobic bacteria, viruses, fungi) may be obtained, and smears from the blisters may be stained for bacteria, dermatophytes, or the multinucleate giant cells of herpes virus infections. For noninfectious vesiculobullous diseases, a skin biopsy is often a useful test.

8. **How should a skin biopsy of a vesiculobullous eruption be performed?**
   The lesion for biopsy should be an early lesion, to avoid secondary changes that might make the diagnosis more difficult. A small, intact blister is a good choice, as the entire lesion and some of the surrounding skin can be removed in one piece. If a punch biopsy technique is used, it is important to avoid rupturing the blister. A small excisional biopsy is a good choice and minimizes the possibility of rupturing the blister. The specimen should be placed in 10% formalin and processed for routine histologic examination. Clinical information, including the age and sex of the patient, a description of the lesions, associated symptoms, and any exacerbating factors, should be provided, along with a differential diagnosis based on the clinical examination.

9. **When are special tests necessary to diagnose blistering diseases of the skin?**
   In addition to routine histology, a skin biopsy for direct immunofluorescence is often helpful in diagnosing the immunobullous diseases (Table 10-4). Direct immunofluorescent technique uses fluorescent, tagged antibodies that are

Table 10-3. Characteristic Distribution of Vesiculobullous Diseases

DISEASE	CHARACTERISTIC DISTRIBUTION
Acrodermatitis enteropathica	Acral, periorificial
Allergic contact dermatitis	Reflects pattern of contact; often linear
Bullous dermatophyte infection	Feet, hands
Bullous diabeticorum	Distal extremities
Bullous pemphigoid	Flexural areas, lower extremities
Cicatricial pemphigoid	Eyes, mucous membranes
Dermatitis herpetiformis	Elbows, knees, buttocks
Erythema multiforme	Acral areas, palms, soles, mucosa
Hailey-Hailey disease	Intertriginous areas, neck
Hand, foot, and mouth disease	Mouth, palms, fingers, soles
Herpes zoster	Dermatomal distribution
Linear IgA bullous dermatosis (childhood type)	Groin, buttocks, perineum
Pemphigus vulgaris	Oral mucosa, other sites
Pemphigus foliaceus	Head, neck, trunk

Table 10-4. Direct Immunofluorescence Findings of Vesiculobullous Diseases

DISEASE	TARGET ANTIGEN	DIRECT IMMUNOFLUORESCENCE FINDINGS
Bullous pemphigoid	BP180, BP230	Linear C3, IgG at DEJ
Bullous SLE	COL7A1	Linear/granular IgG, other Igs at DEJ
Cicatricial pemphigoid	BP180, LAM5, and others	Linear C3, IgG, IgA at DEJ
Dermatitis herpetiformis	eTG	Granular IgA, C3 in upper dermis (see Fig. 10-1)
Epidermolysis bullosa acquisita	COL7A1	Linear IgG, IgA, other Igs at DEJ
Herpes gestationis	BP180	Linear C3, IgG at DEJ
Linear IgA bullous dermatosis	BP180, COL7A1, LAD	Linear IgA, C3 at DEJ
Pemphigus foliaceus	DSG1	IgG, C3 in intercellular spaces
Pemphigus vulgaris	DSG3 (mucous membrane only) DSG3 and DSG1 (mucous membrane and skin)	IgG, C3 in intercellular spaces
IgA pemphigus	DSC1, DSG1, DSG3	IgA in intercellular spaces
Paraneoplastic pemphigus	DSG1, DSG3, DP1, DP2, BP180, BP230, EP, PP, γ-catenin, plectin, 170 kD, DSC2, DSC3	IgG, C3 in intercellular spaces, DEJ
Porphyria cutanea tarda	None (not antibody mediated)	Homogenous IgG at DEJ and around vessels
Anti–p200 pemphigoid	200-kD antigen	IgG, C3 at DEJ
Anti–p105 pemphigoid	105-kD antigen	IgG, C3 at DEJ

DEJ, Dermal–epidermal junction; Ig, immunoglobulin; C3, third complement component.

directed against IgG, IgA, IgM, C3, and fibrin; these antibodies fluoresce when illuminated with a fluorescent microscope (Fig. 10-2). For precise diagnosis of the inherited forms of epidermolysis bullosa, electron microscopy studies may be necessary. Other tests are indicated in specific circumstances, such as urine porphyrin tests when porphyria cutanea tarda is being considered, and zinc levels when acrodermatitis enteropathica is possible.

Zillikens D: Diagnosis of autoimmune bullous skin diseases, *Clin Lab* 54:491–503, 2008.

10. How are specimens obtained for direct immunofluorescence?

Generally, this specialized testing would be ordered by a dermatologist, as the selection of an appropriate laboratory and proper handling of the tissue are essential to an accurate result. For most immunobullous diseases, tissue for direct immunofluorescence testing is obtained from skin next to a blister, and it is either frozen immediately in liquid nitrogen or placed in a transport medium such as Michel's media. It should never be placed in formalin; direct immunofluorescence testing involves identifying immunoglobulins and complement deposited in the skin. These molecules may be altered by formalin.

11. For which vesiculobullous diseases are indirect immunofluorescence helpful?

It is most commonly used in pemphigus vulgaris (less commonly in bullous pemphigoid), epidermolysis bullosa acquisita, and cicatricial pemphigoid. This procedure identifies antibodies present in the circulation; therefore, serum is submitted for evaluation. It is most commonly used to obtain an antibody titer to help monitor disease activity. Again, only a few laboratories perform this testing routinely, so consultation with the laboratory prior to obtaining the specimen is recommended to ensure appropriate handling of the specimen. Enzyme-linked immunosorbent assay (ELISA) testing for these same serum antibodies has now become commercially available and is both sensitive and specific. ELISA has largely replaced indirect immunofluorescent studies as the study of choice for antibody titers and for detecting certain antibodies such as BP180, BP230, desmoglein 1, and desmoglein 3 in blistering diseases.

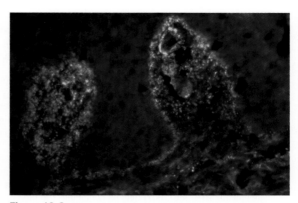

Figure 10-2. Direct immunofluorescence of skin demonstrating linear granular IgA along the basement membrane zone and in the papillary dermis in a patient with dermatitis herpetiformis. (Courtesy of the Fitzsimons Army Medical Center teaching files.)

12. List the most common blistering diseases due to external agents.

- **Allergic contact dermatitis:** Direct contact with allergens may cause an acute, pruritic vesicular eruption in the areas of contact. When it is due to plants such as poison ivy, the pattern is often linear, corresponding to areas where the the skin brushes the plant. The diagnosis can usually be made on the basis of history and clinical findings, particularly exposure to the offending agent. Skin biopsy for routine histologic examination may be helpful in difficult cases (see also Chapter 9).
- **Bullous drug eruptions:** A number of drugs can produce characteristic vesiculobullous eruptions through toxic, immunologic, idiopathic, or phototoxic/photoallergic mechanisms (see also Chapter 14).
- **Miliaria crystallina:** Superficial, fragile vesicles develop as eccrine sweat ducts become obstructed. Predisposing factors include high fever and occlusion, as well as sunburn. Clinical findings are usually diagnostic, but occasional cases require a skin biopsy.
- **Blisters caused by physical agents:** Heat, cold, chemicals, friction, pressure, and radiation (second-degree sunburn) may induce blisters. These can generally be identified readily by history and physical examination.
- **Bullous arthropod bites:** Small blisters around ankles, clothing constrictures, exposed skin areas, pet ownership, travel, or outdoor activities.
- **Bullous impetigo:** Fragile blisters, often ruptured with leading edge scale, with a positive culture for *Staphylococcus* or *Streptococcus*.

13. Name examples of drugs that can cause vesiculobullous eruptions.

See Table 10-5.

Table 10-5. Drugs That Can Cause Vesiculobullous Eruptions

ERUPTION	OFFENDING DRUG(s)
Bullous pemphigoid	Tetracycline, furosemide, ibuprofen and other nonsteroidal antiinflammatory drugs (NSAIDs), captopril, penicillamine, and other antibiotics
Erythema multiforme	Anticonvulsants, barbiturates, sulfonamides, NSAIDs, antibiotics
Linear IgA bullous dermatosis	Vancomycin, lithium, captopril, antibiotics
Phototoxic drug eruption	Psoralens, thiazides, furosemide, fluoroquinolones, doxycycline (and other TCNs), sulfonamides
Porphyria-like drug eruption	Furosemide, tetracycline, naproxen
Toxic epidermal necrolysis and Stevens-Johnson syndrome	Anticonvulsants, sulfonamides, NSAIDs, allopurinol, antiretrovirals

TCNs, tetracyclines.

14. What is epidermolysis bullosa?

This is a group of diseases with inherited defects in the skin that result in blistering spontaneously or after minor trauma. Many subtypes have been described (Table 10-6):

- **Epidermolysis bullosa simplex,** an autosomal dominant trait, begins at birth or early in childhood, with blisters due to mild trauma that heal without scarring.
- **Junctional epidermolysis bullosa** also typically begins at birth and may present with generalized blistering. The blisters occur at the dermal–epidermal junction and are due to molecules involved in anchoring the epidermis to the dermis. This type of epidermolysis bullosa may be inherited as an autosomal recessive trait.
- **Dystrophic epidermolysis bullosa** may be autosomal dominant or recessive in inheritance. It ranges from mild to severe blistering that can be disfiguring. It is due to a defect in the dermal anchoring fibrils (type VII collagen).

For all types of epidermolysis bullosa, skin biopsies for routine histology (sometimes with immunoperoxidase stains to type IV collagen to detect the level of the split), as well as electron microscopy, are often required for diagnosis. Referral to a center specializing in epidermolysis bullosa is optimal, and also the National Epidermolysis Bullosa Registry (telephone: 919-966-2007) may be contacted. The mechanobullous diseases are covered in detail in Chapter 6.

15. Describe the other genetic blistering diseases.

- **Acrodermatitis enteropathica:** This condition may be autosomal recessive or acquired and is due to a deficiency of zinc. Cutaneous findings include scaling and vesicles in a periorificial and acral distribution associated with alopecia. Diarrhea is often present. This disorder occurs in infants, especially premature infants, and alcoholics (acquired form) or other patients with impaired gastrointestinal absorption of zinc. Skin biopsy and serum zinc levels are helpful diagnostic tests. Deficiencies of essential fatty acids and amino acids may also cause acrodermatitis enteropathica.
- **Bullous congenital ichthyosiform erythroderma (epidermolytic hyperkeratosis):** This autosomal dominant disease presents with diffuse erythema at birth, with later development of flaccid bullae, and still later with furrowed hyperkeratosis. The defect is in keratins 1 and 10. The diagnosis is by skin biopsy and family history, in addition to clinical findings and disease course.
- **Hailey-Hailey disease (benign familial pemphigus):** In this autosomal dominant disorder, blisters, erosions, and crusts develop in the intertriginous areas. These may begin early in life or later. The intraepidermal blisters form secondary to a loss of cohesion between keratinocytes (acantholysis). The underlying defect is in *ATP2C1,* which encodes a calcium pump. Secondary bacterial infections are common. A diagnosis is established by routine skin biopsy.
- **Incontinentia pigmenti:** This X-linked disease is seen predominantly in females; affected males usually die in utero. It begins in neonatal life, with vesicles occurring in a whorled pattern. Later, verrucous lesions develop, and finally, hyperpigmented patches appear. Skin biopsy is a helpful diagnostic test.

16. List the vesiculobullous diseases caused by metabolic disorders.

- Bullous diabeticorum (bullous eruption of diabetes mellitus)
- Pellagra
- Porphyria cutanea tarda
- Necrolytic erythemas
- Acrodermatitis enteropathica

17. Describe the clinical findings in bullous diabeticorum.

Bullous diabeticorum is characterized by tense bullae that arise spontaneously on the distal extremities in patients with both insulin-dependent and non–insulin-dependent diabetes. The course is chronic and recurring. The diagnosis is made by the clinical findings and skin biopsy. Although the histologic findings are not specific, they may help to rule out other bullous diseases.

Table 10-6. Subtypes of Epidermolysis Bullosa

DISEASE	DEFECT	LEVEL OF SPLIT
EB simplex	Keratins 5 and 14	Basal keratinocytes
EB simplex with muscular dystrophy EB simplex with pyloric atresia EB simplex, Ogna type EB simplex, Dowling-Meara type	Plectin	Intracytoplasmic plaque of hemidesmosome
Junctional EB, Herlitz Junctional EB, non-Herlitz (GABEB) Junctional EB with pyloric atresia	Laminin components α3, β3, α2 BP180 (COLXVIIa1) Laminin components α3, β3, γ2 Integrins α6, β4	Lamina densa/lucida interface Lamina lucida Lamina densa/lucida interface Lamina lucida/hemidesmosome
Dystrophic EB	Type VII Collagen (COL VIIa1)	Sublamina densa

18. What is the cause of pellagra?

Pellagra is a nutritional disorder caused by a deficiency of niacin, which results in dermatitis, dementia, and diarrhea. The dermatitis may occur in a photodistribution, consisting of vesicles, papules, erosions, and hyperpigmentation. The diagnosis is by clinical findings, as biopsy is nondiagnostic. In developed countries, patients at risk for pellagra include alcoholics and those on isoniazid therapy.

Key Points: Vesiculobullous Disorders

1. Vesiculobullous disorders can often be distinguished by the clinical history, distribution, and location of the split (superficial versus deep blister).
2. Vesiculobullous disorders often require biopsies of intact blisters for diagnosis.
3. Direct immunofluorescence of perilesional skin is required in many cases to rule in or exclude autoimmune bullous disorders.
4. Remember that drug eruptions may mimic many of the vesiculobullous disorders.

19. What is the difference between porphyria cutanea tarda and pseudoporphyria?

Porphyria cutaneous tarda is clinically characterized by skin fragility, tense blisters, scarring, and milia in sun-exposed areas, particularly the dorsal hands (Fig. 10-3). Patients have decreased levels of uroporphyrinogen decarboxylase, sometimes due to alcoholic liver disease or to drugs such as estrogen and iron. Hypertrichosis may develop on the face. The diagnosis is established by skin biopsy for routine histology, as well as porphyrin studies, including a 24-hour urine collection for uroporphyrins. Other porphyrias, including variegate porphyria and hereditary coproporphyria, may present with identical cutaneous findings, and should be separated from porphyria cutanea tarda on the basis of associated clinical findings and complete porphyrin studies. Direct immunofluorescence of the skin may be a helpful test for porphyria but does not distinguish one type from another. Pseudoporphyria demonstrates similar cutaneous findings but porphyrin studies are normal. It is associated with uremia, hemodialysis, and some drugs, especially, nonsterioidal antiinflammatory drugs (NSAID)s.

LaDuca JR, Bouman PH, Gaspari AA: Nonsteroidal anti-inflammatory drug-induced pseudoporphyria: a case series *J Cutan Med Surg* 6:320–326, 2002, Epub.

20. What are the necrolytic erythemas?

Necrolytic erythemas are a group of cutaneous diseases of diverse metabolic origin that share certain histopathologic features. Such conditions include acrodermatitis enteropathica, glucagonoma syndrome, necrolytic acral erythema, Hartnup's disease, and several other rare conditions.

21. What is the difference between bullous pemphigoid and cicatricial pemphigoid?

Bullous pemphigoid (IgG directed against BP180 and BP230) is a chronic autoimmune bullous disease that most commonly affects older adults. The primary lesions may be urticarial plaques or tense bullae (Fig. 10-4). Lesions occur particularly on the flexural surfaces but may be widespread. Blisters form crusts and may heal with pigmentary changes, but not scarring. The oral mucosa is sometimes affected, but lesions in this area are usually minor. Cicatricial pemphigoid (IgG or IgA directed against multiple antigens at the basement membrane zone, including BP180) is a chronic autoimmune blistering disorder associated with scarring of mucosal surfaces. It primarily affects the elderly, with some patients having blisters on the cutaneous surface. In both diseases, the diagnosis is established by correlating the clinical findings with routine histologic examination of lesional skin, direct immunofluorescence of perilesional skin, and indirect immunofluorescence or ELISA testing of serum.

Zenzo G, Marazza G, Borradori L: Bullous pemphigoid: physiopathology, clinical features and management, *Adv Dermatol* 23:257–288, 2007.

22. How do pemphigus vulgaris and pemphigus foliaceus differ?

Pemphigus vulgaris (IgG directed against DSG3 and DSG1) is a chronic blistering disease that typically affects adults and usually begins in the oral mucosa. Flaccid vesicles and bullae develop on the face, scalp, neck, chest, groin, and intertriginous areas. These are often tender rather than pruritic. Generalized involvement may occur, and pemphigus vulgaris may be life-threatening. Pemphigus foliaceus (IgG directed against DSG1 only) is a more

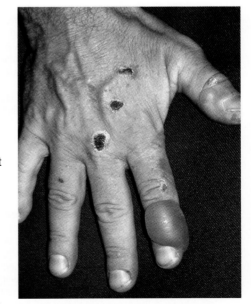

Figure 10-3. Porphyria cutanea tarda. Tense bullae and increased skin fragility manifesting hemorrhagic crusts on the back of a hand. (Courtesy of the Fitzsimons Army Medical Center teaching files.)

superficial form of pemphigus and is generally not as severe as the vulgaris type. Patients develop very superficial vesicles and bullae, typically on the scalp, face, upper chest, and back. Because the blisters are very superficial, they often rupture, and secondary changes of scale, crust, and erosions may be the only findings present. For both varieties, the diagnosis is made by routine histologic exam of an early blister, as well as by direct immunofluorescence of perilesional skin and indirect immunofluorescence of patient serum.

23. Linear IgA bullous dermatosis occurs in two different clinical situations. What are they?

One occurs in early childhood and has been termed **chronic bullous disease** of childhood. Pruritic, urticarial blisters, often sausage-shaped or like a string of pearls, develop on the buttocks and perineal areas, as well as the trunk and extremities (Fig. 10-5). Mucosal lesions are common. The adult form often occurs in the elderly and may be associated with drugs such as vancomycin. Skin lesions may resemble bullous pemphigoid or dermatitis herpetiformis. Diagnosis is by routine histologic exam of an early blister, direct immunofluorescence of perilesional skin, or indirect immunofluorescence to detect IgA antibodies directed against the basement membrane zone of skin.

Dellavalle RP, Burch JM, Tayal S, et al: Vancomycin-associated linear IgA bullous dermatosis mimicking toxic epidermal necrolysis, *J Am Acad Dermatol* 48: S56–S57, 2003.

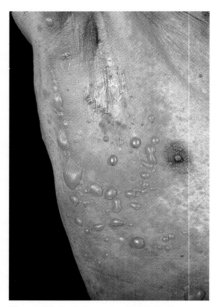

Figure 10-4. Bullous pemphigoid. Erythematous, urticarial plaques with multiple vesicles and bullae are seen. Many of the blisters are tense.

24. Describe the clinical findings in dermatitis herpetiformis.

Dermatitis herpetiformis is an autoimmune disease due to IgA autoantibodies directed against tissue transglutaminase. Dermatitis herpetiformis, an extremely pruritic condition, most commonly begins in early adult life and is characterized by symmetrically distributed papules and vesicles that develop on the elbows, knees, buttocks, extensor forearms, scalp, and, sometimes, face and palms (Fig. 10-6). In some patients, the lesions are generalized and severe. Patients may have an associated gluten-sensitive enteropathy, though it is seldom symptomatic. The diagnosis is established by routine histologic exam of an early blister and direct immunofluorescence of nonlesional skin (IgA is seen in the dermal papillae) (see Fig. 10-2). Scratching may destroy all intact blisters for skin biopsy, and thus direct immunofluorescence may be a particularly helpful diagnostic test. Serologic testing for antiendomysial/eTG antibodies and antigliadin antibodies is also a useful screening test.

Alonso-Llamazares J, Gibson LE, Rogers RS 3rd: Clinical, pathologic, and immunopathologic features of dermatitis herpetiformis: review of the Mayo Clinic experience. *Int J Dermatol* 46:910-919, 2007.

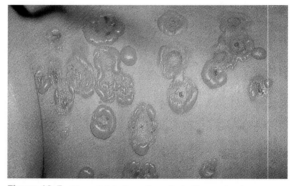

Figure 10-5. Linear IgA bullous dermatosis. Tense, circular, sausage-shaped bullae in a child.

25. Does herpes gestationis have anything to do with herpes viruses?

No. Herpes gestationis, also called gestational pemphigoid, is a rare, autoimmune blistering disease with IgG autoantibodies directed against BP180 (type XVII collagen), which is an important component of the hemidesmosome. It is seen in pregnant women, typically beginning in the second trimester. Lesions often begin in the periumbilical area and may initially be urticarial. Later, tense vesicles and bullae develop, which may resemble bullous pemphigoid. The disease may flare after delivery and may recur in

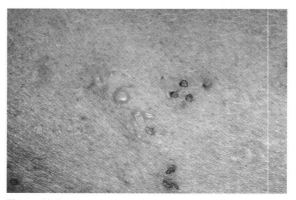

Figure 10-6. Dermatitis herpetiformis. Typical grouped vesicles and excoriations. The lesions are so intensely pruritic that in some patients only excoriations are seen. (Courtesy of the Fitzsimons Army Medical Center teaching files.)

subsequent pregnancies. The pregnancy should be monitored, because premature births as well as small-for-gestational-age infants have occurred in some patients. The diagnosis is made from clinical findings, routine histology of an early blister or urticarial lesion, and direct and indirect immunofluorescence tests.

26. What is bullous systemic lupus erythematosus?

Bullous SLE is a rare blistering eruption that has been reported primarily in patients with established SLE. In most cases, autoantibodies are directed against type VII collagen that is found in the basement membrane zone. Vesicles and bullae may develop on inflamed or noninflamed skin. In some patients, the lesions may resemble bullous pemphigoid, and in others, epidermolysis bullosa acquisita. The diagnosis is made on the basis of clinical findings, routine histologic exam (which may show findings similar to those seen in dermatitis herpetiformis), and immunofluorescence studies including direct, indirect, and a special split-skin indirect immunofluorescence test.

Harris-Stith R, Erickson QL, Elston DM, David-Bajar K: Bullous eruption: a manifestation of lupus erythematosus, *Cutis* 72:31–37, 2003.

27. What is epidermolysis bullosa acquisita?

Epidermolysis bullosa acquisita is an autoimmune bullous disease with autoantibodies directed against type VII collagen in the basement membrane zone. In this disease, vesicles and bullae follow trauma and tend to occur on areas with frictional trauma, such as the fingers, knees, and elbows. Mucosal lesions are common. As with bullous SLE, diagnosis is by clinical findings, routine histology, direct immunofluorescence, indirect immunofluorescence, and split-skin indirect immunofluorescence testing.

Lehman JS, Camilleri MJ, Gibson LE: Epidermolysis bullosa acquisita: concise review and practical considerations, *Int J Dermatol* 48:227–235, 2009.

1. How does a pustule differ from a vesicle or bulla?

A pustule is a purulent vesicle or bulla. Whereas a vesicle contains clear or translucent fluid, a pustule is filled with neutrophils or, less commonly, eosinophils. Pustules are one of the primary lesions in skin. Most pustular eruptions begin as pustules, but others may pass through a transitory stage in which they appear vesicular (vesiculopustules).

2. How are pustules classified?

Pustules may be classified on the basis of where the acute inflammatory cells accumulate (e.g., subcorneal, follicular), pathogenesis (e.g., infectious, autoimmune), predominant inflammatory cells (e.g., neutrophils, eosinophils), and clinical presentation (Table 11-1). Pustules may be unilocular or multilocular.

3. What is the most common pustular skin eruption?

Acne vulgaris, although not all lesions in this condition are pustular (Fig. 11-1). The infectious pustular eruptions are also common (see Chapter 27).

4. Name the different types of pustular psoriasis. How do they differ?

Pustular psoriasis may be broadly subdivided into localized and generalized forms. Localized pustular psoriasis may occur on any site and may also occur within plaques of classic psoriasis. Distinctive variants include acrodermatitis continua of Hallopeau (Fig. 11-2A), which is characterized by pustules and crusting of the distal fingers and toes, and localized pustular psoriasis of the palms and soles (Fig. 11-2B). It is unclear whether pustular eruptions confined to the palms and soles represent a form of localized psoriasis or a different disease called pustular bacterid. Variants of generalized pustular psoriasis include generalized pustular psoriasis of von Zumbusch, exanthematic generalized pustular psoriasis, and impetigo herpetiformis. The von Zumbusch variant presents as generalized pustules in patients with preexisting plaque-type psoriasis or erythrodermic psoriasis. Exanthematic generalized pustular psoriasis arises suddenly without preceding psoriasis (Fig. 11-2C). Impetigo herpetiformis is associated with pregnancy. Hypocalcemia is also frequently present.

5. Do any factors precipitate generalized pustular psoriasis?

The most important inciting factor is the administration of systemic corticosteroids. In a study of 104 patients, corticosteroids were implicated as the precipitating factor in 37 patients (36%). This association is one of the primary reasons that psoriasis is not treated with systemic corticosteroids. Less common precipitating factors included infection (13%), hypocalcemia (9%), pregnancy (3%), and other drugs (e.g., terbinafine).

Baker H, Ryan TJ: Generalized pustular psoriasis: a clinical and epidemiologic study of 104 cases, *Br J Dermatol* 80:771–793, 1968.

6. Is pustular psoriasis treated differently than classic plaque-type psoriasis?

Most treatments that are used on classic plaque-type psoriasis can also be used for the management of pustular psoriasis. The retinoids, especially acitretin, are particularly effective in pustular psoriasis and are the treatment of choice for generalized pustular psoriasis. More recently, isolated cases have been successfully treated with topical biologic agents such as tacrolimus or parental biologic agents such as infliximab and adalimumab.

Rodriquez GF, Fagundo GE, Cabrera-Oaz R, et al: Generalized pustular psoriasis successfully treated with topical tacrolimus, *Br J Dermatol* 152:587–588, 2005.

Ghate JV, Alspaugh CD: Adalimumab in the management of palmoplantar psoriasis, *Dermatol Online J* 15:15, 2009.

7. What is pustular bacterid?

Pustular bacterid (of Andrews) is a controversial clinical eruption. Most dermatologists consider it to be a form of pustular psoriasis localized to the palms and soles. As originally defined by Andrews, pustular bacterid is a pustular eruption of the palms and soles in which the patient has no history or other clinical signs of psoriasis. The lesions are induced by low-grade bacterial infection in occult or evident foci, such as the teeth, tonsils, or gallbladder. The pustular eruption totally resolves with eradication of the infection. A later study has noted that injected *Candida* antigen aggravated up to 37% of patients with this disorder, suggesting that this phenomenon may not be restricted to bacterial infections. The recent recognition of bacterial "superantigens" provides a possible immunologic mechanism for induction of this disorder.

Stevens DM, Ackerman AB: On the concept of bacterids (pustular bacterid, Andrews), *Am J Dermatopathol* 6:281–286, 1984.

Table 11-1. Classification of Pustules

PATHOGENESIS	SITE OF ACCUMULATION
Autoimmune	
IgA pemphigus	Subcorneal
Infectious	
Arthropod reactions	Intraepidermal
Candidiasis	Subcorneal
Furuncle/carbuncle	Follicular
Impetigo	Subcorneal
Hot tub (pseudomonal) folliculitis	Follicular
Kerion (tinea capitis)	Follicular
Pityrosporum folliculitis	Follicular
Vaccinia infection/vaccination	Intraepidermal
Inherited	
Pustular psoriasis	Subcorneal, intraepidermal
Reiter's syndrome	Subcorneal, intraepidermal
Drug eruptions	
Acneiform drug-induced eruptions	Follicular
Toxic erythema with pustules	Subcorneal
Halogenodermas	Intraepidermal
Miscellaneous	
Acne necrotica miliaris	Follicular
Acne vulgaris	Follicular
Erythema toxicum neonatorum	Follicular
Folliculitis decalvans	Follicular
Infantile acropustulosis	Subcorneal, intraepidermal
Miliaria pustulosa	Sweat duct
Pustular bacterid	Intraepidermal
Rosacea	Follicular
Subcorneal pustular dermatosis	Subcorneal
Transient neonatal pustular dermatosis	Subcorneal

8. Why do some consider pustular bacterid a form of localized pustular psoriasis of the palms and soles?

The argument is based on the observation that some patients with pustular eruptions of the palms and soles also have typical psoriasis elsewhere. The clinical appearance and histologic findings of the palmar lesions are identical to those of pustular bacterid. Some dermatologists prefer the term palmar and plantar pustulosis as a noncommittal name for this entity.

9. What is subcorneal pustular dermatosis (Sneddon-Wilkinson disease)?

Subcorneal pustular dermatosis is a rare, benign, chronic, relapsing dermatosis that was described by Sneddon and Wilkinson in 1956. It most commonly affects middle-aged women, although any age group, including children, may be affected. The lesions typically occur in the flexural and intertriginous areas, where they present as superficial vesiculopustules or pustules that often assume annular or gyrate patterns. The lesions may demonstrate peripheral extension and resolve with variable crusting and scaling. Typically, patients are otherwise healthy, but there are isolated case reports of an associated seronegative rheumatoid-like arthritis.

Ratnarathorn M, Newman J: Subcorneal pustular dermatosis (Sneddon-Wilkinson disease) occurring in association with nodal marginal zone lymphoma: a case report, *Dermatol Online J* 14:6, 2008.

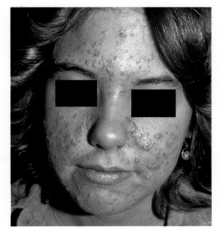

Figure 11-1. Gram-negative pustular acne vulgaris. (Courtesy of the Fitzsimons Army Medical Center teaching files.)

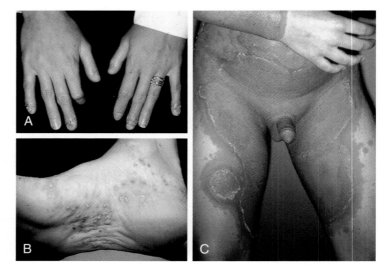

Figure 11-2. Pustular psoriasis. **A,** Acrodermatitis continua of Hallopeau demonstrating extensive crusting and nail dystrophy. **B,** Chronic pustular eruption of the sole of the foot. **C,** Generalized pustular psoriasis demonstrating marked erythema with numerous pustules. (Courtesy of Fitzsimons Army Medical Teaching files.)

10. Discuss the pathogenesis of subcorneal pustular dermatosis.

The pathogenesis of subcorneal pustular dermatosis is unknown; although some cases have been associated with plasma cell dyscrasias. Even the nosology is controversial. While many authors accept this condition as a distinct entity, a few consider it to be synonymous with, or a variant of, pustular psoriasis. Histologically, both entities demonstrate a subcorneal vesicle filled with neutrophils. The strongest points against the relationship of subcorneal pustular dermatosis and psoriasis are that the former has a distinct clinical presentation, patients do not have preceding plaque-type psoriasis, and they are not likely to develop classic psoriasis during the course of their disease. Some drugs such as lithium carbonate may exacerbate subcorneal pustular dermatosis by increasing neutrophil migration into lesions.

11. How is subcorneal pustular dermatosis treated?

Subcorneal pustular dermatosis cannot be cured, but it can be managed. The disease is uncommon enough that good therapeutic studies comparing different treatment modalities are not available. Anecdotal reports have described excellent therapeutic results with dapsone and acitretin. Less frequently used therapies include oral prednisone, topical corticosteroids, sulfapyridine, vitamin E, and ultraviolet B therapy.

Marliere V, Beylot-Barry M, Beylot C, Doutre M: Successful treatment of subcorneal pustular dermatosis (Sneddon-Wilkinson disease) by acitretin: report of a case, *Dermatology* 199:153–155, 1999.

12. What is superficial IgA pemphigus?

Recently, it has been demonstrated that some cases of what were formerly classified as subcorneal pustular dermatosis may demonstrate intraepidermal IgA between the keratinocytes. Most authorities feel that cases with intraepidermal IgA on direct immunofluorescence should be reclassified as superficial IgA pemphigus (Fig. 11-3). It has been demonstrated that the IgA autoantibodies are directed against desmocollin 1 and possibly desmocollins 2 and 3, which are molecules that are important for normal adhesion between keratinocytes.

Düker I, Schaller J, Rose C, et al: Subcorneal pustular dermatosis-type IgA pemphigus with autoantibodies to desmocollins 1, 2, and 3, *Arch Dermatol* 145: 1159–1162, 2009.

13. What are the cutaneous findings in reactive arthritis (Reiter's disease)?

The classic triad of reactive arthritis (Reiter's disease) consists of nongonococcal urethritis, conjunctivitis, and arthritis. However, this triad is present in only 40% of the cases at the time of presentation, and the mucocutaneous findings are helpful in establishing the diagnosis. The mucocutaneous findings include a

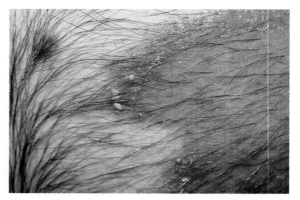

Figure 11-3. Isolated pustule and annular lesions demonstrating scale-crust superficial pustules in a patient with IgA pemphigus. In the past, this would have been considered to be subcorneal pustular dermatosis.

nonspecific stomatitis, nail changes (subungual hyperkeratosis and onycholysis), circinate balanitis, and keratoderma blennorrhagicum. Keratoderma blennorrhagicum is present in about one third of cases and presents as pinpoint erythematous papules that progress to pustules and hyperkeratotic papules and plaques. These are most commonly seen on the bottom of the feet but may also occur on the scalp, elbows, knees, buttocks, and genitalia. Histologically, the findings are identical to the pustules seen in pustular psoriasis.

Wu IB, Schwartz RA: Reiter's syndrome: the classic triad and more, *J Am Acad Dermatol* 59:113–121, 2008.

14. Which drugs are commonly associated with pustular drug eruptions?

Drugs may produce different patterns of pustular drug eruptions, including aggravation of preexisting pustular eruptions such as psoriasis or subcorneal pustular dermatosis. Primary pustular drug eruptions can be classified as acneiform, halogenodermas, and toxic erythema with pustules.

- Acneiform drug eruptions: Systemic corticosteroids (steroid acne), phenytoin, lithium, iodides, bromides, isoniazid (Fig. 11-4)
- Halogenodermas: Iodides, bromides, and fluorides may produce both acneiform drug eruptions and nonfollicular pustules (Fig. 11-5)
- Drug-induced toxic erythema with pustules (acute generalized exanthematous pustulosis): A drug eruption that presents as fever, malaise, and diffuse erythema studded with small pustules; caused by numerous medications including co-trimoxazole, erythromycin, hydroxychloroquine, streptomycin, terbinafine, and cephalosporins

Momin SB, Del Rosso JQ, Michaels B, Mobini N: Acute generalized exanthematous pustulosis: an enigmatic drug-induced reaction, *Cutis* 83:291–298, 2009.

15. What is acne necrotica miliaris?

This chronic folliculitis of the scalp, which primarily affects middle-aged men, presents as follicular-based pustules that quickly develop into perifollicular crusts and scale. The eruption may be asymptomatic or pruritic. If the lesions are pruritic, secondary excoriations may predominate. Acne necrotica miliaris does not result in permanent scarring or hair loss. Most patients respond to low-dose tetracycline, which may need to be continued for years.

16. What is folliculitis decalvans?

Folliculitis decalvans (Quinquaud's disease) is a rare, scarring alopecia of unknown etiology. Clinically, it presents as follicular-based pustules that may assume annular or circinate configurations. The pustules rapidly form crusts; in many patients, the crusts may predominate. The hairs are permanently lost, leaving patches of atrophic hairless skin. Treatment is generally unsatisfactory; topical corticosteroids and oral antibiotics are typically used. Anecdotal reports have described isolated success with oral rifampin or oral zinc sulfate.

17. Discuss the pathogenesis of miliaria pustulosa.

All forms of miliaria result from the retention of sweat secondary to occlusion of the sweat ducts. The pathogenesis of miliaria pustulosa is not entirely understood, but it is believed that heat and occlusion result in the proliferation of surface bacteria that produce toxins that damage the acrosyringium (intraepidermal portion of the eccrine sweat duct). Depending on the level of occlusion, different patterns of disease are produced. If significant numbers of neutrophils are attracted to the acrosyringium, a flaccid pustule develops, producing miliaria pustulosa. If the disease is less severe or the inflammatory response muted, then only an erythematous papule is present, producing the clinical lesion called miliaria rubra (heat bumps, prickly heat). If the damage to the acrosyringium is entirely mechanical, such as occurs following a sunburn, the inflammatory response is minimal and small superficial vesicles are formed at the acrosyringium, producing the variant referred to as miliaria crystallina.

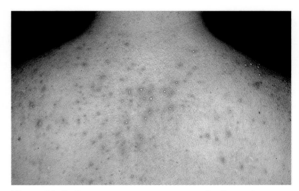

Figure 11-4. Corticosteroid-induced acne manifesting as the explosive onset of numerous follicular-based papules and pustules.

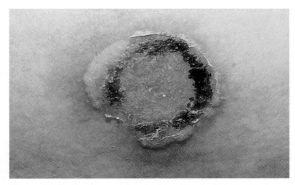

Figure 11-5. Annular pustular eruption of the back secondary to oral potassium iodide (iododerma).

18. How is miliaria pustulosa treated?

Once miliaria pustulosa has developed, there is no satisfactory treatment except removing the patient from the hot and humid environment. Occlusive wear that may have aggravated the condition should also be eliminated. Anecdotally, some dermatologists have tried weak solutions of salicylic acid to produce exfoliation or tape stripping of the stratum corneum to remove the obstruction to sweating, but there are no studies to document the efficacy of these treatments. Some patients may require weeks or even months to establish normal sweating after severe attacks.

19. What is the differential diagnosis of a pustular eruption in a neonate?

- Erythema toxicum neonatorum
- Transient neonatal pustular melanosis
- Incontinentia pigmenti (more commonly vesicular)
- Neonatal acne
- Miliaria pustulosa
- Staphylococcal infection
- Herpes simplex (more commonly vesicular)
- Candidiasis
- Congenital syphilis

Key Points: Neonatal Pustular Eruptions

1. Neonates are frequently born with pustular lesions, with the majority of them being transient.
2. The pathogenesis of neonatal pustular eruptions includes hormonal (neonatal acne), infectious (herpes simplex infection, candidiasis, staphylococcal infection, congenital syphilis), occlusive (miliaria rubra), or idiopathic (transient neonatal pustular melanosis, erythema toxicum neonatorum).
3. Most cases can be clinically differentiated based on the clinical distribution.
4. Problematic cases should be evaluated by diagnostic studies to include examining the blister contents with Wright's stain to look for the primary inflammatory cell type (neutrophils versus eosinophils) and balloon cells to exclude herpes virus infection and Gram stains to rule out bacteria and *Candida* infection.

---

20. How do erythema toxicum neonatorum and transient neonatal pustular melanosis differ?

Erythema toxicum neonatorum (ETN) and transient neonatal pustular melanosis (TNPT) are both benign vesiculopustular disorders of unknown etiology that present during the first few days of life. ETN does not demonstrate a racial predilection and is very common, with up to 20% of neonates being affected. Clinically, it usually presents as macular erythema that usually affects the face initially; approximately 10% to 20% of cases develop pustules within the center of the areas of macular erythema. Biopsies of the pustules demonstrate an acute superficial folliculitis composed primarily of eosinophils. Peripheral eosinophilia may be present in 20% of cases. The lesions resolve without permanent sequelae in 7 to 10 days. Epidemiologically, TNPT differs from ETN in that it occurs in about 5% of black neonates but in <1% of white neonates. Clinically, it presents as vesiculopustules that are not associated with surrounding erythema. The vesiculopustules resolve within 48 hours and are followed by hyperpigmented macules that may take 3 months to resolve. In contrast to ETN, biopsies demonstrate subcorneal pustules that are not follicular based, and the primary inflammatory cells are neutrophils. Peripheral eosinophilia is absent. Both conditions are benign and self-limited. Treatment is not recommended.

Marchini G, Ulfgren AK, Lore K, et al: Erythema toxicum neonatorum: an immunohistochemical analysis, *Pediatr Dermatol* 18: 177–187, 2001.

Merlob P, Metzker A, Reisner SH: Transient neonatal pustular melanosis, *Am J Dis Child* 136:521–522, 1982.

21. What is infantile acropustulosis?

Infantile acropustulosis, also referred to as acropustulosis of infancy, is an inflammatory disease first described in 1979. Most case reports have been in black infants from the southern United States, but it has also been reported in other racial groups and countries including Scandinavia. Clinically, the condition is characterized by recurrent crops of 1- to 2-mm intensely pruritic vesiculopustules on the extremities (Fig. 11-6). Histologically, there are well circumscribed intraepidermal pustules filled with neutrophils. Most cases spontaneously resolve by 2 years of age.

22. What causes infantile acropustulosis?

The etiology and pathogenesis are unknown. It has been postulated that this condition represents a

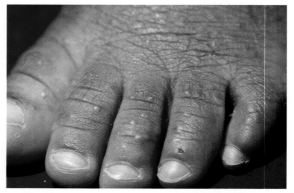

Figure 11-6. Infantile acropustulosis demonstrating typical, pruritic acral pustules in a black child.

nonspecific host response to arthropod bites. In support of this, some infants with scabies demonstrate similar acral vesiculopustules.

23. What is the best treatment of infantile acropustulosis?

Nothing works very well. The disease is self-limited; it usually disappears spontaneously by age 2 years. Patients with severe pruritus can be treated with high doses of antihistamines. Some patients respond to potent topical corticosteroids, while rare patients may require treatment with oral dapsone.

Mancini AJ, Frieden IJ, Paller AS: Infantile acropustulosis revisited: history of scabies and response to topical corticosteroids, *Pediatr Dermatol* 15:337–341, 1998.

LICHENOID SKIN ERUPTIONS

Whitney A. High, MD, JD, MEng

1. How do lichenoid eruptions differ from other papulosquamous conditions?

Lichenoid skin eruptions represent a subcategory of papulosquamous skin disease. While most papulosquamous eruptions present with scaling papules, lichenoid eruptions differ in that the scale is often subtle, and papules tend to remain small and discrete. On occasion, confluent plaques may form.

2. What does "lichenoid" mean?

The term *lichenoid* has at least three commonly accepted applications/definitions:

- Originally, the term lichenoid referred to a clinical resemblance of such eruptions to lichens (complex organism consisting of a symbiotic relationship between a fungus and an alga).
- Lichen planus (LP) is the prototypical disease within this category, and eruptions sharing clinical features with LP may be described as "lichenoid."
- Lichenoid also refers to a specific histologic tissue reaction pattern manifesting as a "bandlike" infiltrate of mononuclear inflammatory cells (predominantly lymphocytes) immediately subjacent to the dermal–epidermal junction, typical of LP.

3. What is the most common lichenoid skin disease?

Lichen planus is a relatively common disorder, accounting for about 1% of all patient visits to dermatology clinics. The disease most often affects middle-aged adults. Although LP is thought to have no consistent gender predilection, some studies have found women to be more often affected than men. A recent meta-analysis regarding the incidence of oral lichen planus found an overall age-standardized prevalence of 1.27% (0.96% in men and 1.57% in women).

Katta R: Lichen planus, *Am Fam Physician* 61:3319–3324, 2000.
Carrozzo M: How common is oral lichen planus? *Evid Based Dent* 9:112–113, 2008.

4. What anatomic locations are most often affected by Lichen planus?

LP may affect both the skin and mucosa. Examination of both areas is essential when the diagnosis of LP is suspected. The frequency of involvement for these areas is somewhat controversial. In general, patients with mucosal disease may not demonstrate skin lesions, but 50% or more of patients with cutaneous disease will demonstrate mucosal lesions. Flexural areas, such as the wrists and ankles, are often involved. Other sites of preferential involvement include the neck, buttocks, sacrum, anogenital region, penis, and buccal or vaginal mucosa.

5. Describe the characteristic primary skin lesions of Lichen planus.

LP is a disease characterized by "P-words":

- Plentiful
- Pruritic
- Polished
- Purple
- Polygonal
- Planar
- Papules

Primary lesions of the skin are 1 to 5 mm, flat-topped, violaceous, shiny papules (Fig. 12-1). While papules are often clustered, individual lesions tend to be discrete, with angulated (polygonal) borders. Wickham's stria, a lacy white network present on the surface of the papules, is often of great diagnostic value.

6. What are the characteristic oral findings of Lichen planus?

Mucosal lesions of LP differ from cutaneous lesions through demonstration of Wickham's stria in the absence of a papular component. A white, reticulated, "netlike" pattern is often present upon the buccal mucosa, the tongue, or other mucosal surfaces (Fig. 12-2). Other mucosal forms may be ulcerative. Some experts believe that some cases of oral LP may be associated with mercury-containing dental amalgams, although the evidence is not conclusive, and still others believe this is a separate category of disease, more aptly termed a mercury-associated lichenoid stomatitis.

Dissemond J: Oral lichen planus: an overview, *J Dermatol Treat* 15:136–140, 2004.
Bruce AJ, Rogers RS 3rd: Lichenoid contact stomatitis, Arch Dermatol 140:1524–1525, 2004.

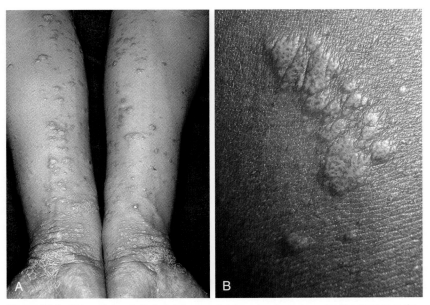

Figure 12-1. Lichen planus. **A,** Typical violaceous, flat-topped, polygonal papules. The location on the volar wrist is characteristic. **B,** Note the Wickham's striae. (Courtesy of James E. Fitzpatrick, MD.)

7. Describe the isomorphic response of Lichen planus.

The isomorphic response (Koebner phenomenon) refers to development of new lesions as a response to external trauma. This phenomenon is characteristic of both LP and psoriasis, among other more rare conditions. In LP, linear aggregates of typical papules may be induced by scratching or rubbing (Fig. 12-3).

8. What causes Lichen planus?

The cause of LP is unknown. Etiologic hypotheses include hypersensitivity reactions, viral infection (particularly hepatitis C), or autoimmune mechanisms. Case reports have linked LP to viral hepatitis, neurologic disease, and severe psychic trauma. Other autoimmune diseases such as vitiligo, inflammatory bowel disease, and autoimmune thyroiditis are seen with increased frequency in those with LP. Lichenoid eruptions (otherwise identical to idiopathic LP) may be seen as a reaction

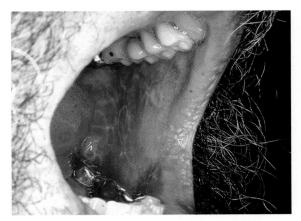

Figure 12-2. Lichen planus, showing reticulated leukoplakia of the buccal mucosa. (Courtesy of James E. Fitzpatrick, MD.)

to drugs or as a manifestation of graft-versus-host disease following allogeneic bone marrow transplantation. Oral disease and, to a lesser degree, cutaneous LP have been associated with hypersensitivity to dental amalgams. In actuality, most LP occurs in otherwise healthy people without an identifiable cause.

9. What are the less common presentations of Lichen planus?

Nail changes occur in about 10% to 15% of patients and include longitudinal ridging, irregular pitting, nail plate splitting, nail loss, and pterygium formation with severe onychodystrophy, including "20-nail dystrophy" (Fig. 12-4). Desquamative vaginitis may occur. Clinical and histologic variants of LP include annular (Fig. 12-5), hypertrophic, ulcerative, vesiculobullous, follicular, and actinic induced. LP may also involve the scalp, yielding a scarring alopecia known as lichen planopilaris.

Bhattacharya M, Kaur I, Kumar B: Lichen planus: a clinical and epidemiological study, *J Dermatol* 27:576–582, 2000.
Karthikenyan K, Jeevankumar B, Thappa DM: Bullous lichen planus of the glans penis, *Dermatol Online J* 9:31, 2003. (Readers can go to this online journal and read about bullous lichen planus in more detail and also see clinical photographs.)

10. How is 20-nail dystrophy related to Lichen planus?

The etiology of 20-nail dystrophy is controversial. This destructive nail disorder affects mostly children, and it is not commonly associated with cutaneous lesions. Typically, all nails show excessive longitudinal ridging, with thin, brittle, opalescent nails. While some experts consider LP to be a possible etiology, other studies utilizing nail biopsy have demonstrated a spongiotic pattern of inflammation rather than a lichenoid process. The condition often results in permanent nail loss, and urgent consultation with a nail specialist is indicated.

Yokozeki H, Niiyama S, Nishioka K: Twenty-nail dystrophy (trachyonychia) caused by lichen planus in a patient with gold allergy, *Br J Dermatol* 52:1087–1089, 2005.

11. Is Lichen planus associated with systemic diseases?

LP has been associated with numerous disorders, but such relationships often engender controversy. Associated conditions include viral hepatitis, chronic active hepatitis, primary biliary cirrhosis, diabetes mellitus, internal malignancy, and autoimmune or connective tissue disease. The relationship to infection with hepatitis C (HCV) is controversial. The latest metaanalysis concluded that the association exists in some regions (East/Southeast Asia, South America, the Middle East, and Europe) but not in others (North America, South Asia, and Africa). At present, it is recommended that patients with LP be queried about major risks factors (IV drug use or sex with IV drug users) or minor risk factors (history of blood transfusion, male sex, and age 30 to 49 years) and that those with significant risk be screened for HCV antibodies.

Bigby, M: The relationship between lichen planus and hepatitis C clarified, *Arch Dermatol* 145:1048–1050, 2009.

12. What is the prognosis of Lichen planus?

The duration of disease activity is related to the site of involvement. Isolated mucosal involvement portends a more chronic course, perhaps lasting decades. Additionally, patients with oral LP are at increased risk of squamous cell carcinoma arising within chronic lesions. Conversely, isolated cutaneous involvement typically resolves spontaneously within 1 to 2 years. Patients with both mucosal and cutaneous lesions typically have an intermediate prognosis. Certain clinical subtypes, such as ulcerative, palmoplantar, and actinic LP, are more persistent and recalcitrant to treatment. Twenty percent of patients may relapse after an initial clearing.

Carbone M, Arduino PG, Carrozzo M, et al: Course of oral lichen planus: a retrospective study of 808 northern Italian patients, *Oral Dis* 15:235–243, 2009.

13. What is the primary symptom of Lichen planus?

The pruritus of LP is often intense. Nearly all patients report some itching. Interestingly, the pruritus of LP often maintains a special quality that will induce rubbing, rather than scratching, for relief. Such rubbing may account for the polished appearance of the lesions. If excoriation occurs, new lesions are likely to develop within wounds (Koebnerization).

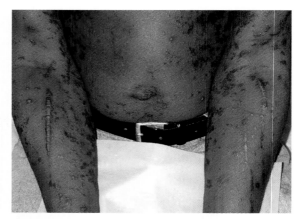

Figure 12-3. Lichen planus with Koebner phenomenon. Note the linear distribution of secondary lesions that develop in sites of excoriation. (Courtesy of Whitney A. High, MD.)

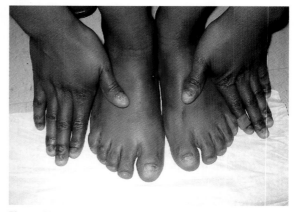

Figure 12-4. Twenty-nail dystrophy secondary to lichen planus. Note that all twenty nails demonstrate varying degrees of nail dystrophy. (Courtesy of Whitney A. High, MD.)

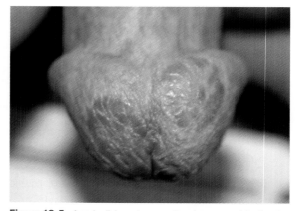

Figure 12-5. Annular lichen planus on the glans was originally misdiagnosed as squamous cell carcinoma until its annular quality was noted by the dermatologist. (Courtesy of Whitney A. High, MD.)

14. Describe the characteristic histopathologic features of classic Lichen planus.

- The stratum corneum is thickened (hyperkeratotic), but is largely devoid of retained keratinocytic nuclei (essentially no parakeratosis).
- The granular layer is focally accentuated ("wedge-shaped" hypergranulosis).
- The Malpighian layer (stratum spinosum and stratum granulosum) is irregularly thickened, demonstrating a "sawtooth" acanthosis, with occasional necrotic keratinocytes in the superficial dermis (Civatte bodies).
- The basal layer is disrupted and appears lost or flattened ("interface reaction").
- The dermal–epidermal junction is vacuolated and obscured by a "bandlike" lymphocytic inflammatory infiltrate. This pattern of infiltration is so typical of LP, it is referred to as a "lichenoid infiltrate."

15. How is lichen planus treated?

Topical corticosteroids and oral antihistamines are used to ameliorate the pruritus in mild cases. Hypertrophic lesions may not respond to topical treatment and instead may require intralesional corticosteroids. The optimal treatment of severe disease is difficult to determine since the studies regarding treatment have been primarily anecdotal or consist of small series. The most commonly used treatment is systemic corticosteroids, but variable degrees of success have also been reported with topical calcineurin inhibitors (tacrolimus and pimectrolims), psoralen plus ultraviolet A (PUVA) light therapy, narrow-band ultraviolet B (UVB) light therapy, oral retinoids (isotretinoin and acitretin), griseofulvin, methotrexate, cyclosporine, sulfasalazine, and thalidomide.

Omidian M, Ayoobi A, Mapar M, et al: Efficacy of sulfasalazine in the treatment of generalized lichen planus: randomized double-blinded clinical trial on 52 patients, *J Eur Acad Dermatol Venereol*, Feb 10, 2010 (Epub ahead of print).

16. What conditions enter the differential diagnosis of an "Lichen planus-like" eruption?

Lichenoid drug eruptions may be indistinguishable from idiopathic LP. Any exogenous ingestant, or rarely a topical chemical, may be causative. Common etiologic agents are listed in Table 12-1. Other potables, such as alcoholic liqueurs containing gold particles, have been implicated in lichenoid eruptions. Contact with certain chemicals, particularly those involved with photodeveloping, may result in a lichenoid contact dermatitis. Clues suggesting a lichenoid drug eruption include an atypical distribution or lack of mucosal involvement. Histopathologic clues to a drug-induced eruption include significant parakeratosis and eosinophils within the inflammatory infiltrate.

Ellgehausen P, Elsner P, Burg G: Drug-induced lichen planus, *Clin Dermatol* 16:325–332, 1998.

17. Are Lichen planus and systemic lupus erythematosus related?

Systemic lupus erythematosus (SLE) has been diagnosed in patients with LP, and an "LP-SLE overlap" syndrome has been described. Papulosquamous lesions of SLE, particularly those of acral areas, may resemble LP, but other features of SLE are usually present, allowing for discrimination.

Nagao K, Chen KR: A case of lupus erythematosus/lichen planus overlap syndrome, *J Dermatol* 33:187–190, 2006.

18. Are Lichen planus and bullous pemphigoid related?

Lichen planus pemphigoides is a rare skin disease that presents with overlapping features of LP and bullous pemphigoid. It is characterized by bullous lesions arising on lichen planus–like papules and also upon uninvolved skin. While the condition may arise *de novo*, particularly in children, it may also be induced by medications including: cinnarizine, captopril, ramipril, simvastatin, PUVA, antituberculous medications, and some Chinese herbs.

Cohen DM, Ben-Amitai D, Feinmesser M, Zvulunov A: Childhood lichen planus pemphigoides: a case report and review of the literature, *Pediatr Dermatol* 26:569–574, 2009.

Xu HH, Xiao T, He CD, et al: Lichen planus pemphigoides associated with Chinese herbs, *Clin Exp Dermatol* 34:329–332, 2009.

Table 12-1. Common Etiologic Drug Classes in LP-like Drug Eruptions

Antihypertensives	Antimalarials	Miscellaneous
Beta-blockers	Chloroquine	Sulfonylureas
ACE inhibitors	Quinacrine	Chlorpropamide
Thiazides	**Anticonvulsants**	Allopurinol
Furosemide	Carbamazepine	Penicillamine
Methyldopa	Phenytoin	Sildenafil
Antimicrobials	**Neurologic agents**	Misoprostol
Acyclovir	Benzodiazepines	
Isoniazid	Phenothiazines	
Tetracyclines	**Lipid-lowering agents**	
Antiinflammatory agents	Lovastatin	
Nonsteroidal anti-inflammatory drugs	Fluvastatin	
Gold salts	**Biologic response modifiers**	
Sulfones	Tumor necrosis factor α antagonists (infliximab, etanercept, adalimumab)	
	Imatinib mesylate	

19. Why is graft-versus-host disease a consideration in Lichen planus-like eruptions?

Graft-versus-host disease (GVHD) is a complication of allogeneic bone marrow transplantation. In GVHD, the immune effector cells of the donor bone marrow (the "graft") react against antigens of the recipient tissues (the "host"). The resultant eruption may be indistinguishable, both clinically and histopathologically, from that of LP. Lichenoid GVHD reaction is often more generalized than is classic LP, and the history would certainly be suggestive. GVHD resulting from solid-organ transplantation is exquisitely rare.

Johnson ML, Farmer ER: Graft-versus-host reactions in dermatology, *J Am Acad Dermatol* 38:369–392, 1998.

Key Points: Lichen Planus

1. The primary lesion of lichen planus is a flat-topped, pruritic, purple, polygonal papule.
2. Lichen planus, in addition to affecting skin, can also affect the oral or vaginal mucosal surface, nails, or hair.
3. Lichen planus frequently demonstrates the isomorphic response (Koebner phenomenon), which refers to the development of new lesions in site of minor trauma.
4. Lichen planus may be clinically and histologically mimicked by numerous drugs (lichenoid drug eruptions).

---

20. Describe the primary lesion of lichen nitidus.

Lichen nitidus (LN) manifests as innumerable, 1- to 2-mm, round or polygonal, flat-topped, shiny, flesh-colored papules occurring in well-circumscribed areas upon the extremities, abdomen, or penis (Fig. 12-6). Rarely, mucosal or nail changes are present.

Al-Mutairi N, Hassanein A, Nour-Eldin O, Arun J: Generalized lichen nitidus, *Pediatr Dermatol* 22:158–160, 2005.

21. What are the other clinical features of lichen nitidus?

LN is uncommon relative to LP. It too has no gender, age, or race predilection. It may affect any age but it is more common in children and young adults. The eruption is typically idiopathic, chronic, and, fortunately, asymptomatic. An isomorphic response may be demonstrated. The disease is most often self-limited and resolves spontaneously over months to

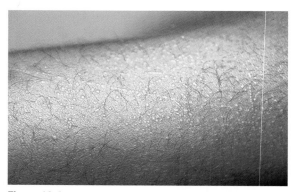

Figure 12-6. Lichen nitidus, with numerous 1- to 2-mm, shiny, flat-topped papules. Note the linear lesions secondary to the isomorphic phenomenon.

years. There are no well recognized disease associations. Rarely, medications have been implicated. Response to treatment, generally limited to mild topical corticosteroids, is poor. Reassurance and education are often the best therapy.

22. Does lichen nitidus demonstrate a lichenoid infiltrate upon biopsy?

No. While LN appears "lichenoid" clinically, the histopathologic findings are granulomatous in nature. Typically, the epidermis demonstrates central atrophy, while peripheral epidermal rete ridges extend into the papillary dermis in "clawlike" fashion, surrounding a granulomatous aggregate of lymphocytes and histiocytes.

23. What is lichen striatus?

Lichen striatus is an uncommon idiopathic dermatosis that presents as a linear plaque, most often on the extremity or neck of a child or, less commonly, an adult. The condition consists of a coalescent group of flesh or rose-colored lichenoid papules (Fig. 12-7). The resultant linear plaque may form a band several centimeters wide and may course the entire length of the extremity.

Patrizi A, Neri I, Fiorentini C, et al: Lichen striatus: clinical and laboratory features of 115 children, *Pediatr Dermatol* 21:197–204, 2004.
Taniguchi Abagge K, Parolin Marinoni L, Giraldi S, et al: Lichen striatus: description of 89 cases in children, *Pediatr Dermatol* 21:440–443, 2004.

24. Discuss the natural history and prognosis of lichen striatus.

Lichen striatus develops rapidly over a period of weeks. Pruritus is common, but may be minimal. Spontaneous resolution within several months is characteristic. Patients with minimal pruritus require only reassurance. Recalcitrant or intensely pruritic cases may respond to topical corticosteroids.

25. What is lichen simplex chronicus?

Lichen simplex chronicus (LSC) is not a disease but rather a reaction of the skin to chronic friction from rubbing or scratching. LSC may be superimposed upon normal skin, but it is often a secondary condition of chronically inflamed skin. The clinical appearance, termed *lichenification*, is characteristic, regardless of the underlying etiology. Relative thickening of the skin, with accentuation of the normal skin lines, is typical. Closely set lichenoid papules may be discerned at the periphery. Frequently, the lichenified plaque maintains a dusky violaceous hue.

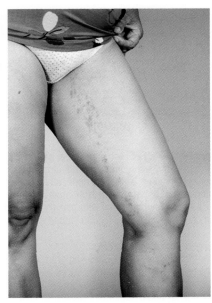

Figure 12-7. Lichen striatus. Linear plaque composed of violaceous, slightly hyperpigmented papules confined to the lower extremity of a young adult. Most cases occur in children. (Courtesy of the Fitzsimons Army Medical Center teaching files.)

26. How is lichen simplex chronicus treated?

LSC is a self-perpetuating dermatosis, and it will persist until the initiating stimulus is eliminated. Interruption of the "itch-scratch cycle" is requisite to resolution. A short course of medium- or high-potency topical corticosteroids is typically employed. Covering the plaque is often important, as this acts as a physical barrier to continued frictional trauma and also acts as an occlusive adjunct for the topical preparation. Patients who express insight into the cause of their condition fare better. Resultant postinflammatory dyspigmentation may last for years, even after the changes of lichenification have resolved.

GRANULOMATOUS DISEASES OF THE SKIN

James E. Fitzpatrick, MD

1. What is meant by "granulomatous diseases of the skin"?

Quite simply, the granulomatous disorders of the skin comprise a broad category of diseases that are characterized by the accumulation of activated macrophages with an epithelioid appearance in the dermis or subcutaneous tissue. A granuloma is a distinct aggregate composed of epithelioid macrophages with or without multinucleated giant cells. These aggregates are typically surrounded by a rim of lymphocytes with plasma cells being variably present. Macrophages develop from bone marrow–derived monocytes that leave the circulation and enter the skin.

2. Explain the role of histiocytes in granulomas.

Many references use the confusing term histiocyte when discussing granulomas. Histiocyte may be used interchangeably with macrophage or monocyte, but the term is not specific and may be applied also to transformed lymphocytes (e.g., histiocytic lymphoma), fibroblasts that demonstrate phagocytosis (e.g., fibrous histiocytoma, reticulohistiocytoma), and antigen-presenting cells (e.g., histiocytosis X). Some authorities eschew the use of this term because it is not specific.

3. What is the difference between an immune granuloma and a foreign body granuloma?

Immune granuloma formation is a local tissue response to a poorly soluble substance that is capable of inducing a cell-mediated immune response (e.g., cutaneous tuberculosis). The persistent presence of a poorly soluble substance in the skin causes the activation of T cells, which secrete cytokines such as interleukin-2 (Il-2) to activate additional T cells and interferon-2 (IFN-2), which transform macrophages into epithelioid macrophages and multinucleated giant cells. In contrast, foreign body granulomas, typically are the result of larger aggregates of inert foreign material that cannot be phagocytized by a single macrophage (e.g., wood splinter). In general, granulomas are produced by infectious agents, foreign bodies, or alterations in the host immune system.

4. List some common granulomatous diseases that affect the skin.

See Table 13-1.

Table 13-1. Agents and Diseases That Can Produce Granulomas

Infectious Agents

Fungi	*Bacteria*	*Miscellaneous Infections*
Blastomycosis	Actinomycosis	Leishmaniasis
Candidiasis	Cat scratch fever	Protothefocosis (algae infection)
Chromomycosis	Granuloma inguinale (donovanosis)	
Coccidioidomycosis	Mycobacterial infections	
Cryptococcosis	Nocardiosis	
Histoplasmosis	Syphilis	
Sporotrichosis	Tularemia	

Foreign Body Agents

Exogenous	*Endogenous*	*Miscellaneous Diseases*
Aluminum	Bone	Actinic granuloma
Cosmetic fillers	Calcium	Crohn's disease
Hair	Cholesterol	Granuloma annulare
Insect parts	Keratin	Granulomatous cheilitis
Paraffin	Hair	Granulomatous rosacea
Silica	Sebum	Lupus miliaris disseminatus faciei
Splinters	Urate crystals	Necrobiosis lipoidica
Starch		Rheumatoid nodule
Sutures		Sarcoidosis
Talc		
Tattoo pigment		

5. Can granulomas be recognized clinically?

Sometimes. Granulomas usually present as dermal nodules, although epidermal changes can be present. Foreign body granulomas may demonstrate a central erosion or ulceration secondary to an attempt by the body to extrude the foreign material through an elimination tract. Granulomas often present as nonspecific erythematous nodules; however, they also may present as dermal nodules with an "apple-jelly hue" that is highly suggestive of an underlying granulomatous process. This apple-jelly hue can frequently be better appreciated by using diascopy (applying pressure to the lesion with a glass slide).

6. How do endogenous "foreign" bodies cause granulomas?

Endogenous substances produce a granulomatous reaction when they come in contact with the dermis or subcutaneous fat. For example, one of the most common foreign body reactions occurs when an epidermoid cyst wall ruptures and its keratin contents come in contact with the dermis. Normally, the keratin within the cyst is protected from the dermis by the cyst's epithelial lining. However, when a cyst ruptures, the keratin is exposed to the dermis and, being a poorly soluble substance, it produces a granulomatous response.

A second mechanism occurs when endogenous substances that are normally soluble crystallize into large aggregates, which then provoke a granulomatous foreign body reaction (e.g., uric acid crystals in gouty tophi and calcium in calcinosis cutis).

7. What are the sources of the exogenous foreign body agents?

See Table 13-2 and Fig. 13-1.

8. Do cosmetic fillers ever produce foreign body granulomas?

Yes. Numerous cosmetic fillers, including products made from collagen (Fig. 13-2), silicone, hyaluronic acid, methacrylate, and polyalkylimide, have been reported to produce foreign body granulomas. In some cases the cosmetic results have been very poor and difficult to correct. The number of reported cases is rapidly increasing as the cosmetic

Table 13-2. Sources of Foreign Bodies

AGENT	SOURCE
Silicone	Breast implants, joint prostheses, soft tissue injections, hemodialysis tubing
Silica	Soil and rock (very abundant), glass
Paraffin (oils)	Cosmetic injection (historically), factitial injection, grease gun injury
Starch	Surgical gloves contaminating wounds
Graphite	Pencil lead (see Fig. 13-1A)
Thorns	Roses, cactus, yucca (see Fig. 13-1B)
Hair	Barbers, dog groomers, sheep shearers
Talc	IV drug use, wound contamination
Aluminum	Adjuvant in DPT immunizations
Zirconium	Deodorant sticks
Beryllium	Metal, ceramic, and electronic industries; fluorescent lamp workers (historically, as this ceased in 1951)

DPT, Diphtheria-pertussis-tetanus, IV, intravenous.

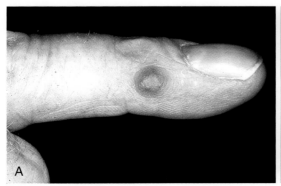
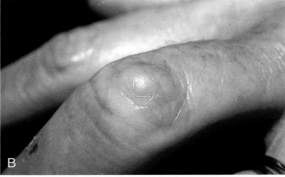

Figure 13-1. A, Typical graphite granuloma due to pencil lead injury. **B,** Skin-colored nodule due to yucca thorn embedded in the skin for several years.

filler industry has rapidly expanded in the last decade and larger numbers of patients are receiving injections for cosmetic fillers.

Sanchis-Bielsa JM, Bagán JV, Poveda R, Salvador I: Foreign body granulomatous reactions to cosmetic fillers: a clinical study of 15 cases, *Oral Surg Oral Med Oral Pathol Oral Radiol Endod* 109:237–241, 2009.

Winslow CP: The management of dermal filler complications, *Facial Plast Surg* 25:124–128, 2009.

9. Can the cause of a foreign body reaction be diagnosed histologically?

Sometimes. Often, a tattoo granuloma may retain some color or pigment that can help with the diagnosis. Silicone, paraffin, and other oils are often accompanied by fibrosis and a characteristic "Swiss cheese" appearance. The Swiss cheese–like holes are actually cavities formerly filled with the oily material that is lost during tissue processing. Also, some foreign bodies are birefringent under polarized light (e.g., talc, starch, silica, and some types of sutures).

Parada MB, Michalany NS, Hassun KM, et al: A histologic study of adverse effects of different cosmetic skin fillers, *Skinmed* 4:345–346, 2005.

10. What is sarcoidosis?

The Seventh International Conference on Sarcoidosis gave the following definition:

"Sarcoidosis is a multisystem granulomatous disorder of unknown etiology. It most commonly affects young adults and presents most frequently with bilateral hilar lymphadenopathy, pulmonary infiltration, and skin or eye lesions. The course and prognosis may correlate with the mode of onset. An acute onset with erythema nodosum heralds a self-limiting course and spontaneous resolution, whereas an insidious onset may be followed by relentless, progressive fibrosis."

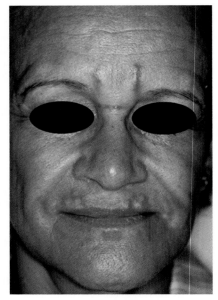

Figure 13-2. Patient with foreign body reaction to cosmetic filler demonstrating erythematous papules and linear lesions at the site of bovine collagen injection. (Courtesy of the Fitzsimons Army Medical Center teaching files.)

11. How often is the skin involved in sarcoidosis?

The skin is involved in 20% to 35% of patients. These findings may be divided into specific and nonspecific lesions. Specific lesions demonstrate sarcoid granulomas on histology, while nonspecific lesions demonstrate some other reactive change.

Lodha S, Sanchez M, Prystowksy S: Sarcoidosis of the skin: a review for the pulmonologist, *Chest* 136:583–596, 2009.

12. Describe the specific cutaneous findings in sarcoidosis.

The most common cutaneous findings are small papules that may be skin-colored, red, violaceous, yellow-brown, brown, or hypopigmented. The surface is typically smooth but variable scale or umbilication may be present. Papules are most commonly found around eyelids, nasal alae and nasolabial folds, and malar and neck regions (Fig. 13-3).

The second most common specific skin lesions are plaques that may assume an annular configuration. Like the papules, the plaques may be skin-colored, red, violaceous, yellow-brown, brown, or hypopigmented and the surface may be smooth or demonstrate variable scale. Plaques are usually more recalcitrant to therapy. Plaques with marked overlying vascular dilatation are termed **angiolupoid sarcoidal plaques**.

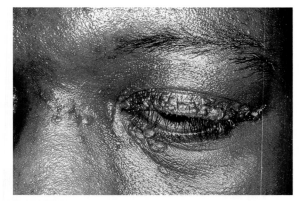

Figure 13-3. Typical numerous periocular papules in a patient with sarcoidosis.

Uncommon types of specific cutaneous lesions include subcutaneous nodules, involvement of scars and tattoos, erythroderma, ulcerations, verrucous lesions, dystrophic nails, scarring alopecia, and pustular lesions.

13. What is lupus pernio?

This distinct form of cutaneous sarcoidosis presents as purplish plaques around the nose, ears, lips, face, and fingers (Fig. 13-4). It is usually an insidious process with slow progression that results in scarring, fibrosis, and deformity. It rarely involutes spontaneously and is associated with bony involvement specifically and systemic disease in general.

Spicknall K, English JC 3rd, Elston DM: Lupus pernio, *Cutis* 79:289–290, 2007.

14. Describe the nonspecific cutaneous lesions of sarcoidosis.

The most common nonspecific cutaneous lesion is erythema nodosum, which may be present in 13% to 20% of patients. Clinically and histologically, it is identical to erythema nodosum associated with other conditions. Less common nonspecific cutaneous lesions include acquired ichthyosis (Fig. 13-5A), calcinosis cutis, erythema multiforme, and nail clubbing.

15. Does sarcoidosis ever present in the skin without extracutaneous involvement?

Yes. Even though sarcoidosis is defined as a multisystem disorder, some patients present with lesions that are clinically and histologically identical to sarcoidosis without any evidence of involvement of other organ systems. It is possible that some of these patients have involvement of other organ systems but it is minimal and asymptomatic. In other cases, the skin lesions predate the discovery of involvement of other organ systems.

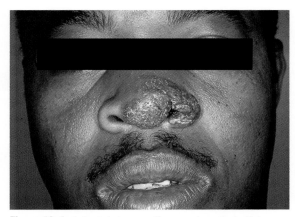

Figure 13-4. Indurated plaque on the nose of a patient with lupus pernio.

16. What is Löfgren's syndrome?

This is the classic acute presentation of sarcoidosis. It consists of bilateral hilar adenopathy, fever, arthralgias, erythema nodosum, and uveitis (Fig. 13-5B). Sarcoidosis that presents in this manner has an approximately 80% chance of resolving within 2 years.

17. What is Heerfordt's syndrome?

Heerfordt's syndrome or uveoparotid fever is a variant of sarcoidosis presenting as uveitis, facial nerve palsy, fever, and parotid gland swelling. Central nervous system involvement is also more common in this presentation.

18. How should cutaneous sarcoidosis be treated?

Treatment of cutaneous sarcoidosis should always be tempered by the fact that 60% to 80% of cases resolve without treatment in 1 to 2 years, especially those patients who present with Löfgren's syndrome. For patients with mild cutaneous disease, potent topical corticosteroid (e.g., clobetasol) or intralesional corticosteroid is the treatment of choice. For patients with extensive cutaneous involvement or systemic disease, prednisone is the treatment of choice. Antimalarials have also been shown to be effective in the chronic plaque form of cutaneous sarcoidosis, and these can be a useful alternative to prednisone. Miscellaneous treatments reported to be of benefit in select patients include

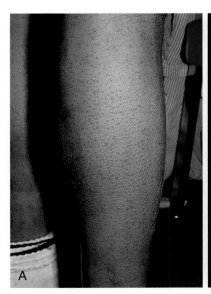

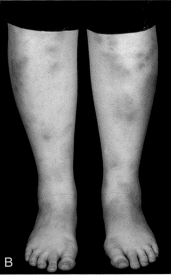

Figure 13-5. A, Acquired ichthyosis in a patient with sarcoidosis. **B,** Patient with Löfgren's syndrome demonstrating tender red subcutaneous lesions characteristic of erythema nodosum.

azathioprine, doxycycline, isotretinoin, levamisole, methotrexate, minocycline, thalidomide, tetracycline, adalimumab, and infliximab.

Doherty CB, Rosen T: Evidence-based therapy for cutaneous sarcoidosis, *Drugs* 68:1361–1383, 2008.

Key Points: Cutaneous Sarcoidosis

1. Cutaneous sarcoidosis occurs in 20% to 35% of patients with sarcoidosis.
2. Cutaneous sarcoidosis may be the first sign of sarcoidosis.
3. Lupus pernio is a distinct variant of cutaneous sarcoidosis that presents as purplish plaques around the nose, ears, lips, face, and fingers. It is associated with more severe bony disease.
4. Löfgren's syndrome consists of bilateral hilar adenopathy, fever, arthralgias, erythema nodosum, and uveitis.
5. Heerfordt's syndrome or uveoparotid fever is a variant of sarcoidosis presenting as uveitis, facial nerve palsy, fever, and parotid gland swelling.

19. What is the typical presentation of granuloma annulare?

Granuloma annulare (GA) typically presents with violaceous or flesh-colored dermal papules arranged in an annular or semiannular configuration (Fig. 13-6A). The lesions may be solitary or multiple. Most commonly, it affects the dorsum of the hands or feet, but it can also occur on the forearms, arms, legs, or thighs. It tends to affect children or young adults with a 2:1 female preponderance. Several less common variants of granuloma annulare include the macular and erythematous forms, subcutaneous nodules (Fig. 13-6B), actinically induced lesions, perforating type, and disseminated form. Biopsies of GA demonstrate a characteristic palisaded granuloma associated with collagen destruction (necrobiotic granuloma) and increased dermal mucin.

Arroyo MP: Generalized granuloma annulare, *Dermatol Online J* 9:13, 2003. (Online journal to which the reader can link, see the paper, clinical photograph, and histology.)

20. Do any systemic associations occur with granuloma annulare?

Patients who present with localized lesions that are few in number have no systemic associations, and no workup needs to be done. However, several studies have suggested an association between the disseminated form of GA and diabetes mellitus. Therefore, an appropriate workup should be done in these patients.

21. What is the typical course of granuloma annulare?

In the classic localized form of GA, the tendency is for spontaneous resolution. Recurrences are fairly common, but the recurrences tend to resolve more quickly than the original lesions. Most studies note that at 2 years postonset of GA, 50% to 80% of patients will be lesion free. However, patients who present with disseminated lesions tend to have a much more protracted course and are frequently less responsive to therapy.

22. How is granuloma annulare treated?

Since GA may spontaneously resolve, expectant observation is certainly a good treatment option. Numerous therapies have been anecdotally reported to be successful, including radiotherapy, cryotherapy, laser, psoralen plus ultraviolet light (type A, [PUVA]), ultraviolet A-1 (UVA-1), niacinamide, isotretinoin, salicylates, potassium iodide, dapsone, antimalarials, cyclosporin, and chlorambucil. None has met with overwhelming success. The treatment of choice at this time is strong topical corticosteroids with or without occlusion or intralesional corticosteroids. Corticosteroid therapy

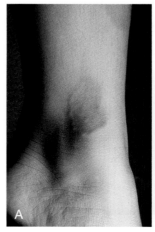
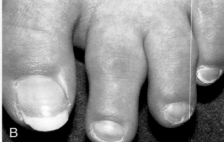

Figure 13-6. A, Typical lesion of granuloma annulare demonstrating raised annular lesions without scale. **B,** Subcutaneous granuloma annulare of proximal second toe.

usually makes the lesions resolve, but potent preparations are necessary to get a good response and may produce secondary thinning of the skin.

23. What is actinic granuloma?

Actinic granuloma, also called annular elastolytic giant cell granuloma, is a granulomatous process that tends to occur in older patients on sun-exposed skin of the face, arms, and neck. Clinically, the lesions are annular and resemble GA, although some cases demonstrate subtle atrophy in the center of the lesion (Fig. 13-7). Histologically, it is also similar to GA in that it demonstrates necrobiotic granulomas, but it differs in that it is usually more superficial, demonstrates more foreign body giant cells and prominent elastophagocytosis (macrophages engulfing and breaking down elastic fibers), and mucin is not increased. Some authorities consider it to be a variant of GA but the majority favors it being a disease *sui generis*. The treatment is the same as for GA but should also include sun protection.

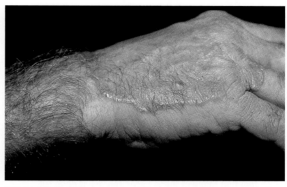

Figure 13-7. Actinic granuloma demonstrating large annular lesion on sun-exposed skin.

Stein JA, Fangman B, Strober B: Actinic granuloma, *Dermatol Online J* 13:19, 2007.

24. Are rheumatoid nodules really a granulomatous disorder?

Yes. Rheumatoid nodules demonstrate sharply demarcated, palisading granulomas with macrophages surrounding areas of fibrinoid degeneration of collagen deep in the dermis or subcutis. A similar histologic picture can be seen in GA, necrobiosis lipoidica, and rheumatic fever nodules.

The differentiation of rheumatoid nodule from deep GA is difficult but possible in most cases. GA demonstrates increased dermal mucin, while rheumatoid nodules demonstrate marked fibrinoid

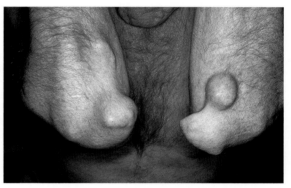

Figure 13-8. Unusually large dermal and subcutaneous rheumatoid nodules in a patient with severe rheumatoid arthritis. (Courtesy of the Fitzsimons Army Medical Center teaching files.)

change that is very eosinophilic. Some cases of deep GA cannot be differentiated histologically and require clinical correlation.

25. Where do rheumatoid nodules typically occur?

These are typically present as asymptomatic, firm, fixed, or mobile subcutaneous nodules adjacent to bony structures. The most common site is the elbow (Fig. 13-8). Other common locations include the extensor aspects of the fingers, flexor sheath tendons in the palms, Achilles tendons, ischial tuberosities, and sacrum. Rheumatoid nodules occur in approximately 25% of patients with rheumatoid arthritis.

García-Patos V: Rheumatoid nodule, *Semin Cutan Med Surg* 26:100–107, 2007.

26. What causes rheumatoid nodules?

The pathogenesis is not understood, but the evidence suggests that rheumatoid arthritis occurs in genetically susceptible patients after an arthritogenic microbial antigen exposure. The identity of the microbial trigger has not been established, although considerable attention has been placed on the Epstein-Barr virus. Once the process is initiated, a complex autoimmune disease develops characterized by increased numbers of CD4+ T cells in the joint, which also activate B cells that produce autoantibodies (primarily IgM) to the Fc portion of autologous IgG. The antigen that provokes the autoimmune response has not been fully established, but research is focusing on type 2 collagen, human cartilage glycoprotein-39, human stress protein BiP, and several different heat shock proteins. How this autoimmune response produces rheumatoid nodules is not clear.

Bodman-Smith MD, Corrigall VM, Berglin E, et al: Antibody response to the human stress protein BiP in rheumatoid arthritis, *Rheumatology* (Oxford) 43:1283–1287, 2004.

Sawada S, Takei M: Epstein-Barr virus etiology in rheumatoid synovitis, *Autoimmune Rev* 4:106–110, 2005.

27. What is accelerated nodulosis?

Accelerated nodulosis is the rapid onset of rheumatoid nodules that develops in a small subset of patients treated with methotrexate. The nodules typically regress following discontinuation of the methotrexate and recur with rechallenge. Although several theories have been proposed, the pathogenesis is not understood.

Williams FM, Cohen PR, Arnett FC: Accelerated cutaneous nodulosis during methotrexate therapy in a patient with rheumatoid arthritis, *J Am Acad Dermatol* 39:359–362, 1998.

28. Are rheumatoid nodules specific for rheumatoid arthritis?

No. They are not pathognomonic for rheumatoid arthritis. They are seen in 5% to 7% of patients with systemic lupus erythematosus and in a rare condition in children called benign pseudorheumatoid nodules, in which the nodules grow rapidly and then spontaneously involute. These children are usually rheumatoid factor–negative, and some authorities feel that many of these cases represent deep GA. Another rare presentation is rheumatoid nodulosis, in which patients present with multiple rheumatoid nodules about the hands. They are rheumatoid factor–positive but have a remarkably benign course.

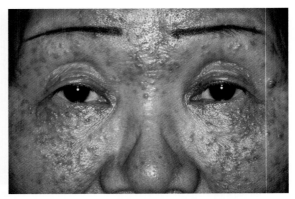

Figure 13-9. Lupus miliaris disseminatus faciei. Numerous red to reddish-brown papules of the central face. (Courtesy of the Walter Reed Army Medical Center teaching files.)

McGrath MH, Fleischer A: The subcutaneous rheumatoid nodule, *Hand Clin* 5:127–135, 1989.

29. Do patients with lupus miliaris disseminatus faciei have lupus erythematosus?

No. Lupus miliaris disseminatus faciei is a chronic granulomatous disorder of the face of unknown cause. Clinically, it presents as multiple brown to brownish-red to brownish-yellow papules of the face (Fig. 13-9), especially the central face and ears. The cause of this mysterious granulomatous disease is unknown, although some dermatologists consider it to be a variant of granulomatous rosacea. Histologically, it is composed of sarcoidal or, more commonly, caseating granulomas that sometimes demonstrate connections to hair follicles.

Sehgal VN, Srivastava G, Aggarwal AK, et al: Lupus miliaris disseminatus faciei. Part II: an overview, *Skinmed* 4:234–238, 2005.

DRUG ERUPTIONS

Alexandra Theriault, MD

1. **A patient presents to your office with a 10-page typed out medical history. She states that she is "allergic" to twenty different medicines. Is she likely to have drug allergies or drug intolerances to most of these drugs?**
   Drug intolerance. Drug intolerances account for 90% of adverse drug reactions. An adverse reaction to a drug is an undesirable and usually unanticipated response independent of the intended therapeutic purpose of the medication. An adverse drug reaction may be either immunologic (i.e., drug allergy) or nonimmunologic (i.e., drug intolerance).

2. **Name some nonimmunologic drug reactions.**
   - Nonimmunologic activation of effector pathways, such as direct release of histamine from mast cells and basophils by aspirin, nonsteroidal antiinflammatory drugs (NSAIDs), opiates, polymyxin B, d-tubocurarine, and radiocontrast media
   - Overdosage
   - Cumulative toxicity, such as the accumulation of drugs or metabolites in the skin (e.g., argyria with the use of silver nitrate spray)
   - Normal pharmacologic effects of the drug that are not the primary therapeutic objective (e.g., alopecia following chemotherapy)
   - Drug interactions (e.g., administration of ketoconazole may lead to higher levels of cyclosporine and increased toxicity)
   - Metabolic changes, such as warfarin producing a hypercoagulable state that results in warfarin necrosis
   - Exacerbation of preexisting dermatologic diseases (e.g., lithium can exacerbate acne, psoriasis, and subcorneal pustular dermatosis)
   - Ecologic changes, such as antibiotics that reduce the bacteriologic flora, predisposing the patient to candidal infections
   - Inherited enzyme or protein deficiencies (e.g., the phenytoin hypersensitivity syndrome occurs in patients deficient in epoxide hydrolase, an enzyme required for metabolism of a toxic epoxide derived from phenytoin)
   - Jarisch-Herxheimer phenomenon secondary to bacterial endotoxins and microbial antigens that are liberated from antimicrobial treatment (e.g., a patient with syphilis develops fever, tender lymphadenopathy, arthralgias, and urticaria while being treated with penicillin)

   Stern RS, Wintroub BU: Cutaneous reactions to drugs. In Freedberg IM, Eisen AZ, Wolff K, editors: *Fitzpatrick's dermatology in general medicine*, ed 5, New York, 1999, McGraw-Hill, pp 1633–1642.

3. **What is the most common manifestation of an adverse drug reaction?**
   Cutaneous reactions are the most common adverse drug reaction and produce a wide range of manifestations: pruritus, maculopapular eruptions, urticaria, angioedema, phototoxic and photoallergic reactions, fixed drug reactions, erythema multiforme, vesiculobullous reactions, and exfoliative dermatitis. Drug-attributed skin reactions are seen in 2% to 5% of inpatients and >1% of outpatients.

   Hunzicker T, Kuzi UP, Braunschweig S, et al: Comprehensive hospital drug monitoring (CHDM): adverse skin reactions, a 20-year survey, *Allergy* 524:388–393, 1997.

4. **How does a cutaneous drug eruption typically present?**
   - Exanthem maculopapular or morbilliform: 46%
   - Urticaria and angioedema: 26%
   - Fixed drug eruptions: 10%
   - Erythema multiforme: 5%
   - Stevens-Johnson syndrome: 4%

Key Points: Drug Eruptions

1. Consider a fixed drug eruption in a patient who presents with bullous or hyperpigmented lesions that are recurrent at the same site.
2. Consider a drug reaction in any patient who presents with an abrupt-onset, symmetrical, cutaneous reaction.
3. Consider a photoinduced drug reaction in a patient presenting with an erythematous, cutaneous reaction involving sun-exposed areas.
4. The clinical signs of a potentially life-threatening drug eruption include: high fever, dyspnea or hypotension, angioedema and tongue swelling, palpable purpura, skin necrosis, blistering, mucous membrane erosions, confluent erythema, and lymphadenopathy.

- Exfoliative dermatitis: 4%
- Photosensitivity reactions: 3%
- Anaphylaxis: 1.5%
- Toxic epidermal necrolysis: 1.3%

5. How should a suspected drug reaction be evaluated?

Six variables should be evaluated:
- Previous experience or relative reaction rates of a given drug
- Rule out alternative etiologies, such as exacerbation of a previous dermatosis or a new skin disease unrelated to the drug
- Timing of events (most drug reactions occur within 1 to 2 weeks of initiation of therapy)
- Drug levels
- Reaction to dechallenge (most drug reactions clear within 2 weeks of discontinuing drug)
- Response to rechallenge is most definitive

6. Which commonly used drugs are most likely to produce a cutaneous reaction?

See Table 14-1.

7. Can preexisting diseases enhance the chance of getting a maculopapular skin eruption when using amoxicillin or ampicillin?

Amoxicillin or ampicillin produces a maculopapular eruption in about 5% of patients taking these drugs (Fig. 14-1). In patients with infectious mononucleosis, the risk of developing a maculopapular eruption increases to 69% to 100%. In chronic lymphocytic leukemia, the incidence is 60% to 70%. Some studies report that maculopapular eruptions are more common in patients who are also taking allopurinol, but this is not accepted by all authorities. The pathogenesis for this phenomenon is unknown.

8. What infectious disease increases the chance of a cutaneous adverse reaction to trimethoprim-sulfamethoxazole?

Acquired immunodeficiency syndrome (AIDS). The normal incidence of cutaneous reactions to trimethoprim-sulfamethoxazole is 3%, but this increases to 29% to 70% in patients with AIDS. Incidence of morbilliform drug reactions is tenfold higher in human immunodeficiency virus (HIV)–infected persons.

9. Which feared drug eruption results in sloughing of the entire skin surface and mucous membranes?

Toxic epidermal necrolysis (TEN) is one of the most severe cutaneous drug eruptions. The skin is initially erythematous and tender but quickly sloughs off in large sheets like "wet wallpaper" (Fig. 14-2). The condition can progress very rapidly, with one of seven patients losing their entire epidermis in 24 hours. Without an epidermis, the body has difficulty keeping fluids in and bacteria out. Despite aggressive supportive care, the mortality rate ranges from 11% to 35%, with the majority of deaths being attributed to sepsis.

The best therapy is to discontinue all likely drugs if possible, make sure the patient is well hydrated, and continually assess the patient for signs of secondary infection. Severe cases are best handled in burn units. The use of systemic corticosteroids and the use of intravenous immunoglobulin (IVIG) remain very controversial.

10. Why do some patients get toxic epidermal necrolysis?

The etiology is not completely understood, but recent evidence has found a genetic predisposition in at least some classes of drugs (e.g., association of aromatic antiepileptic drugs and HLA-B*1502 in the Han Chinese). It is likely that continued research will uncover more ties to a genetic predisposition. The molecular and immunologic events are still not fully elucidated; however, the recent demonstration of very high levels of soluble FasL interacting with Fas, which is expressed on the keratinocytes in toxic epidermal necrolysis, may provide insight into the pathophysiology of this life-threatening disorder. In one series, 77% of cases were clearly established as drug-induced. Since the average patient with TEN is on 4.4 drugs, identifying the offending drug can be problematic.

Table 14-1. Drugs Most Likely to Produce a Cutaneous Reaction

DRUG	REACTIONS PER 1000 PATIENTS
Amoxicillin	51.4
Trimethoprim-sulfamethoxazole	47
Ampicillin	42
Ipodate sodium	27.8
Whole blood	28
Cephalosporins	13

Frequent offenders include allopurinol, ampicillin, amoxicillin, carbamazepine, NSAIDs, phenobarbital, phenytoin, sulfonamides, and carbamazepine.

Abe R: Toxic epidermal necrolysis and Stevens-Johnson syndrome: soluble Fas ligand involvement in the pathomechanisms of these diseases, *J Dermatol Sci* 52:151–159, 2008.

Chung WH, Hung SI, Chen YT: Genetic predisposition of life-threatening antiepileptic-induced skin reactions, *Expert Opin Drug Saf* 9:15–21, 2010.

11. What is the difference between erythema multiforme major, Stevens-Johnson syndrome, and toxic epidermal necrolysis?

This is a critical and important question that is difficult to answer because this nosological nightmare continues to be controversial. The short version of these distinctions is as follows:

- **Erythema multiforme major** is best defined as presentation with targetoid skin lesions that are typical of erythema multiforme, with a more severe variant that is more likely to demonstrate oral lesions, fever, and systemic symptoms. While this variant can be drug-induced, it is more commonly induced by infections such as herpes simplex and *Mycoplasma*. Some dermatologists consider this to be in the spectrum of Stevens-Johnson syndrome. Microscopically, the keratinocytes are being damaged by lymphocytes (satellite cell necrosis).

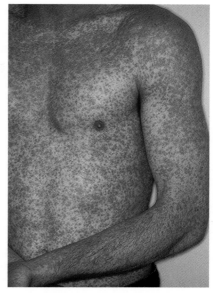

Figure 14-1. Amoxicillin-induced maculopapular (morbilliform) drug eruption in a patient with infectious mononucleosis. In most studies, morbilliform drug eruptions are the most common cutaneous side effect. (Courtesy of Scott D. Bennion, MD.)

- **Stevens-Johnson syndrome** is most commonly defined as presentation with widespread targetoid lesions that are a flat and atypical when compared to the more defined lesions of erythema multiforme. Lesions are also more frequently purpuric. As in the case of erythema multiforme major, the patients may have fever and systemic symptoms. In contrast to erythema multiforme major, the lesions are more likely to become confluent and develop large areas of blisters and detachment of the epidermis. While some cases are idiopathic or induced by infections, the majority are drug induced. Histologically, the findings are identical to erythema multiforme in that the keratinocytes demonstrates satellite cell necrosis. Some dermatologists arbitrarily define this condition as affecting less than 30% of the body surface, and some authorities even recognize a Stevens-Johnson syndrome/toxic epidermal necrosis overlap syndrome.

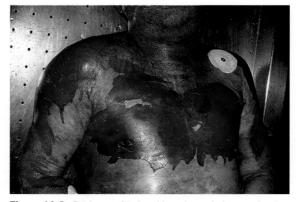

Figure 14-2. Fatal case of toxic epidermal necrolysis secondary to captopril. The skin characteristically sloughs off in large sheets. (Courtesy of James E. Fitzpatrick, MD.)

- **Toxic epidermal necrosis** is best defined as a blistering disorder with extensive detachment of the skin that is almost always drug induced, although there are exceptions. Many of the drugs that produce classic Stevens-Johnson syndrome also produced toxic epidermal necrolysis. Targetoid lesions are not usually present but if present are atypical. Microscopically, biopsies are cell poor and cells usually appear to become necrotic without evidence of satellite cell necrosis, suggesting a soluble factor. Some dermatologists arbitrarily differentiate this from Stevens-Johnson syndrome if more than 30% of the cutaneous surface is involved, although many dermatologists feel that toxic epidermal necrolysis and Stevens-Johnson syndrome represent a spectrum of disease.

12. What drugs are typically associated with Stevens-Johnson syndrome?

Commonly implicated drugs include allopurinol, amoxicillin, ampicillin, barbiturates, carbamazepine, gold, NSAIDs, phenobarbital, phenytoin, and sulfonamides. *Mycoplasma pneumoniae* and other infections are also well documented to produce Stevens-Johnson syndrome (Fig. 14-3).

13. Which type of drug reaction can result in a quick death?

Systemic anaphylaxis, which is IgE mediated, may present with variable findings, including mild pruritus, erythema, urticaria, asthma, circulatory collapse, laryngeal edema, and death. When a patient gives a history of reaction to a drug, the health care provider must ask for details about the previous reaction, particularly seeking a history of urticaria, breathing problems, collapse, and hospitalization.

14. What class of drugs is the most common cause of anaphylaxis?

Beta-lactam antibiotics. Anaphylactic reactions occur in 1 to 5 per 10,000 administrations of penicillin. Most allergic reactions to beta-lactam antibiotics produce urticaria and angioedema, but 10% may result in life-threatening hypotension, bronchospasm, or laryngeal edema. Approximately 1% of all anaphylactic reactions are fatal. Fatal reactions may occur within minutes of parenteral administration of these drugs.

15. Name the drugs most likely to induce urticaria.

Angiotensin-converting enzyme (ACE) inhibitors, gamma-globulin, NSAIDs, penicillins, and sulfonamides. Urticaria produced by drugs is clinically indistinguishable from urticaria produced by other allergens. Aspirin can exacerbate a preexisting urticaria. If possible, aspirin should be discontinued and not utilized in patients with active urticaria.

Mathelier-Fusade P: Drug-induced urticarias, *Clin Rev Allergy Immunol* 30:19–23, 2006.

16. How is drug-induced urticaria mediated?

Urticaria may be produced by both nonimmunologic and immunologic mechanisms. Drugs such as codeine, morphine, amphetamine, hydralazine, quinine, vancomycin, and x-ray contrast media produce urticaria by the nonimmunologic release of histamine by mast cells. Allergic urticaria may be due to a type I (Coombs and Gell) reaction mediated by IgE, causing the release of histamine. This usually develops within minutes to hours (usually within 1 hour) after giving the offending drug, and may precede or be associated with anaphylaxis. Urticaria may also be produced by a type III reaction mediated by antigen-antibody complexes. In contrast to type I reactions, which occur within hours, type III urticaria usually develops 1 to 3 weeks after beginning the drug. The clinical appearance of urticaria is often mistaken for erythema multiforme.

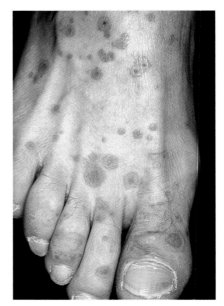

Figure 14-3. Classic lesions of erythema multiforme secondary to co-trimoxazole, demonstrating targetoid appearance. (Courtesy of James E. Fitzpatrick, MD.)

17. A 45-year-old white man comes to the emergency room with large areas of nonpitting edema over the face, eyelids, neck, tongue, and mucous membranes, which developed 6 hours ago. Ten days earlier, he started a new drug for hypertension. What is the most likely cause of his reaction?

The clinical description is that of a patient who has angioedema. An ACE inhibitor, such as captopril, enalapril, or lisinopril, is the most likely antihypertensive drug to produce this reaction. A recent study reported that 35% of 17 patients seen for angioedema during a 5-year period were on ACE inhibitors. In another study, 77% of patients experienced the reaction within 3 weeks of starting treatment.

18. A patient is evaluated for a several-day history of fever, malaise, urticaria, arthralgias, lymphadenopathy, and a peculiar erythema along the sides of his palms and soles. He has been started on several new medications in the last few weeks. What is the most likely diagnosis?

The patient most likely has a serum sickness–like drug eruption caused by immune complexes and complement activation. The diagnostic cutaneous finding is the characteristic erythema on the sides of the palms and soles, a finding seen in 75% of cases of serum sickness–like drug eruptions. Other typical findings include fever and malaise (100%), urticaria (90%), arthralgias (50% to 67%), and lymphadenopathy (13%). Glomerulonephritis is common in serum sickness reactions in animals but uncommon in humans. Reactions occur 7 to 21 days after the drug is given but may occur with the first administration of the drug. Commonly implicated drugs include beta-lactam antibiotics, sulfonamides, thiouracil, cholecystographic dyes, and hydantoin.

19. A man complains of a recurrent burning eruption on his penis. He develops a single blister over the glans penis that heals over 1 to 2 weeks with hyperpigmentation. This same pattern has happened on three occasions in the last 2 years. What does he have?

The history is characteristic of a fixed drug eruption. Fixed drug eruptions are cutaneous reactions that recur at the same site with each administration of the drug, typically within 6 to 48 hours of initiation of the causative agent. Characteristically, it occurs on the face or genitalia but may occur anywhere (Fig. 14-4). It is a well demarcated erythematous lesion that often blisters and heals with hyperpigmentation. Drugs commonly associated include phenolphthalein in laxatives, sulfonamides, β-lactam antibiotics, tetracycline, barbiturates, gold, oral contraceptives, diazepam, and aspirin. Foods have also been implicated in fixed drug reactions.

Gendernalik SB, Galeckas KJ: Fixed drug eruptions: a case report and review of the literature, *Cutis* 84:215–219, 2009.

20. How does drug-induced lupus erythematosus (LE) differ from idiopathic systemic lupus erythematosus (SLE)?

Drug-induced LE is generally milder than idiopathic SLE. Drug-induced LE usually manifests as fever, malaise, pleuritis, pneumonitis, and arthralgias. Skin, mucous membrane, central nervous system findings, and renal disease are more commonly seen in idiopathic SLE. The antinuclear antibodies in drug-induced LE are usually antihistone and single-stranded DNA antibodies, whereas idiopathic SLE is associated with double-stranded DNA and Sm antibodies. Drug-induced LE usually resolves simply by stopping the drug. Drug-induced LE constitutes 5% to 10% of all cases of SLE. Less commonly patients may have drug-induced subacute cutaneous lupus erythematosus with anti-Ro/SSA antibodies or classic systemic lupus with drug-induced double-stranded DNA antibodies.

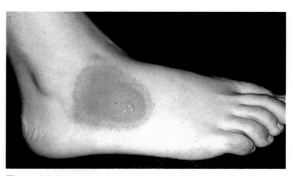

Figure 14-4. Sulfonamide-induced fixed drug eruption of the ankle manifesting an erythematous plaque and focal blisters. (Courtesy of James E. Fitzpatrick, MD.)

21. What drugs are usually associated with drug-induced LE?

Of patients treated continuously with procainamide, 90% develop antinuclear antibodies after 2 years, and 10% to 20% develop symptoms of LE. Other commonly implicated drugs include hydralazine, isoniazid, chlorpromazine, procainamide, hydantoin, d-penicillamine, methyldopa, quinidine, and minocycline.

Marzano AV, Vezzoli P, Crosti C: Drug-induced lupus: an update on its dermatologic aspects, *Lupus* 18:935–940, 2009.

22. Which drug is usually associated with erythema nodosum?

Erythema nodosum, which is a form of panniculitis that characteristically presents as tender erythematous nodules over the shins, is most commonly associated with oral contraceptives. Sulfonamides, bromides, iodides, tetracycline, penicillin, and 13-cis retinoic acid have also been associated with erythema nodosum.

23. What drugs are associated with lichenoid drug eruptions?

Lichenoid drug eruptions clinically and histologically resemble lichen planus. The lesions are usually multiple, purple, discrete, flat-topped polygonal papules and plaques. As in the case of lichen planus, this reaction may also affect or even be limited to the oral mucosa. This differs from other drug reactions in that it may take weeks to years following administration of the drug to develop the lesions. Sulfonamides (especially thiazide diuretics), gold, captopril, propranolol, and antimalarials are the most common drugs that produce these reactions. It may take months for the rash to resolve following discontinuation of the drug.

Woo V, Bonks J, Borukhova L, Zegarelli D: Oral lichenoid drug eruption: a report of pediatric case and review of the literature, *Pediatr Dermatol* 26:458–464, 2009.

24. Name the drugs most likely to produce cutaneous hyperpigmentation and discoloration.

Drugs produce cutaneous hyperpigmentation and discoloration by different mechanisms. The two main mechanisms of hyperpigmentation and discoloration are drug deposition (e.g., heavy metals) and stimulation of melanocytic activity (Table 14-2; Fig. 14-5).

Table 14-2. Drugs Producing Changes in Skin Pigmentation

COLOR	DRUG
Slate-gray	Chloroquine Hydroxychloroquine (see Fig. 14-5A) Minocycline (see Fig. 14-5B) Phenothiazines
Slate-blue	Amiodarone
Blue-gray	Gold (chrysoderma)
Yellow	Beta-carotene Quinacrine
Red	Clofazimine
Brown (hyperpigmentation)	Adrenocorticotropic hormone (ACTH) Bleomycin Oral contraceptives Zidovudine

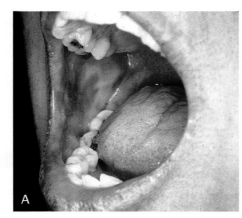
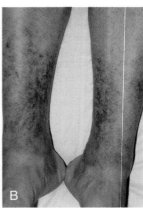

Figure 14-5. A, Hydroxychloroquine-induced slate-gray pigmentation of the buccal mucosa. **B,** Minocycline-induced slate-gray pigment of lower legs. The minocycline is complexed with the extravascular hemosiderin from stasis dermatitis, which accounts for the distinctive distribution. (Courtesy of the Fitzsimons Army Medical Center teaching files.)

25. What drugs can produce subepidermal bullae and erosions on the dorsum of the hands?

The description is characteristic of the eruption seen in porphyria cutanea tarda and, less commonly, in variegate porphyria and hereditary coproporphyria. This reaction is called pseudoporphyria since the porphyrin levels are normal (Fig. 14-6). Tetracycline, nalidixic acid, oral contraceptives, cyclosporine, furosemide and other sulfonamides, dapsone, NSAIDs, 5-fluorouracil, isotretinoin, and pyridoxine are most likely to induce pseudoporphyria.

LaDuca JR, Bouman PH, Gaspari AA: Nonsteroidal anti-inflammatory drug-induced pseudoporphyria: a case series, *J Cutan Med Surg* 6:320–326, 2002.

26. Name two drugs that commonly exacerbate porphyria cutanea tarda.

Ethanol and estrogens.

27. A 30-year-old white woman is evaluated with a new case of "acne." Over the last few days, she has suddenly developed erythematous follicular papules and pustules over her upper trunk. She was admitted 3 weeks earlier with an acute

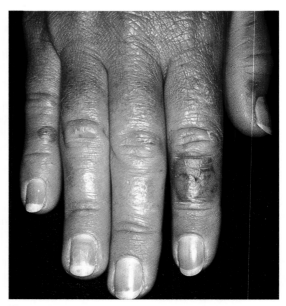

Figure 14-6. Tetracycline-induced pseudoporphyria demonstrating hemorrhagic blisters and erosions over the back of the hand. (Courtesy of James E. Fitzpatrick, MD.)

exacerbation of SLE that is now improving. What is the most likely diagnosis?

Steroid acne is the most likely diagnosis. Her history indicates a high probability that she was started on corticosteroids during the admission. Steroid acne typically presents with inflammatory papules and pustules, but comedones and cysts are typically absent. In contrast to acne vulgaris, steroid acne preferentially involves the trunk and demonstrates lesions in the same stage of development. Other drugs associated with similar eruptions include lithium, isoniazid, bromides, and iodides. Many chemotherapeutic agents have also been associated with acneiform reactions. These include cetuximab, dactinomycin, erlotinib, fluoxymesterone, gefitinib, medroxyprogesterone, and vinblastine.

Roe E, Garcia Muret MD, Marcuello E, Capdevila J, et al: A description and management of cutaneous side effects during cetuximab or erlotininb treatments: a prospective study of 30 patients, *J Am Acad Dermatol* 2:151–158, 2001.

28. A middle-aged man who is a dialysis patient presents to your clinic with a "woody" appearance to his legs. He had an MRI with gadolinum-containing contrast a few months prior. What might he be suffering from?

Nephrogenic systemic fibrosis (formerly called nephrogenic fibrosing dermopathy). Nephrogenic systemic fibrosis is an uncommon disease with cutaneous manifestations that include induration, thickening, and hardening of the skin, most commonly on the extremities. The pathophysiology is related to the exposure of patients with renal insufficiency to gadolinium-based contrast agents.

High HA, Ayers RA, Cowper SE: Gadolinium is quantifiable within the tissue of patients with nephrogenic systemic fibrosis, *J Am Acad Dermatol* 56:710–712, 2007.

29. Describe a typical presentation of warfarin necrosis.

The patient is typically a woman who has been given a loading dose of warfarin (Coumadin). Between 3 and 5 days after starting the drug, the patient develops one or more lesions over the thighs, buttocks, or breasts. Initially painful and red, the lesions rapidly become necrotic with hemorrhagic bullae and an erythematous edge (Fig. 14-7). A necrotic eschar rapidly develops.

Rapid recognition of the characteristic lesions in the typical situation is the key to reducing tissue destruction. Therapy includes discontinuing warfarin, administering vitamin K to reverse the effect of warfarin, giving heparin as an anticoagulant, and administering monoclonal antibody-purified protein C concentrate. Therapy may also include debridement, grafting, and even amputation. Warfarin necrosis has frequently been associated with low levels of protein C. Most authorities recommend that the warfarin should be discontinued.

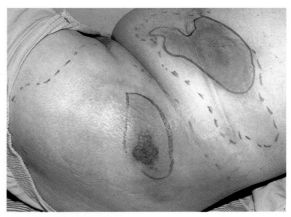

Figure 14-7. Characteristic lesions of warfarin necrosis, demonstrating early necrosis and hemorrhagic bullae surrounded by a ring of erythema.

30. Name and describe the two types of photoinduced drug eruptions.

Phototoxic drug reactions and photoallergic drug reactions. Phototoxic reactions occur within minutes to hours after exposure to both the drug and light and occur in all individuals given the specific drug and ultraviolet (UV) exposure. The rash clinically resembles a sunburn and stinging is a prominent feature. Photoallergic drug reactions are mediated by type IV delayed hypersensitivity and occur 24 to 48 hours after UV exposure. Clinically, the lesions are on sun-exposed sites, but are not as well demarcated as phototoxic reactions. They are also eczematous and pruritic.

31. What drugs commonly cause phototoxic drug reactions?

Amiodarone, chlorpromazine, demeclocycline (Fig. 14-8), doxycycline, psoralens, and tetracycline.

32. What drugs commonly cause photoallergic drug reactions?

Griseofulvin, quinine, quinolones, sulfonamides, phenothiazines, quinidine, hydrochlorothiazides, piroxicam, and pyridoxine.

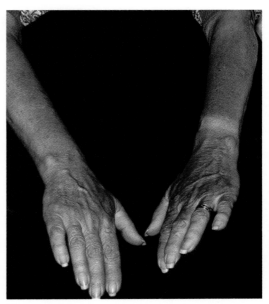

Figure 14-8. Demeclocycline-induced phototoxic reaction on the dorsum of the hands. (Courtesy of James E. Fitzpatrick, MD.)

33. What is AGEP? How does it present?

AGEP is an acronym for **a**cute **g**eneralized **e**xanthematous **p**ustulosis. Patients present with an abrupt onset of a generalized, scarlatiniform, erythematous exanthem associated with numerous small, sterile, nonfollicular pustules (Fig. 14-9). There may be associated fever, prostration, and leukocytosis. In one study, 17% of patients had a personal history of psoriasis. The lesions typically occur within a few days of initiating the offending drug. Beta-lactam antibiotics are the most common culprits followed by macrolides and mercury. The reaction is typically short lived. Resolution usually occurs within 1 to 2 weeks of discontinuing the offending agent and is accompanied by widespread skin desquamation.

Roujeau JC, Bioulac-Sage P, Bourseau C, et al: Acute generalized exanthematous pustulosis. Analysis of 63 cases, *Arch Dermatol* 127:1333–1338, 1991.

34. You have been treating a patient for severe, scarring acne with an oral medication for the last three months. Her acne looks great but now she is starting to lose hair. What drug are you most likely using?

Isotretinion. Other more common agents linked to alopecia are ACE inhibitors, allopurinol, anticoagulants, azathioprine, bromocriptine, beta-blockers, cyclophosphamide, didanosine, hormones, indinavir, NSAIDs, phenytoin, methotrexate, and valproate.

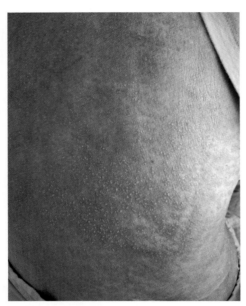

Figure 14-9. Acute generalized exanthematous pustulosis due to amoxicillin, demonstrating typical small pustules on a background of erythema. (Courtesy of James E. Fitzpatrick, MD.)

VASCULITIS

Curt P. Samlaska, MD, and James E. Fitzpatrick, MD

1. How are vasculitic disorders defined and classified?

Vasculitis is defined as inflammation of blood vessels. Vasculitis may be confined to the skin; however, the majority of cases of cutaneous vasculitis are part of multisystemic disorders that in addition to involving skin also involve other organ systems. Classification is problematic due to the lack of standardization and definition. The most accepted classification scheme for systemic vasculitis syndromes is based on the size of the involved blood vessels, as shown in Table 15-1. Subclassification of these syndromes is based on clinical and histologic criteria that have been determined to be suggestive of a specific disorder. The American College of Rheumatology Subcommittee on Classification of Vasculitis has determined classification criteria for many of these disorders (see Table 15-1). This classification system is excellent for systemic vasculitis but it omits some forms of vasculitis that are confined to the skin.

2. Are there specific serologic markers for any of these vasculitic disorders?

Yes. Antimyeloperoxidase antibodies directed against cytoplasmic components of neutrophils have been used to help identify patients with segmental necrotizing glomerulonephritis and some types of systemic vasculitis. Antibodies directed against serine proteinase 3 that is found in the cytoplasm of neutrophils (c-ANCA) have been detected in 66% to 90% of patients with active Wegener's granulomatosis. Patients with pulmonary-renal syndrome who have antibodies directed against cytoplasmic myeloperoxidase, in neutrophils that produce a peripheral antineutrophil cytoplasmic pattern (p-ANCA), are most likely to have microscopic polyangiitis.

Harper L, Savage CO: Pathogenesis of ANCA-associated systemic vasculitis, *J Pathol* 190:349–359, 2000.

3. What is a leukocytoclastic vasculitis?

Patients with leukocytoclastic vasculitis, also referred to as leukocytoclastic angiitis and allergic or necrotizing vasculitis, present with characteristic purpuric papules, most frequently involving the extremities, known as palpable purpura (Fig. 15-1). Biopsies of cutaneous leukocytoclastic vasculitis demonstrate an intense perivascular infiltrate composed of intact and fragmented neutrophils (nuclear dust) that focally infiltrate the vessel wall producing fibrinoid changes and/or necrosis. These damaged vessels frequently demonstrate extravasation of erythrocytes and may also demonstrate thrombosis.

Kluger N, Francès C: Cutaneous vasculitis and their differential diagnoses, *Clin Exp Rheumatol* 27(1 Suppl 52):S124–S138, 2009.

4. What are some important precipitating causes of small vessel leukocytoclastic vasculitis?

- **Infections:** Bacterial (streptococcal infections, bacterial endocarditis), viral (parvovirus B19, HIV, hepatitis A–C), mycobacterial (Hansen's disease, tuberculosis), fungal *(Candida albicans)*, protozoan *(Plasmodium malariae)*, helminthic *(Schistosoma haematobium, S. mansoni, Onchocerca volvulus)*
- **Drugs:** Aspirin, sulfonamides, penicillins, barbiturates, amphetamines, propylthiouracil

Table 15-1. Classification of Systemic Vasculitides

VESSEL SIZE	VASCULITIC SYNDROME
Large vessel vasculitis	Giant cell (temporal) arteritis Takayasu arteritis
Medium vessel vasculitis	Polyarteritis nodosa (classic PAN) Kawasaki disease
Small vessel vasculitis	Wegener's granulomatosis Churg-Strauss syndrome Microscopic polyangiitis (polyarteritis) Henoch-Schönlein purpura Essential cryoglobulinemic vasculitis Cutaneous leukocytoclastic vasculitis

Adapted from Jennette JC, Falk RJ, Andrassy K, et al: Nomenclature of systemic vasculitides: proposal of an International Consensus Conference, *Arthritis Rheum* 37:187–192, 1994. Adopted by the Chapel Hill Consensus Conference on the Nomenclature of Systemic Vasculitis, 1994.

- **Malignancies:** Lymphomas, colonic carcinoma, hairy cell leukemia, multiple myeloma, lung cancer, renal cell carcinoma, prostate cancer, breast cancer, head and neck cancer

In the majority of cases of leukocytoclastic vasculitis, the precipitating antigen cannot be identified.

Veraldi S, Mancuso R, Rizzitelli G, et al: Henoch-Schönlein syndrome associated with human parvovirus B19 primary infection, *Eur J Dermatol* 9:232–233, 1999.

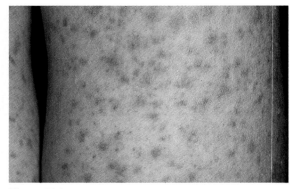

Figure 15-1. Leukoclastic vasculitis secondary to ampicillin. Typical lesions of palpable purpura are seen.

5. What is Henoch-Schönlein purpura?

Henoch-Schönlein purpura is a variant of leukocytoclastic vasculitis characterized by the deposition of immune complexes containing IgA in small vessels with the most commonly affected vessels being in the skin, kidney, and gastrointestinal tract. The precipitating antigen is not identifiable in all cases but many cases are associated with streptococcal or viral infections. It is usually seen in young children although any age can be affected. The classic four components of the syndrome include cutaneous palpable purpura, colicky abdominal pain, arthralgias and/or arthritis and kidney involvement.

González LM, Janniger CK, Schwartz RA: Pediatric Henoch-Schönlein purpura, *Int J Dermatol* 48:1157–1165, 2009.

6. What is the mnemonic that can help remember the clinical features of Henoch-Schönlein purpura?

The mnemonic PAPAH (pä-pä) can be used to remember the clinical features of HSP: **p**urpura, **a**bdominal **p**ain, **a**rthralgias, **h**ematuria. Some patients with abdominal involvement demonstrate significant melena or less commonly develop intussusception of the bowel. While more than 40% of patients demonstrate at least some degree of renal involvement, primarily manifesting as hematuria and proteinuria, only 1% develop chronic renal impairment. Less commonly, other organs such as the brain or lungs can be involved.

7. What is "acute hemorrhagic edema of infancy" and how does it differ from Henoch-Schönlein purpura?

Acute hemorrhagic edema of infancy, which also called "cockade purpura," is also an IgA-mediated immune complex leukocytoclastic vasculitis that affects small cutaneous vessels. This variant almost always affects young children (median age is 11 months), and like Henoch-Schönlein purpura, it is usually associated with a preexisting upper respiratory infection. It differs in that the primary cutaneous clinical lesions are typically indurated, edematous plaques with variable hemorrhage that are less likely to ulcerate. The lesions frequently affect the head and neck region and extremities (Fig. 15-2). The children typically do not demonstrate significant involvement of the gastrointestinal tract, joints or kidneys and do not develop permanent sequelae.

Fiore E, Rizzi M, Ragazzi M, et al: Acute hemorrhagic edema of young children (cockade purpura and edema): a case series and systematic review, *J Am Acad Dermatol* 59:684–695, 2008.

8. What are cryoglobulins?

Cryoglobulins are abnormal circulating IgG and IgM immunoglobulins that precipitate at low temperatures and redissolve at 37° C. Cryoglobulins are frequently found in patients with paraproteinemias, such as multiple myeloma and macroglobulinemia. Mixed cryoglobulinemia, with more than one antibody class involved, has been reported in systemic lupus erythematosus, rheumatoid arthritis, Sjögren's syndrome, and hepatitis B and C infection.

Trejo O, Ramos-Casals M, Garcia-Carrasco M, et al: Cryglobulinemia: study of etiologic factors and clinical and immunologic features in 443 patients from a single center, *Medicine* (Baltimore) 80:252–262, 2001.

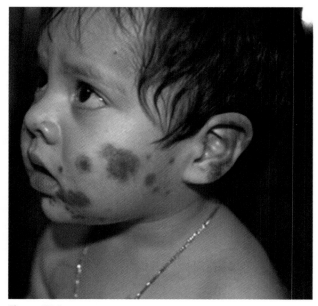

Figure 15-2. Acute hemorrhagic edema of a young child demonstrating hemorrhagic indurated plaques of the head. As seen here, the ears and cheeks are frequently involved. (Courtesy of the Joanna Burch Collection.)

9. Can cryoglobulins produce a vasculitis?

Yes. Some authorities consider cryoglobulinemic leukocytoclastic vasculitis to be a distinct subset of leukcytoclastic vasculitis, and it is often discussed separately. Cryoglobulinemic vasculitis is most commonly associated with type II cryoglobulins (monoclonal immunoglobulins, usually IgM, with rheumatoid factor binding activity to the Fc portion of polyclonal IgG) and type III cryoglobulins (mixed polyclonal immunoglobulins that usually bind to IgG). Type I immunoglobulins (monoclonal immunoglobulin, most commonly IgM) are more likely to present as occlusive infarctive lesions without an associated infiltrate, although rare cases of vasculitis have been reported. Hepatitis B and C are emerging as major causes of mixed cryoglobulinemia. Clinically, patients with cryoglobulinemic leukocytoclastic vasculitis resemble those having classic adult leukocytoclastic vasculitis, except that the lesions are more commonly associated with cold exposure and are more commonly confined to acral areas where the body temperature is lower.

10. What is Churg-Strauss syndrome?

Churg-Strauss syndrome (allergic granulomatosis) is an uncommon multisystemic vasculitis that is characterized with asthma, eosinophilia, extravascular granulomas, and positive ANCA titers. The main systemic features of Churg-Strauss syndrome are summarized in Table 15-2. Pulmonary involvement and eosinophilia helps discriminate Churg-Strauss syndrome from polyarteritis nodosa. The primary cutaneous lesions most commonly consist of palpable purpura involving the extremities, although some patients may also demonstrate fixed papules or plaques or even subcutaneous nodules. Cutaneous lesions have been reported in 45% to 70% of patients. Cutaneous involvement should be considered an important feature when present; biopsies in addition to demonstrating vasculitis of small blood vessels, frequently demonstrate large numbers of eosinophils and, less commonly, may demonstrate extravascular granulomatous inflammation.

Table 15-2. Clinical Features of Churg-Strauss Syndrome	
FINDING	SENSITIVITY
Asthma	100%
Blood eosinophilia >10%	95%
Paranasal sinus abnormalities	86%
Mononeuropathy or polyneuropathy	75%
Pulmonary infiltrates	40%
Extravascular (perivascular) eosinophils	14%
History of seasonal allergies	—

11. What were those features again?

To recall the diagnostic criteria for Churg-Strauss syndrome, remember the mnemonic **BEAN SAP**: **b**lood **e**osinophilia, **a**sthma, **n**europathy, **s**inus abnormalities, **a**llergies, and **p**erivascular eosinophils. The American College of Rheumatology has recently established these six criteria for the diagnosis of Churg-Strauss syndrome, with the presence of four of these six criteria yielding a diagnostic sensitivity of 85% and a specificity of 99.7%.

12. What is Wegener's granulomatosis?

Wegener's granulomatosis is an uncommon multisystem vascultitis that is characterized by vasculitis and necrotizing granulomatosis inflammation that most commonly affects the upper respiratory tract, lungs, and kidneys. It has been estimated that the prevalence in the United States is approximately 3 per 100,000 individuals.

13. What are the features needed to establish a diagnosis of Wegener's granulomatosis.

There are four criteria for establishing the diagnosis of Wegener's granulomatosis:
- Abnormal urinary sediment (red cell casts or >5 red blood cells/high-power field)
- Abnormal findings of chest radiographs (nodules, cavities, or fixed infiltrates)
- Oral ulcers or nasal discharge
- Granulomatous inflammation on biopsy

The presence of two or more of the four criteria gives a diagnostic sensitivity of 88% and a specificity of 92%. The majority of patients with active disease also demonstrate a positive c-ANCA; however, although supportive of this diagnosis, it is not specific because patients with Churg-Strauss syndrome, microscopic polyarteritis, and polyarteritis nodosa may also demonstrate elevated c-ANCA titers.

de Groot K, Gross WL: Wegener's granulomatosis, *Lupus* 7:285–291, 1998.

14. Is there an easy way to remember these diagnostic criteria?

Simply remember the mnemonic **ROUGH**:
- Chest **R**adiograph
- **O**ral ulcers

- **U**rinary sediment
- **G**ranulomas
- **H**emoptysis

Hemoptysis during illness has been added as a fifth criterion.

15. List the cutaneous findings in Wegener's granulomatosis.

- Leukocytoclastic vasculitis (Fig. 15-3A)
- Papules (Fig. 15-3B)
- Petechiae
- Ulcerative lesions (Fig. 15-3C)
- Urticaria
- Erythema
- Purpura
- Pyoderma gangrenosum

None of these cutaneous findings is specific for Wegener's granulomatosis.

16. Wegener's granulomatosis and Churg-Strauss syndrome seem very similar. How do you distinguish between them?

It is often difficult to distinguish between Wegener's granulomatosis and Churg-Strauss syndrome due to the presence of nasal, sinus, and pulmonary involvement in both diseases and the fact that all the classic features are rarely found in a single patient. There are many situations in which the features of systemic vasculitides overlap, and these are referred to as overlap vasculitis syndromes, similar to the overlap syndromes reported for other rheumatologic conditions.

The use of cytoplasmic antineutrophil cytoplasmic antibodies (c-ANCA) for differentiating between these two disorders is helpful (c-ANCA is usually present in high titers in Wegener's but not in Churg-Strauss), but is not included in the current diagnostic criteria for either syndrome. The presence or absence of other features should confirm the diagnosis in most cases (Table 15-3).

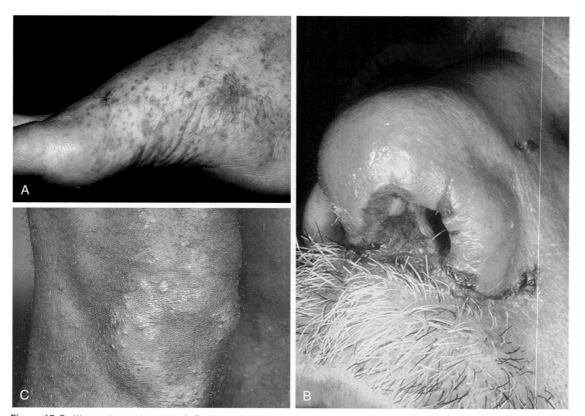

Figure 15-3. Wegener's granulomatosis. **A,** Fatal case demonstrating purpuric lesions. The patient was c-ANCA-positive. **B,** Nasal erosions and ulceration. **C,** Nonspecific papules on the knee in a patient with limited Wegener's granulomatosis involving the sinuses and the skin. (Courtesy of James E. Fitzpatrick, MD.)

Table 15-3 Wegener's Granulomatosis versus Churg-Strauss Syndrome

	WEGENER'S	CHURG-STRAUSS
Asthma	−	+
Blood eosinophilia	−	+
Perivascular eosinophils on biopsy	−	+
Hemoptysis	+	−
Microhematuria	+	−

Key Points: Antineutrophil Cytoplasmic Antibodies

1. Antineutrophilic cytoplasmic antibodies directed against serine proteinase 3 produce a distinct granular cytoplasmic staining pattern (c-ANCA).
2. c-ANCA is found in up to 90% of patients with Wegener's granulomatosis. High titers often correlate with increased disease activity.
3. Antineutrophilic cytoplasmic antibodies directed against myeloperoxidase produces a distinct perinuclear cytoplasmic pattern (p-ANCA).
4. p-ANCA is found in up to 70% of patients with microscopic polyarteritis nodosa and up to 50% of patients with Churg-Strauss syndrome.

17. What forms of treatment are available for Wegener's granulomatosis and Churg-Strauss syndrome?

Systemic corticosteroids are the mainstay for treatment of most forms of systemic vasculitis, and it is the most common treatment used in Churg-Strauss syndrome. Corticosteroids alone are often not effective in Wegener's granulomatosis, and most patients require cyclophosphamide in combination with corticosteroids for effective control. This is one of the most important reasons for distinguishing between these two disorders.

Koldingsnes W, Gran JT, Omdal R, Husby G: Wegener's granulomatosis: long-term follow-up of patients treated with pulse cyclophosphamide, *Br J Rheumatol* 37:659–664, 1998.

Stein SL, Miller LC, Konnikov N: Wegener's granulomatosis, *Pediatr Dermatol* 15:352–356, 1998.

18. What are the major organs involved in classic (systemic) polyarteritis nodosa (PAN)?

Kidneys, heart, liver, gastrointestinal (GI) tract, and peripheral nerves. PAN, in its classic form, is a multisystem, segmented necrotizing inflammation of small- and medium-sized muscular arteries. Signs and symptoms are nonspecific and constitutional, reflecting the organ involvement. Pulmonary arteries are typically not involved. The mean age of onset is 48 years, with a male:female ratio of about 4:1. Diagnosis is established by demonstrating vasculitic changes on biopsy of involved organs or by demonstrating typical aneurysms of medium-sized vessels on angiography.

Ishiguro N, Kawashima M: Cutaneous polyarteritis nodosa: a report of 16 cases with clinical and histopathological analysis and a review of the published work, *J Dermatol* 37:85–93, 2010.

19. How is classic polyarteritis nodosa different from Kawasaki disease?

Both disorders affect medium-sized vessels. PAN produces a necrotizing inflammation of medium-sized and/or small arteries without producing glomerulonephritis or vasculitis in arterioles, capillaries, or venules. Patients with Kawasaki disease are most often children with mucocutaneous lymph node syndrome (adenopathy, glossitis, cheilitis, conjunctivitis, etc.) with arteritis involving large (often resulting in coronary arteritis, coronary artery aneurysms, and myocardial infarctions), medium-sized, and small arteries.

20. What is primary cutaneous polyarteritis nodosa?

As the name implies, this is polyarteritis nodosa that is essentially confined to the skin, although it is not uncommon for patients to experience fever, arthralgias, and mysositis. The cutaneous lesions are most commonly located on the lower extremity and manifest as painful subcutaneous nodules that may resemble erythema nodosum, or demonstrate a characteristic "star-burst" appearance (Fig. 15-4). This diagnostic appearance is due the arteritis following the bifurcations of the small- and medium-sized arteries. Secondary changes that may be present include associated livedo reticularis and ulceration. In contrast to systemic polyarteritis nodosa, peripheral gangrene is not seen. Laboratory studies are generally normal except for variable mild leukocytosis and an elevated erythrocyte sedimentation rates (ESR).

21. What is the primary difference between microscopic polyangiitis and PAN?

The distinguishing feature for these two systemic disorders is primarily based on the size of the vessel that is affected. Patients with microscopic polyangiitis have involvement of small arterioles, whereas individuals with classic PAN have involvement of medium-sized arteries. Some authors consider microscopic polyarteritis a subset of PAN, although others consider it a distinct form of vasculitis.

Homas PB, David-Bajar KM, Fitzpatrick JE, et al: Microscopic polyarteritis: report of a case with cutaneous involvement and antimyeloperoxidase antibodies, *Arch Dermatol* 128:1223–1228, 1992.

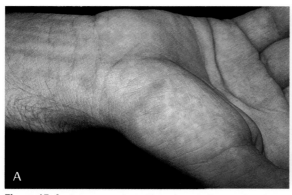
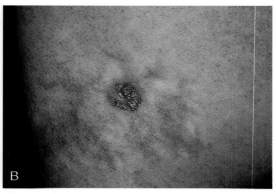

Figure 15-4. Cutaneous polyarteritis nodosa. **A,** Characteristic linear erythematous lesion. Note the Y-shaped bifurcation. **B,** Reticulated hyperpigmented lesion with an associated ulceration. (Courtesy of James E. Fitzpatrick, MD.)

22. What is the difference between giant cell (temporal) arteritis and Takayasu arteritis?

Both disorders affect large vessels. Takayasu's arteritis manifests with a progressive granulomatous inflammation of the aorta and its major branches and most frequently afflicts patients aged <50 years. Giant cell arteritis usually affects patients >50 years old with a granulomatous vasculitis that can also involve the aorta and its major branches. However, giant cell arteritis shows a predilection for the extracranial branches of the carotid artery, particularly the temporal artery, which can progress to visual loss and blindness if not treated with systemic steroids. Patients with giant cell arteritis may occasionally demonstrate unilateral alopecia, cutaneous ulceration or atrophy of the scalp due to loss of the blood supply to the skin.

Nordborg C, Nordborg E, Petursdottir V: Giant cell arteritis. Epidemiology, etiology, and pathogenesis, *APMIS* 108:713–724, 2000.

23. What is erythema elevatum diutinum?

Erythema elevatum diutinum is a rare form of small vessel vasculitis that is confined to the skin. This chronic disorder is characterized by persistent, elevated, erythematous plaques and/or nodules, with a predilection for overlying joint spaces, such as the fingers, wrists, elbows, knees, ankles, and toes (Fig. 15-5). The lesions are usually painful. Biopsies of developed lesions demonstrate a chronic leukocytoclastic vasculitis with extensive tissue fibrosis. There may be an associated IgA or, less commonly, an IgG monoclonal gammopathy (immune complex disease) and an association with inflammatory bowel disease, rheumatoid arthritis, systemic lupus erythematosus, streptococcal infection, IgA monoclonal gammopathy, multiple myeloma, myelodysplasia, celiac disease, relapsing polychondritis, and human immunodeficiency virus (HIV) infection. Some patients have shown a dramatic response to dapsone.

Farley-Loftus R, Dadlani C, Wang N, et al: Erythema elevatum diutinum, *Dermatol Online J* 14(10):13, 2008.

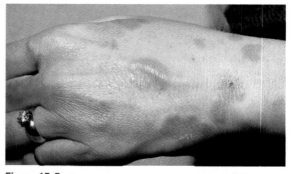

Figure 15-5. Erythema elevatum diutinum. Violaceous painful plaques on the dorsum of the hands. (Courtesy of the Fitzsimons Army Medical Center teaching files.)

24. Are there any other obscure disorders known to dermatologists, but little known to other subspecialties, that could be classified as vasculitis?

Yes— granuloma faciale, which is an uncommon, chronic, benign, small vessel vasculitis that most commonly affects middle-aged adults. While sun-exposed skin on the face is the area most commonly affected, it has also been reported to appear on

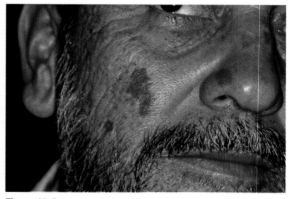

Figure 15-6. Granuloma faciale demonstrating purplish indurated plaques of the nose and cheeks. (Courtesy of the Joanna Burch Collection.)

extrafacial sites including the trunk and upper and lower extremities. The lesions are characteristically solitary but can be multiple. The primary lesion is a papule, nodule, or plaque that varies in size from millimeters to several centimeters (Fig. 15-6). The overlying epidermis is characteristically smooth with the follicular orifices being accentuated producing a characteristic "peau de orange" appearance. The color is highly variable and varies from yellowish to amber to brown to red to violaceous. Most lesions are asymptomatic, although occasional patients may complain of mild pruritus or burning. Once present, the lesions typically persist for years or decades, and progressive enlargement of lesions is not uncommon. The pathogenesis of this peculiar form of cutaneous vasculitis is unknown.

Thiyanaratnam J, Doherty SD, Krishnan B, Hsu S: Granuloma faciale: case report and review, *Dermatol Online J* 15(12):3, 2009.

DEPOSITION DISORDERS

Lisa E. Maier, MD, and Lori Lowe, MD

1. How is "deposition disorder" defined?

Deposition disorders comprise a diverse group of conditions or diseases in which there is accumulation, deposition, or production of substances in the skin. Typically, these substances are products of abnormal metabolism or degenerative phenomena occurring locally or systemically. The major cutaneous deposits may be subdivided into the hyalinoses, mucinoses, and mineral salts.

Touart DM, Sau P: Cutaneous deposition diseases. Part I, *J Am Acad Dermatol* 39:149–171, 1998.

2. What is amyloid?

Amyloid is a protein with distinct tinctorial and ultrastructural properties found as extracellular deposits. It is composed of a nonfibrillary protein known as the amyloid P component and a fibrillary component that is derived from various sources. The amyloid fibril has an antiparallel, β-pleated sheet configuration. Ultrastructurally, amyloid is composed of rigid, nonbranching fibrils measuring 6 to 10 nm in diameter.

3. How is amyloid identified?

With light microscopy, amyloid appears as amorphous, hyaline-like, eosinophilic deposits. Amyloid demonstrates green birefringence with the alkaline Congo red stain, reddish metachromasia with crystal violet, and yellow-green fluorescence with thioflavin-T stain (Fig. 16-1). These stains are not absolutely specific for amyloid, as false-positive results may occur with the other hyaline-like deposition disorders.

4. Name the various types of amyloidosis.

Amyloidosis may be classified according to clinical presentation and type of amyloid fibril protein deposition (Table 16-1). The amyloid in the macular and lichenoid variants is derived from degenerated tonofilaments of keratinocytes. Nodular amyloidosis is formed from light-chain–derived AL protein produced locally by plasma cells. It cannot be distinguished from primary systemic amyloidosis, and therefore, systemic disease should be excluded in all patients with nodular amyloidosis. There are also rare forms of hereditary systemic amyloidoses that have less frequent skin manifestations.

5. What are the cutaneous manifestations of primary or myeloma-associated systemic amyloidosis? How often do they occur?

Cutaneous lesions are seen in about 30% of cases of primary or myeloma-related systemic amyloidosis. The most common skin lesions are petechiae or ecchymoses due to amyloid deposition within blood vessel walls with subsequent fragility and dermal hemorrhage. These are often seen at sites predisposed to trauma, such as the hands or intertriginous areas. Pinching the skin gives characteristic purpuric lesions known as "pinch purpura." Purpura around the eyes may occur spontaneously but is also seen following proctoscopy or vomiting ("postproctoscopic purpura") (Fig. 16-2). Waxy papules, nodules, or plaques may be present. Less common manifestations include sclerodermoid plaques, bullae, alopecia, and nail dystrophy.

6. Name the other organ systems that may be involved in primary or myeloma-associated amyloidosis.

Mucous membrane involvement with macroglossia occurs in 20% of cases. Hepatomegaly is found in about 50% of cases. Cardiac involvement may manifest as a restrictive cardiomyopathy or constrictive pericarditis. Peripheral nerve involvement results in paresthesias, peripheral neuropathy, and median nerve entrapment (carpal tunnel syndrome). Proteinuria is found in 80% to 90% of

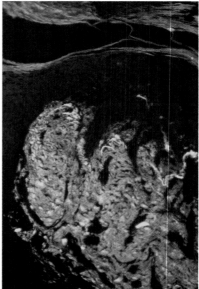

Figure 16-1. Lichen amyloidosis. Thioflavin-T demonstrates strong staining of fluorescent amyloid in the papillary dermis. (Courtesy of James E. Fitzpatrick, MD.)

Table 16-1. Classification of Amyloidosis

CLINICAL DISORDER	AMYLOID PROTEIN PRECURSOR	AMYLOID PROTEIN
Primary systemic amyloidosis	Immunoglobulin light chain	AL
Myeloma-associated amyloidosis	Immunoglobulin light chain	AL
Secondary systemic amyloidosis	Serum amyloid A lipoprotein	AA
Primary localized cutaneous amyloidosis		
Macular amyloidosis	Keratinocyte tonofilaments	–
Lichen amyloidosis	Keratinocyte tonofilaments	–
Nodular amyloidosis	Immunoglobulin light chain (produced locally by plasma cells)	AL

patients at some time during their course. Renal failure usually develops late in the disease course but may be a cause of death.

Prokaeva T, Spencer B, Kaut M, et al: Soft tissue, joint, and bone manifestations of AL amyloidosis: clinical presentation, molecular features, and survival, *Arthritis Rheum* 56:3858–3868, 2007.

Silverstein SR: Primary, systemic amyloidosis and the dermatologist: where classic skin lesions may provide the clue for early diagnosis, *Dermatol Online* J 11:5, 2005.

7. Compare lichen amyloidosis and macular amyloidosis.

Lichen amyloidosis is the most common form of localized cutaneous amyloidosis. Lesions are pruritic, flesh-colored to brown papules, often with overlying scale (Fig. 16-3A). Papules may coalesce into verrucous plaques. The shins are the most common site of

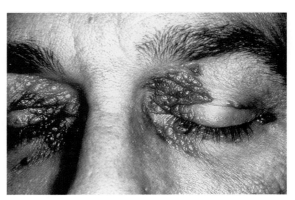

Figure 16-2. Primary systemic amyloidosis. Characteristic periorbital purpuric plaques.

involvement. In macular amyloidosis, pruritic macular hyperpigmentation occurs most commonly in the interscapular area. The chest or extremities are less commonly involved. The lesions have a characteristic reticulate or rippled appearance. Both of these variants of primary localized cutaneous amyloidosis occur more frequently in patients from the Middle East, Asia, and Central and South America. The etiology of both lichen and macular amyloidosis is unclear but thought to be related to chronic scratching or frictional exposure. An autosomal dominant family history may be found in up to 10% of patients with lichen amyloidosis. Lichen amyloidosis is occasionally associated with multiple endocrine neoplasia type 2A.

Tanaka A, Arita K, Lai-Cheong JE, et al: New insight into mechanisms of pruritus from molecular studies on familial primary localized cutaneous amyloidosis, *Br J Dermatol* 161:1217–1224, 2009.

8. How does nodular amyloidosis present? With what is it associated?

Nodular amyloidosis typically presents as solitary or multiple waxy nodules (Fig. 16-3B). Common sites of involvement include the face, scalp, lower extremities, and genitalia. It may be associated with the subsequent development of systemic amyloidosis up to 15% of cases. Rarely, it is found in association with Sjögren's syndrome.

Kalajian AH, Waldman M, Knable AL: Nodular primary localized cutaneous amyloidosis after trauma: a case report and discussion of the rate of progression to systemic amyloidosis, *J Am Acad Dermatol* 57(Suppl 2):S26–S29, 2007.

Yoneyama K, Tochigi N, Oikawa A, et al: Primary localized cutaneous nodular amyloidosis in a patient with Sjögren's syndrome: a review of the literature, *J Dermatol* 32:120–123, 2005.

9. In what setting is secondary systemic amyloidosis seen?

Secondary systemic amyloidosis is associated with chronic systemic disease, such as infection, collagen vascular disease, or neoplasm. Examples of disease associations include tuberculosis, leprosy, osteomyelitis, rheumatoid arthritis, scleroderma, pustular psoriasis, leukemia, and lymphoma.

10. What are the systemic manifestations of secondary systemic amyloidosis?

Organs commonly involved in secondary systemic amyloidosis include the liver, spleen, and kidneys, resulting in hepatosplenomegaly and nephrotic syndrome, respectively. Although skin lesions are generally lacking, biopsy of subcutaneous abdominal fat may demonstrate amyloid deposition.

Hazenberg BP, Bijzet J, Limburg PC, et al: Diagnostic performance of amyloid A protein quantification in fat tissue of patients with clinical AA amyloidosis, *Amyloid* 14:133–140, 2007.

Lachmann HJ, Goodman HJ, Gilbertson JA, et al: Natural history and outcome in systemic AA amyloidosis, *N Engl J Med* 356:2361–2371, 2007.

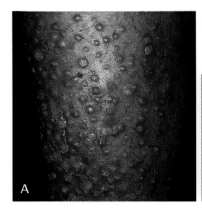
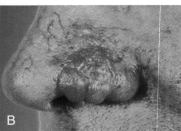

Figure 16-3. A, Lichen amyloidosis. Numerous pruritic, scaly papules on the anterior shin. **B,** Nodular amyloidosis demonstrating large waxy nodule on the nose.

11. What is lipoid proteinosis?

Lipoid proteinosis, also known as hyalinosis cutis et mucosae and Urbach-Wiethe disease, is a rare autosomal recessive genodermatosis in which skin and mucous membranes are infiltrated with a hyaline scleroprotein. The presenting symptom, hoarseness, develops in infancy due to involvement of the vocal cords with hyaline deposits. Bullae, pustules, and crusts, followed by acneiform scars, are seen on the face and extremities. Waxy papules develop along the eyelids, producing a characteristic "string of beads" appearance. Later, verrucous plaques occur on the elbows and knees. Lipoid proteinosis is caused by loss-of-function mutations in the extracellular matrix protein 1 gene (*ECM1*).

Bahhady R, Abbas O, Ghosn S, et al: Erosions and scars over the face, trunk, and extremities, *Pediatr Dermatol* 26:91–92, 2009.

12. What is colloid milium?

Colloid milium is a cutaneous eruption characterized by flesh-colored to yellow-brown translucent papules that may coalesce into plaques. The eruption is most commonly found in adults in areas of chronic sun exposure, but a rare juvenile form is also recognized. Amorphous fissured eosinophilic material in the papillary dermis is seen on histopathology. Excessive sun exposure is a likely etiologic factor in adult colloid milium.

Pourrabbani S, Marra DE, Iwasaki J, et al: Colloid milium: a review and update, *J Drugs Dermatol* 6:293–296, 2007.

13. Which histologic feature or "deposit" is common to all porphyrias?

The porphyrias are a group of diseases resulting from defects in the enzymes that regulate heme biosynthesis. The biochemical and clinical features are different for each type of porphyria, yet all demonstrate similar cutaneous histology with deposits of eosinophilic, hyaline material around blood vessels. This material stains positively with the periodic acid–Schiff stain and represents reduplicated basal lamina or type IV collagen.

14. Which porphyria classically demonstrates the largest deposits? What are its cutaneous features?

Erythropoietic protoporphyria, also termed protoporphyria, has the largest eosinophilic deposits in cutaneous lesions. This autosomal dominant disorder of porphyrin metabolism is caused by a deficiency of the enzyme ferrochelatase (heme synthetase). Symptoms begin in early childhood and include photosensitivity, pruritus, burning, erythema, and edema. Chronic changes include a waxy, "cobblestone" thickening of the skin and shallow scars or pits. Increased protoporphyrin may be identified in the feces and blood, although urinary porphyrins are usually normal.

Lecha M, Puy H, Deybach JC: Erythropoietic protoporphyria, *Orphanet J Rare Dis* 4:19, 2009.

15. Name some of the cutaneous mucinoses.

The mucinoses are a heterogeneous group of disorders characterized by dermal mucin deposition. This mucin is largely hyaluronic acid, an acid mucopolysaccharide, with smaller amounts of chondroitin sulfate and heparin. Disorders resulting in diffuse mucin deposition include generalized myxedema, pretibial myxedema, lichen myxedematosus, scleredema, reticular erythematous mucinosis, and the mucopolysaccharidoses (storage diseases). Mucin deposition may also be focal or localized, as with follicular mucinosis (alopecia mucinosa), cutaneous focal mucinosis, and digital mucous cyst.

Jackson EM, English JC 3rd: Diffuse cutaneous mucinoses, *Dermatol Clin* 20:493–501, 2002.

16. Describe the clinical lesions seen in pretibial myxedema and its disease associations.

Patients with pretibial myxedema develop nodules or diffuse plaques usually on the anterior lower legs, although involvement of other sites has been rarely reported (Fig. 16-4A). The lesions result from large amounts of dermal mucin deposition. Pretibial myxedema is seen in 1% to 4% of patients with Graves' disease and, less commonly, in patients with autoimmune thyroiditis.

Fatourechi V: Pretibial myxedema: pathophysiology and treatment options, *Am J Clin Dermatol* 6(5):295–309, 2005.

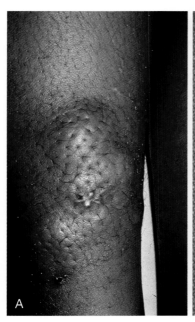 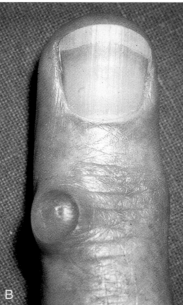

Figure 16-4. A, Pretibial myxedema. Thick plaques on anterior lower legs with peau d'orange change secondary to dermal mucin. **B,** Digital mucous cyst. Dome-shaped cystic nodule overlying the distal interphalangeal joint.

Key Points: Cutaneous Deposition Disorders

1. Amyloid deposition can result in both localized and systemic disease.
2. Pretibial myxedema is associated with Graves' disease.
3. The porphyrias are a group of diseases caused by defects in heme biosynthesis–related enzymes.
4. Lesions of lichen myxedematosus result from an increase in both dermal mucin and fibroblasts.
5. IgG lambda paraproteinemia is the most common serum abnormality associated with scleromyxedema.
6. Lesions of gout result from uric acid deposition in the skin and soft tissues.
7. Calciphylaxis usually occurs in the setting of renal disease.

---

17. Describe the clinical lesions seen in lichen myxedematosus.

In lichen myxedematosus, also known as papular mucinosis, numerous flesh-colored to erythematous, densely grouped lichenoid papules are found primarily on the face and arms. Rare cases have been reported in association with human immunodeficiency virus or hepatitis C infection. In the scleromyxedema variant, lesions coalesce into indurated plaques resulting in diffuse skin thickening. Scleromyxedema can involve internal organs resulting in neurologic, musculoskeletal, gastrointestinal, pulmonary, renal, and cardiovascular sequelae. Lesions of lichen myxedematosus/scleromyxedema result from an increase in both dermal mucin and fibroblasts.

18. What serum abnormality has been associated with scleromyxedema?

Scleromyxedema is nearly always associated with serum paraproteinemia, usually IgG with lambda light chains. Rare cases with kappa light chains have been reported. Waldenström's macroglobulinemia or multiple myeloma may be rarely associated.

Rongioletti F, Rebora A: Updated classification of papular mucinosis, lichen myxedematosus, and scleromyxedema, *J Am Acad Dermatol* 44:273–281, 2001.

19. Describe the clinical lesions in scleredema and its disease associations.

Scleredema presents as a firm, woody induration of the skin typically involving the upper trunk, posterior neck, and shoulders. Histologically, it is characterized by an accumulation of dermal mucin and increased sclerosis of dermal collagen. Scleredema may be seen in several different clinical settings, including postinfection, in association with diabetes mellitus, and in the setting of paraproteinemia.

Boin F, Hummers LK: Scleroderma-like fibrosing disorders, *Rheum Dis Clin North Am* 34:199–220, 2008.

20. What is a digital mucous (myxoid) cyst?

A digital mucous cyst is a common solitary, asymptomatic, semitranslucent, dome-shaped nodule that typically presents in adults and elderly patients on the dorsal finger near the proximal nail fold or distal interphalangeal joint (Fig. 16-4B). It may distort the nail matrix, resulting in a groove in the nail plate. Clear, gelatinous mucoid material can be expressed from the cyst. The pathogenesis is controversial; however, it is often attributed to degenerative changes in the distal interphalangeal joints.

Lin YC, Wu YH, Scher RK: Nail changes and association of osteoarthritis in digital myxoid cyst, *Dermatol Surg* 34:364–369, 2008.

21. What substance is elevated in gout?

Gout is a heterogeneous group of disorders of purine metabolism resulting in elevated levels of uric acid (monosodium urate). Patients have either increased uric acid production or decreased renal excretion. Some risk factors for hyperuricemia include alcohol use, obesity, high purine diets, diabetes, myeloproliferative disorders, renal disease, and/or diuretic therapy.

22. Where is the uric acid deposited in gout? What are the resulting clinical manifestations?

Uric acid crystals in gout are most commonly deposited in the synovium, soft tissues, and skin. The most common site is the synovium of joints, producing acute gouty arthritis. The metatarsophalangeal joint of the great toe is classically involved. Uric acid deposition in the skin and soft tissues results in gouty tophi, which are seen in 20% to 50% of patients. Common sites of involvement include the helix of the ear, elbows, and digits (Fig. 16-5A). These gouty tophi may ulcerate and discharge monosodium urate crystals that appear as a thick chalky material. Under light microscopy, these crystals are needle-shaped and birefringent (Fig. 16-5B).

Thissen CA, Frank J, Lucker GP: Tophi as first clinical sign of gout, *Int J Dermatol* 47(Suppl 1):49–51, 2008.

23. How is gout treated?

Acute attacks of gout may be treated with a variety of agents, including colchicine, nonsteroidal antiinflammatory agents, or systemic corticosteroids. Long-term therapy may include colchicine, allopurinol, probenecid, or urine alkalinization (to increase uric acid solubility).

Eggebeen AT: Gout: an update, *Am Fam Physician* 76:801–808, 2007.

24. How many types of calcinosis cutis are there?

- **Dystrophic calcinosis cutis:** Occurs when there is deposition of calcium salts within inflamed or damaged tissue. Calcium and phosphorus metabolism is normal. It may be localized, such as within acne scars or epidermoid cysts, or widespread. Widespread dystrophic calcinosis cutis most often occurs in association with connective tissue disease, such as dermatomyositis or scleroderma.
- **Metastatic calcinosis cutis:** Is seen with aberrations in calcium or phosphorus metabolism. It usually occurs when the serum calcium-phosphorus product exceeds 60.
- **Idiopathic calcinosis cutis:** Is the term used when no obvious underlying cause can be identified for tissue calcification. As with dystrophic calcification, this variant may be widespread, such as in calcinosis universalis, or localized, as in tumoral calcinosis or scrotal calcinosis.
- **Iatrogenic calcinosis cutis:** Deposition of calcium due to medical agents such as intravenous calcium gluconate, intravenous calcium chloride, calcium alginate dressings, and calcium chloride electrode paste.

25. What underlying medical conditions have been associated with metastatic calcinosis cutis?

- Hyperparathyroidism
- Pseudohypoparathyroidism

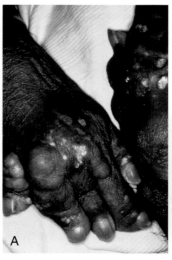
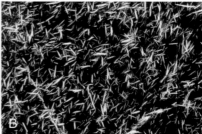

Figure 16-5. A, Gouty tophi. Tophaceous deposits of gout overlying digits. **B,** Aspirate from gouty tophus demonstrating diagnostic birefringent gout crystals with polarization. (Courtesy of the Fitzsimons Army Medical Center teaching files.)

- Vitamin D toxicity
- Milk-alkali syndrome
- Sarcoidosis
- Destructive bone disease
- Malignancies
- Chronic renal failure

26. What is calciphylaxis and who develops it?

Calciphylaxis is a type of metastatic calcification in which there is calcification of the walls of small- and medium-sized blood vessels in the dermis and subcutis resulting in infarction of the overlying skin. Clinically, patients develop livedo reticularis–like mottling, painful hard plaques, and necrotic ulcers. It is usually seen in the setting of chronic renal failure and secondary hyperparathyroidism (Fig. 16-6). Calciphylaxis, however, has uncommonly been reported with normal levels of calcium and phosphate and in the absence of renal disease.

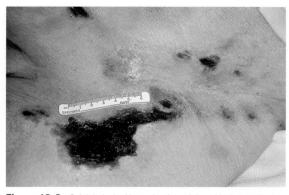

Figure 16-6. Calciphylaxis. Necrosis of overlying skin in a patient with chronic renal failure.

Daudén E, Oñate MJ: Calciphylaxis, *Dermatol Clin* 26:557–568, 2008.

27. What is osteoma cutis?

Osteoma cutis is the deposition of bone within cutaneous tissues. Primary osteoma cutis involves normal skin and can be associated with several syndromes including Albright hereditary osteodystrophy, fibrodysplasia ossificans progressiva, and congenital platelike osteomatosis. Secondary osteoma cutis or metaplastic ossification occurs in association with or secondary to trauma, inflammatory skin conditions, or neoplasia. Miliary osteoma cutis of the face presents as multiple, small, firm papules on the face, typically in women afflicted with acne, although it may also arise on normal skin.

Touart DM, Sau P: Cutaneous deposition diseases. Part II, *J Am Acad Dermatol* 39:527–544, 1998.

PHOTOSENSITIVE DERMATITIS

Todd T. Kobayashi, MD, Lt Col, USAF, MC, and Kathleen M. David-Bajar, MD

1. What is the definition of photosensitivity?

Although there is not a definition accepted by all, most dermatologists define photosensitivity as the development or exacerbation of a skin eruption and/or symptoms (including pruritus or pain) following exposure to sunlight. In some instances, a patient may not specifically relate the eruption to sun exposure, usually due to a delay in the onset of signs or symptoms following sun exposure. Thus, if a skin eruption is photodistributed, even without a definite history of exacerbation following sun exposure, many dermatologists classify it as a photosensitive dermatosis. Some photosensitivity reactions (e.g., phototoxic drug reactions) are very similar to sunburn but occur with less intense sun exposure than would normally be required to induce sunburn in that individual.

Millard TP, Hawk JL: Photosensitivity disorders: cause, effect and management, *Am J Clin Dermatol* 3:239–246, 2002.

2. What is the difference between a phototoxic reaction and a photoallergic reaction?

A **phototoxic reaction** (Fig. 17-1) is an exaggerated "sunburn" reaction where skin cells are damaged directly by electromagnetic radiation through the production of free radicals, toxic metabolites, heat, or by direct damage to DNA, augmented by external chemicals. It may occur within minutes to hours of exposure, though it may also be delayed for a day or two. A phototoxic reaction can be produced in anyone given a high enough dose of ultraviolet (UV) light and a phototoxic chemical. It can happen on first-time exposure without a need for sensitization.

A **photoallergic reaction** only occurs in sensitized individuals when electromagnetic radiation (usually ultraviolet light, but sometimes visible light) interact with an endogenous (Fig. 17-2A) or exogenous (Fig. 17-2B) chemical, converting it to an allergen that the person's immune system recognizes as an allergen (requires more than one exposure). Photoallergic reactions typically occur 1 to 3 days after exposure (with the exception of solar urticaria, which is immediate). Phototoxic reactions tend to be well demarcated in the areas of exposure. Photoallergic reactions are also photodistributed, but often have extension of the cutaneous reaction onto covered areas or even distant sites in an autoeczematous type of eruption. Sometimes chemicals may produce both a phototoxic and photoallergic phenomenon.

3. What is the clinical appearance of a photodistributed eruption?

A photodistributed eruption affects the skin in a characteristic distribution, affecting the convex surfaces of face, external areas of forearms and arms, dorsal hands, V-area of upper chest, lateral sides and posterior of neck, and any other area exposed to the sun. It characteristically spares the ocular/eyelid area, beneath the nose and lower lip, inframandibular chin/neck, and inner parts of arms and forearms, and clothing covered sites. In photocontact dermatitis, the affected areas are those areas with exposure to both sunlight and the causative topical agent.

4. Name some of the most common topical phototoxic and photoallergic agents and their action spectrums.

The action spectrum for almost all topical phototoxic and photoallergic reactions is UVA, rarely UVB and visible light. Some of the most common topical agents are listed in Table 17-1.

5. Name some of the most common systemic phototoxic and photoallergic agents and their action spectrums.

As in the case of the topical agents, the action spectrum for almost all systemic phototoxic and photoallergic reactions is UVA, rarely UVB and visible light. Some of the most common systemic agents are listed in Table 17-2.

Stein, KR, Scheinfeld, NS: Drug-induced photoallergic and phototoxic reactions, *Expert Opin Drug Saf* 6:431–443, 2007.

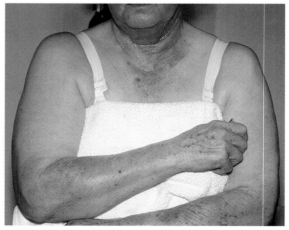

Figure 17-1. Phototoxic drug eruption. Sunburn-like erythema on the cheeks, neck, V-area of the chest, and dorsal forearms.

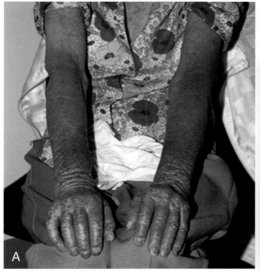
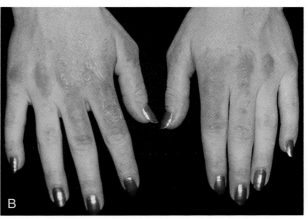

Figure 17-2. A, Photoallergic drug eruption due to oral compazine demonstrating marked erythema and swelling of the dorsum of the hands, arms, and V of the chest. (Courtesy of the John L. Aeling, M.D. Collection.) **B,** Photoallergic contact dermatitis. Erythema of the dorsal hands and fingers due to a sunscreen containing para-aminobenzoic acid (PABA).

Table 17-1. Topical Agents Causing Phototoxic and Photoallergic Reactions

PHOTOTOXIC CHEMICALS	PHOTOALLERGIC CHEMICALS
Benzocaine	Sunscreens: oxybenzone, benzophenone, etc.
Benzoyl peroxide (UVB)	Fragrances: methylcoumarin, musk ambrette, sandalwood oil
Coal tar	NSAIDs
Erythromycin	Oxicams: ampiroxicam, droxicam, meloxicam, piroxicam, tenoxicam
Halogenated salicylanilides	Prioprionic acid derivatives: benzophenone, dexketoprofen, ketoprofen,
Hydrocortisone	piketoprofen, suprofen (UVA and UVB), tiaprofenic acid, diclofenac
Ketoprofen	Antimicrobials: bithionol, chlorhexadine, fenticlor, hexachlorophene
Porphyrins (visible light and UVB)	Phenothiazines: chlorpromazine, promethazine
Psoralens	Miscellaneous
	Acyclovir
	Dibucaine
	Halogenated salicylanilides (UVA and UVB)
	Hydrocortisone

Table 17-2. Systemic Agents Causing Phototoxic and Photoallergic Reactions

PHOTOTOXIC	PHOTOALLERGIC
Antimicrobials Tetracyclines: demeclocycline, dimethylchlorotetracycline, doxycycline, lymecycline, minocycline, tetracycline Quinolones: ciprofloxacin, enoxacin, fleroxacin, levofloxacin, lomefloxacin (UVA and UVB), nalidixic acid, pefloxacin, sparfloxacin Griseofulvin Voriconazole	**NSAIDs:** piroxicam, celecoxib, ketoprofen **Sulfur-containing medications:** hydrochlorothiazide, sulfacetamide (UVB), sulfadiazine (UVB), sulfapyradine (UVB), sulfonamides (UVB), sulfonylureas **Antimalarials:** chloroquine unknown, hydroxychloroquine (UVB), quinidine, quinine
Sulfur-containing medications: bumetanide, furosemide, hydrochlorothiazide, sulfonamides (UVB), sulfonylureas **NSAIDs:** proprionic acid derivatives: benzophenone, carprofen, ketoprofen, nabumetone, naproxen, suprofen (UVA and UVB), tiaprofenic acid **Antimalarials:** chloroquine unknown, hydroxychloroquine (UVB), quinidine	**Antimicrobials:** chloroamphenicol unknown, enoxacin, lomefloxacin (UVA and UVB), sulfonamides Griseolfulvin **Phenothiazines:** chlorpromazine, dioxopromethazine, perphenazine, thioridazine
Miscellaneous: amiodarone, atorvastatin (UVB), calcium-channel blockers, chlorpromazine, prochlorperazine, porphyrins (UVB and visible), psoralens, retinoids (UVA and UVB), St. John's wart (hypericin)	**Miscellaneous:** amantadine, dapsone unknown, diphenhydramine (UVB), flutamide (UVA and UVB), pilocarpine, pyridoxine, ranitidine

6. Give some examples of unique phototoxic reactions.

- Pseudoporphyria (nonsteroidal antiinflammatory drugs, especially naproxen)
- Photoonycholysis (tetracyclines, fluoroquinolones, and psoralen)
- Hyperpigmentation (amiodarone, tricyclics, diltiazem, minocycline, hydroxychloroquine, gold, silver)
- Lichenoid eruptions (quinine, quinidine, gold, calcium channel blockers, idiopathic actinic lichen planus)
- This may also be considered a photoallergic syndrome as the immune system is involved
- Phytophotodermatitis (furocoumarins in yarrow, parsley, celery, parsnips, milfoil, lime, grasses)
- Tar (roofers and road workers)
- Radiation recall reaction (methotrexate or other antimetabolite given after radiation or sunburn, which reproduces or exaggerates the burn reaction)

7. What are some scenarios in which the skin may be more sensitive to ultraviolet radiation?

- Isotretinoin and retinoids (thinning of the stratum corneum)
- 5-Fluorouracil (5-FU) (antimetabolite affecting DNA repair)
- Methotrexate (MTX) (antimetabolite affecting enzymatic recovery after UV damage)
- Postprocedure (peels, resurfacing, dermabrasion, etc.) causing thinning of the stratum corneum and increased keratinocyte turnover

8. What are the important questions to ask a patient with suspected photosensitivity?

- How long does it take for the skin reaction to develop following light exposure? Some reactions (e.g., solar urticaria) occur within minutes following sun exposure, while others (e.g., chronic cutaneous lupus erythematosus) may take weeks to develop.
- Have you ever had a similar skin reaction to light? Some reactions (e.g., polymorphous light reaction) tend to be recurrent or seasonal, while others may be one-time events (e.g., photosensitive drug reaction).
- Is there a family history of similar skin reactions to light? Some photosensitive disorders are familial (e.g., erythropoietic protoporphyria) or occur more frequently in certain racial groups (e.g., actinic prurigo in Native Americans).
- What do you put on your skin? Numerous products (soaps, perfumes, sunscreens) may produce photoallergic contact dermatitis in some individuals.
- What medications do you take by mouth? Numerous drugs, both prescription and nonprescription, can occasionally produce photosensitive reactions.
- Are there any associated cutaneous symptoms? Pruritus is a typical complaint associated with certain diseases (such as photoallergic contact dermatitis), while pain or burning is more commonly associated with phototoxic disorders (e.g., erythropoietic protoporphyria).
- Do you have any other symptoms? Some photosensitive dermatoses are confined to the skin, while others (e.g., systemic lupus erythematosus) are associated with internal involvement.

9. What are the most common causes of photosensitive dermatoses?

Medications, both systemic and topical, are frequent causes of photosensitivity. Polymorphous light eruption is the most common cause of chronic photodermatitis, but often is a diagnosis of exclusion.

10. What is persistent light reactivity?

In persistent light reactivity, photodermatitis believed to be triggered by topical or systemic drugs persists long after the presumed causative agent has been discontinued. These unfortunate patients may be sensitive to a broad range of light, even visible light, and patients may be totally incapacitated by this disease. **Chronic actinic dermatitis** and **actinic reticuloid** are related diseases involving persistent and severe photodermatitis and occur primarily in older men (Fig. 17-3). Some believe that the primary event in these conditions is a photocontact dermatitis (photoallergic dermatitis) which persists due to chronic low-grade exposure, and in rare cases, even progressing to an "antigen-driven" form of mycosis fungoides, though this is controversial.

Key Points: Photosensitive Dermatitis

1. Phototoxic reactions clinically and symptomatically resemble sunburn while photoallergic reactions resemble dermatitis.
2. Over 350 drugs have been reported to produce photosensitive reactions.
3. Photosensitive drug reactions may occur in either the UVA or UVB spectrum. Because UVA passes through window glass, patients may develop photosensitive drug reactions even while they are in their homes or cars.
4. Photosensitivity is a component of several genetic disorders characterized by defective DNA repair (such as xeroderma pigmentosum) or enzymatic deficiencies leading to the accumulation of phototoxic porphyrins.

---

11. What is polymorphous light eruption (PMLE)?

PMLE is a common, chronic photoeruption that typically begins in the first three decades of life. There may be a positive family history of sunlight sensitivity. Patients characteristically report the onset of skin disease beginning with sun exposure in spring or early summer. Patients sometimes demonstrate gradual improvement with continuing sun exposure, a phenomenon termed "hardening." The specific skin lesions of PMLE may be of numerous (polymorphous) types, but one or two morphologic types usually predominate in individual patients. These include erythematous macules, patches, papules, plaques (Fig. 17-4), and vesicles and bullae. Lesions are photodistributed, often on the face and neck, chest, and dorsal arms and hands. The lips may also be involved. The etiology of PMLE is unknown, and most patients with PMLE do not have antinuclear antibodies. Patients with PMLE have been reported to be sensitive to ultraviolet B (UVB), ultraviolet A (UVA), or both. Synonyms include benign summer light eruption and juvenile spring eruption.

Dummer R, Ivanova K, Scheidegger EP, Burg G: Clinical and therapeutic aspects of polymorphous light eruption, *Dermatology* 207:93–95, 2003.

12. How is PMLE diagnosed?

PMLE is a clinical diagnosis, based on the history of a recurrent photoeruption, usually occurring each spring or early summer, with a consistent skin biopsy. There is no individual clinical, histologic, or laboratory finding that can establish a diagnosis of PMLE. Thus, it is important to exclude other causes of photosensitive dermatoses, such as lupus erythematosus and photodrug eruptions. Generally, the skin biopsy is helpful in this regard. In addition to routine histology, other negative tests include direct immunofluorescence testing of lesional skin (to exclude cutaneous lupus erythematosus), testing for antinuclear antibodies (including anti–Ro/SS-A antibodies), and a porphyrin screen (to rule out erythropoietic protoporphyria). Light testing may demonstrate a lowered minimal erythema dose (MED), that is, the dose of ultraviolet light required to produce erythema is less than one would predict on the basis of skin type (Fig. 17-5).

13. How is PMLE treated?

Sunscreens and other sun-protective measures are helpful, but a number of cases are not controlled with such measures. Topical steroids, β-carotene, antimalarials, and hardening with psoralen plus UVA (PUVA; see Chapter 55) are alternatives that may be successful.

14. What is actinic prurigo?

Actinic prurigo has historically been considered to be a variant of PMLE and has even been called hereditary PMLE of Native Americans. In recent years, however, most references have used the term actinic prurigo. In this population, the family history is usually positive, although sporadic cases do occur. Actinic prurigo may also occur in other ethnic groups (Fig. 17-6). Patients are more likely to demonstrate involvement of the lips (cheilitis).

Hojyo-Tomoka MT, Vega-Memije ME, Cortes-Franco R, Dominguez-Soto L: Diagnosis and treatment of actinic prurigo, *Dermatol Ther* 16:40–44, 2003.

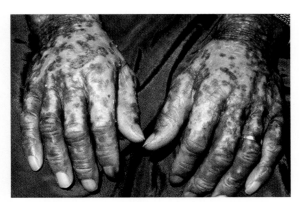

Figure 17-3. Actinic reticuloid. Elderly man with chronic, highly pruritic photosensitivity with erythema, scale, pigmentary changes, and lichenification of the skin. (Courtesy of the Fitzsimons Army Medical Center teaching files.)

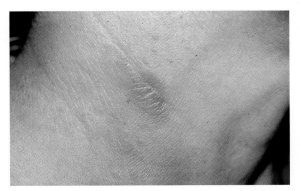

Figure 17-4. Polymorphous light eruption. Erythematous, scaly plaque on the lateral neck, which tended to recur each spring.

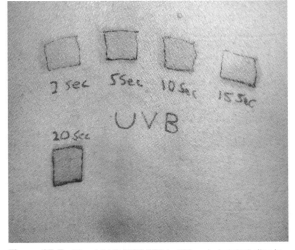

Figure 17-5. Ultraviolet B (UVB) (290 to 320 nm) phototest sites in a patient with polymorphous light eruption demonstrating marked photosensitivity. These test sites were read at 48 hours. (Courtesy of the Fitzsimons Army Medical Center teaching files.)

15. What is solar urticaria?

Urticaria, or hives, may be triggered by ultraviolet or even visible light. The urticarial papules or plaques usually develop on exposed areas within minutes of sun exposure and are accompanied by pain or pruritus. Rarely, systemic reactions leading to anaphylactic shock can occur. Solar urticaria is a photoallergic reaction (type I hypersensitivity response) and is most likely IgE mediated, though direct degranulation of mast cells may also be a pathogenic mechanism.

Ryckaert S, Roelandts R: Solar urticaria: a report of 25 cases and difficulties in phototesting, *Arch Dermatol* 134:71–74, 1998.

16. Discuss the differential diagnosis of photodermatoses in infants or young children.

In the neonatal period, photodermatoses are uncommon, probably due in part to the minimal degree of exposure to sunlight. However, cutaneous lesions of neonatal lupus erythematosus typically occur very early in life and are often photoexacerbated. These patients develop erythematous, often annular plaques, usually distributed on the face and scalp. Cardiac conduction defects may also be seen. Nearly all of these infants and their mothers have circulating anti–Ro/SS-A antibodies and, less commonly, anti–La/SS-B antibodies. The differential diagnosis also includes several genodermatoses that may present as photosensitivity early in life. Other childhood photodermatoses include polymorphous light eruption, photodrug eruptions, photocontact dermatitis, hydroa aestivale, hydroa vacciniforme, erythropoietic protoporphyria, and cutaneous lupus erythematosus (Table 17-3).

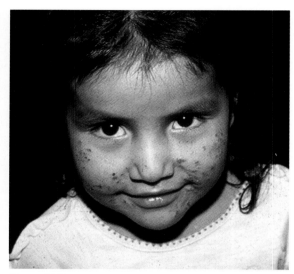

Figure 17-6. Actinic prurigo. Native American child with pruritic photosensitive dermatitis of nose, cheeks, and chin. Note that she also has a low-grade cheilitis on her lower lip. (Courtesy of the Fitzsimons Army Medical Center teaching files.)

17. How do hydroa aestivale and hydroa vacciniforme differ?

These rare, vesiculopapular photoeruptions of unknown etiology occur in childhood. Lesions occur primarily on the face, especially the ears, nose, and cheeks, and on the chest and dorsal hands. Hydroa aestivale occurs more commonly in females and is not associated with scarring. Hydroa vacciniforme is more common in males and heals with shallow, vacciniform scars. There may be an association with Epstein-Barr virus (EBV) in hydroa vacciniforme. Some consider both of these diseases variants of PMLE.

18. Which porphyrias are associated with photodermatoses?

The most common porphyria with prominent cutaneous findings is porphyria cutanea tarda (PCT). There is a delay in the onset of lesions following sun exposure; thus, many PCT patients do not specifically complain of photosensitivity. The cutaneous changes seen in PCT may also be seen in other porphyrias, including variegate porphyria and hereditary coproporphyria; in pseudoporphyrias associated with hemodialysis; and with certain medications, such as furosemide, nalidixic acid, tetracycline, and naproxen (referred to as pseudoporphyria).

More acute photosensitivity is seen in erythropoietic protoporphyria, congenital erythropoietic porphyria, and erythropoietic coproporphyria and is manifested by burning and stinging within minutes of exposure, followed by erythema, blistering, and scarring if severe.

19. Describe the cutaneous changes in porphyria cutanea tarda.

Skin fragility with minor trauma is a common complaint, particularly over the dorsal fingers and hands. Skin lesions are usually found on the dorsal hands, fingers, and feet and sometimes on the face and upper trunk. Tense vesicles and bullae develop in these sites and heal with erosions, scarring, atrophy, milia, and pigmentary changes (Fig. 17-7). Hypertrichosis and thickened, sclerotic plaques may develop on the face and chest. Patients may not relate the skin changes to sun exposure, but on questioning, they often have a history of worsening in the summer months or following other periods of intense sun exposure.

20. What causes porphyria cutanea tarda?

The porphyrias are due to specific enzyme deficiencies that lead to accumulation of porphyrins. Porphyrins absorb light in the 400- to 410-nm (Soret band) range, in the lower range of visible light. This absorbed light energy is then transferred to cellular structures or to molecular oxygen, causing damage to tissues.

PCT is due to a deficiency of the enzyme uroporphyrinogen decarboxylase. There are two main categories of PCT patients, acquired and hereditary. Patients with acquired PCT have the enzyme deficiency in the liver only and often

Table 17-3. Genodermatoses Associated with Photosensitivity

DISEASE	SKIN FINDINGS	INHERITANCE	OTHER
Xeroderma pigmentosum	Lentigines, skin cancers, photoaging	Autosomal recessive	Photophobia, keratitis, corneal opacification and vascularization, neurologic abnormalities: hyporeflexia, deafness, seizures (most common in groups A and D; do not usually occur in XP variant). XP variant patients usually have no neurologic problems. Complementation groups A to G: defective global genomic nucleotide excision repair (GG-NER) of UVR-induced DNA damage (e.g., pyrimidine dimers) from any part of the genome
Cockayne's syndrome	Photosensitivity without pigmentary changes or increased risk of skin cancer. Scaly facial photodermatitis	Autosomal recessive	Loss of adipose tissue, prominent ears, dental caries, thinning of skin and hair. Hypogonadism, stooped posture, joint contractures, short stature with extremely thin body habitus ("cachectic dwarfism"), microcephaly, mental retardation, deafness. Calcification of basal ganglia, demyelination, pigmentary retinal degeneration, osteoporosis. Cockayne's syndrome (CS) cells are defective in the repair of pyrimidine dimer photoproducts and oxidative DNA base modifications typically induced by UVB and UVA, respectively. Two complementation groups: CS-A (mutations in *ERCC8*) and CS-B (mutations in *ERCC6*); identical phenotypes. Mutations in *XPB*, *XPD*, and *XPG* genes have been associated with combined XP/CS phenotypes
Trichothiodystrophy	Ichthyosis, brittle hair. Hair shaft: alternating light and dark bands ("tiger tail banding"), trichoschisis, trichorrhexis nodosa	Autosomal recessive	PIBI(D)S: photosensitivity, ichthyosis, brittle hair, intellectual impairment, decreased fertility, short stature. Other features: microcephaly, receding chin, protruding ears. Mutations in *XPD*, *XPB*, general transcription factor IIH polypeptide 5 (*GTF2H5* or *TFB5*), and *C7orf11*
UV-sensitive syndrome (UVsS)	Photosensitivity, solar lentigines	Autosomal recessive	Similar to CS: defective TC-NER, normal GG-NER; however, unlike CS, patients with UVsS only have defective in repair of UVB-induced photoproducts (not repair of oxidative damage). Two complementation groups: mutations in *ERCC6*, and an undefined gene.
Bloom's syndrome	Malar erythema and telangiectasias, café-au-lait macules, hypopigmentation	Autosomal recessive	Elongated face with malar hypoplasia and prominent nose, short stature, diabetes mellitus, recurrent infections. Small at birth, severe growth retardation, respiratory infections, malignancy. Increased frequency of leukemia, lymphoma, GI adenocarcinoma. Men: sterile; women: reduced fertility. Normal intelligence. Decreased IgA, IgM, sometimes IgG. Mutations in BLM (*RECQL3*), resulting in chromosomal instability (increased sister chromatid exchanges, chromosomal breakage and rearrangement). Quadriradial configurations in lymphocytes and fibroblasts are diagnostic.

Continued

Table 17-3. Genodermatoses Associated with Photosensitivity—cont'd

DISEASE	SKIN FINDINGS	INHERITANCE	OTHER
Rothmund-Thomson syndrome	Erythema, edema and vesicles on the cheeks and face during the first few months of life, followed by poikiloderma that also typically affects the dorsal aspect of the hands/forearms and the buttocks. Sparse hair (scalp, eyebrows, eyelashes), hypoplastic nails, acral keratoses (in adolescents and adults)	Autosomal recessive syndrome	Cataracts, usually normal intelligence, and cerebellar ataxia. Short stature, skeletal (e.g., radial ray defects, osteoporosis) and dental abnormalities, juvenile cataracts, chronic diarrhea/vomiting during infancy, pituitary hypogonadism (may be associated with midface hypoplasia/ "saddle nose"). Osteosarcoma (10%230%), squamous cell carcinoma (,5%; often acral). Normal immune function, intelligence, and lifespan (in the absence of malignancy). Mutations in *RECQL4*; protein product is a DNA helicase. Genomic instability may account for propensity for malignancies.
Hartnup's disease	Pellagra-like eruption	Autosomal recessive	Intermittent ataxia, which may be accompanied by nystagmus and tremors. Psychiatric disturbances and other nonspecific neurologic abnormalities have been reported in some patients, but significant mental retardation is not a feature. Defective renal and intestinal neutral amino acid transport. Marked aminoaciduria and tryptophan deficiency.
Kindler syndrome	Poikiloderma, trauma-induced skin blistering, mucosal inflammation	Autosomal recessive	Subtype of epidermolysis bullosa (EB). Loss-of-function mutations in the *FERMT1* gene. Clinical overlap between Kindler syndrome and dystrophic EB. Unlike other forms of EB, Kindler syndrome is characterized by impaired actin cytoskeleton-extracellular matrix interactions and a variable plane of blister formation at or close to the dermal–epidermal junction.

Data from Online Mendelian Inheritance in Man (OMIM). McKusick-Nathans Institute of Genetic Medicine, Johns Hopkins University (Baltimore, MD) and National Center for Biotechnology Information, National Library of Medicine (Bethesda, MD). Available at: http://www.ncbi.nlm.nih.gov/omim/.

have attacks triggered by agents such as alcohol, estrogen, hexachlorobenzene, and iron. PCT may also develop in patients with chronic liver disease (e.g., hepatitis C infection or hemochromatosis). In hereditary PCT, uroporphyrinogen decarboxylase is deficient in most tissues, not just the liver. Both heterozygous and homozygous inheritances of enzyme deficiencies have been described.

21. How is porphyria cutanea tarda diagnosed?

Fluorescent spectrophotometric analysis of plasma is a rapid screen for porphyria. Plasma is exposed to an excitation wavelength of 400 to 410 nm, and the emission peaks are measured. A sharp emission peak at 619 nm confirms a porphyrin disorder. To differentiate the specific porphyrins further, a 24-hour urine specimen is submitted for porphyrin studies. In PCT, the major porphyrins elevated in urine are uroporphyrin I and 7-carboxylporphyrin III. In addition, stool porphyrins should be tested; PCT patients have normal levels of protoporphyrins but increased isocoproporphyrins in the stool.

22. How is variegate porphyria distinguished from porphyria cutanea tarda?

Variegate porphyria (VP) may produce cutaneous lesions that are indistinguishable from those seen in PCT, but patients with VP have increased levels of protoporphyrins in their stool and only moderately increased urine porphyrins. Unlike PCT patients, VP patients often have acute attacks of porphyria (gastrointestinal pain and neurologic deficits) similar to those seen in patients with acute intermittent porphyria, and thus it is important to distinguish VP from PCT.

23. What treatments are used in porphyria cutanea tarda?

- Eliminate any agents that may trigger PCT, such as alcohol.
- Protect from both ultraviolet and visible light.

- Phlebotomy is most often the treatment of choice. Phlebotomy is believed to work by decreasing excessive iron stores. Removal of about 500 mL of whole blood is done at periodic intervals as tolerated, until the hemoglobin level is about 10 to 11 gm/dL or until side effects are experienced.
- Low-dose hydrochloroquine or hydroxychloroquine therapy is an alternate treatment that requires very close monitoring for hepatotoxicity.

24. What are the cutaneous findings in erythropoietic protoporphyria?

Patients with erythropoietic protoporphyria usually have complaints beginning in childhood, though cases presenting in adult life are well documented. Photosensitivity may be severe, with almost immediate burning and stinging of the exposed skin following sun exposure. Erythema, edema, hivelike lesions, vesicles, and purpura may then develop, particularly on the nose, cheeks, and dorsal hands (Fig. 17-8). With time, these areas develop atrophic, waxy scars. The skin over the knuckles may become thickened, wrinkled, and shiny, giving the appearance of very aged hands.

25. How is a diagnosis of erythropoietic protoporphyria made?

Erythropoietic protoporphyria is believed to be due to a deficiency of the enzyme ferrochelatase. Red blood cells (RBCs) and feces show increased levels of protoporphyrins. In addition, if fresh RBCs are examined with a fluorescence microscope, 5% to 30% of RBCs will fluoresce a coral red color. This fluorescence is transient and light sensitive; thus, RBCs should be collected and examined in a dark room.

Murphy GM: Diagnosis and management of the erythropoietic porphyrias, *Dermatol Ther* 16:57–64, 2003.

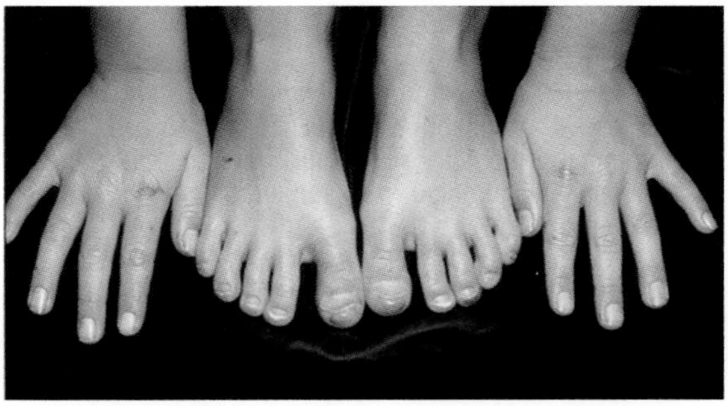

26. What treatments are used in erythropoietic protoporphyria?

Therapy is primarily preventative, aimed at protecting the skin from ultraviolet and visible radiation. Beta-carotene capsules given orally have anecdotally been shown to ameliorate the disease.

Alemzadeh R, Feehan T: Variable effects of beta-carotene therapy in a child with erythropoietic protoporphyria, *Eur J Pediatr* 163:547–549, 2004.

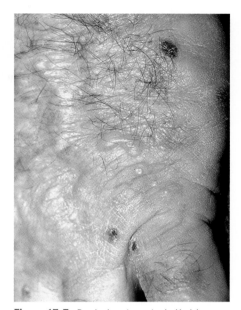

Figure 17-7. Porphyria cutanea tarda. Vesicles, crusts, and milia on the hand of a patient with alcohol-triggered PCT.

Figure 17-8. Erythropoietic protoporphyria. Young child with intense photosensitivity of hands and feet (associated with wearing sandals) manifesting as tense blisters, crusting, and very early thickening of the skin. (Courtesy of the Fitzsimons Army Medical Center teaching files.)

27. Do any other medical problems occur in patients with erythropoietic protoporphyria?

About 11% of patients with erythropoietic protoporphyria have a mild anemia of unknown etiology. Cholelithiasis is seen and may occur at a very early age. Liver disease is common but only rarely leads to fatal hepatic failure.

28. Name some other photorelated disorders.

Sunburn, immediate pigment darkening versus tanning, cutaneous and some systemic immunosuppression, vitamin D3 synthesis, actinic keratoses (AKs), skin cancers, photoaging, solar elastosis, solar lentigo, ephelide, poikiloderma of Civatte, Favre-Racouchot syndrome, colloid milium, erosive pustular dermatosis of the scalp, middermal elastolysis, actinic granulolma (annular elastolytic granuloma), giant cell arteritis, and brachioradial pruritus.

1. Are some disorders of pigmentation markers for systemic disease?

Yes. Examples include the following:
- Generalized depigmentation: Albinism
- Generalized hyperpigmentation: Addison's disease
- Ash-leaf hypopigmented macules: Tuberous sclerosis
- Axillary and inguinal freckles: Neurofibromatosis
- Lentigines: Peutz-Jeghers syndrome

2. How do you diagnose a pigmentation disorder?

The clinical history is the most important aspect of the investigation of a pigmentation disorder. It should focus on the time of onset (such as at birth, during childhood, or later in life) and a family history. Other facts to be determined include any associated illness or symptoms, drug ingestion, chemical exposure, occupation, and exposure to sunlight, artificial ultraviolet light, heat, or ionizing radiation. Finally, a careful review of systems should be performed, followed by a skin examination.

3. What are the important elements of a skin examination of a patient with a pigmentation disorder?

The entire skin surface should be evaluated with attention to the color, shape, and distribution of the lesion(s). Lesion **color** helps to place the disorder into a specific category to aid in narrowing the diagnostic possibilities. The **shape** of a lesion is sometimes diagnostic. Linear areas of depigmentation, often in areas of trauma, are suggestive for vitiligo, whereas ash-leaf–shaped hypopigmented macules suggest tuberous sclerosis. **Distribution** of pigmentary changes also helps in diagnosis. Symmetrical depigmentation on the arms, legs, and/or torso suggests vitiligo. Increased pigmentation of the oral mucosa, axillae, and palmar creases is associated with Addison's disease.

Other diagnostic tests: Wood's lamp examination is sometimes helpful. Skin biopsy, with or without special stains for melanin (silver nitrate or the Fontana-Masson stain), determines epidermal melanocyte number and the extent and location of epidermal and dermal pigmentation.

4. What is a Wood's lamp?

A hand-held black light. A Wood's lamp emits light in a narrow spectrum of long-wave ultraviolet to short-wave visible light. Hypopigmented areas appear lighter, and depigmented areas appear pure white. Furthermore, epidermal hyperpigmentation is enhanced (appears darker), whereas dermal hyperpigmentation is not enhanced.

LEUKODERMA: PARTIAL OR COMPLETE LOSS OF SKIN PIGMENTATION

5. Name some heritable forms of leukoderma.

- **Albinism** is a group of autosomal recessive disorders characterized by generalized depigmented or hypopigmented skin and decreased visual acuity and nystagmus secondary to alterations in the formation of melanin.
- **Waardenburg's syndrome** is an autosomal dominant disorder associated with congenital deafness, heterochromic irides, amelanotic skin macules, white forelock, laterally displaced medial canthi, and widening of the nasal root.
- **Hermansky-Pudlak syndrome** is rare autosomal recessive disorder in which affected individuals suffer from generalized hypopigmentation, excessive bleeding due to platelet abnormalities, and lysosomal defects leading to ceroid accumulation in most body tissues.

Dessinioti C, Stratigos AJ, Rigopoulous D, Katsambas AD: A review of genetic disorders of hypopigmentation: lessons learned from the biology of melanocytes, *Exp Dermatol* 18:741–749, 2009.

6. Name the skin disorder that manifests with complete loss of skin pigmentation.

Vitiligo is a depigmenting disorder due to loss of epidermal melanocytes. There are both familial and nonfamilial forms, and the overall incidence is 1% in the United States. Vitiligo has been reported to be associated with autoimmune disorders, including thyroid disease and diabetes mellitus type 1. The pathogenesis is not totally understood. Curiously enough, patients have both circulating antimelanocyte antibodies and skin-homing melanocyte-specific cytotoxic T lymphocytes. How these two portions of the immune system interact to result in melanocyte destruction is not understood. Vitiligo affects all races and affects both sexes equally.

Halder RM, Chappell JL: Vitiligo update, *Semin Cutan Med Surg* 28:86–92, 2009.

7. Describe the clinical appearance of the skin lesions in vitiligo.

Typically, lesions of vitiligo are stark white with a well-demarcated border and no other skin changes. Sometimes, the border is hyperpigmented and rarely erythematous. Areas commonly affected are the periorbital, perioral, and anogenital areas, as well as the elbows, knees, axillae, inguinal folds, and forearms. Frequently, lesions of vitiligo develop symmetrically on the trunk and extremities (Fig. 18-1A). Vitiligo also causes depigmentation of hair (leukotrichia). Less commonly vitiligo is focal or segmental (Fig. 18-1B).

8. When does vitiligo have its onset?

The peak incidence occurs in the third decade of life, but 50% of cases occur before age 20. Vitiligo has been reported in all age groups with onset as early as birth and as late as 81 years.

9. Do any factors influence the onset of vitiligo?

The patient presenting with vitiligo usually describes asymptomatic areas of skin that have rapidly lost all pigment. Rarely does the patient recall an associated illness, but skin trauma is commonly reported to cause vitiligo lesions. One caveat: Vitiligo occurs only in patients predisposed to the condition. Thus skin trauma will not induce vitiligo in nonpredisposed individuals.

10. Is vitiligo treatable?

Yes. Vitiligo repigments in small part from the border and mostly from the hair follicle. Localized vitiligo may be treated with high-potency topical steroids, topical tacrolimus and pimecrolimus, as well as topical calcipotriene. For more generalized vitiligo, narrow-band ultraviolet light B (UVB, 311 nm) is now the treatment of choice. It must be administered 2 to 3 times weekly for many months. All patients with vitiligo should use sunscreens to protect depigmented skin from sun damage.

Lotti T, Buggiani G, Troiano M, et al: Targeted and combination treatments for vitiligo. Comparative evaluation of different current modalities in 458 subjects, *Dermatol Ther* 21(Suppl 1):S20–S26, 2008.

Key Points: Normal Skin Pigmentation: A Combination of Four Pigments in the Epidermis and Dermis

1. Oxygenated hemoglobin (red) in the arterioles and capillaries.
2. Deoxygenated hemoglobin (blue) in the venules.
3. Any ingested carotenoids or incompletely metabolized bile (yellow).
4. Epidermal melanin (brown), which is synthesized by epidermal melanocytes. Melanin is the most important pigment in determining skin color.

Key Points: Racial Differences in Pigmentation

1. Pigmentation is determined by the type of melanin synthesized and the amount distributed to the surrounding keratinocytes.
2. Fair-skinned people produce a light brown form of melanin (pheomelanin), and distribute only small amounts to surrounding keratinocytes.
3. Melanocytes of darkly pigmented individuals produce a dark brown form of melanin (eumelanin), and distribute large amounts of it to neighboring keratinocytes.
4. All of the skin colors in between are due to a mixture of light brown pheomelanin and dark brown eumelanin.

Key Points: Pigmentation Disorders

1. Most patients, over a lifetime, will suffer from a pigmentation disorder.
2. Fortunately, the most common pigmentation disorders are benign, self-limited, and reversible. For example, one of the most common develops following a cutaneous inflammatory reaction, when the skin is either more darkly pigmented (postinflammatory hyperpigmentation) or less pigmented (postinflammatory hypopigmentation) than surrounding normal skin.
3. Postinflammatory changes in pigmentation slowly revert to normal over several months.
4. The two major types of cutaneous dyspigmentation are leukoderma and melanoderma. Patients with leukoderma present with areas of skin that appear lighter than surrounding normal skin, whereas patients with melanoderma have skin that appears darker than normal.
5. The major forms of cutaneous dyspigmentation can be broken down into subtypes, depending on whether there is alteration in melanocyte number or pigment content of the skin.

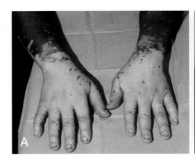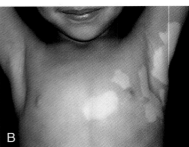

Figure 18-1. Vitiligo. **A,** African-American man with vitiligo. Note the complete loss of skin pigmentation of the hands and wrists. **B,** Segmental vitiligo. (Courtesy of James E. Fitzpatrick, MD.)

Key Points: Sun-tanning

1. Sunlight stimulates human epidermal melanocytes to increase melanin synthesis and stimulates increased melanocyte transfer of melanosomes to keratinocytes. This melanocyte response to sunlight is called *tanning*.
2. The action spectrum of sunlight that causes tanning is the ultraviolet spectrum (wavelengths 290 to 400 nm).
3. Excess sunlight exposure causes abnormal melanocyte function, resulting in areas of melanocyte overproduction of melanin and increased melanocyte proliferation.
4. Overproduction of melanin in a localized area causes the development of brown macules called *freckles*.
5. Skin lesions that are made up of increased numbers of keratinocytes and melanocytes with increased melanin synthesis are called *solar lentigines*.

11. What is piebaldism?
Piebaldism is an uncommon autosomal dominant depigmentation disorder that is characterized by a white scalp forelock and hyperpigmented macules within areas of skin depigmentation. Piebaldism is due to mutations on the *KIT* protooncogene that is located on chromosome 4. A normal KIT receptor is required for normal development and migration of melanocytes. Melanocytes migrate during embryologic development in a dorsal-to-ventral direction; melanocytes in piebaldism fail to properly migrate to ventral skin surfaces, such as the forehead, abdomen, and volar arms and legs. For this reason, depigmented areas in piebaldism predominate on ventral skin surfaces. Patients are otherwise healthy. There is no treatment available for piebaldism.

12. What is albinism?
Albinism is a group of inherited disorders of the melanin pigment system. All forms are autosomal recessive. In oculocutaneous albinism type 1 (OCA1), there is a defect in the enzyme tyrosinase with an absence in melanin synthesis. Generally, albinism presents as depigmented or hypopigmented skin and hair, nystagmus, photophobia, and decreased visual acuity (Fig. 18-2). There are four different forms of oculocutaneous albinism. Some forms affect the skin, hair, and eyes (oculocutaneous albinism); other forms primarily affect the eyes (ocular albinism). There is no treatment available for albinism.

13. How does albinism differ from the other inherited leukodermas?
The common feature of vitiligo, piebaldism, and the rarer leukoderma syndromes is a decrease or total absence of epidermal melanocytes. By comparison, patients with albinism have a normal epidermal melanocyte number, but the melanocytes synthesize inadequate amounts of melanin.

14. Can disorders of amino acid metabolism cause leukoderma?
Yes. See Table 18-1.

15. How do chemicals cause skin depigmentation or skin hypopigmentation?
Monobenzyl ether of hydroquinone (MBEH) and para–substituted phenols (PSP) cause skin depigmentation by destroying melanocytes. It is believed that both MBEH and PSP are taken up by melanocytes and metabolized into toxic products that kill the melanocytes. Hydroquinone, a commonly used skin-lightening agent, causes decreased melanin synthesis by competing with tyrosine and dihydroxyphenylalanine for the enzyme tyrosinase. With hydroquinone bound to its active site, tyrosinase is unable to synthesize melanin. Other chemicals, such as arsenic, mercaptoethyl amines, chloroquine, hydroxychloroquine, and corticosteroids, act to metabolically suppress melanocytes, resulting in decreased melanin synthesis and skin lightening. In most cases, the effects of these chemicals are reversible.

16. Can patients with nutritional disorders suffer from leukoderma?
Yes. Patients suffering from protein loss or deficiency diseases, including kwashiorkor, intestinal malabsorption, and nephrotic syndrome, often manifest with facial, truncal, and extremity hypopigmentation. The hypopigmentation is believed to be due to dysregulation of normal melanogenesis secondary to lack of amino acid precursors for melanin synthesis and for normal melanin polymer formation. Normal pigmentation returns following treatment of the nutritional disorder.

17. What disorders should the clinician consider in a patient with hypopigmented macules and patches?

Tuberous sclerosis, nevus depigmentosus, hypomelanosis of Ito, sarcoidosis, discoid lupus erythematosus, cutaneous T-cell lymphoma, eczema, psoriasis, secondary syphilis, leprosy, and tinea versicolor.

18. What is tuberous sclerosis?

Tuberous sclerosis, an autosomal dominant disorder with an incidence of 1/6000 births, is a multifaceted disorder that causes tumors in nearly every organ in the body. See Chapter 5, Neurocutaneous Disorders.

19. What is nevus depigmentosus?

Nevus depigmentosus consists of single or multiple hypopigmented macules or patches that grow proportionally with the patient. The trunk is the most commonly affected body area. However, nevus depigmentosus has been reported to occur on the extremities, buttocks, and face, and may be localized, segmental, or, less often, systematized. Most lesions present by age 3 years with the remainder (about 7%) presenting later in childhood. Lesion morphology varies from circumscribed irregular, oval, or round macules or patches to a unilateral band or streak with a "splashed paint" appearance arranged along one or more Blaschko line. Lesional skin has normal melanocyte number but reduced numbers of melanosomes in melanocytes and surrounding keratinocytes. The etiopathogenesis has not been fully established.

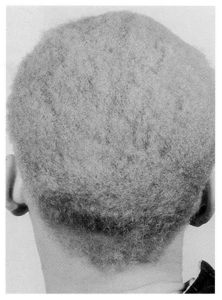

Figure 18-2. Albino African-American boy with generalized hypopigmentation.

20. How does nevus depigmentosus compare to hypomelanosis of Ito?

Some experts believe nevus depigmentosus to be a less severe form of hypomelanosis of Ito. The skin lesions of hypomelanosis of Ito very closely resemble those of nevus depigmentosus. However, hypomelanosis of Ito lesions are larger and more widespread. Moreover, 15% to 25% of hypomelanosis of Ito patients suffer from disorders of the central nervous system, eyes, hair, teeth, and musculoskeletal system. There is no single molecular mechanism underlying hypomelanosis of Ito. Some authorities believe that hypomelanosis of Ito should be referred to as linear and whorled nevoid hypomelanosis.

21. Which infectious disorders can have associated leukoderma?

Secondary syphilis, pinta, yaws, onchocerciasis, and leprosy. The inflammatory reaction associated with these diseases alters melanocyte homeostasis, with resultant decreased melanin synthesis and transfer to keratinocytes.

22. Describe the pigmentation changes seen with the treponematoses.

- **Secondary syphilis:** Hypopigmented macules can be found on the neck, shoulders, upper chest, and axillae in patients with secondary syphilis (due to *Treponema pallidum*). The hypopigmented neck lesions have been termed the "necklace of Venus."

Table 18-1. Inherited Disorders of Amino Acid Metabolism with Related Leukoderma

DISORDER	AFFECTED AMINO ACID	INCIDENCE	INHERITANCE	MANIFESTATIONS
Phenylketonuria	Phenylalanine	1:10,000	AR	Hypopigmentation of hair, eyes, and skin; mental retardation if not treated early
Histidinemia	Histidine	1:12,000	AR	Hypopigmentation, mental retardation
Homocystinuria	Methionine	1:58,000 to 1:1,000,000 depending on geographic region	AR	Hypopigmentation of skin, hair, and eyes; CNS abnormalities; skeletal abnormalities (Marfan's syndrome–like); thromboembolic disease

AR, Autosomal recessive.

- **Pinta:** Pinta is a chronic nonvenereal disease caused by *T. carateum* that is endemic in Central and South America. The primary lesion, at the site of inoculation, is a hypopigmented patch or plaque on the arm, leg, or torso. Secondary pinta lesions (pintides) are at first erythematous, then become hyper- and hypopigmented. Later in the disease, pinta lesions become more uniformly hypopigmented.
- **Yaws:** Yaws is a nonvenereal disease caused by *T. pallidum* subspecies pertenue that is common in children in impoverished, very warm, tropical areas of Africa. It may also be seen in Southeast Asia, the Pacific Islands, and tropical America. The primary lesion heals as an atrophic hypopigmented scar. Secondary yaws often heals without dyspigmentation, but the gummatous tertiary yaws lesions localized to the lower extremities, volar wrists, and dorsal hands are depigmented.

23. What cutaneous lesions are seen with Hansen's disease?

Hansen's disease, or leprosy, is a chronic infectious disease caused by *Mycobacterium leprae*. *M. leprae* infects the skin and peripheral nerves and in some patients may produce anesthetic, hypopigmented patches, plaques, or nodules. Patients with indeterminate and tuberculoid leprosy have one or few lesions, whereas patients with lepromatous leprosy have many lesions. Lesions may repigment following antibiotic cure.

24. Why is lesional skin of tinea versicolor frequently hypopigmented?

Tinea (pityriasis) versicolor is caused by overgrowth of the normal skin flora of several species of yeast in the genus *Malassezia* (*Pityrosporum*) including *M. globosa, M. sympodialis, M. furfur, M. obtusa,* and *M. slooffiae.* In its pathogenic hyphal form, *Malassezia* secretes an enzyme that breaks down epidermal unsaturated fatty acids to azelaic acid, which inhibits melanocyte tyrosinase. Tinea versicolor is common in tropical and temperate climates and is found in all races and age groups. The typical lesion is a scaly, slightly erythematous macule or patch located on the proximal anterior and posterior torso (Fig. 18-3). Tinea versicolor may be either hypopigmented or hyperpigmented.

Prohic A, Ozegovic L: *Malassezia* species isolated from lesional and non-lesional skin in patients with pityriasis versicolor, *Mycoses* 50:58–63, 2007.

MELANODERMA: ABNORMAL DARKENING OF THE SKIN

25. What are lentigines? What heritable disorders manifest these?

Lentigines are brown to dark brown, 1- to 5-mm macules that may occur on any cutaneous surface. They resemble freckles, but on biopsy, these lesions have increased numbers of melanocytes and increased melanocyte and basal keratinocyte pigmentation.

A benign condition characterized by the rapid development of hundreds of lentigines widespread over the skin surface in adolescents or young adults has been described. However, the presence of multiple lentigines at a young age is suggestive of autosomal dominant disorders, especially Moynahan's syndrome or Peutz-Jeghers syndrome (Fig. 18-4).

26. Why is it important to identify patients with Peutz-Jeghers syndrome?

Patients with Peutz-Jeghers syndrome have widespread cutaneous lentigines that involve the arms, legs, torso, digits, lips, buccal mucosa, palate, tongue, and eyelids. In addition, they suffer from gastrointestinal (GI) polyps, usually in the small bowel, which, by the second decade of life, can become symptomatic with diarrhea, hemorrhage, obstruction, or intussusception. Malignant degeneration of GI polyps has been reported, with carcinomas developing most commonly in the large intestine but also in the small intestine and stomach.

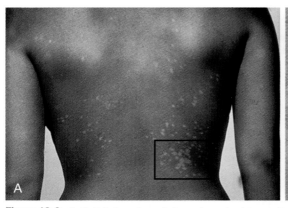 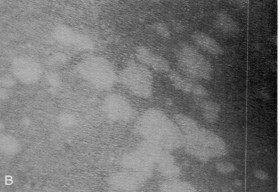

Figure 18-3. A, Multiple hypopigmented macules and patches on the torso of a woman with tinea versicolor. **B,** Enlargement of area in **A** outlined by rectangle.

27. Describe the clinical manifestations of Moynahan's syndrome.

Patients with Moynahan's syndrome have hundreds of lentigines on the face, trunk, and extremities. Less commonly they may also demonstrate café-au-lait macules (Fig. 18-5). The mnemonic **LEOPARD** has been applied to the clinical symptoms associated with this syndrome:

- **L**entigines
- **E**lectrocardiographic conduction defects
- **O**cular hypertelorism
- **P**ulmonic stenosis
- **A**bnormal genitalia
- Growth **R**etardation
- Sensorineural **D**eafness

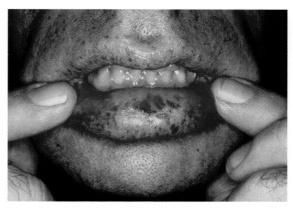

Figure 18-4. A 45-year-old man with numerous hyperpigmented macules of Peutz-Jeghers syndrome.

28. Are there pigmentation disorders associated with neurofibromatosis?

Yes. Common pigmented lesions of neurofibromatosis 1 (NF1, von Recklinghausen's disease) are café-au-lait macules (CALM) and inguinal and axillary freckling. CALM are, as the name would imply, flat, tan to light brown lesions located anywhere on the body; these range from a few millimeters to several centimeters in diameter. Greater than 90% of CALM of NF1 are present at birth or appear within the first year of life.

CALM are relatively common, and a patient must have six or more for the diagnosis of NF1 to be considered. If six or more are present, the absolute number of CALM does not correlate with the development of other systemic problems associated with NF1. NF1 is a relatively common autosomal dominant disorder that occurs in 1:3000 live births.

29. Do any other disorders manifest with CALM?

Yes. In 1937, Albright reported a syndrome consisting of osteitis fibrosa disseminata, endocrine dysfunction with precocious puberty in females, and CALM. The CALM of Albright's syndrome differ from those of NF1 by being larger and occurring predominantly on the forehead, posterior neck, sacrum, and buttocks. CALM of Albright's syndrome tend to be unilateral and do not cross the midline, whereas CALM of NF1 exist in a random, generalized pattern. CALM of Albright's syndrome appear at or soon after birth.

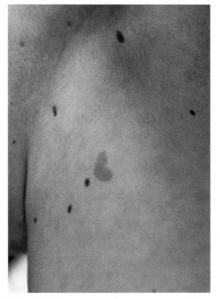

Figure 18-5. LEOPARD syndrome. Numerous oval, flat, brown lentigines and a solitary café-au-lait macule. (Courtesy of the William L. Weston, M.D. collection.)

30. What is Becker's melanosis?

Becker's melanosis (also known as Becker's pigmented hairy hamartoma or Becker's nevus) is a benign pigmented lesion that develops in the second or third decade of life with a male:female ratio of 5:1. There is no predominance of race, and one large study reported a prevalence of 0.52% in males between ages 17 and 26 years. Greater than 80% of lesions occur on the trunk, appearing as a tan to dark brown patch with an irregular border ranging in size from 100 to 500 cm^2. Excess hair growth has been reported in 56% of cases. With onset in the teen years and young adulthood, Becker's melanosis is easily differentiated from a congenital nevus and CALM of Albright's syndrome, which are present at birth. Once fully developed, Becker's melanosis remains stable for the life of the patient.

31. What is a nevus spilus?

Nevus spilus is a CALM that contains darkly pigmented, 1- to 3-mm–diameter macules or papules. The lesion is present at birth and can involve any cutaneous surface. The darkly pigmented macules and papules of nevus spilus are junctional or compound nevi.

32. Do any natural factors stimulate human epidermal pigmentation?

Yes. The following factors have been reported to enhance melanocyte growth and pigmentation:

- Melanocyte-stimulating hormone
- Insulin-like growth factor
- Adrenocorticotropic hormone
- Stem cell factor
- Endothelin-1
- Nerve growth factor
- Basic fibroblast growth factor
- Leukotriene C4 and B4
- KIT ligand (formerly steel factor)
- Leukemia inhibitory factor
- Hepatocyte growth factor
- Granulocyte-macrophage colony–stimulating factor

Hirobe T: Role of keratinocyte-derived factors involved in regulating the proliferation and differentiation of mammalian epidermal melanocytes, *Pigment Cell Res* 18:2–12, 2005.

33. What drugs are used to stimulate skin pigmentation? How do they work?

The psoralens or furocoumarins, potent photosensitizing drugs, have been used for thousands of years to stimulate skin pigmentation. The most commonly used agent in dermatology for skin photosensitization is 8-methoxypsoralen (8-MOP). The exact mechanism of skin photosensitization is not known, but 8-MOP is preferentially taken up by epidermal cells, where it binds to cell membranes and is concentrated within cell nuclei. Upon photoactivation, 8-MOP causes alteration in cell membrane signaling and forms covalent bonds with DNA that lead to the formation of psoralen-DNA adducts. Together, the altered cell membrane signaling and psoralen-DNA adducts incite a cascade of events that stimulate melanocyte melanin synthesis and melanin transfer to keratinocytes, resulting in increased skin pigmentation.

34. Can other drugs cause increased skin pigmentation?

Yes. Arsenicals, busulfan, 5-fluorouracil, cyclophosphamide, topical nitrogen mustard (mechlorethamine), and bleomycin most commonly cause increased skin pigmentation. The mechanisms by which these drugs cause hyperpigmentation are unknown, but it is possible that the drug or a metabolite either directly stimulates epidermal melanocytes to increase melanin synthesis or indirectly stimulates metabolic pathways that cause increased epidermal melanization.

Litt J, editor: *Litt's drug eruption reference manual*, ed 15, New York, 2009, Informa Healthcare.

35. Can endocrine and metabolic disorders cause altered skin pigmentation?

Yes. Addison's disease is the prototype disorder with diffuse hypermelanosis associated with pigment accentuation in mucous membranes, skin folds, palmar creases, and pressure points (elbows, knees, knuckles, and coccyx). Adrenocorticotropic hormone (ACTH) or melanocyte-stimulating hormone (MSH)–producing tumors can cause increased skin pigmentation. Similarly, systemic administration of ACTH and MSH may cause skin hyperpigmentation. Pregnancy and estrogen therapy can cause hyperpigmentation, usually of the nipples and anogenital skin. Additionally, a masklike hyperpigmentation, called melasma, can develop on the forehead, temples, cheeks, nose, and upper lip in pregnant women and women receiving estrogen therapy.

Patients with porphyria cutanea tarda can have profound hyperpigmentation of sun-exposed skin associated with facial hirsutism. Nutritional disorders, such kwashiorkor, pellagra, and intestinal malabsorption, can cause skin hyperpigmentation along with areas of hypopigmentation.

36. Can forms of radiation other than ultraviolet radiation cause increased skin pigmentation?

Yes. Thermal (infrared) and ionizing radiation skin injury can result in hyperpigmentation, probably due to melanocyte-stimulating inflammatory mediators and immune cytokines released in response to injury from these different forms of radiation.

BLUE-GRAY DYSPIGMENTATION

37. Are there other types of dyspigmentation besides leukoderma and melanoderma?

Yes. Blue-gray skin discoloration can develop from melanin in dermal melanocytes, dermal melanin deposition, or nonmelanin dermal dyspigmentation (Table 18-2).

38. Name the different types of hyperpigmentation due to excess numbers of dermal melanocytes.

Mongolian spot, nevus of Ota, and nevus of Ito.

39. Differentiate a nevus of Ota from a nevus of Ito.

Nevus of Ota (oculodermal melanocytosis) is an acquired disorder of dermal melanocytosis with an age of onset in early childhood or young adulthood. Less than 1% of Asiatic individuals are affected, and non-Asiatic races are affected

Table 18-2. Classification of Dermal Hyperpigmentation

INCREASED MELANOCYTE NUMBER	INCREASED MELANIN	NONMELANIN PIGMENTS
Genetic		
Mongolian spot	–	–
Nevus of Ota	–	–
Nevus of Ito	–	–
Chemical or Drug		
–	Fixed drug eruption	Silver
–	–	Mercury
–	–	Bismuth
–	–	Gold
–	–	Antimalarials
–	–	Phenothiazines
–	–	Minocycline
–	–	Amiodarone
–	–	
Endocrine or Metabolic		
–	Chronic nutritional deficiency	–
–	Melasma	Ochronosis
Physical		
–	Erythema ab igne	–
Inflammation and Infection		
–	Macular amyloidosis	–
–	Erythema dyschromicum perstans	–
–	Postinflammatory hyperpigmentation	–

even less frequently. Females are affected five times more frequently than males, with color hues ranging from dark brown, to purplish-brown, to blue-black. In its most common form, it involves the periorbital skin of one eye, although bilateral forms can occur, and pigmentation can extend to involve the temple, forehead, periorbital cheek, nose areas, and ocular structures (Fig. 18-6).

A variant of nevus of Ota, called nevus of Ito, can occur over the shoulder and neck region and has the same natural history as nevus of Ota.

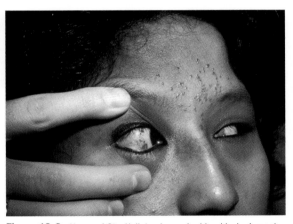

Figure 18-6. Nevus of Ota. Unilateral macular blue-black pigment affecting the forehead, cheek, and ocular mucosa. (Courtesy of the Fitzsimons Army Medical Center teaching files.)

40. **What types of hyperpigmentation are due to dermal melanin deposition?**
    - **Macular amyloidosis:** Brownish-gray macules on the torso or extremities
    - **Fixed drug eruption:** Reddish-brown to blue-gray macule, with erythema, edema, scale, and sometimes blisters (see Chapter 14)
    - **Erythema ab igne:** Blue-gray patches, sometimes with erythema and scale
    - **Erythema dyschromicum perstans:** Erythematous, ash-gray macules and patches
    - **Postinflammatory hyperpigmentation:** Brown to gray macules and patches (Fig. 18-7)

41. **How does erythema ab igne occur?**
    Erythema ab igne is a skin reaction to thermal injury. Chronic heating pad use is a common cause of this disorder. Usually, the affected area has a netlike pattern of blue-gray discoloration, sometimes with associated erythema and scale. Patients often complain that the affected area burns, stings, or itches. Treatment requires discontinuing heating pad use. Skin dyspigmentation slowly resolves over several months to a year, although permanent dermal scarring and hyperpigmentation can result.

42. **Are there any metabolic disorders associated with nonmelanin skin dyspigmentation?**
    Yes. Ochronosis (alkaptonuria) is a rare autosomal recessive inherited deficiency of homogentisic acid oxidase that results in accumulation of homogentisic acid in connective tissue, where it causes a dark brown to bluish-gray

dyspigmentation. Commonly affected skin areas include the pinna, tip of the nose, sclera, extensor tendons of the hands, fingernails, and tympanic membranes. Less commonly, blue macules develop on the central face, axillae, and genitalia.

Homogentisic acid also is deposited in the bones and articular cartilage, causing ochronotic arthropathy that results in premature degenerative arthritis. Overall, the course of ochronosis is progressive dyspigmentation and articular degeneration with no successful treatment available.

43. What pigmentation disorders are associated with heavy-metal deposition in the dermis?

Silver, mercury, bismuth, arsenic, and gold can cause brown to blue-gray discoloration due to metal deposition in the dermis. Silver, mercury, and bismuth toxicity result in blue-gray discoloration of the skin, nails, and mucosa. Silver toxicity (argyria) is most prominent in sun-exposed areas. Chrysoderma is an uncommon brown skin pigmentation that develops following parenteral gold administration and is most prominent in sun-exposed areas.

44. What drugs can deposit in the dermis and cause pigmentary changes?

Amiodarone (Fig. 18-8), bleomycin, busulfan, chloroquine, chlorpromazine, clofazimine, minocycline, ifluoperazine, thioridazine, and zidovudine cause blue-gray pigmentation of the skin and mucosa.

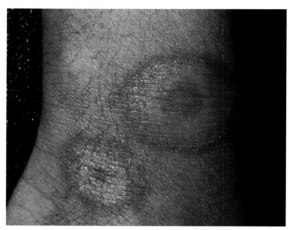

Figure 18-7. Two target-shaped patches of postinflammatory hyperpigmentation on the dorsal wrist of a woman following resolution of erythema multiforme.

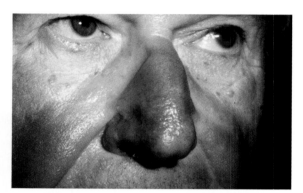

Figure 18-8. Amiodarone-induced photodistributed blue-gray hyperpigmentation. (Courtesy of the Fitzsimons Army Medical Center teaching files.)

PANNICULITIS

Heidi Gilchrist, MD and James W. Patterson, MD

CHAPTER 19

1. What is panniculitis?

Panniculitis represents infiltration of subcutaneous tissue by inflammatory cells, neoplastic cells, or both. This condition presents clinically as a deep induration or swelling of the skin. Associated signs and symptoms may include erythema, ulceration, drainage, warmth, and pain. Under certain circumstances, induration or nodularity may be present without significant inflammation or may persist after the inflammation has largely subsided.

2. Name the various types of panniculitis. How are they classified?

Although no single classification seems to be totally satisfactory, disorders tend to be grouped by a combination of histopathologic features and etiologies (Table 19-1). **Septal panniculitis** refers to a predominance of inflammation involving the connective tissue septae between fat lobules, whereas **lobular panniculitis** indicates predominant involvement of the fat lobules themselves. **Lipodystrophy** and **lipoatrophy** may be end-stage changes of the fat brought about by several different etiologies, including inflammation, trauma, or metabolic or hormonal alterations.

3. What is erythema nodosum?

Erythema nodosum (Fig. 19-1) consists of an eruption of erythematous, tender nodules— typically over the pretibial areas but occasionally elsewhere—that is regarded as a hypersensitivity response to some antigenic challenge. It is typically an acute process lasting 3 to 6 weeks, but a more chronic form can occur. Some experts consider the condition termed **subacute nodular migratory panniculitis** (Vilanova's disease) to be a chronic variant of erythema nodosum.

Requena L, Yus ES: Panniculitis. Part I. Mostly septal panniculitis, *J Am Acad Dermatol* 45:163–683, 2001.

4. What is the pathogenesis of erythema nodosum?

Erythema nodosum is usually considered to represent a delayed hypersensitivity response that reflects a common reaction pattern to a wide variety of eliciting factors. The subcutaneous septa in well-developed lesions often contain granulomas, and recent work has shown a strong correlation between genetic polymorphisms of tumor necrosis factor–α and erythema nodosum (TNF-α promotes granuloma formation). Reactive oxygen intermediates may be involved in the tissue damage and inflammation that accompany erythema nodosum.

Labunski S, Posern G, Ludwig S, et al: Tumor necrosis factor-alpha promoter polymorphism in erythema nodosum, *Acta Derm Venereol* 81:18–21, 2001.

5. List some of the common underlying conditions associated with erythema nodosum.

Streptococcal infection of the upper respiratory tract and medications (especially oral contraceptives, sulfonamides, penicillins, bromides, and iodides) are among the most common known causes. Other triggers include deep fungal

---

Table 19-1. Major Forms of Panniculitis

Septal Panniculitis	**Traumatic Panniculitis**
Erythema nodosum	**Infectious Panniculitis**
Subacute nodular migratory panniculitis	**Malignancy**
Scleroderma panniculitis	**Other Changes of the Fat**
Lobular and Mixed Panniculitis	Lipodystrophy
Nodular vasculitis (erythema induratum)	Lipoatrophy
Lupus panniculitis	Lipohypertrophy
Other types of connective tissue panniculitis	
Metabolic Derangements	
Altered melting/solidification points of fat	
Sclerema neonatorum	
Subcutaneous fat necrosis of the newborn	
Pancreatic (enzymatic) fat necrosis	
Alpha-1 antitrypsin deficiency panniculitis	

infections (such as coccidioidomycosis), *Yersinia* infection, pregnancy, sarcoidosis, inflammatory bowel disease, and leukemia. Many episodes are idiopathic: A cause is not identified in one third to one half of cases.

6. How should a biopsy of erythema nodosum be obtained?

The specimen should be obtained from the most fully developed (central) portion of the lesion (Fig. 19-2). It is absolutely critical that the biopsy be deep enough to incorporate subcutaneous fat. Incisional biopsies that include a generous horizontal expanse of subcutis are preferred to small punch biopsies.

7. What are the characteristic microscopic features of erythema nodosum?

The typical histologic features include a predominantly septal panniculitis with a slight spillover of inflammatory cells into the fat lobules. Cell types may include lymphocytes, neutrophils, and eosinophils, especially in acute disease. In older lesions, small granulomas (Miescher's granulomas) are sometimes observed within connective tissue septa. Perivascular infiltrates are common, but true vasculitis with destruction of vessel walls is not observed.

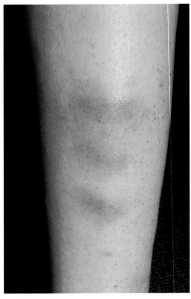

Figure 19-1. Typical lesion of erythema nodosum on the leg. Erythema nodosum heals without scarring. (Courtesy of James E. Fitzpatrick, MD.)

8. How is erythema nodosum treated?

Treatment of the underlying disorder, if known, is of primary importance. Salicylates or nonsteroidal antiinflammatory drugs, bed rest, and potassium iodide (particularly in chronic forms of the disease) are usually considered to be first-line therapies while colchicine, dapsone, hydroxychloroquine, and prednisone are second-line therapies used in recalcitrant cases.

9. What is nodular vasculitis?

This form of panniculitis most commonly occurs on the posterior lower legs (Fig. 19-3), as opposed to the classically anterior location of erythema nodosum. Ulceration and drainage sometimes occur.

10. What causes nodular vasculitis?

It was originally considered a hypersensitivity reaction to tuberculosis and termed **erythema induratum of Bazin.** Studies confirm that in many cases *Mycobacterium tuberculosis* DNA can be detected in the lesions by polymerase chain reaction (PCR); however, nodular vasculitis can also be idiopathic or associated with other infectious agents (*Nocardia*, hepatitis C) or drugs (propylthiouracil). These cases with nontuberculous etiologies are sometimes termed **erythema induratum of Whitfield**.

Baselga E, Margall N, Barnadas MA, et al: Detection of *Mycobacterium tuberculosis* DNA in lobular granulomatous panniculitis (erythema induratum-nodular vasculitis), *Arch Dermatol* 133:457–462, 1997.

Key Points: Panniculitis

1. Given the similar clinical appearance among panniculitides, histopathologic characterization is often critical for a correct diagnosis.
2. An incisional biopsy with a wide base in the fat is far more likely to be diagnostic than a deep shave or punch biopsy.
3. The biopsy should be taken from the most indurated lesion; if that lesion has an ulcer, the biopsy should avoid the ulcer base.
4. If the lesions are ulcerated or suppurated, consider tissue culture at the time of the biopsy.

Key Points: Erythema Nodosum

1. Erythema nodosum is the most common cause of panniculitis.
2. Erythema nodosum lesions typically last 3 to 6 weeks but frequently recur.
3. Erythema nodosum can occur at any age and can be located at any site on the body; classically, however, it is a disease most frequently found in women in their 20s to 40s and is mainly located on the anterior shins.
4. Spontaneous ulceration does not occur in erythema nodosum; if present, suspect another diagnosis such as erythema induratum, thrombophlebitis, polyarteritis nodosa, α-1 antitrypsin deficiency, necrobiosis lipoidica, pancreatic panniculitis, ulcerative sarcoidosis, or infection.
5. One should always consider the possibility that the presence of erythema nodosum reflects a reaction to a drug, a remote focus of infection, pregnancy, inflammatory bowel disease, malignancy, or sarcoidosis.

11. Describe the microscopic features of nodular vasculitis.

Nodular vasculitis presents as a lobular panniculitis with a mixed infiltrate that may be granulomatous. Vasculitis of a medium-sized artery or vein is present deep in the fat. Caseous necrosis is present in up to 50% of cases. Although necrosis can occur in cases not associated with tuberculosis, it may be more common in lesions that are positive for *Mycobacterium tuberculosis*–complex DNA.

Boonchai W, Suthipinittharm P, Mahaisavariya P: Panniculitis in tuberculosis: a clinicopathologic study of nodular panniculitis associated with tuberculosis, *Int J Dermatol* 37:361–363, 1998.

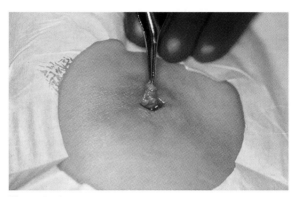

Figure 19-2. Appropriate wedge biopsy technique for panniculitis as shown in a case of erythema nodosum. The biopsy extends from the epidermis to a wide base in the subcutaneous fat. (Courtesy of Kenneth E. Greer, MD.)

12. What is the differential diagnosis of nodular vasculitis?

Clinical clues to an association with tuberculosis include constitutional symptoms, elevated erythrocyte sedimentation rate, an abnormal chest x-ray, or a positive tuberculin skin test. Both polyarteritis nodosa and superficial thrombophlebitis also show vasculitis involving medium-sized vessels in the subcutis. In both conditions, the inflammation is more specifically directed toward the vessel, and extensive lobular inflammation obscuring the vessel changes is uncommon. The clinical findings are also quite different in these two disorders (e.g., hypertension, renal, and central nervous system disease in systemic polyarteritis; association with internal malignancy in superficial migratory thrombophlebitis). In one author's experience (JWP), true examples of nodular vasculitis are seldom seen, but this might change with the recent rise in number of cases of tuberculosis associated with human immunodeficiency virus.

13. How should nodular vasculitis be treated?

Treatment should be directed toward any underlying infection, especially tuberculosis. Studies have demonstrated the responsiveness of mycobacteria-associated lesions to multidrug antituberculous therapy. Symptomatic care includes bed rest, bandages, antiinflammatory agents, and avoidance of potential aggravating factors such as smoking. In more severe non-tuberculous cases, potassium iodide, dapsone, colchicine, antimalarials, tetracyclines, and prednisone can be used.

Mascaró JM Jr, Baselga E: Erythema induratum of Bazin, *Dermatol Clin* 26:439–445, 2008.

14. What are the clinical features of lupus panniculitis?

Lupus panniculitis, also termed **lupus profundus,** consists of erythematous or flesh-colored subcutaneous nodules. The lesions occur on the face, upper outer arms, shoulders, and trunk, including the breasts. They sometimes show overlying follicular plugging, epidermal atrophy, and hyperpigmentation—changes associated with cutaneous (discoid) lupus erythematosus (Fig. 19-4). The overlying skin can be "bound down" to the subcutaneous nodule or plaque, resulting in an obvious depression in the skin surface.

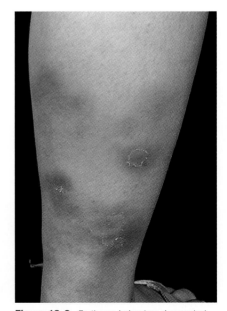

Figure 19-3. Erythema induratum demonstrating characteristic indurated subcutaneous nodules. Spontaneous ulceration is common. (Courtesy of James E. Fitzpatrick, MD.)

15. Describe the microscopic features of lupus panniculitis.

There is typically a mixed septal and lobular panniculitis with a predominance of lymphocytes in a patchy or diffuse and/or perivascular distribution. Nodular aggregates of lymphocytes surrounded by plasma cells may be present; there may even be formation of lymphoid follicles with germinal centers. Interstitial mucin deposition and hyalinization of the fat also occur. Overlying epidermal changes associated with cutaneous lupus erythematosus may be seen in close to one half of cases.

Ng PP, Tan SH, Tan T: Lupus erythematosus panniculitis: a clinicopathologic study, *Int J Dermatol* 41:488–490, 2002.

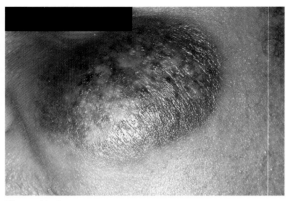

Figure 19-4. Lupus panniculitis on the face, manifested by a large tender nodule. Directly overlying the panniculitis is a lesion of discoid lupus erythematosus. (Courtesy of Kenneth E. Greer, MD.)

16. What is the significance of diagnosing lupus panniculitis?

Panniculitis may be a presenting finding of either cutaneous or systemic lupus erythematosus, or rarely of dermatomyositis or other autoimmune diseases. A small percentage of patients presenting with lupus panniculitis fulfill criteria for systemic lupus erythematous, and other complications have been reported, such as the development of antiphospholipid antibody syndrome. Antinuclear antibodies are common, and occasionally other circulating antibodies are detected, such as antineutrophil cytoplasmic antibodies. Because of the unusual clinical locations of lupus panniculitis, the true diagnosis may not be suspected for months or years. Early biopsy and direct immunofluorescence study of these lesions may provide the first clues to the diagnosis of lupus erythematosus and allow for early institution of appropriate therapy. Treatments for the panniculitis include intralesional corticosteroids, systemic antimalarials, and dapsone.

17. Are sclerema neonatorum and subcutaneous fat necrosis of the newborn the same thing?

No, but in both conditions, there are varying degrees of sclerosis of the subcutaneous fat of newborns. **Sclerema neonatorum** is very rare and occurs in premature, hypothermic infants with underlying medical problems. It is characterized by diffusely cold, rigid, boardlike skin; neonatal death is common. In **subcutaneous fat necrosis of the newborn** (Fig. 19-5A), relatively discrete, firm subcutaneous nodules develop several weeks after birth in an otherwise healthy baby. Hypercalcemia may be present, causing seizures and nephrocalcinosis, but the overall prognosis for survival and resolution of the lesions is excellent.

Ladoyanni E, Moss C, Brown RM, Ogboli M: Subcutaneous fat necrosis in a newborn associated with asymptomatic and uncomplicated hypercalcemia, *Pediatr Dermatol* 26:217–219, 2009.

18. How similar are the microscopic features of sclerema neonatorum and subcutaneous fat necrosis of the newborn?

Both conditions show needle-shaped clefts within lipocytes, presumably representing triglyceride crystals that have been dissolved during tissue processing. Sclerema neonatorum tends to show thickened fibrous septa and little

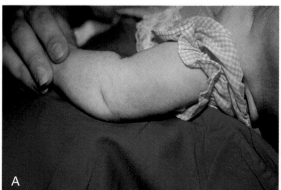
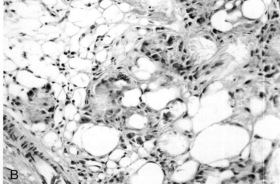

Figure 19-5. A, Subcutaneous fat necrosis of the left upper arm in an otherwise healthy infant. **B,** Biopsy of subcutaneous fat necrosis demonstrating characteristic fat destruction with needle-shaped clefts that induce a foreign body reaction consisting of macrophages and multinucleated giant cells. (Courtesy of James E. Fitzpatrick, MD.)

inflammation, while subcutaneous fat necrosis shows a substantial lobular panniculitis with a foreign body reaction to the needle-shaped clefts (Fig. 19-5B).

19. Why do these disorders occur in neonates and infants?

Neonatal fat has an increased ratio of saturated to unsaturated fatty acids, which results in higher melting and solidification points for stored fat. This, plus other possible metabolic defects, leads to crystal formation, fat necrosis, and inflammation when the fat is subjected to stresses such as ischemia or trauma.

20. What is pancreatic fat necrosis?

Subcutaneous nodules occur on the legs (Fig. 19-6) or elsewhere associated with acute or chronic pancreatitis or pancreatic carcinoma. Visceral fat may also be involved. Although immune mechanisms may play a role in producing this form of fat necrosis, the weight of evidence favors the effects of circulating pancreatic lipase, amylase, and trypsin on subcutaneous fat. The frequent co-occurrence of arthritis with joint fluid analysis revealing free fatty acids is a clinical reminder of the systemic effects of these pancreatic enzymes. Treatment is directed toward the underlying pancreatic disease.

Preiss JC, Faiss S, Loddenkemper C, et al: Pancreatic panniculitis in an 88-year-old man with neuroendocrine carcinoma, *Digestion* 66:193–196, 2002.

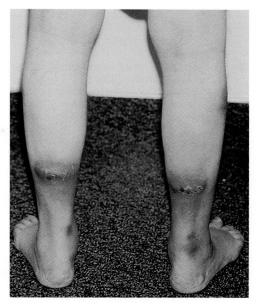

Figure 19-6. Pancreatic fat necrosis showing classic involvement of the lower legs. Note the desquamation on the patient's right posterior leg, suggesting that spontaneous discharge is likely.

21. Are there any characteristic histopathologic features of pancreatic fat necrosis?

The changes are rather unique and include necrosis of the fat with formation of lipocyte remnants with thick, shadowy walls ("ghost cells") and pools of basophilic material that represent saponification of fat by calcium salts.

22. What is the role of α-1 antitrypsin deficiency in the development of panniculitis?

Since the mid-1970s, it has become apparent that patients with this inherited proteinase inhibitor deficiency, especially those most severely affected and having the homozygous PiZZ phenotype, are prone to develop painful hemorrhagic subcutaneous nodules (Fig. 19-7) that ulcerate and drain. Without α-1 antitrypsin, the activity of neutrophil elastase is unchecked. It is believed that in such individuals a variety of triggering factors, such as trauma, may initiate a sequence of events that includes unchecked complement activation, inflammation, endothelial cell damage, and tissue injury. Microscopic clues to the diagnosis include diffuse neutrophilic infiltration of the reticular dermis, and liquefactive necrosis of the dermis and the subcutaneous septa, with resultant separation of fat lobules. Treatment options include dapsone, systemic corticosteroids, plasma exchange therapy, and, more recently, parenteral administration of a proteinase inhibitor.

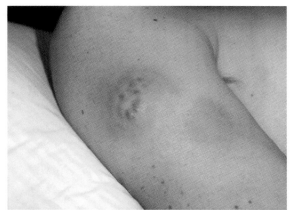

Figure 19-7. Alpha-1 antitrypsin deficiency panniculitis showing foci of hemorrhage in the center of the lesion. (Courtesy of Kenneth E. Greer, MD.)

Chowdhury MM, Williams EJ, Morris JS, et al: Severe panniculitis caused by ZZ alpha-1-antitrypsin deficiency treated successfully with human purified enzyme (Prolastin), *Br J Dermatol* 147:1258–1261, 2004.

23. Name some types of trauma that can produce panniculitis.

Numerous forms of trauma, either accidental or purposeful, can produce painful subcutaneous nodules or plaques. These include cold injury ("popsicle panniculitis" on the cheeks of children), injection of foreign substances such as oils or medications (Fig. 19-8), or blunt force trauma. There are some unique microscopic clues for each of these types of injury, so biopsy is particularly helpful when traumatic panniculitis is suspected. Polarization microscopy is one simple test for detecting the presence of refractile foreign material in tissue sections. The therapeutic challenge lies mainly in finding and removing the source of the injury that has produced the panniculitis.

24. Which infectious organisms can produce panniculitis?

Panniculitis can result from localized or generalized infection caused by gram-positive and gram-negative bacteria, mycobacteria (Fig. 19-9A), *Nocardia, Cryptococcus* (Fig. 19-9B), *Candida,* and *Fusarium* species. Other organisms that have been associated with panniculitis include streptococci, *Toxocara, Trypanosoma,* and *Borrelia burgdorferi* (as a manifestation of Lyme disease).

Immunosuppressed patients appear to be particularly at risk for infection-induced panniculitis. Microscopic features vary and can occasionally mimic other forms of panniculitis. However, findings that should suggest the possibility of infection include mixed

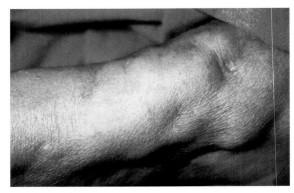

Figure 19-8. Sclerosing panniculitis with lipoatrophy caused by repeated injection of pentazocine. (Courtesy of Kenneth E. Greer, MD.)

septal-lobular involvement, neutrophilic infiltration, vascular proliferation and hemorrhage, and sweat gland necrosis. Special stains and culture studies are crucial to making the correct diagnosis and instituting appropriate antimicrobial therapy.

Patterson JW, Brown PC, Broecker AH: Infection-induced panniculitis, *J Cutan Pathol* 16:183–193, 1989.

25. Describe the role of malignancy in producing panniculitis.

Malignant infiltrates can sometimes produce subcutaneous nodules that mimic other forms of panniculitis. Malignancies that are capable of producing panniculitis-like lesions include poorly differentiated carcinomas, lymphomas (Fig. 19-10), multiple myeloma, and leukemias. Microscopic clues to the recognition of malignant infiltrates include a monotonous cell population and/or cytologic atypia, "lining up" of atypical cells between collagen bundles,

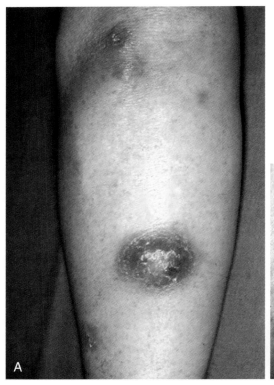

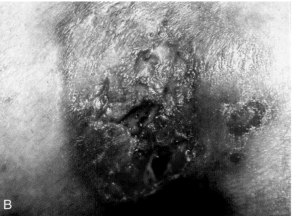

Figure 19-9. A, Panniculitis caused by *Mycobacterium marinum*. The classic linear appearance of the lesions denotes local lymphangitic spread, common in cutaneous infections with this organism. **B,** Ulceronecrotic panniculitis secondary to *Cryptococcus neoformans*. Skin disease is most often due to hematogenous spread of primary pulmonary infection. (Courtesy of Kenneth E. Greer, MD.)

and minimal alteration of connective tissue in the presence of dense cellular infiltration. Also, forms of more traditional inflammatory panniculitis can accompany malignancy, including erythema nodosum, migratory thrombophlebitis, and pancreatic fat necrosis. Therefore, diagnosis again is heavily dependent on biopsy.

Cassis TB, Fearneyhough PK, Callen JP: Subcutaneous panniculitis-like T-cell lymphoma with vacuolar interface dermatitis resembling lupus erythematosus panniculitis, *J Am Acad Dermatol* 50:465–469, 2004.

26. What is lipodystrophy?

Lipodystrophy generally refers to a paucity or complete absence of subcutaneous fat, sometimes due to redistribution. It can be generalized or localized, inherited or acquired. Lipodystrophy can be idiopathic, but is often associated with inherited syndromes, endocrine abnormalities such as insulin-resistant diabetes mellitus, complement

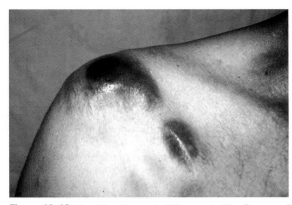

Figure 19-10. B-cell lymphoma mimicking panniculitis. (Courtesy of Kenneth E. Greer, MD.)

abnormalities (Fig. 19-11A), or autoimmune disease. It is well recognized that highly active antiretroviral therapy (highly active antiretroviral therapy [HAART], particularly protease inhibitors) causes a distinctive redistribution of subcutaneous fat with accumulation of fat in abdominal and cervical areas and wasting of the face and extremities.

Koutkia P, Grinspoon S: HIV-associated lipodystrophy: pathogenesis, prognosis, treatment, and controversies, *Annu Rev Med* 55: 303–317, 2004.

27. What is lipoatrophy?

This term is sometimes used interchangeably with lipodystrophy, but it is more commonly used to describe a focal loss of subcutaneous fat. Probably the most common form of lipoatrophy is postinflammatory in nature and can occur following several types of panniculitis. Microscopically, lipoatrophy features "collapse" of fat lobules, with a reduced

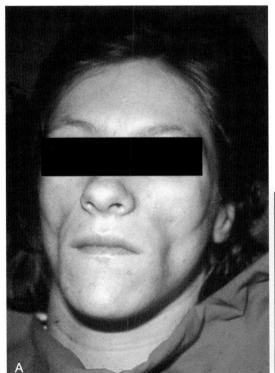

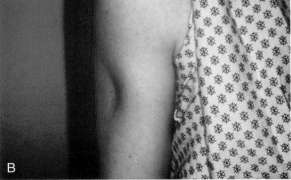

Figure 19-11. A, Acquired partial lipodystrophy with associated C3 nephritic factor. Note the prominent wasting of the facial fat in this patient. **B,** Localized lipoatrophy associated with injection of medication. (Courtesy of Kenneth E. Greer, MD.)

number of variably sized lipocytes and development of numerous capillaries in a mucinous background stroma. Localized lipoatrophy also occurs following injection of medications, especially corticosteroids (Fig. 19-11B). A variety of plastic surgical procedures has been used to improve or correct lipoatrophy.

28. What is lipohypertrophy?

Lipohypertrophy, which manifests as induration of involved skin, occurs in some individuals due to repeated injections of insulin. This effect is apparently independent of the source of insulin, and can even occur with human recombinant insulin. Growth hormone injections have also resulted in lipohypertrophy. In lipohypertrophy, lipocytes are enlarged and appear to encroach upon the midportion of the dermis. Rotation of insulin injection sites is a key to management of lipohypertrophy, both to prevent or minimize the hypertrophic changes and to assure adequate insulin absorption.

Chernausek SD, Backeljauw PF, Frane J, et al: Long-term treatment with recombinant insulin-like growth factor (IGF)-I in children with severe IGF-I deficiency due to growth hormone insensitivity, *J Clin Endocrinol Metab* 92:902–910, 2007.
Chowdhury TA, Escudier V: Poor glycemic control caused by insulin-induced lipohypertrophy, *Br Med J* 327:383–384, 2003.

29. Discuss the approach to use when attempting to diagnose an "unknown" case of panniculitis.

- Careful history and physical examination are of greatest importance, emphasizing the location of the eruption, as well as its timing in relation to any possible drug ingestion, infection, or trauma.
- Laboratory studies should be guided by the clinical history but might include cultures of distant sites (e.g., for possible streptococcal pharyngitis in erythema nodosum), antinuclear antibody determination (to rule out lupus panniculitis), or measurement of α-1 antitrypsin levels (for evaluation of proteinase inhibitor–deficiency panniculitis).
- Skin biopsy can be of tremendous benefit, and recognition of established microscopic patterns of disease can be complemented by special stains and polarization microscopy.
- Immunohistochemistry can be useful in selected cases where malignancy is a possibility, and x-ray microanalysis is a specialized test that can be used to determine the identity of foreign material in cases of traumatic panniculitis.

ALOPECIA

Leonard C. Sperling, MD

CHAPTER 20

1. How is alopecia classified?

Alopecia (hair loss) can be divided into: 1) disorders of the hair shaft and 2) all other forms of hair loss. Abnormalities of the hair shaft can produce alopecia because the shafts are fragile and "break off." The other forms of alopecia can be divided into cicatricial (scarring) and noncicatricial alopecia. In cicatricial alopecia, hair is lost permanently. Both cicatricial and noncicatricial alopecia can be divided into diffuse and patterned hair loss. In diffuse hair loss, hair thins evenly from all parts of the scalp, and discrete "bald spots" do not occur. In patterned alopecia, certain areas of the scalp are affected more than others.

Eudy G, Solomon AR: The histopathology of noncicatricial alopecia, *Semin Cutan Med Surg* 25:35–40, 2006.
Sperling LC, Cowper SE: The histopathology of primary cicatricial alopecia, *Semin Cutan Med Surg* 25:41–50, 2006.

2. What are some common types of patterned hair loss?

- **Patchy:** Multiple scattered lesions
- **Moth-eaten:** Myriad, diffusely distributed, small lesions
- **Ophiasis:** Hair loss around periphery of the scalp
- **Male pattern baldness:** Symmetrical hair loss predominantly affecting the top (vertex) of the scalp

3. Can cicatricial and noncicatricial alopecia be differentiated clinically?

In the setting of alopecia, cicatricial means that there has been permanent destruction of hair follicles, and they have been replaced by fibrous tissue. Usually, an obvious scar, such as that seen after wounding, is not evident, but there is a loss of follicular openings that gives the scalp a smooth and shiny appearance (Fig. 20-1). The texture of the scalp may remain soft and supple, although sometimes induration or firmness is palpable.

4. What causes common balding?

People who become bald have hair follicles that are genetically programmed to miniaturize under the influence of postpubertal androgens. Probably, several genes (inherited from both mother and father) influence the severity of balding. Until very late in the balding process, the number of hairs does not decrease, but the hairs become progressively smaller until they are no longer visible to the naked eye. Except in very marked and long-standing balding, very fine, short hairs can be seen exiting from follicular orifices if a magnifying lens is used.

Randall VA: Androgens and hair growth, *Dermatol Ther* 21(5):314–328, 2008.

5. How effective are medical treatments for common balding?

About one third of balding patients who use topical minoxidil solution experience significant (cosmetically obvious) hair regrowth. Any regrowth that occurs is only maintained while the drug is used. If therapy is stopped, hair density reverts to its pretreatment state. Oral finasteride, a 5α-reductase inhibitor, is somewhat more effective, and can be used in combination with topical minoxidil.

Rogers NE, Avram MR: Medical treatments for male and female pattern hair loss, *J Am Acad Dermatol* 59(4):547–566, 2008.

6. Is common balding in women managed differently than in men?

Women whose balding is a manifestation of hyperandrogenism (excessive production of circulating androgens) may benefit from therapy directed at the cause of hyperandrogenism. Polycystic ovarian disease, late-on-set congenital adrenal hyperplasia, Cushing's syndrome, and adrenal and ovarian neoplasms are potential causes of hyperandrogenism. In the absence of elevated circulating androgens, nonspecific therapy directed at suppressing ovarian androgen production or blocking the peripheral effect of androgens is sometimes tried. Oral contraceptive agents (to suppress ovarian androgen production) and spironolactone are most often utilized for this purpose. Topical minoxidil solution is also useful, but oral finasteride is seldom used in women.

7. What are the surgical options for treatment of balding?

Men, and occasionally women, can achieve permanent cosmetic improvement by undergoing a hair transplantation procedure. Hair follicles from the occipital area (donor site) are moved to the balding area (recipient site). The procedure is tedious and expensive, but the cosmetic results can be quite good. Various other surgical procedures, including scalp reductions (which involve excising the bald areas) and scalp flaps, are sometimes used in selected patients.

8. Discuss the common causes of circular bald spots.

Although many forms of alopecia can result in a circular bald patch, the most common causes are tinea capitis and alopecia areata. **Tinea capitis** is a superficial fungal infection with a predilection for children, especially black children. The surface of the skin is scaly and sometimes inflamed, and small dark stubs of hair ("black dots") may be scattered within the affected area. In this condition, the hair shaft is invaded and replaced by myriad circular fungal spores. In the United States, *Trichophyton tonsurans* is usually the culprit. A circular, scaly, or crusted bald spot on the scalp of a black child should be considered to be tinea capitis until proven otherwise (Fig. 20-2A).

Alopecia areata also commonly affects children, but adults more often develop the condition. In alopecia areata, the affected areas may be totally hairless, but the scalp surface looks otherwise normal, without scaling and minimal, if any, erythema. A few short hairs may be present in the bald spot; these "exclamation mark" hairs tend to taper and lose pigment as they approach the scalp and may appear to float on the surface of the scalp (Fig. 20-2B).

9. What is alopecia totalis?

Alopecia areata may cause one or many bald spots. If it affects the entire scalp, it is called **alopecia totalis** (Fig. 20-3). If the entire body is affected, it is referred to as **alopecia universalis**.

10. How is alopecia areata treated?

When a solitary lesion of alopecia areata is small (<5 cm in diameter), no treatment may be needed. The prognosis for such a lesion is excellent, and spontaneous regrowth often occurs. Intralesional corticosteroids, and sometimes potent topical corticosteroids, may hasten regrowth. Larger or more numerous lesions carry a more guarded prognosis. Intralesional

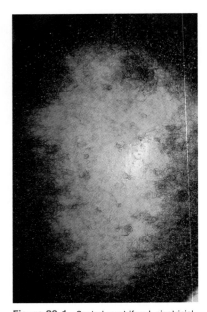

Figure 20-1. Central, centrifugal, cicatricial alopecia, a common form of hair loss in the African-American population. In this patient, the smooth skin, devoid of most follicular openings, reflects light like a mirror.

corticosteroid injections are often begun. For extensive hair loss involving 30% to 100% of the scalp surface, a short (e.g., 3-month) course of systemic corticosteroids (usually prednisone) may be tried. If hair regrowth does not resume or if hair loss recurs once corticosteroids are stopped, the prognosis is poor. The use of systemic corticosteroids to treat extensive alopecia areata is controversial. Appropriate risk-versus-benefit considerations must be carefully analyzed.

Although spontaneous regrowth may occur even in alopecia totalis, no therapy has been found to be consistently safe and effective for severe disease. For now, topical immunotherapy with chemicals causing allergic contact dermatitis (e.g., diphencyprone) seems to offer the most hope.

Hordinsky M, Caramori A: Alopecia areata. In McMichael A, Hordinsky M, editors: *Hair and scalp diseases*, New York, 2008, Informa Healthcare, pp 91–105.

11. How is tinea capitis treated?

Although topical antifungal agents work well for tinea corporis, they are of little value in treating tinea capitis. Systemic antifungal agents are required to eradicate the spores that invade affected hair shafts. A course of treatment generally takes 1 to 3 months. **Griseofulvin** is the treatment of choice because it is safe and effective, rarely causing significant side effects. Ultramicrosized formulations of griseofulvin can be given in half the dose required with microsized forms of the drug. Fungal resistance to griseofulvin is rare. For the few patients whose tinea capitis is resistant to griseofulvin,

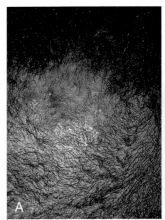
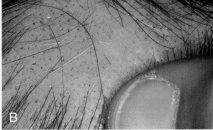

Figure 20-2. A, Tinea capitis. A large bald patch studded with small inflammatory papules surrounded by smaller, similar lesions. Close examination may reveal "black dots" scattered within the bald area. **B,** A patch of alopecia areata showing several "exclamation mark hairs."

or who cannot tolerate griseofulvin because of side effects (such as headache or gastrointestinal upset), terbinafine and itraconazole are acceptable alternatives.

Andrews MD, Burns M: Common tinea infections in children, *Am Fam Physician* 77(10):1415–1420, 2008.

12. What is trichotillomania?
Compulsive hair pulling or plucking.

13. Who is most likely to be affected by trichotillomania?
The typical patient is an adolescent girl, although the condition can affect children of both sexes as well as adults. In trichotillomania, hairs are forcibly plucked out of the scalp by the patient, usually as a mechanism for relieving tension or stress. Less often, trichotillomania is a manifestation of psychosis or an obsessive-compulsive neurosis. Although the patient may deny plucking, the often bizarre shape of the bald area, combined with the presence of short hairs of various lengths within the area of thinning, suggest the diagnosis (Fig. 20-4). The diagnosis may be confirmed by a scalp biopsy demonstrating diagnostic features, or by creating a "hair growth window." This test is performed by weekly shaving of an involved area to prevent plucking; the hair will recover and regain normal density within the shaved area, resembling a "five o'clock shadow."

Buescher L, Resch D: The biopsychosocial aspects of hair disease. In McMichael A, Hordinsky M, editors: *Hair and scalp diseases*, New York, 2008, Informa Healthcare, pp 267–275.

Tay YK, Levy ML, Metry DW: Trichotillomania in childhood: case series and review, *Pediatrics* 113(5):e494–e498, 2004.

14. Why do cancer patients lose their hair?
Cancer patients are susceptible to two forms of diffuse hair loss. **Anagen effluvium** is a direct effect of anticancer treatment. Patients receiving radiation therapy to the scalp or systemic chemotherapy can shed all or most of their hair within a few weeks of starting treatment. This hair loss is a direct effect of the chemotherapy or radiotherapy on the hair follicle, whose rapidly dividing cells are very susceptible to injury. When the hair matrix (the epithelial root that produces the hair shaft) is exposed to radiation or chemical toxins, it can only produce a thinned hair shaft that eventually tapers to a point (Fig. 20-5A). This marked tapering makes the shaft extremely fragile, and the hair shaft can literally be combed away or broken off by minor trauma. Unless the dose of radiation or chemotherapy is very high, regrowth of hair occurs once therapy is stopped.

In **telogen effluvium** the metabolic and emotional "stress" of severe, debilitating illness causes many of the actively growing (anagen) hairs to enter the shedding (telogen) phase of hair growth prematurely. The hairs remain in telogen for about 3 months before they are finally shed (Fig. 20-5B), so there is always a "lag" time between the onset of severe disease and actual hair loss. Seldom is more than 50% of the hair shed in telogen effluvium, so patients develop thin hair but do not become completely bald. If the patient recovers and is no longer debilitated, hairs reenter the actively growing phase and the hair regrows.

Kligman AM: Pathologic dynamics of human hair loss: I. Telogen effluvium, *Arch Dermatol* 83:175–198, 1961.

15. In what other clinical settings can a telogen effluvium occur?
Normally, about 10% of scalp hairs are in the telogen (preshedding) phase at any given time. Whenever an abnormally large number of otherwise normal telogen hairs are present, a telogen effluvium occurs. There are several clinical situations in which a telogen effluvium is found, including severe illness such as metastatic cancer, but any serious illness or major surgical procedure can also result in a telogen effluvium. The most common form of telogen effluvium occurs in women about 3 months after giving birth. In addition, virtually all newborn infants develop a telogen effluvium during the first 6 months of life, which is why many babies have more hair at birth than at 3 to 4 months after birth.

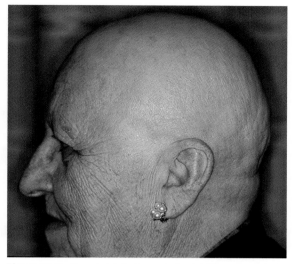

Figure 20-3. Alopecia totalis demonstrating total loss of scalp hair and most of eyebrows. (Courtesy of James E. Fitzpatrick, MD.)

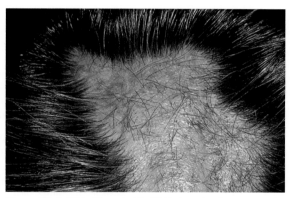

Figure 20-4. Trichotillomania. The highly irregular shape, sharp circumscription, and presence of "broken off" hairs of various lengths are typical of this condition.

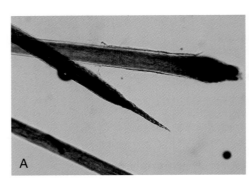
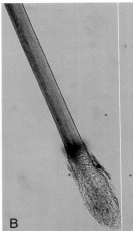

Figure 20-5. Hair loss in cancer therapy. **A,** Anagen effluvium. The shaft tapers down to a pencil-like point and easily separates from the follicle. **B,** Normal telogen hair. About 50 to 100 telogen hairs such as these normally shed during the course of the day. Much higher numbers are shed during a telogen effluvium.

Causes of telogen effluvium can be summarized as follows:
- Physiologic effluvium of the newborn
- Postpartum
- Postfebrile (e.g., malaria)
- Severe infection
- Debilitating chronic illness
- Postsurgical (major procedure or major trauma)
- Hypothyroidism and other endocrinopathies
- Crash or liquid protein diets; starvation
- Drugs: Retinoids, anticoagulants, anticonvulsives, antithyroid, heavy metals

Sperling LC: Hair and systemic disease, *Dermatol Clin* 711–726, 2001.

16. To what forms of hair loss are black patients susceptible?
- Black children are particularly prone to acquiring tinea capitis.
- Hair shaft fragility disorders are also common among African-American women because of certain hair grooming techniques using chemical hair "relaxers." These products are effective in straightening kinky or curly hair but are caustic and, with continued use, the hair shaft becomes frayed. The foci of fraying have a special appearance termed trichorrhexis nodosa, which looks like the bristles of two paint brushes that have been pushed together (Fig. 20-6). The hair shafts easily fracture at the points of trichorrhexis nodosa, leaving abnormally short hair shafts behind. Patients have scalp hair of very uneven length and may complain that their hair "falls out" with combing or "won't grow." In fact, their hair is growing but breaking off.

17. Discuss the mechanism of central, centrifugal, cicatricial alopecia (CCCA).
The most common form of cicatricial alopecia in black patients was once called "hot comb alopecia" but is now called *central, centrifugal, cicatricial alopecia* (CCCA). The condition more often affects adult women than men and typically causes hair loss that is most severe on the central crown of the scalp and slowly progresses centrifugally (see Fig. 20-1). When the bald patches are carefully examined, a few normal hairs may be found, but most follicular openings have been completely obliterated, suggesting a cicatricial process. Scattered inflammatory, perifollicular papules may be found in the peripheral zone where hair thinning has just begun. Scalp biopsy confirms that hair follicles are completely destroyed and replaced with fibrous tissue. "Hot combs" are rarely used nowadays for straightening hair, so hot comb alopecia is a misnomer. It is uncertain whether hair care products are primarily responsible for hair loss in these patients, but chemical relaxers and other cosmetics may exacerbate the condition.

Sperling LC, Solomon AR, Whiting DA: A new look at scarring alopecia, *Arch Dermatol* 136:235–242, 2000.

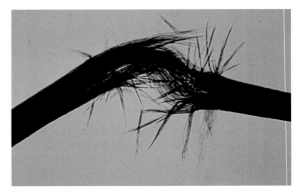

Figure 20-6. Trichorrhexis nodosa fracture in a woman using chemical hair straightners.

18. Name some medications that cause hair loss.

Anticancer medications, colchicine, thallium (rat poisons and insecticides), antiepileptic drugs (phenytoin, valproic acid, and carbamazepine), anticlotting drugs (heparin and coumarin), and retinoids (acitretin).

Bergfeld W: Telogen effluvium. In McMichael A, Hordinsky M, editors: *Hair and scalp diseases*, New York, 2008, Informa Healthcare, pp 119–135.
Brodin M: Drug-related alopecia, *Dermatol Clin* 5:571–579, 1987.

Key Points: Alopecia

1. A circular, scaly, or crusted bald spot on the scalp of a black child should be considered tinea capitis until proven otherwise.
2. Women whose balding is a manifestation of hyperandrogenism (excessive production of circulating androgens) may benefit from therapy directed at the cause of hyperandrogenism.
3. When a solitary lesion of alopecia areata is small, no treatment may be needed. The prognosis for such a lesion is excellent, and spontaneous regrowth often occurs.
4. In trichotillomania, hairs are forcibly plucked out of the scalp by the patient, usually as a mechanism for relieving tension or stress.
5. The most common form of cicatricial alopecia in black patients is called *central, centrifugal, cicatricial alopecia.* It is not caused by cosmetic practices, but chemical relaxers may exacerbate the condition.

---

19. What is alopecia mucinosa?

This term actually refers to two entirely different causes of hair loss. The conditions have in common a similar histologic finding—**follicular mucinosis,** the accumulation of mucin (acid mucopolysaccharides) within the follicular epithelium, resulting in hair damage and hair loss.

The first form of alopecia mucinosa is a benign condition found in young and otherwise healthy individuals. One or more oval or circular hairless patches or plaques are present, which can be hypopigmented or erythematous and may be scaly, eczematous, or studded with minute papules. The condition usually involves the head, neck, upper arms, or upper torso. Spontaneous resolution usually occurs in months to years.

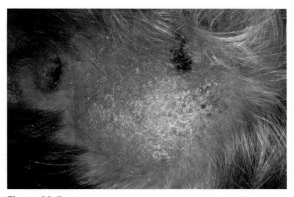

Figure 20-7. Alopecia mucinosa occurring in a patient with mycosis fungoides. (Courtesy of Fitzsimons Army Medical Center teaching files.)

The second form of alopecia mucinosa occurs in patients with mycosis fungoides, a form of cutaneous T-cell lymphoma. Patients are usually elderly, and numerous, often large, hairless, erythematous, and indurated plaques are found (Fig. 20-7). Histologically, follicular mucinosis is present, but an atypical lymphocytic infiltrate that often invades the epidermis and follicles is also seen. This atypical cellular infiltrate allows for the diagnosis of mycosis fungoides. The hairless lesions and histologic follicular mucinosis are merely manifestations of the underlying lymphoma.

Gibson LE, Brown HA, Pittelkow MR, Pujol RM: Follicular mucinosis, *Arch Dermatol* 138(12):1615, 2002.

20. What is meant by the term "moth-eaten alopecia"?

"Moth-eaten alopecia" is a form of noncicatricial, patterned hair loss in which there are myriad small foci of alopecia scattered over the scalp (Fig. 20-8). This pattern of alopecia is described as the classic form of alopecia seen in patients with secondary syphilis. However, other etiologies, such as alopecia areata and systemic lupus erythematosus, can result in the same pattern of hair loss. Furthermore, hair loss in syphilis can be diffuse as well as moth-eaten.

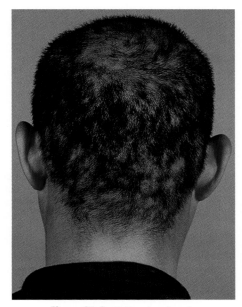

Figure 20-8. Moth-eaten alopecia.

ACNE AND ACNEIFORM ERUPTIONS

Joanna M. Burch, MD, and John L. Aeling, MD

1. How common is acne?

Acne vulgaris is the most common dermatologic disorder, affecting between 40 and 50 million individuals of all ages in the United States. Eighty-five percent of people between the ages of 12 and 24 years will have some acne. Direct costs related to acne, including factors such as loss of productivity and related depression, exceed $2.2 billion annually in the United States.

Bhambri S, Del Rosso JQ, Bhambri A: Pathogenesis of acne vulgaris: recent advances, *J Drug Dermatol* 8:615–617, 2009.
White GM: Recent findings in the epidemiologic evidence, classification, and subtypes of acne vulgaris, *Arch Dermatol* 39:S34–S37, 1998.

2. What is the pathophysiology of acne?

The pilosebaceous unit, made up of a follicle (pore), sebaceous gland, and a vellus hair, is the target organ affected in acne. The face, chest, and back are areas with the greatest concentration of pilosebaceous follicles, corresponding to the areas most commonly affected by acne lesions. The primary lesion of acne is the microcomedo. This is the result of obstruction of the sebaceous follicles by sebum and abnormally differentiated and desquamated keratinocytes that may produce large comedones (Fig. 21-1). The four main pathophysiologic factors in acne vulgaris are:

- Inflammation (recent evidence indicates that inflammatory events precede the hyperkeratinization of the follicle)
- Sebaceous gland hyperplasia with excess sebum production
- Altered follicular epithelial growth and differentiation
- *Propionibacterium acnes* colonization of the follicle

Theboutot D, Gollnick H, Bettoli V, et al: New insights into the management of acne: an update from the Global Alliance to Improve Outcomes in Acne Group, *J Am Acad Dermatol* 60:S1–S50, 2009.
Smolinski KN, Yan AC: Acne update, *Curr Opin Pediatr* 16:385–391, 2004.

3. What are the acne subtypes.

Acne presents in many forms and variations. The most common form is acne vulgaris, which is classified according to the predominant lesion type as comodonal, papular, pustular, nodular, or cystic. It can be graded as mild, moderate, or severe (Fig. 21-2). Other clinical subtypes of acneiform skin lesions include:

- Neonatal acne
- Infantile acne
- Perioral dermatitis
- Acne rosacea
- Acne excoriée
- Acne mechanica
- Acne conglobata
- Pyoderma faciale
- Acne fulminans
- Drug-induced acne
- Favre-Racouchot syndrome

4. How does the composition of sebum contribute to the formation of acne?

The major constituent of sebaceous lipid is triglyceride, which makes up over 50% of the lipid; wax esters account for 25%, squalene 15%, and there are small amounts of cholesterol esters and free cholesterol. Increased sebum production is characteristic of patients with acne, but the seborrhea itself is not sufficient to produce acne. Desaturation of the fatty acids in sebum may lead to the development of acne lesions. Lipoperoxidases characterize the sebum of acne patients, and this, along with other qualitative changes in the sebum lipids, induce alteration of keratinocyte differentiation and induce interleukin-1 (IL-1) secretion, leading to follicular hyperkeratinization.

Kurokawa I, Danby FW, Ju Q, et al: New developments in our understanding of acne pathogenesis and treatment, *Exp Dermatol* 18:821–832, 2009.
Downing DT, Stewart ME, Wertz PW, et al: Essential fatty acids and acne, *J Am Acad Dermatol* 14:221–225, 1986.

5. Does stress exacerbate acne?

Yes, it seems to. Many patients report that emotional stress makes their acne worse. In one survey of 4576 consecutive patients with various dermatologic problems, 55% of those with acne reported that episodes of emotional stress were closely related to exacerbation of their acne. A prospective cohort study, published in 2003, of 22 university students with acne during exams showed increased acne severity that was significantly associated with increased stress levels. Another study in high school students also found that increased stress correlated with increased acne severity. There did not seem to be an increase in sebum production during times of stress in this study. New data regarding the physiology of sebaceous glands indicate that these skin organs have receptors for numerous neuropeptides (NPs), and these receptors modulate inflammation, proliferation, and sebum production and composition, as well as androgen metabolism in human sebocytes. Further elucidation of these neural skin connections may help our understanding of the connection between stress and acne.

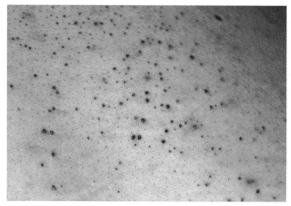

Figure 21-1. Numerous microcomedones and comedones in patient with acne. (Courtesy of the William L. Weston, M.D. Collection.)

Chiu A, Chon SY, Kimball AB: The response of skin disease to stress: changes in the severity of acne vulgaris as affected by examination stress, *Arch Dermatol* 139:897–900, 2003.

Koo, JYM, Smith LL: Psychologic aspects of acne, *Pediatr Dermatol* 8:185–188, 1991.

Yosipovitch G, Tang, M, Dawn AG, et al: Study of psychological stress, sebum production and acne vulgaris in adolescents, *Acta Derm Vereneol* 87:35–39, 2007.

6. Does diet affect acne?

Minimally. Association between diet and acne has long been postulated. Arguments for such an association include the observations that acne prevalence is low in rural, nonindustrialized societies and increases with the adoption of a Western diet. A study published in 1971 rechallenged patients with large amounts of foods that reportedly exacerbated their acne without showing any significant change in acne severity. In another study, 1925 patients kept food diaries and found milk to be most commonly associated with their acne flares. A study showing no association between chocolate bar consumption and acne has been criticized for several reasons most recently, because the chocolate bars given to subjects during the study did not contain milk, in contrast to the average chocolate bar of the time. To further examine the role of diet and acne, especially dairy consumption, a recent study examined data from the Nurses Health Study (NHS) II to see if there was a positive association between milk in the teenage diet and acne. Intake of milk during adolescence was associated with a history of teenage acne. The association was more marked for skim than whole milk. Interestingly, soda, French fries, chocolate candy, and pizza were not significantly associated with acne. The authors hypothesized that the hormonal content, not the fat in milk, may be responsible for the acne. Two other large studies have reported a similar positive

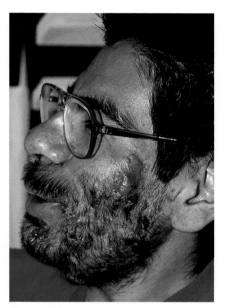

Figure 21-2. Severe inflammatory cystic acne vulgaris.

association between milk intake and acne. Smith, Mann, Braue, et al. enrolled 43 men with moderate acne, ages 15 to 25, in a trial randomized to a low glycemic index diet or a high glycemic–index diet. The men on the low glycemic–index diet lost significantly more weight and had significantly improved acne over the other group. The relative contribution of the high glycemic–load diet on acne pathogenesis versus the improvement in insulin and hormone levels with weight loss is unknown.

Adebamowo CA, Spiegelman D, Danby FW, et al: High school dietary intake and teenage acne, *J Am Acad Dermatol* 52:207–214, 2005.

Smith RN, Man NJ, Braue A, et al: The effect of a high-protein, low glycemic-load diet versus a conventional, high glycemic-load diet on biochemical parameters associated with acne vulgaris: a randomized, investigator-masked controlled trial. *J Am Acad Dermatol* 57: 247–256, 2007.

Spencer, EH, Ferdowsian HR, Barnard ND: Diet and acne: a review of the evidence, *Int J Dermatol* 48:339–347, 2009.

7. When can teenagers with acne expect their acne to resolve?

Acne affects approximately 8% of adults aged 25 to 34, and 3% aged 35 to 44. Most teenage boys can anticipate clearing of their acne between 20 and 25 years of age. For women, the news is not so good. The majority of patients with adult acne, including adult-onset acne, are women. This can last up to and beyond age 40.

Goulden V, Stables GI, Cunliffe WJ: Prevalence of facial acne in adults, *J Am Acad Dermatol* 41:577–580, 1999.

8. Discuss the topical therapy of acne vulgaris.

The single most important topical medications used to treat acne are retinoids. We now have numerous topical preparations to choose from that are less irritating and decrease the most common complaint associated with class of acne therapy. These include adapalene (Differin), tazarotene (Tazorac), and tretinoin (Avita, Retin-A, Retin-A Micro). Twelve weeks of use is required for maximum benefit. Retinoids are the only drugs that normalize keratinization within the follicular infundibulum and prevent comodone formation. *Propironibacterium acnes,* the anaerobic bacterium associated with acne pathogenesis, stimulates the innate immune response via Toll-like receptors (TLRs). This sets off an inflammatory cascade of cytokines. Retinoids are known to downregulate TLRs and inhibit downstream inflammatory transcription factors. Recent recommendations from a global alliance to improve outcomes in acne recommended that retinoid-based combination therapy (retinoid plus antimicrobial or benzoyl peroxide) be the first-line treatment for most forms of acne vulgaris. Retinoids have been shown to maintain improvement achieved with this initial combination therapy.

Other topical treatments include benzoyl peroxide (BPo), topical antibiotics (erythromycin, clindamycin, and sodium sulfacetamide), α-hydroxy acids, salicylic acid, and azelaic acid. Antibiotic resistance of *P. acnes* has become more common. More than half of patients undergoing therapy with a topical antibiotic will develop resistance. No bacterial resistance has been reported with topical benzoyl peroxide. The following are recommendations for preventing bacterial resistance in the treatment of acne: combining antimicrobials with a retinoid and BPo, limiting the duration of antimicrobial therapy, not using antimicrobials as monotherapy, and avoiding concurrent use of oral and topical antibiotics, especially if chemically different.

Theboutot D, Gollnick, H, Bettoli V, et al: New insights into the management of acne: an update from the Global Alliance to Improve Outcomes in Acne Group, *J Am Acad Dermatol* 60:S1–S50, 2009.

9. Discuss oral antibiotic use in acne vulgaris.

Antibiotics are indicated in patients with inflammatory lesions (red papules, pustules, or nodules) of moderate to severe grade. Antibiotics appropriate for use in acne are the tetracyclines and the macrolides, with trimethoprim/sulfamethoxasole as a distant alternative. Antibiotics reduce the numbers of *P. acnes* in the follicles and also have numerous antiinflammatory effects.

Antibiotics should *never* be used as monotherapy in acne. There is a significant problem with antibiotic resistance, and only two of the four main pathophysiologic mechanisms of disease are being addressed. Oral antibiotics should be combined with a keratolytic such as a topical retinoid and topical benzoyl peroxide. Oral therapy will take 4 to 8 weeks to show significant improvement. After adequate clinical response in 3 to 6 months, the dose should be tapered in an attempt to provide maintenance with topical medications.

Espersen F: Resistance to antibiotics used in dermatological practice, *Br J Dermatol* 139:4–8, 1998.

10. Will the oral antibiotics used in acne interfere with the efficacy of oral contraceptives (OCs) to prevent pregnancy?

Probably not. Whether the contraceptive efficacy of OCs is adversely affected by antibiotics such as penicillins, sulfonamides, and tetracyclines is highly controversial. Tetracycline, doxycycline, ampicillin, and metronidazole have been shown in pharmacokinetic studies not to decrease contraceptive steroid levels. When contraceptive failure rates of dermatology patients on OCs and antibiotics were compared to patients who take OCs but not antibiotics, no difference was found. However, there is a theoretical risk, and this should be discussed with female patients taking both antibiotics and OCs.

11. Discuss the use of OCs in the treatment of acne.

OCs most often used today to treat acne are a combination of ethinyl estradiol and a progestin. The only OCs officially approved by the Food and Drug Administration (FDA) for use in acne are Ortho-TriCyclen (Ortho-McNeil Pharmaceutical, Raritan, NJ), Estrostep (Parke-Davis, Detroit, MI), and, most recently, YAZ (Bayer Healthcare Pharmaceuticals, Montville, NJ). The second- and the third-generation progestins combined with an estrogen are the most appropriate choices for the treatment of acne because they have the lowest androgenic activity (Table 21-1). Multiple studies suggest that OCs are significantly better than placebo in the treatment of mild to moderate acne. The trials comparing different OCs are somewhat conflicting. OCs work by suppressing the endogenous production of androgens, reducing free testosterone, and increasing sex hormone–binding globulin. Patients should be screened for risk factors associated with OCs prior to beginning this therapy (see Table 21-1). The World Health Organization and the American College of Obstetricians and Gynecologists no longer require pelvic exam before initiating OC therapy in most healthy female patients of childbearing age.

Arowojulo AO, Gallo MF, Lopez LM, et al: Combined oral contraceptive pills for treatment of acne, *Cochrane Database Syst Rev* 8;(3): CD004425, 2009.

Frangos JE, Alvaian CN, Kimball AB: Acne and oral contraceptives: update on women's health screening guidelines, *J Am Acad Dermatol* 58:781–786, 2008.

Sawaya ME: Antiandrogens and androgen inhibitors, In Wolverton SE, editor: *Comprehensive dermatologic drug therapy*, ed 2, Philadelphia, 2007, Saunders, pp 430–432.

12. When should a patient be started on isotretinoin therapy?

Isotretinoin is the mainstay of therapy for severe acne. It is indicated for patients with severe, scarring, nodulocystic acne and those with moderate to severe acne who have failed an adequate trial (3 to 6 months) of conventional

Table 21-1. Combination Oral Contraceptives for Acne

ESTROGEN	PROGESTIN	BRAND NAMES	OTHER INFORMATION
Ethinyl estradiol	Desogestrel	Apri, Cyclessa, Desogen, Ortho-Cept	3rd-generation progestin
Ethinyl estradiol	Gestodene	N/A (not available in U.S.)	3rd-generation progestin
Ethinyl estradiol	Norgestimate	Mononessa, Ortho Cyclen, Orthotricylcen, Orthotricy-clen Lo, Sprintec, Trinessa	3rd-generation progestin
Ethinyl estradiol	Norethindrone	Brevicon, Estrostep, Junel, Modicon, Necon, Nelova, Norethin, OrthoNovum, Ovcon-35, TriNorinyl	2nd-generation progestin
Ethinyl estradiol	Ethynodiol diacetate	Demulen, Ovulen, Zovia	2nd-generation progestin
Ethinyl estradiol	Levonorgestrel	Alesse, Aviane, Empresse, Levlen, Levlite, Lovora, Nordette, Portia, TriLevlen, Triphasil, Trivora	2nd-generation progestin
Ethinyl estradiol	Drospirenone	Yasmin, YAZ	New progestin that is an analog of spironolactone Has antiandrogenic and antimineralocorticoid properties

therapy (retinoid and/or benzoyl peroxide [BP] plus an oral antibiotic). Isotretinoin is also beneficial for patients with severe hidradenitis suppurativa, acne rosacea, and gram-negative acne who are unresponsive to conventional therapy. However, it is not as effective in these diseases as it is in severe acne vulgaris, and relapses are more frequent. The recommended dose is 1.0 mg/kg/day for 20 to 24 weeks. Isotretinoin should be used as monotherapy for acne vulgaris.

Goldsmith LA, Bolognia JL, Callen JP, et al: American Academy of Dermatology Consensus Conference on the Safe and Optimal Use of Isotretinoin: summary and recommendations, *J Am Acad Dermatol* 50:900–906, 2004.

13. What are the side effects of isotretinoin?

Isotretinoin is a potent teratogen. Of the pregnancies that have occurred in patients taking isotretinoin, one third have resulted in spontaneous abortion, one third ended in therapeutic abortion, and of the one third that continued to term, 20% showed a major fetal malformation, including those of the brain, heart, and ears. Many of these patients, who had a pregnancy while taking isotretinoin, were pregnant when the drug was started. When considering treatment with isotretinoin in females of childbearing age, the FDA requires documentation of two negative pregnancy tests. Contraceptive counseling must be done and documented on the patient's chart, and two forms of birth control are recommended for the duration of therapy plus 6 weeks posttherapy. Therapy should be started on the third day of the menstrual cycle with a negative pregnancy test to ensure that the patient is not pregnant when therapy is initiated. Beginning in March 2006, the FDA requires all patients, prescribers, and dispensers of isotretinoin to be registered with the internet-based iPLEDGE program (www.iPLEDGEprogram.com).

Other side effects of isotretinoin include dry skin, lips, and eyes, dry mucous membranes with nosebleeds, headache (including rare instances of pseudotumor cerebri), muscle and backaches, hypertriglyceridemia, increased liver function tests, and depression (see next question). These should be discussed in detail with the patient prior to starting therapy and documentation of the discussion made in the chart. There are also several case reports of inflammatory bowel disease (IBD) being triggered by isotretinoin use. A review of adverse events reported to the United States FDA Medwatch scheme over a 5-year period (1997 to 2002) revealed 85 cases of IBD, of which the causal association with isotretinoin was considered probable or highly probable in 73% of cases.

Reddy D, Siegel CA, Sands BE, et al: Possible association between isotretinoin and inflammatory bowel disease, *Am J Gastroenterol* 101:1569–1573, 2006.

14. What about depression and suicide with isotretinoin?

A number of case reports and case series appear in the literature that link depression, suicide, and suicidal ideation to isotretinoin use. In several of these cases, cessation of the drug resulted in improvement of the depressive symptoms and rechallenge caused recurrence of depression. Between 1982 and 2000, the FDA received reports of 394 cases of depression and 37 suicides occurring in patients exposed to isotretinoin. However, depression is more common in the age group affected by acne than in the general population. To complicate matters further, there is evidence that acne itself has significant psychological effects, and there are case reports of improvement in depression scores of acne patients during and after treatment with isotretinoin. Epidemiologic studies to date have not shown a causal relationship between isotretinoin and depression and suicide. Because depression and suicide are serious matters, careful monitoring of patients undergoing therapy with isotretinoin for signs/symptoms of depression and suicidal ideation is advisable.

Magin P, Pond D, Smith W: Isotretinoin, depression, and suicide: a review of the evidence, *Br J Gen Pract* 55:134–138, 2005.

15. Discuss light and laser therapy of acne vulgaris.

One of the important pathogenic mechanisms of acne is *Propionibacterium acnes* growth in the follicle. *P. acnes* produces porphyrins, which can be activated by visible light, inducing a photodynamic reaction that kills the bacteria. Several studies have shown improvement in acne utilizing visible light, especially in the blue light spectrum (400 to 420 nm) where these porphyrins are most strongly activated. Blue and red (660 nm) light combined has also been used, as well as light in the yellow and green spectrum (500 to 600 nm). Several studies have shown improvement in acne lesions with relatively few side effects. However, clearing seems to be variable among patients and relapse rates are high.

Photodynamic therapy utilizes a lower-power visible light source in which the effectiveness is amplified by the use of a topical photosensitizing agent, most often aminolevulinic acid (ALA). Photodynamic therapy tends to have more side effects, such as burning at the sites of treatment and postinflammatory hyperpigmentation. Existing studies suggest promise for this therapy, with sustained improvement in acne for up to 20 weeks after several treatments.

Several laser devices have been employed and studied in the treatment of acne. There are a few small studies evaluating the 1450-nm diode laser was used to target and destroy sebaceous glands. Due to differences in treatment regimen and other allowed acne treatment, no comparisons can be made between studies.

Elman M, Lebzelter J: Light therapy in the treatment of acne vulgaris, *Dermatol Surg* 30:139–146, 2004.

Theboutot D, Gollnick, H, Bettoli V, et al: New insights into the management of acne: an update from the Global Alliance to Improve Outcomes in Acne Group, *J Am Acad Dermatol* 60:S1–S50, 2009.

Key Points: Acne

1. In acne, the pilosebaceous unit is the target of disease. The microcomedone is the earliest lesion.
2. Combination therapy including a retinoid plus benzoyl peroxide (BPo) or an antimicrobial agent is the preferred approach for almost all patients with acne. A topical keratolytic (benzoyl peroxide or topical retinoids) should *always* be used with a topical or oral antibiotic in treating inflammatory acne.
3. Topical retinoids should be first-line agents in the maintenance therapy of acne.
4. Bacterial resistance to BPo does not occur. Using BPo concomitantly with antimicrobial therapy for acne (as a leave-on or as a wash) is effective in limiting antibiotic resistance. Benzoyl peroxide for 5 to 7 days between antibiotic courses may reduce resistant organisms on the skin.
5. Drug-induced acne is caused most often by anabolic and corticosteroids. It is differentiated from acne vulgaris by its sudden onset, distribution mainly on the upper trunk, and its monomorphous pustular appearance without comedones.

---

16. What is SAPHO syndrome?

This syndrome combines **s**ynovitis, **a**cne, **p**ustulosis, **h**yperostosis, and **o**steitis. It is a disorder characterized by noninfectious osteoarticular inflammatory lesions and a variety of skin abnormalities demonstrating aseptic, neutrophil-rich pseudoabscesses. In adults, chronic multifocal osteomyelitis is a classic manifestation. Skin findings include palmoplantar or other forms of pustulosis, severe acne, or psoriasis. The acne associated with this syndrome is most often acne conglobata, with highly inflammatory comedones, nodules, abscesses, and draining sinuses located primarily on the trunk, which often heal with significant scarring.

Magrey M, Kahn MA: New insights into synovitis, acne, pustulosis, hyperostosis and osteitis (SAPHO) syndrome, *Curr Rheumatol Rep* 11:329–333, 2009.

17. Is there a difference between neonatal acne and infantile acne?

Yes. Neonatal acne occurs in up to 20% of newborns; it usually develops during weeks 2 to 4 of life (Fig. 21-3). It is more common in males, is relatively mild, and regresses spontaneously in most infants by age 6 months. It is thought to be due to maternal androgens and is not associated with significant scarring or an increased incidence of acne in later life. Infantile acne usually begins between the third and sixth months of life and may persist to age 5 and rarely longer. It is uncommon and occurs more often in males. It can be severe, with nodules, cysts, and significant residual scarring. Endocrine abnormalities and virilizing tumors can be associated. Some studies show an increased incidence of severe acne in later life.

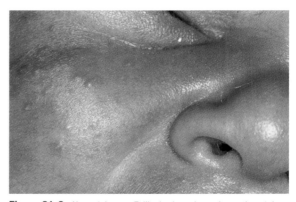

Figure 21-3. Neonatal acne. Follicular-based papules and pustules in a neonate.

18. What is neonatal cephalic pustulosis?

This is a recently recognized entity that may have been labeled in the past as neonatal acne. It appears during the first few days of life in both males and females with erythema, pustules, or papules mainly on the head and neck. It is thought to be an inflammatory reaction to *Malassezia* spp. The monomorphic appearance, absence of comedones, and the lack of a follicular distribution distinguish this entity from neonatal acne. It resolves spontaneously within one week.

19. What is perioral dermatitis?

This common distinctive acneiform skin eruption occurs mainly in women aged 15 to 25 years, but also occurs in children. Perioral dermatitis is characterized by erythema, scaling, and follicular papules that occur around the mouth, nose, and, less frequently, the eyes. The etiology is unknown, but many patients have used mid- or high-potency topical steroids inappropriately. In one study, 20% of children with perioral dermatitis have a family history of rosacea. The treatment includes the cessation of all topical corticosteroids and an 8 to 10 week course of a tetracycline antibiotic. Tetracycline and derivatives should not be used in children under 8 years of age. Oral erythromycin and topical clindamycin are effective substitutes. Recurrences are rare.

20. Do any drugs cause or aggravate acne?

A wide range of drugs have been reported to cause or aggravate acne, although many of these associations are isolated case reports (Table 21-2).

21. How does steroid acne differ from acne vulgaris?

Steroid acne has a sudden onset, the lesions are monomorphic (all lesions at the same stage of development), and comedones are absent. It occurs primarily on the upper trunk, less frequently on the face, and clears when the drug is withdrawn.

22. What is pyoderma faciale?

This is an acute, ferocious skin disease of women aged 15 to 40. It strikes like a hurricane, often in patients with no previous history of acne. It most commonly involves the central face but may affect the upper trunk. It is characterized by severe pustules, nodules, cysts, and draining sinus tracts (Fig. 21-4). Many of the patients have a history of flushing,

Table 21-2. Drugs That Cause or Aggravate Acne

Steroid hormones	**Halogens**
Topical corticosteroids	Iodides
Systemic corticosteroids	Bromides
Anabolic steroids	Halogenated hydrocarbons
Some progestins	**Antituberculous drugs**
Testosterone	Isoniazid
Antidepressants	**Miscellaneous drugs**
Lithium	Thiourea
Amineptine	Thiouracil
Antiepileptic drugs	PUVA
Phenytoin	
Trimethadione	

PUVA, Psoralen plus ultraviolet light, type A.

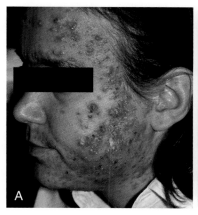 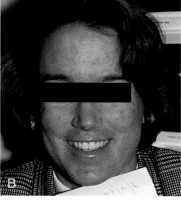

Figure 21-4. Pyoderma faciale. **A,** This fulminant eruption developed when the patient was tapered off systemic corticosteroids. **B,** Same patient after treatment with a tapered course of prednisone and Accutane. The eruption did not recur.

and some authors regard it as a severe variant of acne rosacea. It has been reported in some patients during pregnancy or immediately postpartum.

23. How do you treat pyoderma faciale?

This is one of the few times that oral steroids should be used to treat acne. Prednisone in a dose of 40 to 60 mg daily tapered over 3 to 4 weeks is indicated. Isotretinoin should be started in a dose of 1 mg/kg/day in conjunction with the prednisone and continued for 4 to 6 months. Once the disease has been brought under control, it rarely, if ever, recurs.

Plewig G, Jansen T, Kligman AM: Pyoderma faciale, *Arch Dermatol* 128:1611–1617, 1992.

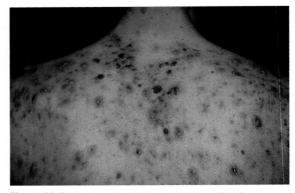

Figure 21-5. A male patient with acne fulminans. Note the ulcerative lesions on the upper back.

24. What is acne fulminans?

This rare systemic disease is seen predominately in young men. Its clinical features include fever, polyarthritis, leukocytosis, malaise, weight loss, anorexia, and severe, acute cystic and often ulcerative acne lesions. It occurs primarily on the upper trunk, but lesions may also be seen on the buttocks, proximal extremities, neck, and face (Fig. 21-5). The etiology is unknown, but it is thought to be immunologically mediated. It has been described in young men, particularly soldiers, who are introduced into a tropical environment where they are exposed to high humidity, temperature, and the friction of wearing a backpack. Like pyoderma faciale, it usually responds well to treatment with isotretinoin and oral prednisone.

25. What is hidradenitis suppurativa?

Hidradenitis is a chronic, suppurative, recurring inflammatory disease that affects apocrine gland–bearing sites. The axilla and groin are most frequently involved, but the disease is also seen on the perineum, buttocks, neck, and scalp (Fig. 21-6). It is more common in females and begins after puberty. It is characterized by inflammatory nodules, abscess formation, scarring, and sinus tract formation.

26. How do you treat hidradenitis suppurativa?

This frustrating chronic disease is treated by measures that reduce friction and moisture. Weight reduction, loose undergarments, topical antiseptic soaps, and topical aluminum chloride are helpful in some patients.

- Acute exacerbations can be treated with systemic antibiotics. Problem cases should have bacterial cultures and sensitivities taken, although not all cultures grow pathogenic bacteria. The chronic use of topical clindamycin proves beneficial in some patients.
- Chronic inflammatory nodules can be treated with intralesional steroids. Systemic retinoids may help some patients but are not as effective as when used to treat severe acne vulgaris, and relapses are quite common.
- Severe refractory hidradenitis is best treated by complete surgical excision of the involved area. Incision and drainage should be minimized because it often leads to chronic sinus tract formation. Carbon dioxide laser stripping with secondary intention healing has been used as well.
- Newer treatments, such as the anti–TNF-α biologics and photodynamic therapy, have had mixed success.

Revuz J: Hidradenitis supperativa, *J Eur Acad Dermatol Venereol* 23:985–998, 2009.

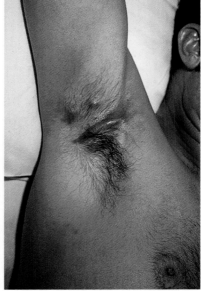

Figure 21-6. Hidradenitis suppurativa of the axilla with cysts and draining sinus tracts.

27. Discuss acne rosacea.

Acne rosacea is a chronic skin disease that most commonly occurs between the ages of 30 and 50 years, although it can be seen in adolescents and elderly patients. The course is typically chronic with remissions and relapses. It is characterized by flushing, telangiectasia, papules, and pustules, and in severe late-stage disease, patients may develop chronic facial lymphedema and rhinophyma. It is usually symmetrical and is most commonly seen on the convex areas of the face, including the nose, cheeks, forehead, and chin (Fig. 21-7). Blepharitis, conjunctivitis, and keratitis are common associations.

The etiology of rosacea is unknown. Genetic factors seem to play a role in that the disease is more common in persons of Celtic ancestry and less common in blacks. Factors that stimulate flushing, such as hot beverages, alcohol, ultraviolet light exposure, and emotional factors, frequently exacerbate the disease. A rosacea-like eruption can be induced by the topical application of fluorinated corticosteroids and tacrolimus ointment to the face.

Powell FC: Rosacea, *N Engl J Med* 352:793–803, 2005.

28. How is acne rosacea treated?

Trigger factors that produce flushing should be avoided. These triggers vary greatly from patient to patient. Both oral and topical metronidazole are effective. Topical erythromycin, azelaic acid cream, and sodium sulfacetamide have also been shown to be effective treatments. Tetracycline, doxycycline, minocycline erythromycin are effective systemic therapies for rosacea. Subantimicrobial doses of doxycycline (40 mg extended release tablet) have been shown to decrease papulopustules in rosacea via antiinflammatory effects. Combined with topical azelaic acid or metronidazole there seems to be a synergistic effect.

Oral isotretinoin is helpful for severe resistant cases, but the drug is not as effective as when used for severe cystic acne, and relapses are more common. Oral antibiotics have little effect on flushing, telangiectasia, lymphedema, or rhinophyma. Isotretinoin may provide some benefit for early rhinophyma, but severe rhinophyma is best treated by surgical paring or electrosurgery. Persistent telangiectasia can be treated by a tunable dye vascular laser with good cosmetic results.

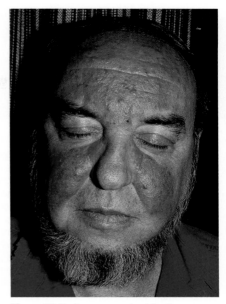

Figure 21-7. Acne rosacea involving the convex surfaces of the face.

Fowler JF Jr: Combined effect of anti-inflammatory dose doxycycline (40-mg doxycycline, USP monohydrate controlled-release capsules) and metronidazole topical gel 1% in the treatment of rosacea, *J Drugs Dermatol* 6: 641–645, 2007.

29. What is Favre-Racouchot syndrome?

This describes the development of multiple open comedones located on the inferolateral aspect of the orbital rim in elderly patients. It is associated with marked solar elastosis of the surrounding skin.

AUTOIMMUNE CONNECTIVE TISSUE DISEASES

Todd T. Kobayashi, MD, Lt Col, USAF, MC, and Kathleen M. David-Bajar, MD

1. Discuss the skin changes of lupus erythematosus.

Skin changes occur very frequently in lupus erythematosus (LE) and are second in frequency only to musculoskeletal complaints in this condition, occurring in about 85% of patients. It is useful to classify the eruptions seen in LE as to their possible diagnostic and prognostic significance. Skin lesions that are diagnostic of LE have been called lupus-specific eruptions. Skin biopsies of these lesions show characteristic histopathologic changes of cutaneous LE. Further classification of the lupus-specific eruptions into subtypes of cutaneous LE is also useful, as some lesions of cutaneous LE are more strongly associated with systemic lupus erythematosus.

Lupus patients also develop many skin changes that are not specific for LE, termed lupus-nonspecific eruptions (Table 22-1). These eruptions do not help to establish a diagnosis of LE, but they may still be very important to note, as specific systemic findings may be associated with them. For example, cutaneous lesions of palpable purpura in a patient with LE are not lupus-specific, that is, such lesions may be seen in patients who do not have LE; however, they may be associated with vasculitic lesions of the kidney or central nervous system (CNS), and thus they have significance in the evaluation and treatment of lupus.

Walling HW, Sontheimer RD: Cutaneous lupus erythematosus: issues in diagnosis and treatment, *Am J Clin Dermatol* 10:365–381, 2009.

2. What is acute cutaneous lupus erythematosus (ACLE)?

ACLE presents as an acute malar or more generalized photodistributed eruption. The malar erythema has been described as a "butterfly rash," since the pattern across the cheeks resembles the wings of a butterfly (Fig. 22-1). Nearly all patients presenting with ACLE will have systemic lupus erythematosus (SLE), often in an acute flare. ACLE is usually transient, improving when the SLE improves, and generally does not result in scarring of the skin. A common diagnostic pitfall is the confusion of rosacea with the malar rash of ACLE. Rosacea is common; it is photo-exacerbated. Nonspecific joint symptoms are common, and 5% of the normal population will have a positive antinuclear antibody (ANA) test, often leading to a misdiagnosis of ACLE. Remember, a patient with ACLE is most often in an acute flare and will be "sick," whereas a rosacea patient will have a chronic history and no systemic symptoms beyond their baseline "aches and pains."

3. Are there any common skin eruptions that may be confused with acute cutaneous lupus erythematosus?

Many patients have complaints of erythema of the face due to a wide variety of conditions, but not all of them are photoinduced. The differential diagnosis of photosensitive eruptions of the face is not as broad and includes polymorphous light eruption, photoreactions to systemic medications and topical products, and certain types of porphyria (see Chapter 17). In addition, certain facial eruptions, such as rosacea, occasionally may be triggered or worsened by sun exposure. ACLE is an important cutaneous finding since it is strongly associated with SLE. Thus, patients with ACLE will have additional systemic complaints relating to SLE and will nearly always have a positive ANA test.

4. What is subacute cutaneous lupus erythematosus (SCLE)?

This type of cutaneous LE was first described and characterized in the late 1970s. These patients have an eruption that is more persistent than that of ACLE, lasting weeks to months or longer. The lesions of SCLE consist of scaly, superficial, inflammatory macules, patches, papules, and plaques that are photodistributed, particularly on the upper chest and back, lateral neck, and

Table 22-1. Classification of Cutaneous Disease in Lupus Erythematosus

LUPUS-SPECIFIC ERUPTIONS	LUPUS-NONSPECIFIC ERUPTIONS
Acute cutaneous lupus erythematosus (ACLE) (Malar rash of lupus; macular or papular photodistributed eruption; lupus hairs) Subacute cutaneous lupus erythematosus (SCLE) (Annular, serpiginous, psoriasiform, or pityriasiform) Chronic cutaneous lupus erythematosus (CCLE) (Discoid lupus erythematosus (DLE), hypertrophic DLE, tumid LE, chilblain LE, lupus mucinotic nodules) Lupus panniculitis Bullous eruption of systemic lupus erythematosus (SLE) Neonatal lupus erythematosus (NLE)	Nonscarring alopecia Telangiectasia Livedo reticularis and retiform purpura Palpable purpura (leukocytoclastic vasculitis) Periungual erythema Urticarial vasculitis Raynaud's syndrome Photosensitivity

dorsal arms and forearms. Several different morphologic types of SCLE have been described: annular, serpiginous, and two types of papulosquamous lesions, psoriasiform and pityriasiform (Fig. 22-2). Some patients have more than one morphologic type of lesion.

Sontheimer RD: Subacute cutaneous lupus erythematosus: 25-year evolution of a prototypic subset (subphenotype) of lupus erythematosus defined by characteristic cutaneous, pathological, immunological, and genetic findings, *Autoimmun Rev* 4:253–263, 2005.

5. Do patients with SCLE have SLE?

About one half of patients with SCLE will have four or more criteria for the classification of SLE, though most SCLE patients do not have serious renal or CNS lupus erythematosus. Typically, they have skin disease, photosensitivity, and musculoskeletal complaints. Dry eyes and dry mouth are also common. Some patients with SCLE experience severe manifestations of SLE, and thus all SCLE patients should be monitored for systemic disease.

6. How do you make a diagnosis of SCLE?

SCLE is a clinical diagnosis based on the presence of a typical photodistributed eruption and a skin biopsy consistent with cutaneous LE. Direct immunofluorescence testing may also be helpful. In addition to granular deposition of immunoreactants at the dermal–epidermal junction, particulate deposition of IgG within the epidermis has been described in SCLE. Most patients with SCLE have circulating antibodies to Ro/SS-A (Sjögren's syndrome A) and, less commonly, to La/SS-B (Sjögren's syndrome B). These antibodies are not demonstrable in all patients with SCLE; thus, their absence does not exclude this diagnosis. Additionally, a negative ANA does not exclude the diagnosis of SCLE, and some patients may have positive titers to Ro/SS-A or La/SS-B but test negative for ANA.

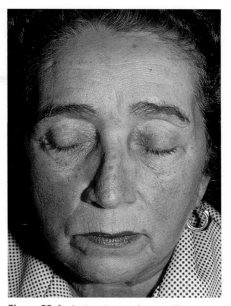

Figure 22-1. Acute cutaneous lupus erythematosus. Note the classic malar erythema ("butterfly rash").

7. What is the initial workup of SCLE?

Once a diagnosis of SCLE is made, it is important to evaluate for the presence of SLE:

- History and physical examination data should be gathered to identify manifestations of SLE in other organ systems.
- Laboratory testing should be directed by findings on the history and physical exam but will generally include a complete blood count with differential, urinalysis, serum chemistries including renal function tests, and an ANA panel to include anti–Ro/SS-A, anti–La/SS-B, and anti–native DNA antibodies. Complement determinations may be ordered since some SCLE patients have partial or complete complement deficiencies.
- A medication history is very important since SCLE may be triggered or worsened by a number of medications, especially thiazide diuretics (Table 22-2). Some physicians recommend avoiding estrogens and sulfonamides in any patient with LE.

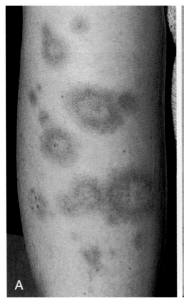

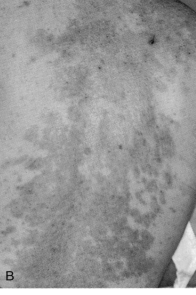

Figure 22-2. Subacute cutaneous lupus erythematosus. **A,** Annular lesions on the upper arms. **B,** Erythematous papules and plaques on the back.

Table 22-2. Medications Associated with Subacute Cutaneous Lupus Erythematosus

Adalimumab	Glyburide	Nifedipine	Procainamide
Aldactone	Gold	Nitrendipine	Ranitidine
Captopril	Griseofulvin	Omeprazole	Simvastatin
Cilazapril	Hydrochlorothiazide	Oxprenolol	Spironolactone
Cinnarizine	Infliximab	Penicillamine	Sulfonylureas
Diltiazem	Interferon-α, -β	Phenytoin	Taxotere
Docetaxel	Leflunomide	Piroxicam	Terbinafine
Etanercept	Naproxen	Pravastatin	Verapamil

8. How is SCLE managed?

Cutaneous complaints are often of most concern to these patients, and thus dermatologists are generally the physicians managing this disease. Broad-spectrum sunscreens and sun-protective measures, including lifestyle changes and clothing, are perhaps the most important initial measures. Some patients respond to topical steroids, although potent topical steroids are usually required. Oral antimalarial therapy is also beneficial in many patients. Less commonly used treatments include dapsone, gold, immunosuppressive drugs, retinoids, and systemic steroids.

9. What is chronic cutaneous lupus erythematosus?

There are several types of cutaneous LE that are very persistent, termed *chronic cutaneous lupus erythematosus*. Discoid lupus erythematosus (DLE) is the most common of these chronic forms of cutaneous LE. An unusual variant of DLE with thick keratotic scale is referred to as hypertrophic DLE. Tumid LE is a variant where scale and other epidermal changes are absent. Lupus panniculitis and lupus mucinotic nodules are other forms of chronic cutaneous LE.

10. Describe the skin changes of discoid lupus erythematosus.

DLE is a chronic inflammatory disease consisting of fixed, indurated, erythematous papules and plaques that are often distributed on the head and neck, although any cutaneous region can be affected (Fig. 22-3A). Without intervention, DLE lesions may last for many years and are associated with extensive scarring, a feature that helps distinguish DLE from SCLE. When DLE occurs on the scalp, permanent scarring alopecia may result. Pigmentary changes, both hyperpigmentation and hypopigmentation, are also frequently associated with lesions of DLE. Epidermal changes, including scale, keratotic plugging of the hair follicles, and sometimes crusting, are also generally present. The external ears are often involved in DLE (Fig. 22-3B); thus, this area should be carefully examined in patients with suspected DLE.

11. Do patients with DLE develop systemic lupus erythematosus?

If the initial workup of a patient with localized lesions of DLE does not reveal evidence of SLE, the risk of developing SLE is about 5%. If lesions are generalized, the risk is slightly higher. However, DLE lesions are not uncommon in patients with an established diagnosis of SLE. About 25% of SLE patients will develop lesions of DLE at some time in the course of their disease (Table 22-3).

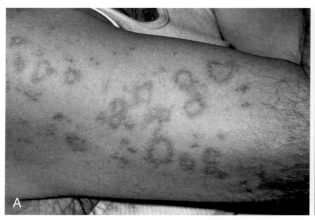
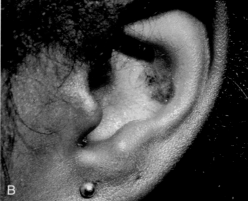

Figure 22-3. Discoid lupus erythematosus. **A,** Fixed, erythematous, scaly discoid plaques of DLE with central atrophy on the upper arms. **B,** DLE lesion in the concha of the ear. Hypopigmented and hyperpigmented areas, erythema, and scarring are present. (Panel A courtesy of the John L. Aeling, M. D. Collection.)

Table 22-3. Comparison of Lupus-Specific Eruptions

DISEASE	DURATION	% OF PATIENTS WITH SLE	PHOTOSENSITIVE
ACLE	Hours–weeks	99%	Yes
SCLE	Weeks–months	50%	Yes
CCLE	Months–years	5%	50%

12. How is discoid lupus erythematosus treated?

As with other types of cutaneous LE, sunscreens and sun-protective measures are the foundation of therapy. Potent topical steroids and intralesional corticosteroids are often helpful. Antimalarial drugs are also used. Less often, therapy with gold, immunosuppressive medications, or systemic corticosteroids is offered.

Wozniacka A, McCauliffe DP: Optimal use of antimalarials in treating cutaneous lupus erythematosus, *Am J Clin Dermatol* 6:1–11, 2005.

13. What is minocycline-induced lupus?

This condition has been reported in patients taking minocycline for acne. Most patients are young females who have taken minocycline chronically. The most common symptom is symmetric polyarthralgia, but other findings such as fatigue, fever, elevated liver enzymes, pneumonitis, and anemia have also been reported. Lupus-specific skin eruptions, such as acute cutaneous LE or discoid LE, have not been reported. Nearly all patients will have a positive screening ANA test. Once minocycline is discontinued, most patients have resolution of symptoms.

14. What is lupus panniculitis?

In lupus panniculitis, inflammation involves the subcutaneous tissue, resulting in inflamed nodules that often resolve with depressed scars. Lesions tend to favor the proximal extremities and trunk, which is a clinical clue differentiating this form of panniculitis from other forms of panniculitis. There may be overlying lesions of DLE. When lupus panniculitis occurs with an overlying DLE lesion, it may be called lupus profundus. About one half of patients with lupus panniculitis have four or more criteria for the classification of SLE. The diagnosis is confirmed by an adequate excisional biopsy. Small punch biopsies are not adequate to rule out other causes of panniculitis. Direct immunofluorescence examination may be helpful in establishing the diagnosis. The treatment of choice is antimalarial drugs.

Fraga J, García-Díez A: Lupus erythematosus panniculitis, *Dermatol Clin* 26:453–463, 2008.

15. Describe the bullous eruption of SLE.

This rare blistering eruption has been described primarily in patients with established SLE. The histopathologic findings are quite different from those of other forms of cutaneous LE. Biopsies demonstrate a separation of the epidermis from the dermis and a neutrophil-rich inflammatory cell infiltrate. Antibodies to type VII collagen, a component of anchoring fibrils (see Chapter 1), have been described in some patients with the bullous eruption of SLE. It has been proposed, but not proven, that these antibodies are involved in the pathogenesis of this disease.

16. How is the bullous eruption of systemic lupus erythematosus treated?

These patients typically respond to therapy with oral dapsone. Systemic corticosteroids have also been used.

17. What is neonatal lupus erythematosus (NLE)?

In NLE, infants develop skin disease (50%), heart disease (50%), or both (10%). The skin lesions occur most commonly on the face and head (Fig. 22-4), morphologically resemble SCLE lesions, and are transient, resolving within a few months, but sometimes leaving atrophic lesions. The heart disease usually manifests as isolated complete heart block, although lesser degrees of heart block have been reported. The heart block is generally permanent and may require a pacemaker. About 10% of infants with NLE and heart disease die from cardiac complications. A few infants with NLE also have thrombocytopenia and and/or liver disease.

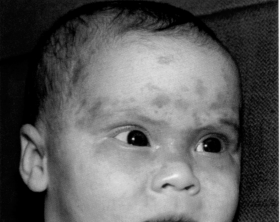

Figure 22-4. Neonatal lupus erythematosus demonstrating sharply defined erythema of the scalp and face. Periocular involvement producing a "raccoon eyes" appearance is common and is strongly suggestive of the diagnosis. (Courtesy of the Fitzsimons Army Medical Center teaching files.)

Nearly all infants with NLE have anti–Ro/SS-A and sometimes anti–La/SS-B antibodies, as will their mothers. A few NLE patients have been reported to have anti-U1RNP antibodies in the absence of anti-Ro or anti-La antibodies. These antibodies are transient and are not detectable after a few months of life. They are of maternal origin, transferred via the placenta.

Lee LA: Neonatal lupus erythematosus, *J Invest Dermatol* 100:9S–13S, 1993.

18. Which tests should be done in an infant with suspected NLE?
Serum from both the infant and mother should be assayed for ANA, and specifically for anti–Ro/SS-A, anti–La/SS-B, and anti-U1RNP antibodies. A skin biopsy for routine histology and direct immunofluorescence is also recommended. The biopsy will show histopathologic and direct immunofluorescence changes similar to those seen in SCLE.

19. Once a diagnosis of NLE is made, what workup should be done?
A physical examination should be performed, including cardiac examination and electrocardiogram. Because of reports of involvement of the liver and platelets, liver function tests and a platelet count should also be done. Additional tests or procedures may be done as indicated by physical findings. Mothers of infants with NLE should also be examined, because some will have or develop SCLE, SLE or symptoms of Sjögren's syndrome.

20. What is the lupus band test?
This direct immunofluorescence test is performed either on lesional skin or on normal, nonlesional skin. Granular deposits of immunoglobulins and complement are detected in a band-like pattern at the dermal–epidermal junction (Fig. 22-5). When this pattern is seen in lesional skin, it supports a diagnosis of cutaneous LE. When found in nonlesional skin, it is suggestive of SLE.

21. What is scleroderma?
Scleroderma is a chronic disease that involves the microvasculature and connective tissue and results in fibrosis. It may be localized, as in morphea, or more generalized and involving visceral organs, as in progressive systemic sclerosis. In morphea, sclerotic, indurated plaques develop that may be solitary, multiple, linear, or generalized. The surface is usually smooth, with the center of the lesion a whitish to brown color (Fig. 22-6), whereas the border of active lesions is often violaceous. Morphea usually involves the skin and subcutaneous tissues but may involve deeper structures, even bone. Patients with morphea generally do not develop systemic sclerosis.

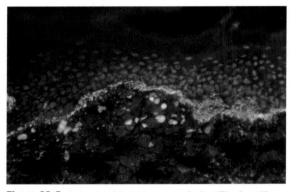

Figure 22-5. Lupus band test. Linear granular bandlike deposition of C1q at the junction between the epidermis and dermis in a patient with discoid lupus erythematosus. (Courtesy of the Fitzsimons Army Medical Center teaching files.)

22. What is the CREST syndrome?
- **C**alcinosis cutis
- **R**aynaud's phenomenon
- **E**sophageal dysfunction (or dysmotility)
- **S**clerodactyly
- **T**elangiectasia

CREST syndrome, or Thibierge-Weissenbach syndrome, is generally considered a type of limited systemic sclerosis. In addition to the cutaneous changes of calcinosis cutis, Raynaud's phenomenon, sclerodactyly, and telangiectasia, these patients often develop hyperpigmentation, particularly in sun-exposed areas (Fig. 22-7). Most patients with the CREST syndrome have circulating antibodies to centromeres, called anticentromere antibodies.

23. Describe the early cutaneous findings in progressive systemic sclerosis (PSS).
The earliest cutaneous complaints of PSS are often swelling of the hands and feet or symptoms associated with Raynaud's phenomenon. Telangiectasia may also develop early in the course

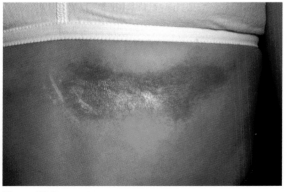

Figure 22-6. Typical well-developed lesion of morphea demonstrating an indurated plaque with both lighter areas and brownish discoloration. This lesion was very firm to palpation. (Courtesy of the Fitzsimons Army Medical Center teaching files.)

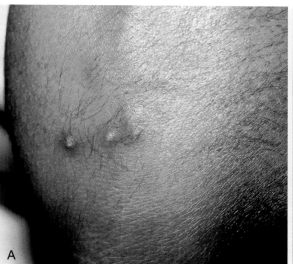

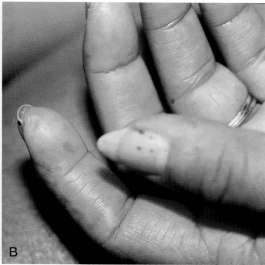

Figure 22-7. CREST syndrome. **A,** Firm, tender, whitish papules of calcinosis cutis on the elbow. **B,** Sclerodactyly and telangiectasia on the fingers.

of disease. The proximal nail folds show changes in the capillaries, including avascular areas (dropout) and marked dilatation. Over time, the skin of the digits becomes thickened and sclerotic (Fig. 22-8). Sclerotic changes are often progressive, involving the face and extremities, and may eventually involve large areas of the body. Other late changes include digital ulcers and even loss of the digits.

24. What is dermatomyositis?

Dermatomyositis is a chronic inflammatory disease involving the skin and skeletal muscles. Its etiology is unknown. Polymyositis is the term used for involvement of the skeletal muscles without cutaneous involvement. The muscle involvement usually presents as proximal muscle weakness, sometimes with pain, and later with muscle atrophy. Muscle involvement may precede, follow, or occur simultaneously with skin disease and, in some instances, may not be detectable, a condition called *amyopathic dermatomyositis*. A number of cutaneous changes are present, including blotchy erythema, erythematous to violaceous papules and plaques particularly on extensor surfaces, poikilodermatous changes, and calcinosis cutis.

Euwer RL, Sontheimer RD: Amyopathic dermatomyositis (dermatomyositis siné myositis): presentation of six new cases and review of the literature, *J Am Acad Dermatol* 24:959–966, 1991.

25. Are there skin changes diagnostic of dermatomyositis?

Two cutaneous findings have been described as pathognomonic of dermatomyositis: Gottron's papules and Gottron's sign. Gottron's papules

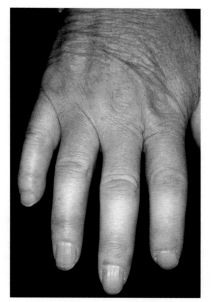

Figure 22-8. Progressive systemic sclerosis. Characteristic sclerodactyly manifesting as tight, shiny, thickened skin. (Courtesy of James E. Fitzpatrick, MD.)

are erythematous to purplish flat papules on the extensor surfaces of the interphalangeal joints. Gottron's sign consists of symmetrical violaceous erythema, sometimes with edema, over the dorsal knuckles of the hands, elbows, knees, and medial ankles (Fig. 22-9A). Other skin findings that are characteristic of dermatomyositis are periorbital edema with a lilac-colored erythema (heliotrope, Fig. 22-9B), periungual telangiectasia with cuticle dystrophy, and a photodistributed violaceous erythema of the forehead; also, sun-exposed areas of the neck, upper chest, shoulders, dorsal arms, forearms, and hands. A diagnostic clue favoring dermatomyositis over lupus erythematosus is the violaceous erythema or papules over the knuckles. Lupus, on the other hand, shows erythema over the dorsal phalanges, but often spares the knuckles.

Callen JP, Wortmann RL: Dermatomyositis, *Clin Dermatol* 24:363–373, 2006.

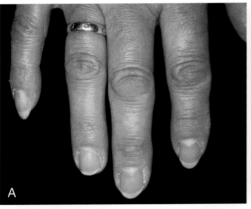
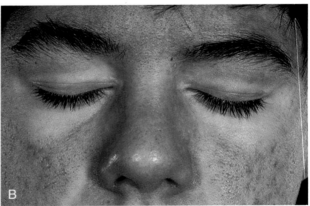

Figure 22-9. Dermatomyositis. **A,** Characteristic violaceous erythema over dorsal knuckles in a patient with associated breast cancer. **B,** Characteristic photodistributed erythema with heliotrope of upper eyelids. (Courtesy of James E. Fitzpatrick, MD.)

Key Points: Dermatomyositis

1. Gottron's papules (erythematous to violaceous papules over the knuckles) are a cutaneous finding that is pathognomonic of dermatomyositis.
2. Patients with dermatomyositis frequently demonstrate lilac-tinged erythema of the upper eyelids that is referred to as a heliotrope sign.
3. Amyopathic dermatomyositis (dermatomyositis siné myositis) is the presence of cutaneous findings of dermatomyositis with no evidence of muscle involvement.
4. Between 10% and 50% of adult patients that present with dermatomyositis have an underlying malignancy.

26. How do you diagnose dermatomyositis?

- Skin biopsy may be helpful, although the histopathologic changes are consistent with, rather than diagnostic of, dermatomyositis.
- Serum levels of muscle enzymes are typically elevated, with the creatine phosphokinase (CPK) level the most reliable indicator of disease activity.
- An electromyogram of an affected muscle will generally be abnormal.
- Biopsy of an affected muscle may be diagnostic, but nonspecific changes are also seen. The use of magnetic resonance imaging has been reported recently to be helpful in identifying muscle groups that would most likely yield significant findings on muscle biopsy.
- Although many patients with dermatomyositis have a positive screening ANA, only a small percentage will have specific ANAs detected, such as anti–Jo-1 or anti–Mi-2.

Dunn CL, James WD: The role of magnetic resonance imaging in the diagnostic evaluation of dermatomyositis, *Arch Dermatol* 129:1104–1106, 1993.

27. Are any diseases associated with dermatomyositis?

Adults with dermatomyositis have been reported to have a variety of malignancies that sometimes follow a clinical course of exacerbation and remission in concert with the dermatomyositis. Screening with a careful history, physical examination and age appropriate laboratory screening tests is recommended in adult patients with dermatomyositis. Female patients should be carefully screened for ovarian cancer.

28. What is the antisynthetase syndrome?

The antisynthetase syndrome is seen in both polymyositis and dermatomyositis patients and is associated with the anti–Jo-1 antibody, in addition to anti-PL7, -PL12, -OJ, and -EJ autoantibodies. In addition to skin and muscle involvement, patients may develop arthritis, Raynaud's syndrome, and interstitial lung disease.

29. What is an overlap syndrome?

Many patients diagnosed with autoimmune rheumatic disease display overlapping features of different connective tissue diseases and cannot be categorized easily into one of the established clinical entities, such as systemic lupus erythematosus, dermatomyositis, or systemic sclerosis. The term "overlap syndrome" has been used to classify these patients and is useful for descriptive purposes, clarifying prognosis and facilitating disease management.

30. What is mixed connective tissue disease?

Mixed connective tissue disease (MCTD) is a disorder characterized by a mixture of other well-defined connective tissue disorders such as systemic lupus erythematosus, progressive systemic sclerosis, dermatomyositis, and even Sjögren's syndrome. Most patients with MCTD have anti-U1RNP ribonuclear protein (U1RNP) antibodies. Patients often present with Raynaud's phenomenon, swelling of the digits (dactylitis), and arthritis. Patients may develop myositis, sclerodermoid lesions of the skin, and, later, sclerodactyly. Interstitial lung disease and renal disease may ensue.

Venables PJ: Mixed connective tissue disease, *Lupus* 15:132–137, 2006.

31. What is the antiphospholipid antibody syndrome?

Antiphospholipid antibodies (anticardiolipin antibodies, lupus anticoagulant antibodies, and anti–β2-glycoprotein I antibodies) are associated with an increased risk of both arterial and venous thrombosis and recurrent spontaneous abortions. Patients may present to the dermatologist with livedo reticularis, retiform purpura, ulcerations, deep venous thrombosis, or superficial thrombophlebitis. Sneddon's syndrome is livedo reticularis/retiform purpura associated with CNS thrombosis (stroke). Catastrophic antiphospholipid antibody syndrome involves multiple other organ systems with thrombosis involving the CNS, lungs, kidneys, gastrointestinal tract, and skin.

32. What are some other connective tissue diseases with cutaneous manifestations?

- **Autoimmune urticaria:** May affect up to 30% or more of chronic idiopathic urticaria patients (>6 weeks duration of urticaria) with associated autoantibodies to the high-affinity IgE receptor or, less frequently, against IgE.
- **Juvenile idiopathic arthritis:** High episodic fever daily for 2 weeks with symmetrical polyarthritis or oligoarthritis, as well as one of the following: exanthem, generalized adenopathy, hepatosplenomegaly, serositis.
- **Adult-onset Still's disease:** Recurrent episodes of high spiking fevers, frequently in the late afternoon; a salmon-pink exanthem that may demonstrate Koebnerization; arthritis with subsequent carpal ankylosis is characteristic.
- **Sjögren's syndrome:** Xerostomia and xerophthalmia; arthritis; petechiae and purpura, urticarial vasculitis, and annular erythema.
- **Relapsing polychondritis:** Patients present with inflammation of the cartilaginous portions of the ear and nose, eventually causing a deformed ear or saddle-nose deformity. Acute involvement of the tracheal cartilage may cause collapse of the airway. Arthritis most often involves the costochondral joints. Other manifestations include audiovestibular damage, heart valve disease, and neurologic, ocular, and renal disease. Patients may die of rupture of the chordae tendineae of the heart valves.
- **Rheumatoid arthritis:** Patients present with arthritis. Cutaneous manifestations include rheumatoid nodules, rheumatoid neutrophilic dermatitis, palisaded neutrophilic and granulomatous dermatitis, leukocytoclastic vasculitis, and pyoderma gangrenosum.

33. What autoantibodies are associated with the different autoimmune connective tissue diseases?

See Tables 22-4, 22-5, and 22-6.

Sheldon J: Laboratory testing in autoimmune rheumatic diseases, *Best Pract Res Clin Rheumatol* 18:249–269, 2004.
D'Cruz, D: Testing for autoimmunity in humans, *Toxicol Lett* 127: 93–100, 2002.

Table 22-4. Autoantibodies Associated with Lupus Erythematosus

AUTOANTIBODY	PREVALENCE	TARGET	CLINICAL ASSOCIATIONS
High Specificity for SLE			
dsDNA	50%–80%	Double-stranded (native) DNA	LE nephritis; useful in monitoring activity of SLE
Sm	15%–20%	Splicesome RNP (ribonucleoprotein particles involved in splicing pre-mRNA)	–
rRNP	30%–40%	Ribosomal P proteins (proteins involved in ribosome function)	Neuropsychiatric LE
Low Specificity for SLE			
ANA	95%–98%		Most common IF patterns: homogeneous, peripheral
ssDNA	70%	Denatured DNA	Possible risk for SLE in DLE patients; also seen in RA, DM/PM, MCTD, SS, SjS, localized scleroderma
C1q	60%	C1q component of complement	Severe SLE, hypocomplementemic urticarial vasculitis
U1RNP	50%	Splicesome RNP	Overlapping features with other CTD; MCTD (100%)

Continued

Table 22-4. Autoantibodies Associated with Lupus Erythematosus—cont'd

AUTOANTIBODY	PREVALENCE	TARGET	CLINICAL ASSOCIATIONS
Ro (SS-A)	30%–90%	hYRNP (quality control function for misfolded RNA molecules)	SCLE (75%–90%), neonatal LE/congenital heart block (99%), SCLE–SjS overlap, SjS
Cardiolipin	50%	Cardiolipin, a negatively charged phospholipid	Recurrent spontaneous abortions, thrombocytopenia, and hypercoagulable state in SLE (cutaneous manifestations include livedo reticularis, leg ulcers, acral infarction/ulceration, hemorrhagic cutaneous necrosis); similar associations in primary antiphospholipid antibody syndrome; clinical associations strongest with IgG class of anticardiolipin
Histones	40%–70%	Histones	Drug-induced SLE, RA
β2 glycoprotein I	25%	An important cofactor for cardiolipin in cardiolipin autoantibody assays	Relatively high risk of thrombosis in SLE and primary antiphospholipid antibody syndrome (95%–100%)
Rheumatoid factor	25%	Fc portion of IgG	Sjögren's (70%–80%), SS (20%–30%), RA (>80%)
La (SS-B)	10%–20%	hYRNP	SCLE (30%–40%), SCLE–SjS overlap, primary SjS (20%)
Ku	10%	DNA end-binding repair protein complex	Overlap with other CTD such as DM/PM, SSc

ANA, Antinuclear antibodies; CTD, connective tissue diseases; DLE, discoid lupus erythematosus; DM/PM, dermatomyositis/polymyositis; IF, immunofluorescence; LE, lupus erythematosus; MCTD, mixed connective tissue disease; PCNA, proliferating cell nuclear antigen; RA, rheumatoid arthritis; RNP, ribonucleoprotein; SCLE, subacute cutaneous lupus erythematosus; SjS, Sjögren's syndrome; SLE, systemic lupus erythematosus; SS, systemic sclerosis.

Table 22-5. Autoantibodies Associated with Inflammatory Dermatomyopathies

AUTOANTIBODY	MEDIAN PREVALENCE	MOLECULAR SPECIFICITY	CLINICAL ASSOCIATION
High Specificity for DM/PM			
155 kDa and/or Se	80%	Uncharacterized polypeptides (nuclear?)	Clinically amyopathic DM, classic DM with malignancy
Jo-1	20%–30%	Histidyl tRNA synthetase	Antisynthetase syndrome
PL-7	3%	Threonyl tRNA synthetase	Antisynthetase syndrome
PL-12	3%	Alanyl tRNA synthetase	Antisynthetase syndrome
OJ	2%	Isoleucyl tRNA synthetase	Antisynthetase syndrome
EJ	2%	Glycyl tRNA synthetase	Antisynthetase syndrome, possibly increased frequency of skin changes
Mi-2	5%–15%	Helicase nuclear proteins	Adult and juvenile myositis, Gottron's papules/sign, shawl sign, periungual telangiectasias, cuticular dystrophy
SRP	5%	Signal recognition particle	Fulminant DM/PM, cardiac involvement
Low Specificity for DM/PM			
ANA (most common IF patterns: speckled, nucleolar)	40%		Clinically amyopathic DM (65%)
ssDNA	40%	Single-stranded DNA	SLE, SSc, localized scleroderma

Table 22-5. Autoantibodies Associated with Inflammatory Dermatomyopathies—cont'd

AUTOANTIBODY	MEDIAN PREVALENCE	MOLECULAR SPECIFICITY	CLINICAL ASSOCIATION
PM-Scl (PM-1)	8%–10%	Ribosomal RNA processing enzyme	Overlap with scleroderma
Ro (especially 52 kDa Ro)	15%	hYRNP	Overlap with SjS, SCLE, neonatal LE/CHB, SLE
U1RNP	10%	Splicesome RNP	Overlap connective tissue diseases
U2RNP	1%	Splicesome RNP	Overlap with scleroderma
Ku	3%	DNA end-binding repair protein complex	Overlap with scleroderma

ANA, Antinuclear antibodies; CHB, congenital heart block; DM/PM, dermatomyositis/polymyositis; IF, immunofluorescence; LE, lupus erythematosus; RNP, ribonucleoprotein; SCLE, subacute cutaneous lupus erythematosus; SjS, Sjögren's syndrome; SLE, systemic lupus erythematosus; SRP, signal recognition; SSc, systemic sclerosis.

Table 22-6. Autoantibodies Associated with Systemic Sclerosis and Scleroderma

AUTOANTIBODY	SS, ALL	SS WITH DIFFUSE CUTANEOUS SCLERODERMA	SS WITH LIMITED CUTANEOUS SCLERODERMA (CREST SYNDROME)	LOCALIZED SCLERODERMA (LINEAR SCLERODERMA; MORPHEA, LOCALIZED AND GENERALIZED)
ANA (most common IF patterns: speckled, nucleolar, centromere)	95%			40%
Centromere (CENP-B)		30%	80%	
Scl-70 (DNA topoisomerase I, which unwinds DNA)		60%–70%	15%	
Fibrillin-1 (major component of microfibrils in the extracellular matrix)		5%	10%	30%
Histones	40%			35%
Rheumatoid factor	25%			25%
ssDNA	10%			50%
Fibrillarin (part of U3RNP complex)	5%			
PM-Scl (good prognosis)	5%			
RNA polymerase I/III (poor prognosis)	5%–20%			
U1RNP	Overlap features with SLE, RA and myositis	5%		
Th/To (RNase MRP/RNase P RNP)		11%	19%	5%

SS, Systemic sclerosis; ANA, antinuclear antibodies; HMG, high-mobility group; IF, immunofluorescence; RNP, ribonucleoprotein.

1. What percentage of the population experiences acute urticaria during their lifetime?

An estimated 15% to 25% of the population will experience at least one episode of urticaria during their lifetime (Fig. 23-1).

Kaplan AP: Urticaria and angioedema. In Adkinson F, Bochner BS, Busse WW, et al, editors: *Middleton's allergy: principles and practices,* ed 7, Philadelphia, 2009, Mosby.

2. How is acute versus chronic urticaria defined?

Classification of urticaria begins with duration and frequency of the rash. Although arbitrary, 6 weeks of nearly daily symptoms has been chosen as the dividing point for differentiating between acute and chronic urticaria.

Ormerod AD: Urticaria: recognition, causes, and treatment, *Drugs* 48:717–730, 1994.

3. What are the common causes of acute urticaria?

Acute urticaria is more common in children and young adults and is most often caused by allergic reactions (e.g., food, drugs, and insect stings) or an acute infection, particularly viral. However, food is rarely a cause of chronic urticaria.

4. Are all urticarial reactions from medications allergic (IgE-mediated) in nature?

No. Some medication reactions may not be truly allergic but may be caused by nonspecific mast cell–releasing or anaphylactoid properties. Common drugs with this mechanism of action include opiates, vancomycin, radiocontrast media (especially, high-osmolar, ionic forms), and nonsteroidal antiinflammatory drugs.

5. What is the cause of most chronic urticaria?

In most patients seen in referral centers, chronic urticaria remains unexplained despite extensive workup. However, the two largest subgroups of chronic urticaria patients have lesions, induced from physical stimuli (e.g., heat, pressure, vibratory, and cold) or with an autoimmune basis.

6. Is chronic urticaria primarily of allergic etiology?

No. In a large series of patients with chronic urticaria, a personal or family history of allergy was no more common than in the general population, suggesting that there is no connection between chronic urticaria and allergy.

7. How common are the physical urticarias?

Of 554 patients with urticaria seen in a university clinic in England, physical urticarias constituted 17.5% of the total; most of the remainder were idiopathic. The most frequent of the physical urticarias were dermographism (8.5%) (Fig. 23-2), cholinergic urticaria (5.1%), and acquired cold urticaria (2.5%).

8. What association has been described between autoantibodies and chronic urticaria?

In two studies, antithyroid microsomal antibodies have been reported in 12% to 14% of patients with chronic urticaria; however, thyroid status did not relate to the occurrence of urticaria and typically hives did not revert when a euthyroid state was achieved. A number of patients with chronic urticaria react to intradermal injection of their own serum by developing a wheal and flare that persists up to 8 hours. Many of these patients have IgG antibodies in their serum that react with the alpha subunit of the high-affinity IgE receptor on mast cells and basophils. In other patients, the IgG antibody appears to react with IgE itself. The frequency of these IgG autoantibodies in patients with chronic urticaria is not yet established but has been reported to be as high as 40% and 10%, respectively, in a referral clinic.

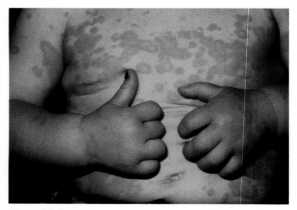

Figure 23-1. Urticaria in a child. Note that some lesions demonstrate an annular appearance. (Courtesy of James E. Fitzpatrick, MD.)

Grattan CEH, Francis DM, Hide M, Greaves MW: Detection of circulating histamine-releasing autoantibodies with functional properties of anti-IgE in chronic urticaria, *Clin Exp Allergy* 21:695–704, 1991.

Hide M, Francis DM, Grattan CEH, et al: Autoantibodies against the high-affinity IgE receptor as a cause of histamine release in chronic urticaria, *N Engl J Med* 328:1599–1604, 1993.

Leznoff A, Sussman GL: Syndrome of idiopathic chronic urticaria and angioedema with thyroid autoimmunity: a study of 90 patients, *J Allergy Clin Immunol* 84:66–71, 1989.

Tong LJ, Balakrishnan G, Kochan JP, et al: Assessment of autoimmunity in patients with chronic urticaria, *J Allergy Clin Immunol* 99:461–465, 1997.

9. What is the "triple response"? Name the components.

The triple response is responsible for producing an urticarial lesion and can classically be produced by injection of an allergen into the skin of a sensitized individual. The three components producing the reaction are as follows:

- Vasodilatation (erythema)
- Increased vascular permeability (wheal)
- Axon reflex (flare)

10. What is the mechanism of the axon reflex?

The axon reflex is produced by stimulation of cutaneous sensory nerve endings, with antidromic conduction of the impulse and release of the neurokinin substance P. Substance P is a vasodilator and it also causes the release of histamine and other mediators from cutaneous mast cells, thus augmenting the urticarial reaction.

11. List five mediators that are capable of directly causing vasodilatation and increased vascular permeability in the skin.

- Histamine
- Prostaglandin D2 (PGD2)
- Leukotriene C4 and D4
- Platelet-activating factor (PAF)
- Bradykinin

12. Name three mediators that may cause vasodilatation and increased vascular permeability indirectly through action on the mast cell.

Substance P, the anaphylatoxins (C3a, C4a, and C5a), and histamine-releasing factors all cause release of mast cell mediators. Of these mediators, only substance P has an additional direct action on blood vessels.

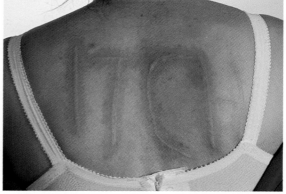

Figure 23-2. Dermographism: Whealing immediately following pressure.

13. Which cells synthesize histamine-releasing factors?

Histamine-releasing factor may be responsible for the release of histamine and other mediators from basophils and/or mast cell. These factors have been described as products of neutrophils, platelets, alveolar macrophages, T lymphocytes, B lymphocytes, and monocytes.

14. What cytokines/chemokines may also be increased in urticarial lesions?

There is evidence for increased production of interleukin-5 (IL-5); eotaxin 1, 2, 3; and Rantes.

15. In what form of physical urticaria are subjects at risk of drowning?

Patients with acquired cold urticaria may have massive mediator release if immersed in cold water. Such release has resulted in drowning, presumably because the patient went into shock from the massive mediator release.

16. How quickly after the application of cold does whealing develop in acquired cold urticaria?

Whealing in cold urticaria does not develop during the exposure to the cold stimulus, but, rather, two minutes after rewarming, and a large hive appears by ten minutes (Fig. 23-3). The delay is probably due to the decrease in cutaneous blood flow during exposure to the cold.

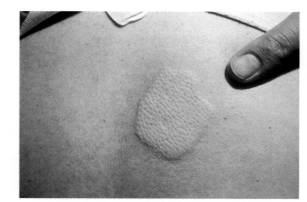

Figure 23-3. Positive ice cube test in a patient with acquired cold urticaria. (Courtesy of James E. Fitzpatrick, MD.)

17. Only one form of urticaria has whealing that is sufficiently characteristic to suggest a specific diagnosis. Which one?

The initial wheals in cholinergic urticaria are quite different from those in other forms of urticaria. They are small, punctate monomorphic (often referred to as pencil-eraser–sized, ~0.5-cm diameter) with a prominent erythematous flare. Over time, they may become confluent, and form larger areas of whealing.

18. Where does cholinergic urticaria usually develop?

On the upper thorax and neck, but it may spread distally to involve the entire body.

19. What are the precipitating events for cholinergic urticaria? By what mechanism do they produce the whealing?

Exercise, warm baths and showers, and emotions are the classic triggers of cholinergic urticaria. There is an elevation of the core body temperature, which is perceived centrally, resulting in efferent cholinergic output to the skin and leading to mast cell degranulation.

20. How are the solar urticarias classified?

Solar urticarias (Fig. 23-4) are classified into six types according to the inciting wavelength:

- **Type I:** 280 to 320 nm
- **Type II:** 320 to 400 nm
- **Type III:** 400 to 500 nm
- **Type IV:** 320 to 500 nm
- **Type V:** 280 to 500 nm
- **Type VI:** 400 nm (protoporphyrin IX)

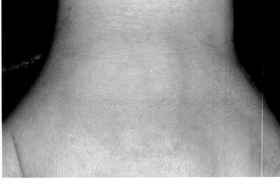

Figure 23-4. Solar urticaria. Phototesting with ultraviolet B (UVB) (290 to 320 nm) wavelength produced urticaria in this patient with a history of sun-induced anaphylaxis. (Courtesy of James E. Fitzpatrick, MD.)

Key Points: Urticaria and Angioedema

1. Acute urticaria is usually from a secondary cause such as an allergic reaction to food, drugs, insect stings, or infection.
2. Chronic urticaria is most often idiopathic and not due to an allergic etiology but has an autoimmune basis in up to 50% of cases.
3. The most common physical urticaria is dermographism, but in chronic urticaria, screen for physical stimuli such as pressure, cold, and heat.
4. In angioedema without urticaria, one should screen for both hereditary and acquired angioedema by obtaining a C4 level.
5. The main medications to control urticaria are antihistamines directed toward blocking the H1 receptor, and there may be added benefit with H2 blockers.

---

21. What is Darier's sign?

Darier's sign is a finding in urticaria pigmentosa. In urticaria pigmentosa, yellow-tan to red-brown macules containing increased numbers of mast cells are scattered over the body. Stroking the skin over the pigmented macules causes an urticarial wheal to form that is limited to the area of the pigmented lesion (Fig. 23-5).

22. How often does aspirin cause or exacerbate urticaria?

Aspirin is rarely a cause of urticaria in an otherwise asymptomatic patient, but many patients with chronic urticaria will have increased whealing if they take aspirin or nonsteroidal antiinflammatory drugs when their disease is active. These same patients are usually able to take aspirin with a much lower risk when their urticaria is inactive, indicating that aspirin is not the cause but a nonspecific exacerbating factor, presumably acting on a pharmacologic basis. Prospective and retrospective data suggest that aspirin administration will cause a flare in 20% to 40% of patients with active urticaria.

Moore-Robinson M, Warin RP: Effect of salicylates in urticaria, *BMJ* 4:262–264, 1967.

23. What is the prognosis of chronic urticaria?

Champion followed 554 patients with urticaria seen at a hospital clinic in England. After 6 months, 50% still had active disease. Of these patients, 40% continued to have at least intermittent symptoms 10 years later. The prognosis was somewhat worse in patients with only angioedema and even poorer if both urticaria and angioedema were present.

Champion RH, Roberts SOB, Carpenter RG, Roger JH: Urticaria and angioedema: a review of 554 patients, *Br J Dermatol* 81:588–597, 1969.

24. Much has been discovered in recent years regarding the histopathology of chronic idiopathic urticaria. What three major types of cells may be encountered in increased numbers in these biopsies?

The characteristic histopathologic finding of nonvasculitic chronic urticaria is a subtle to modest perivascular and interstitial infiltrate. There are increased numbers of lymphocytes. Mast cells are increased some 10-fold, while there is a fourfold increase in mononuclear cells. There is increased histamine in blisters suctioned from chronic urticaria patients. Although eosinophils are often not prominent, increased deposition of the major basic protein of the eosinophil is present in the tissue in 50% of patients, indicating eosinophil involvement in the inflammatory process, although only a fraction of these had evidence of eosinophilic accumulation.

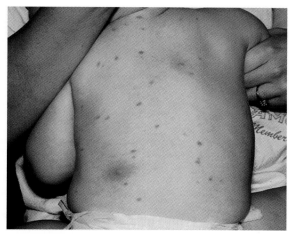

Figure 23-5. Child with urticaria pigmentosa demonstrating multiple tan papules and a positive Darier's sign in two lesions that have been stroked. (Courtesy of James E. Fitzpatrick, MD.)

Elias J, Boss E, Kaplan AP: Studies of the cellular infiltrate of chronic idiopathic urticaria: prominence of T lymphocytes, monocytes, and mast cells, *J Allergy Clin Immunol* 78:914–918, 1986.

Sabroe RA, Poon E, Orchard GE, et al: Cutaneous inflammatory cell infiltrate in chronic idiopathic urticaria: comparison of patients with and without anti-FceRI or anti-IgE autoantibodies, *J Allergy Clin Immunol* 103:484–493, 1999.

Ying S, Kikuchi Y, Meng Q, et al: TH1/TH2 cytokines and inflammatory cells in skin biopsy specimens from patients with chronic idiopathic urticaria: comparison with allergen-induced late phase cutaneous reaction, *J Allergy Clin Immunol* 109:694–700, 2002.

25. In contrast to chronic idiopathic urticaria, what are the typical histologic features of urticarial vasculitis?

Biopsy specimens from patients with urticarial vasculitis typically reveal necrotizing vasculitis of the small venules with deposition of immunoglobulin and complement. In those with low serum complement (hypocomplementemic urticarial vasculitis), polymorphonuclear leukocytes commonly predominate, while in those with normal serum complement, a lymphocytic infiltrate is more typical.

26. Can clinical findings suggest the presence of urticarial vasculitis?

The individual lesions of vasculitis may resemble those of idiopathic urticaria; however, they may feel firmer, tend to persist for greater than 24 hours, and, on clearing, they tend to leave an ecchymotic area due to leakage of red blood cells into the perivascular tissue (Fig. 23-6). Associated systemic symptoms, such as arthralgias and myalgias, are also common. The erythrocyte sedimentation rate is often increased, autoantibodies may be present, and there may be evidence of renal disease.

27. A number of clues in the patient's history may suggest that a patient with recurrent angioedema has the hereditary form. Name some.

Between 75% and 85% of patients with hereditary angioedema (HAE) give a positive family history of similar attacks. The attacks of angioedema themselves are characterized by absence of urticaria and pruritus, both common with idiopathic angioedema. In HAE, episodes of angioedema are often triggered by trauma such as surgery. However,

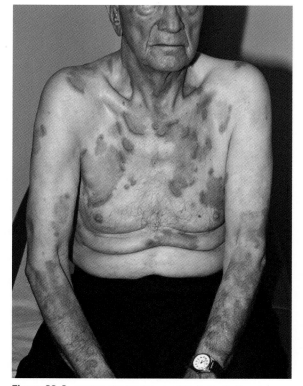

Figure 23-6. Lesions of urticarial vasculitis demonstrating an annular appearance, with some areas showing a violaceous hue due to extravasation of red blood cells. (Courtesy of the JLA Collection.)

such a triggering event may not be evident. Significant upper airway obstruction is seen almost exclusively in HAE, as opposed to ordinary idiopathic angioedema. Attacks of severe abdominal pain are common in HAE, representing edema of the bowel wall. Finally, attacks of HAE typically progress for several days and respond poorly to treatment with antihistamines or epinephrine.

28. Why is C1 esterase deficiency not a part of the differential diagnosis of chronic urticaria?

Hereditary deficiency of C1 esterase inhibitor is the underlying defect in HAE. These individuals have recurring attacks of nonpruritic angioedema but do not have urticaria.

29. Name the recommended screening laboratory test for hereditary angioedema.

Serum C4. C2 is usually within normal limits when the patient is between attacks. In 80% of individuals with HAE, the C1 esterase inhibitor is low; however, the enzyme level can be normal but nonfunctional in 15% to 20% of patients. The normal immunoassay will not detect these patients; a functional assay is required but is usually not readily available and is more expensive than a determination of C4 level.

30. What is the treatment of choice for HAE? How does it work?

HAE is inherited in an autosomal dominant pattern. Attenuated androgens, such as danazol, induce synthesis of normal C1 esterase inhibitor by the liver in these patients. Patients with the functionally abnormal C1 esterase inhibitor also respond, since they too have one normal gene. Pooled C1 inhibitor (prophylaxis) and kallikrien inhibitors for acute attacks are available.

31. How may a patient with HAE be treated prophylactically prior to elective surgery?

Effective prophylactic treatment to prevent attacks of HAE triggered by the trauma of surgery includes epsilon-amino caproic acid, 15 gm/day for 2 to 3 days, or the administration prior to surgery of 2 to 3 units of fresh frozen plasma to restore normal levels of C1 esterase inhibitor.

32. A 60-year-old patient presents with a new onset of attacks of nonpruritic angioedema and a depressed C4 level. What is the first diagnosis you consider?

Acquired C1 esterase inhibitor deficiency. This situation is usually encountered in patients with lymphoma who have a circulating low-molecular-weight IgM, decreased C1 esterase inhibitor level, and low levels of the C1–C4. The mechanism of C1 activation is by reaction with immune complexes or by binding of the C1 to antiidiotypic antibody bound to the immunoglobulin on the surface of the tumor cells. Acquired C1 esterase deficiency has also been reported with connective tissue disorders such as systemic lupus erythematosus, with carcinoma, and with an IgG antibody directed toward C1 esterase inhibitor. In the latter circumstance, the C1 levels are usually normal. Androgen therapy benefits patients with acquired C1 esterase inhibitor deficiency by increasing C1 esterase inhibitor production by the liver.

33. Certain drugs have been identified as being particularly effective for a subset of patients with chronic urticaria or angioedema. What are these drugs, and when is a trial with them indicated?

* Cyproheptadine has been reported to be particularly effective in controlling acquired cold urticaria.
* Corticosteroids and nonsteroidal antiinflammatory drugs prevent the lesions of delayed pressure urticaria, whereas antihistamines are completely without benefit.
* Hydroxychloroquine has been effective in some cases of hypocomplementemic urticarial vasculitis.
* The attenuated androgens, such as danazol and stanozolol, increase synthesis of C1 esterase inhibitor, thereby preventing attacks of hereditary angioedema.

Schocket AL, editor: *Clinical management of urticaria and anaphylaxis,* New York, 1993, Marcel Dekker.

34. What three mediator antagonists have been reported to be useful in symptomatic control of urticaria?

Competitive antagonists of the H1 and H2 histamine receptor and antagonists of leukotriene D4 receptor have been reported to be useful in treating urticaria. The latter two are usually used in conjunction with an H1 antagonist. Recent studies suggest that the nonsedating H1 antagonists are just as effective in treating urticaria as the classic, sedating antagonists.

Bensch GW, Borish L: Leukotriene receptor antagonists in the treatment of chronic idiopathic urticaria (abstract), *J Allergy Clin Immunol* 103:S154, 1999.

Monroe EW, Bernstein DI, Fox RW, et al: Relative efficacy and safety of loratadine, hydroxyzine, and placebo in chronic idiopathic urticaria, *Arzneimittelforschung* 42:1119–1121, 1992.

INFECTIONS AND INFESTATIONS

VIRAL EXANTHEMS

William L. Weston, MD

1. What is the difference between an exanthem and an enanthem?

Any skin rash associated with a viral infection is called an exanthem. If the rash occurs on mucosal surfaces, it is called an enanthem.

2. Which viruses cause exanthems?

Of the hundreds of viruses that infect humans, almost all may produce an exanthem. Some viruses produce an exanthem in most infected persons. These include measles, rubella, the human herpes viruses, and parvovirus B19. A few viruses produce an exanthema in less than 1% of those infected; these include mumps, respiratory syncytial, and equine encephalitis.

Scott LA, Stone M: Viral exanthems, *Dermatol Online J* 9:4, 2003.
Weston WL, Lane AT, Morelli JG: Viral infections. In Weston WL, Lane AT, Morelli JG, editors: *Color textbook of pediatric dermatology*, 4th ed, St Louis, 2007, Mosby, pp 113–138.

3. How do viruses cause exanthems?

In the viral exanthems studied to date, the responsible virus is found within the skin, either in keratinocytes or endothelial cells. It is believed that the virus disseminates to skin during the viremic phase of infection, and the observed exanthem is the result of the host response to the virus.

4. Which viruses cause morbilliform (measles-like) eruptions?

Measles, rubella, enteroviruses, human herpesvirus (HHV) –6 and –7, Epstein-Barr virus (EBV), and cytomegalovirus (CMV) (Fig. 24-1).

Ramsay M, Reacher M, O'Flynn C, et al: Causes of morbilliform rash in a highly immunized English population, *Arch Dis Child* 87:202–206, 2002.

5. Which viruses cause grouped blisters on a red base?

Herpes simplex virus and varicella-zoster virus (Fig. 24-2A).

6. Which viruses cause hand, foot, and mouth disease?

Coxsackie A16, ECHO 71, and other enteroviruses cause hand, foot, and mouth syndrome (Fig. 24-2B).

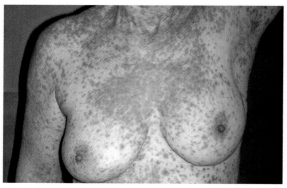

Figure 24-1. Morbilliform viral eruption. Numerous widespread red macules and papules. (Courtesy of the Walter Reed Army Medical Center.)

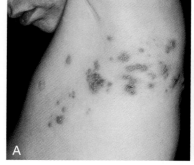
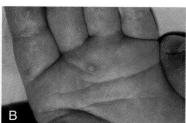

Figure 24-2. A, Grouped vesicles limited to a dermatome in herpes zoster infection. **B,** Discrete palmar vesicle in epidemic hand, foot, and mouth syndrome. (Panel A courtesy of James E. Fitzpatrick, MD.)

Fölster-Hoist R, Kreth HW: Viral exanthems in childhood—infectious (direct) exanthems. Part I: classic exanthems, *J Dtsc Dermaol Ges* 7:309–316, 2009.

7. What is the difference between Gianotti-Crosti syndrome and papular acrodermatitis of childhood?

Gianotti-Crosti syndrome and papular acrodermatitis of childhood are synonyms for a viral eruption characterized by the acute onset of a symmetrical, erythematous papular eruption that is accentuated on the face, extremities, and buttocks (Fig. 24-3). It most commonly occurs in young children between the ages of 1 to 3 years but may occur in younger children or even adolescents.

8. Which are the most common viruses that cause papular acrodermatitis of childhood?

Although originally described in association with infections with the hepatitis B virus, in the United States, it is most commonly associated with EBV infection. Less common causes include CMV, various coxsackieviruses (A16, B4, B5), adenoviruses parvovirus B19, human herpes virus–6, and even viral vaccinations.

Chuh AA, Chan HH, Chiu SS, et al: A prospective case control study of the association of Gianotti-Crosti syndrome with human herpesvirus 6 and human herpesvirus 7 infections, *Pediatr Dermatol* 19:492–497, 2002.

9. Which virus classically causes a lacy eruption?

Parvovirus B19, the cause of erythema infectiosum. Patients also often demonstrate bright erythema of the cheeks that has been described as a "slapped cheek" appearance (Fig. 24-4).

10. Which viruses cause scarlatina (scarlet fever–like) eruptions?

Enteroviruses, adenoviruses, and hepatitis B and C.

11. Which virus causes purpura of the hands and feet?

Parvovirus B19 may cause the purpuric gloves and socks syndrome.

Harel L, Straussberg I, Zeharia A, et al: Papular purpuric rash due to parvovirus B19 with distribution on the distal extremities and face, *Clin Infect Dis* 35:1558–1561, 2002.

12. Do viral exanthems cause petechiae?

Yes. Many viruses do, including ECHO 4, 7, and 9; EBV; measles; rubella; respiratory syncytial virus (RSV); dengue; and parvovirus B19.

13. Can viral exanthems be on one half of the body?

Yes. The unilateral laterothoracic exanthem, seen predominantly in children, can be unilateral at initial presentation. Some cases spread to the contralateral side but often remain accentuated on the side of initial presentation. Although it is believed to be a viral exanthem, a viral cause has not been proven (Fig. 24-5).

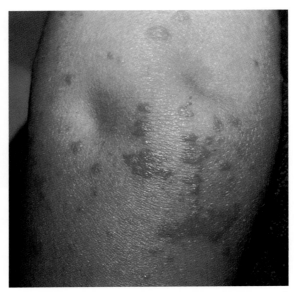

Figure 24-3. Acral-located red papules in papular acrodermatitis of childhood Gianotti-Crosti syndrome.

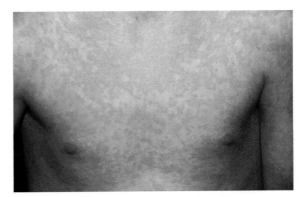

Figure 24-4. Lacy rash of chest in erythema infectiosum.

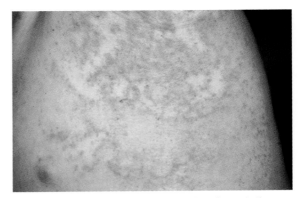

Figure 24-5. Unilateral laterothoracic exanthem demonstrating a lacy appearance.

Drago F, Rampini E, Rebora A: Atypical exanthems: morphology and laboratory investigations may lead to aetiological diagnosis in about 70% of cases, *Br J Dermatol* 147:255–260, 2004.

14. Which disorder most commonly mimics a viral morbilliform eruption?

Drug eruptions (morbilliform drug eruptions) are often clinically indistinguishable from viral morbilliform eruptions. Less commonly, urticaria, arthropod reactions, early guttate psoriasis, and early pityriasis rosea can also be morbilliform.

Lerch M, Pichler WJ: The immunological and clinical spectrum of delayed drug-induced exanthems, *Curr Opin Allergy Clin Immunol* 4:411–419, 2004.

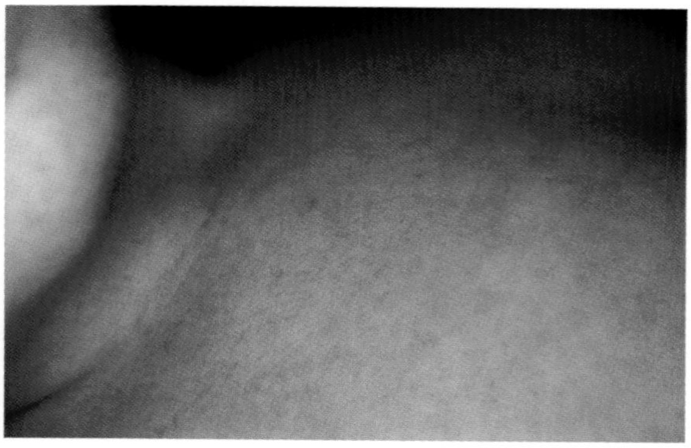

15. What are the clinical features of roseola infantum (exanthem subitum, sixth disease)?

Figure 24-6. Roseola infantum demonstrating subtle, evanescent, erythematous papular exanthem. (Courtesy of the Fitzsimons Army Medical Center teaching files.)

Roseola infantum is a disease that typically presents in infants and very young children as 2 to 5 days of high fever (103° F to 105° F) in an otherwise healthy infant, followed by defervescence and the appearance of pale, small, pink papules that are primarily located on the trunk and head (Fig. 24-6). The exanthem typically lasts from hours to 1 or 2 days. It is most commonly caused by HHV-6 and, less commonly, HHV-7.

Key Points: Viral Exanthems

1. Most viral exanthems are morbilliform (measles-like).
2. The virus is always present within the rash in either the keratinocytes or endothelial cells.
3. Any virus can produce an exanthema, including those that rarely do so.
4. Drug rashes are the most common mimics of viral exanthems.

16. How does sunlight exposure affect a viral exanthem?

The erythema of viral exanthema often becomes more confluent and prominent within sun-exposed areas of skin (photodistributed).

Norval M, El-Fhorr A, Garssen J, et al: The effects of ultraviolet light irradiation on viral infections, *Br J Dermatol* 130:693–695, 1994.

17. What is the STAR complex?

The STAR complex is a viral exanthema associated with sore throat and monoarticular arthritis (**s**ore **t**hroat, **a**rthritis, and **r**ash).

18. Which viruses cause the STAR complex?

Rubella and parvovirus B19; also, rarely, EBV, coxsackie, and enteroviruses.

Jundt JW, Creager AH: STAR complexes: febrile illness associated with sore throat, arthritis, and rash, *South Med J* 86:251–254, 1993.

CHAPTER 25

BULLOUS VIRAL ERUPTIONS

Sylvia L. Brice, MD

1. What do herpes simplex (HSV) virus and varicella-zoster virus (VZV) have in common?
HSV-1, HSV-2, and VZV are all members of the human herpesvirus family. Other members of this family include cytomegalovirus, Epstein-Barr virus, human herpesvirus–6, human herpesvirus–7, and human herpesvirus–8. The human herpesviruses all contain double-stranded DNA, share certain structural features and mechanisms for infection and replication, and have the capacity to establish latent infection in the human host.

Brice S: Viral diseases of the skin. In Rakel RE, Bope ET, editors: *Conn's current therapy*, 58th ed, Philadelphia, 2010, Saunders.

2. What happens during primary HSV infection?
Primary infection refers to an individual's first infection with HSV, either type 1 or 2, at any site. These patients are seronegative initially but subsequently develop HSV-specific antibodies. During primary infection, HSV gains access to the host through the epithelial surface. Following active replication within the skin or mucosa, HSV infects the associated cutaneous neurons and migrates to the sensory root ganglia, where a latent infection is established. Primary HSV infection may be associated with extensive cutaneous lesions, severe pain, and systemic symptoms. However, in many cases, the primary infection is asymptomatic (or unrecognized).

3. What about recurrent infection?
Recurrent HSV infection represents reactivation of the latent virus in the sensory ganglia. "Reactivated" virus particles migrate along the nerves to the site in the skin where the primary infection occurred, with subsequent viral replication and the development of clinical lesions (Fig. 25-1A). The most common sites for recurrent herpes simplex infection are the lips (herpes labialis, "cold sores"), genitalia (herpes genitalis), and sacral area (Fig. 25-1B). Often, individuals experience a prodrome of tingling or burning in the skin prior to the development of visible lesions. Certain factors, such as fever, stress, menses, and sun exposure, may precipitate recurrent infection. The frequency of recurrent infection varies greatly between individuals. In most individuals, clinically evident recurrence becomes less frequent over time.

4. What is the difference between a primary and an initial HSV infection?
When an individual without preexisting antibodies to either HSV-1 or HSV-2 develops an infection with herpes (either type 1 or 2), it is referred to as the primary infection. When an individual with preexisting antibodies to one type of HSV then experiences an infection with the other HSV type, it is referred to as the initial (or initial, nonprimary) infection.

5. How is HSV transmitted?
HSV is transmitted by direct contact of the infected mucocutaneous surface(s) of one individual with the mucosa or skin of another individual. HSV does not survive long outside its normal habitat, and so transmission by contact with fomites is extremely uncommon. It is assumed that HSV-1 is generally transmitted inadvertently during childhood from infected family members, whereas infection with HSV-2 may develop later when individuals become sexually active.

6. How long is incubation period for HSV (i.e., the time from initial infection to appearance of vesicles)?
The time interval between exposure and development of primary disease is estimated to be 3 to 14 days. However, not all cases of primary disease are symptomatic, and so the first evidence of infection may be a recurrent episode, well after the actual exposure. This is important to note, especially in the case of genital infection where the sudden development of "herpes" in one partner in a monogamous couple could create concerns regarding infidelity.

7. Define asymptomatic shedding.
In individuals previously infected with HSV, virus may periodically be present at the site of infection in the absence of clinically evident lesions. This is referred to as asymptomatic shedding. During asymptomatic shedding, the presence of virus may be documented by viral culture or polymerase chain reaction (PCR). Although the viral titer is lower than during clinically active disease, transmission of the virus can nevertheless occur. In fact, contact during periods of asymptomatic shedding is thought to be responsible for many cases of disease transmission.

8. Can you be infected with HSV and not know it?
Yes. Many individuals who give no history of HSV infection are seropositive for HSV-specific antibodies. Using viral culture or PCR, HSV can periodically be recovered from the mouth and/or anogenital region of such individuals (see "asymptomatic shedding" above). Based on the seroprevalence of herpes-specific antibody, 70% to 80% of the

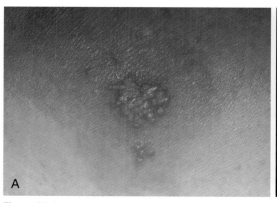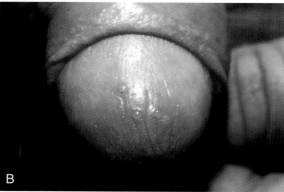

Figure 25-1. A, Classic lesion of recurrent herpes simplex with grouped vesicles on an erythematous base. **B,** Recurrent herpes genitalis. (Courtesy of the Fitzsimons Army Medical Center teaching files.)

population is infected with HSV-1 and 25% to 30% with HSV-2. It is estimated that out of every four individuals with genital herpes, three do not know they are infected.

Xu F, Sternberg MR, Kottiri BJ, et al: Trends in herpes simplex virus type 1 and type 2 seroprevalence in the United States, *JAMA* 296:964–973, 2006.

9. How do HSV-1 and -2 differ?

HSV types 1 and 2 are very closely related, sharing approximately 50% homology in their genetic composition. As expected, many of their viral proteins are also similar (known as type-common), although each type also produces unique proteins (type-specific). Immunohistologic techniques can be used to distinguish these type-specific proteins and differentiate HSV-1 from HSV-2 in clinical situations. Serologic testing that can accurately identify and differentiate antibodies to HSV-1 versus antibodies to HSV-2 is now also available (glycoprotein G type-specific assays). HSV-1 is usually associated with oral herpes and HSV-2 with genital herpes, although each virus can affect both sites. HSV-1 cannot be differentiated from HSV-2 based on the appearance of the skin lesions alone.

10. How do you diagnose HSV infection?

The clinical history of recurrent blisters or erosions in the same site (especially in an oral or genital distribution) is highly suspicious for HSV infection. A prodrome of tingling or burning is also consistent with this diagnosis. On physical exam, the classic lesion is grouped vesicles on an erythematous base (see Fig. 25-1A), but, more often, only nonspecific crusted erosions are seen. To confirm the diagnosis, laboratory assessment may be needed. The gold standard remains viral culture. However, use of many other rapid and sensitive techniques for detection of viral-specific proteins or nucleic acids is often available. For any method of detection, the age of the lesion sampled is critical. Vesicles are optimal but ulcers and erosions, if they are not dry and crusted, may also yield positive results.

11. How is a Tzanck smear performed?

In a Tzanck smear, the base of the suspected herpetic lesion is gently scraped, and the skin or mucosal cells removed are placed on a glass slide. The cells are stained and then examined by light microscopy for evidence of viral-induced cytologic change, including the characteristic multinucleated giant cells. Tzanck smears provide an efficient and inexpensive method of diagnosis, although the results are not always definitive. This technique cannot distinguish HSV-1 from HSV-2 or HSV from VZV.

12. What are the drugs of choice for treatment of HSV?

There are three systemic antiviral agents routinely used for the treatment of HSV: acyclovir, valacyclovir, and famciclovir (Table 25-1). Valacyclovir is the L-valyl ester of acyclovir with a bioavailability 3 to 5 times greater than acyclovir. Famciclovir is the diacetyl-6-deoxy analog of penciclovir. It is well absorbed and has a long intracellular half-life. Both valacyclovir and famciclovir offer the advantage of less frequent dosing compared to acyclovir. All three drugs are generally safe and highly effective because of their very specific antiviral activity. The antiviral drug is preferentially taken up by infected cells, where it must be converted to its active form by the viral enzyme thymidine kinase. The active form preferentially inhibits viral DNA synthesis, with little impact on host cell metabolism.

Cernik C, Gallina K, Brodell RT: The treatment of herpes simplex infections: an evidence-based review, *Arch Intern Med* 168: 1137–1144, 2008.

13. When is chronic suppressive therapy indicated?

Once an episode of recurrent HSV infection (whether oral or genital) has begun, initiation of antiviral therapy often provides only mild symptomatic improvement. If antiviral therapy is initiated during the prodromal phase, the response

Table 25-1. Recommendations for Systemic Antiviral Treatment of Mucocutaneous Herpes Simplex Virus (HSV) Infection*

	DRUG	RECOMMENDED DOSAGE
Genital HSV		
Primary/first episode	Acyclovir	400 mg PO tid or 200 mg PO 5 times per day for 7–10 days (mild to moderate)
	Valacyclovir	5 mg/kg IV q8h for 5 days (severe)
	Famciclovir	1 g PO bid for 7–10 days
		250 mg PO tid for 10 days
Recurrent episode (start at prodrome)	Acyclovir	400 mg PO tid or 200 mg PO 5 times per day for 5 days
	Valacyclovir	500 mg PO bid for 3 days
	Famciclovir	1 g daily for 5 days
		1 g PO bid for 1 day
		125 mg PO bid for 5 days
Chronic suppression	Acyclovir	400 mg PO bid or 200 mg PO tid; adjust up or down according to response (>6 outbreaks per year)
	Valacyclovir	500 mg PO qd (<10 outbreaks per year)
	Famciclovir	1 g PO qd (10 or more outbreaks per year)
		250 mg PO bid (6 or more outbreaks per year)
Orofacial HSV		
Primary/first episode	Acyclovir	15 mg/kg 5 times per day for 7 days
	Valacyclovir	1 g bid for 7 days
	Famciclovir	500 mg bid for 7 days
Recurrent (start at prodrome)	Acyclovir	400 mg PO 5 times per day for 5 days
	Valacyclovir	2 g PO bid for 1 day
	Famciclovir	1500 mg as single dose
Chronic suppression	Acyclovir	400 mg PO bid–tid
	Valacyclovir	500 mg to 1 g PO qd
Orolabial or Genital HSV in Immunosuppressed Patients		
Recurrent/suppressive	Acyclovir	400 mg PO 3 times per day or 5–10 mg/kg IV q8h
	Valacyclovir	500 mg to 1 g PO bid
	Famciclovir	500 mg PO bid

*Dose should be adjusted in the presence of renal insufficiency.
Bid, Twice daily; IV, intravenous; PO, by mouth; qd, daily; tid, three times a day.

may be somewhat better. In patients with frequently recurrent or severe disease, especially with genital herpes, chronic suppressive therapy may be considered. After 1 year on therapy, a "drug holiday" may be given to assess the continued need for treatment, since the natural history of recurrent infection is to decrease in frequency with time.

14. **Are patients with genital herpes at greater risk for becoming infected with the human immunodeficiency virus (HIV)?**
Genital infection with herpes simplex virus–2 increases the risk for HIV infection, even between active episodes. The population of immune cells that remain at the site of genital herpes lesions even after they have healed is thought to provide a favorable environment for acquisition of HIV.

15. **What recommendations can you make to a patient with genital herpes to reduce the risk of transmission to his or her partner?**
At the very least, avoidance of sexual contact during clinically apparent disease (i.e., until lesions are completely dry) is advised. In light of the problem with asymptomatic shedding, the safest practice is the routine use of a condom, even between active episodes. The systemic antiviral agents decrease, but do not eliminate asymptomatic shedding. However, in the case of monogamous but discordant (one partner has genital herpes and the other does not) couples, chronic suppressive therapy taken by the infected partner may reduce the likelihood of transmitting the disease to the uninfected partner.

Gupta R, Warren T, Wald A: Genital herpes, *Lancet* 370:2127–2137, 2007.

16. **Can HSV infect the skin in areas other than around the mouth or anogenital areas?**
HSV infection may involve and recur at any location on the mucocutaneous surface. HSV infection of the hand or fingers, known as herpetic whitlow, is usually the result of autoinoculation from another site of infection (Fig. 25-2A). Herpes gladiatorum is a problem most commonly seen in athletes who participate in close contact sports such as

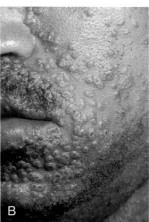
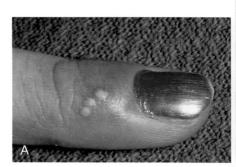

Figure 25-2. A, Herpetic whitlow. **B,** Eczema herpeticum (Kaposi's varicelliform eruption) in a patient with atopic dermatitis. (Panel A courtesy of the Walter Reed Army Medical Center teaching files; panel B courtesy of Scott D. Bennion, MD.)

wrestling. Typically transmitted from active herpes labialis or asymptomatic shedding in oral secretions of an infected opponent, herpes gladiatorum often affects the head, neck, or shoulders. Eczema herpeticum, also known as Kaposi's varicelliform eruption, represents a cutaneous dissemination of HSV (Fig. 25-2B). It may develop as a complication of a localized HSV infection in patients with atopic dermatitis or other underlying skin disease.

17. How does a baby get herpes? Is it a serious problem?

In most cases, transmission of HSV to the neonate occurs by delivery through an infected birth canal. Postpartum acquisition occurs less commonly. Development of primary or initial non-primary genital herpes by the mother at or near the time of delivery poses a significant risk for the infant. However, most cases of neonatal herpes are the result of asymptomatic shedding in women with no known history of genital herpes. The usual onset of neonatal herpes is 5 to 21 days following exposure. Approximately 80% of infected neonates have at least some characteristic skin lesions. Herpes infection in the neonatal period can be devastating because of the inadequate immune response seen in neonates.

Corey L, Wald A: Maternal and neonatal herpes simplex virus infections, *N Engl J Med* 361:1376–1385, 2009.

18. Describe the natural history of varicella.

Varicella, or chickenpox, is the primary infection with varicella-zoster virus (VZV). It is characterized by the appearance of two to three successive crops of diffuse, pruritic vesicles and papules over several days. These lesions then evolve into pustules and crusted erosions, so that lesions in all stages of development are present together (Fig. 25-3). Lesions generally persist for up to 1 week.

Varicella most commonly occurs during childhood. It is highly contagious, both via respiratory secretions and contact with the cutaneous lesions. The incubation period ranges from 10 to 23 days, and the patient is considered contagious from 4 days before the onset of lesions until all lesions have crusted.

Key Points: Herpes Simplex Virus

1. HSV is transmitted by direct contact with the infected skin or mucosal surface.
2. Many cases of primary HSV are asymptomatic so that the first evidence of infection may represent a recurrence.
3. Asymptomatic shedding occurs in both orolabial and genital HSV infection.
4. For laboratory confirmation, either viral culture or an antigen detection technique is recommended.
5. Early initiation of oral antiviral therapy is the key to its success.

19. What is shingles?

Herpes zoster, or "shingles," is the recurrent form of infection with VZV and represents reactivation of the latent virus in the sensory ganglia. The cutaneous eruption consists of painful and/or pruritic vesicles, which tend to follow a unilateral, dermatomal distribution (Fig. 25-4). Prodromal pain may often precede the development of visible lesions. The entire course is usually 2 to 3 weeks in duration. The most common area of involvement for herpes zoster is the trunk (dermatomes innervated by the thoracic nerves), followed by the head (first branch of the trigeminal nerve). Herpes zoster is most typically seen in older and/or immunocompromised individuals.

Whitley RJ: A 70-year-old woman with shingles: review of herpes zoster, *JAMA* 302:73–80, 2009.

20. Can herpes zoster be recurrent?

Approximately 5% of patients with herpes zoster will experience a recurrence, usually in the same dermatome. However, recurrent HSV may also have a "zosteriform" distribution, indistinguishable from herpes zoster both clinically and on Tzanck smear. Although this presentation is not common, the possibility should be entertained, especially when the dermatomes involved are in the orofacial or genital distribution or the patient presents with "recurrent zoster."

21. What is disseminated zoster?

Disseminated zoster is defined as the presence of more than 20 vesicles outside the primary and adjacent dermatomes. It is uncommon in immunocompetent patients, but up to 40% of immunocompromised patients may develop this complication. In these cases, visceral involvement may also occur.

22. Is herpes zoster contagious?

Herpes zoster is the result of reactivation of latent VZV in the sensory ganglia. There is no evidence that a person can develop herpes zoster as a result of contact with patients with either varicella or herpes zoster. However, direct contact with the cutaneous lesions may result in transmission of primary varicella to a susceptible host.

23. What is postherpetic neuralgia?

Postherpetic neuralgia is the most common complication of herpes zoster. It is defined as the presence of pain after skin lesions have healed, or pain lasting more than 3 months after the onset of cutaneous lesions. The pain is often severe and debilitating. Overall, it occurs in 10% to 15% of patients, but the incidence increases dramatically with age so that over half of patients with herpes zoster who are older than 60 years develop postherpetic neuralgia. Other risk factors include prominent prodromal symptoms and moderate or severe pain at presentation. In most cases, postherpetic neuralgia resolves spontaneously within the first 12 months, but it may persist for years.

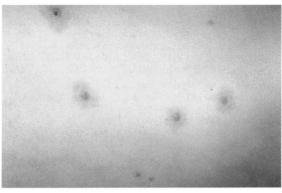

Figure 25-3. Varicella with skin lesions at all stages of development. (Courtesy of Joseph G. Morelli, MD.)

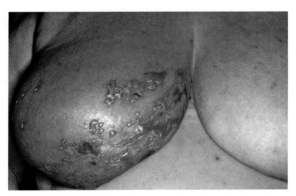

Figure 25-4. Grouped vesicles on an erythematous base in a dermatomal distribution. (Courtesy of the Fitzsimons Army Medical Center teaching files.)

Sampathkumar P, Drage LA, Martin DP: Herpes zoster (shingles) and postherpetic neuralgia, *Mayo Clin Proc* 84:274–280, 2009.

24. How do you diagnose VZV infection?

For varicella, the physical findings of lesions in various stages of development (papules, vesicles, pustules, and erosions), especially with a history of exposure to an individual with varicella (or zoster), is generally enough to make the diagnosis. The diagnosis of herpes zoster is also often made on the basis of physical findings. A Tzanck smear may be useful. If additional laboratory evaluation is indicated, immunohistochemical testing to detect viral-specific antigens in infected cells is recommended. A viral culture may be performed, although culturing VZV is more difficult and takes longer than culturing HSV. Use of PCR has become more commonly available. VZV serology is rarely useful for diagnosis.

25. What is the treatment for varicella?

Generally, symptomatic therapy, such as calamine lotion and oral antihistamines, is all that is required. Acyclovir is not routinely recommended for otherwise healthy children from a cost-effective standpoint. However, for varicella in an adult or immunocompromised individual, prompt initiation of systemic antiviral therapy is advised (Table 25-2). Routine childhood vaccination to prevent varicella is now recommended for children and adolescents who have not been infected. Vaccination is also recommended for susceptible adults, especially those at high risk for exposure.

26. How about herpes zoster?

Herpes zoster is a self-limited disease and in most young, otherwise healthy persons, symptomatic measures (cool compresses, antihistamines, analgesics) are sufficient. However, for persons who are over 50 years of age, have ophthalmic zoster, or are immunocompromised, systemic antiviral therapy is recommended (see Table 25-2). If started within 72 hours of the onset of skin lesions, systemic antiviral therapy reduces the discomfort and duration of the acute infection and may reduce the severity of postherpetic neuralgia.

Table 25-2. Recommendations for Systemic Antiviral Treatment of Varicella-Zoster Virus*

Varicella (start within 24 hours of rash onset) Acyclovir 20 mg/kg (up to 800 mg) PO qid for 5 days (children) Acyclovir 800 mg PO 5 times per day for 7 days (adult) Acyclovir 10–12 mg/kg q8h for 7–10 days
Herpes zoster: Immunocompetent patients Acyclovir 800 mg PO 5 times per day for 7–10 days Valacyclovir 1 g PO tid for 7 days Famciclovir 500 mg PO tid for 7 days
Herpes zoster: Immunosuppressed patients Acyclovir 800 mg PO 5 times per day for 10 days[†] Acyclovir 10 mg/kg/dose IV q8h for 7–10 days[†] Valacyclovir 1 g PO tid for 10 days[†] Famciclovir 500 mg PO tid for 10 days[†]

*Dose should be adjusted in the presence of renal insufficiency.
[†]Continue until there are no new lesions for 48 hours.
IV, Intravenous; PO, by mouth; tid, three times a day.

Key Points: Varicella-Zoster Virus

1. Varicella (chicken pox) is the primary infection.
2. Herpes zoster (shingles) is the recurrent infection.
3. Postherpetic neuralgia is a common complication of herpes zoster, especially in older individuals.
4. Ophthalmologic evaluation and systemic antiviral therapy are recommended for patients with herpes zoster ophthalmicus.
5. The herpes zoster vaccine may substantially reduce the risk for herpes zoster and the development of postherpetic neuralgia in patients age 60 years or older.

27. Should I be concerned about the patient with herpes zoster involving the tip of the nose?

Lesions of herpes zoster involving the tip, side, or root of the nose indicate involvement of the nasociliary branch of the first division of the trigeminal nerve. This is known as Hutchinson's sign and should alert you to the possibility of herpes zoster ophthalmicus (see Fig. 25-4). Ocular disease occurs in 20% to 70% of patients with ophthalmic zoster, and antiviral therapy as well as ophthalmologic evaluation is routinely recommended. The triad of herpes zoster with cutaneous involvement of the auditory canal and auricle, ipsilateral facial palsy, and excruciating ear pain is known as the Ramsay Hunt syndrome and is the result of viral reactivation within the geniculate ganglion.

28. Who should get the herpes zoster vaccine?

A live attenuated zoster vaccine received FDA approval in 2006 and is recommended for individuals age 60 years or older who are not significantly immunosuppressed. The vaccine substantially reduces the risk for herpes zoster and the development of postherpetic neuralgia.

Harpaz R, Ortega-Sanchez IR, Seward JF: Prevention of herpes zoster. Recommendations of the Advisory Committee on Immunization Practices (ACIP), *MMWR* 57:1–30, 2008.

29. What is hand, foot, and mouth disease?

Hand, foot, and mouth disease (HFMD), or vesicular stomatitis with exanthem, is usually seen in infants or young children. Following a brief prodrome of fever, malaise, and sore throat, the characteristic enanthem develops. Red macules, vesicles, and ulcers may be seen on the buccal mucosa, tongue, palate, and pharynx (Fig. 25-5A). Lesions may also occur on the hands and feet (dorsal aspects, as well as the palms and soles) (Fig. 25-5B). HFMD is caused by one of several enteroviruses, most commonly coxsackievirus A16. It is highly contagious and spreads by direct contact via the oral–oral or oral–fecal route. Over the past 10 years, outbreaks of HFMD caused by enterovirus 71 have been reported in Asia and Australia. Although HFMD associated with coxsackievirus A16 infection is typically a mild illness, HFMD caused by enterovirus 71 has shown a higher incidence of neurologic involvement including fatal cases of encephalitis.

30. What is orf?

Human orf, or ecthyma contagiosum, is caused by a parapoxvirus that is usually contracted by direct exposure to infected, or recently vaccinated, sheep or goats. Milkers' nodules are caused by a closely related virus found in cows. The lesions of both orf and milkers' nodules are identical, consisting of dome-shaped, firm bullae that develop an umbilicated crust (Fig. 25-6). One to several lesions develop, usually on the hands and forearms. They generally resolve without therapy in 4 to 6 weeks.

Centers for Disease Control and Prevention (CDC): Orf virus infection in humans—New York, Illinois, California, and Tennessee, 2004–2005, *MMWR* 55(3):65–68, 2006.

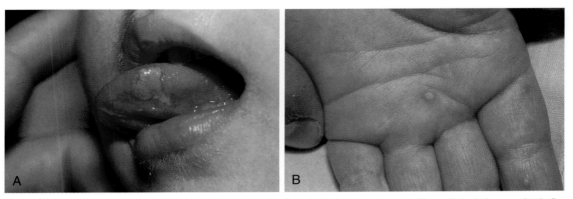

Figure 25-5. Hand, foot, and mouth disease. **A,** Vesicular stomatits. **B,** Typical lesions on palmar skin. The vesicular lesions are classically gray and often elliptical.

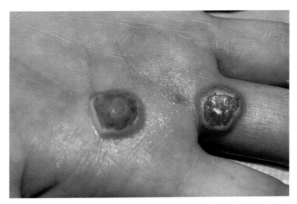

Figure 25-6. Classic lesions of orf demonstrating a central ulceration and necrotic vesiculobullous edge.

WEBSITES

International Herpes Management Forum: www.ihmf.org
National Institute of Allergy and Infectious Diseases: www.niaid.nih.gov
Centers for Disease Control and Prevention: www.cdc.gov

WARTS AND MOLLUSCUM CONTAGIOSUM

Barbara R. Reed, MD

You got to go all by yourself, to the middle of the woods, where you know there's a spunk-water stump, and just as it's midnight you back up against the stump and jam your hand in and say:
   Barley-corn, barley-corn, injun-meal shorts,
   Spunk-water, spunk-water, swaller these warts,
and then walk away quick, 11 steps, with your eyes shut, and then turn around three times and walk home without speaking to anybody. Because if you speak the charm's busted.

—Tom Sawyer to Huck Finn on curing warts in *The Adventures of Tom Sawyer* by Mark Twain

1. What causes warts?
Warts are caused by a virus, the human papillomavirus (HPV). HPV is a circular, double-stranded DNA virus containing approximately 8000 base pairs. There are over 200 known types of HPV, and over 100 have been totally sequenced.

2. Name the common types of warts.
HPV infection is highly specific for epidermis, especially extremities, palms, and soles, but also the scalp and mucosal surfaces such as the mouth, larynx, genital areas, and rectal mucosa. Some types of HPV have a predilection for infection in certain locations in the body (Table 26-1). For example, flat warts are seen mostly on the face and hands of children and are often caused by HPV types 3 and 10 (Fig. 26-1A). Common warts occur most often on the fingers and periungual skin and are commonly due to HPV types 2, 4, and 29 (Fig. 26-1B). Warts in immunosuppressed patients are caused by HPV type 8 and others (Fig. 26-1C).

3. How frequently are the different cutaneous warts seen?
The three types of cutaneous HPV infections are widespread throughout the general population. Common warts, which represent up to 71% of cutaneous warts, occur frequently among school-aged children, with a prevalence of 4% to 20%. Plantar warts are most common among adolescents and young adults and represent about 34% of cutaneous warts. Flat warts are least common (4%) and affect mostly children. Other groups at high risk for cutaneous warts are butchers, meat packers, and fish handlers.

4. Can warts cause cancer?
Certain types of HPV infection have been associated with the development of malignancy. Although bowenoid papulosis is not considered a premalignancy, it may be associated with an increased risk of cervical cancer. Carcinomas of the conjunctiva, cornea, nasal cavities, oral cavity, esophagus, and plantar surface of the foot also have been reported in association with various types of HPV.

Carcinogenic wart types include the following: 16, 18, 31, 33, 35, 39, 45, 51, 52, 56, 58, 59, 68, and 69.

Table 26-1. Clinical Presentation of Common Types of Warts

TYPE OF WART	USUAL LOCATION	COMMON PRESENTATION	COMMON HPV TYPES
Common (verruca vulgaris)	Variable	Flesh-colored, rough, hyperkeratotic papules; single or grouped	2, 4, 29
Plantar, palmar	Soles, palms; may be painful	Thick, hyperkeratotic lesions	1, 2, 4, 10
Flat (verruca planae)	Face, hands, knees	Small, 2–5-mm, flat-topped, hyperpigmented papules; multiple	3, 10
Anogenital (condyloma acuminatum)	Genitalia, anogenital region	Moist, cauliflower-like masses, variably sized; sexually transmitted	6, 11, 42–44

5. What is epidermodysplasia verruciformis (EV)?

EV is a rare, inherited disorder in which cutaneous HPV infection is generalized and persistent. Most cases are autosomal recessive, but autosomal dominant and X-linked dominant forms are also reported. It is caused by mutations in either the *EVER1* or *EVER2* genes. The lesions are either flat warts or reddish-brown plaques, often developing in sun-exposed areas (Fig. 26-2A). Malignant change occurs in about 10% of cases, but metastasis is uncommon. HPV types 5 and 8 are most commonly seen in EV patients, although several other HPV types may also been seen.

Gül U, Kiliç A, Gönül M, et al: Clinical aspects of epidermodysplasia verruciformis and review of the literature, *Int J Dermatol* 46:1069–1072, 2007.

6. What techniques are used to study warts?

Polymerase chain reaction combined with enzyme-linked immunosorbent assay (ELISA), in situ hybridization, or reverse dot-blot hybridization. Nucleotide sequencing may provide further characterization.

7. How does a person become infected with warts?

HPV infection occurs after exposure to humans or animals with HPV infection. The most common mode of transmission is through touch or contact from an individual infected with HPV, although HPV may also survive on inanimate objects

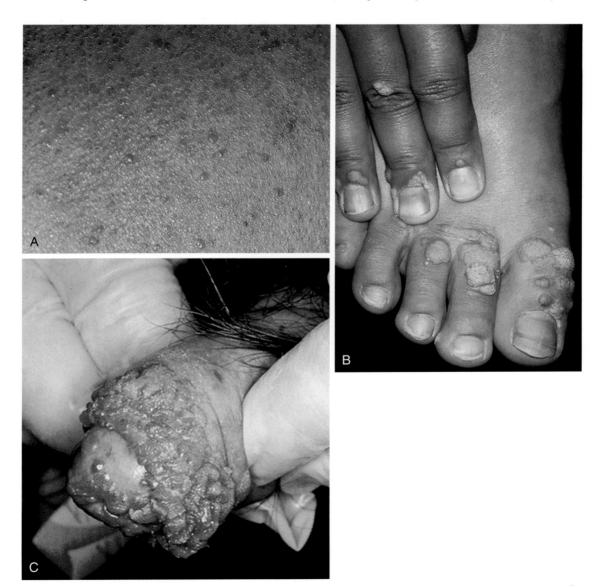

Figure 26-1. Common types of warts. **A,** Flat warts of the face presenting as multiple 1- to 2-mm papules. **B,** Multiple common warts of the hands and feet. **C,** Condyloma acuminatum of the penis presenting as moist cauliflower-like papillomas. (Panels A and B courtesy of James E. Fitzpatrick, MD; panel C courtesy of Scott Norton, MD.)

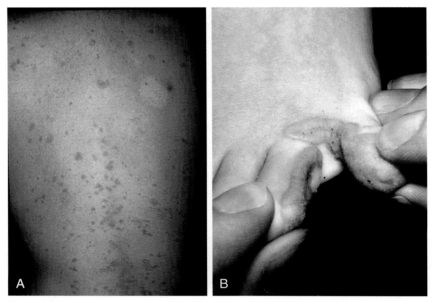

Figure 26-2. A, Multiple reddish-brown macules of the back in a patient with epidermodysplasia verruciformis. **B,** "Kissing" warts produced by inoculation of the toe web space. (Courtesy of James E. Fitzpatrick, MD.)

for unknown amounts of time. Small abrasions or cracks in the skin of exposed persons allow the virus to penetrate. Such infection may commonly occur at a swimming pool, where chlorinated water and rough concrete surfaces may abrade the skin, or at other public places. Genital warts may be transmitted through sexual intercourse. People who work with meat, fish, and poultry also commonly have warts in the hand and forearm area, which are thought to be promoted through microinjuries sustained during processing of animals or fish, as well as from prolonged immersion of the skin in water.

Autoinoculation is another form of transmission. Periungual warts are often found in persons who have a habit of biting their cuticles, for example. Presumably the excoriated areas are more hospitable to virus, but spread of a single common wart is also possible. Flat warts in the beard area or on the legs may be spread by shaving.

8. Do warts spread?

Yes, especially if they are injured. Such injury may happen if the warts are in a location traumatized by shaving or scratching. This reaction is known as the Koebner phenomenon. (The Koebner reaction is also present in skin conditions that have no known viral cause, such as psoriasis and lichen planus.) Close approximation of two surfaces, where one surface is affected and the opposing surface is unaffected, is also associated with an increased likelihood of spreading (e.g., adjacent toe surfaces; Fig. 26-2B).

9. How long is the incubation period of warts?

Unknown. It is estimated to be several weeks to over 1 year.

10. How can warts be prevented?

No one is certain how to avoid the development of warts.

There are now vaccines available to help prevent warts. Gardasil® helps to prevent genital warts in men and women. Cervarix® helps prevent cervical cancer in women.

11. What is the difference between the Gardasil® and Cervarix® HPV vaccines?

Gardasil® is a quadrivalent vaccine with activity against HPV 16 and HPV 18, which are responsible for approximately 70% of all cervical carcinomas. It is also protective against infection with HPV types 6 and 11, which are nononcogenic HPV strains that produce genital warts in both men and women. In contrast, Cervarix® is a bivalent vaccine with proven protection against the oncogenic strains HPV 16 and 18. There is also some evidence that it produces some protection against other oncogenic HPV types, including HPV 31, 33, and 45.

12. Can HPV live in the human body in a dormant state?

HPV is demonstrable by DNA hybridization and polymerase chain reaction in skin that is clinically normal, indicating the likelihood of a latent or subclinical form of HPV. In addition, it is not uncommon for a wart to recur in the same location many years following apparent resolution.

13. Are plantar warts caused by a special kind of virus? Are they more difficult to treat?

The term *plantar wart* refers to a location rather than to a pattern of behavior. Plantar warts are simply warts on the plantar aspect (sole) of the foot. Warts in this location have a unique appearance from being compressed by the pressure of walking.

For reasons that are not entirely clear, plantar warts are more difficult to eradicate. Excision by scalpel or carbon dioxide laser often results in scarring, and recurrence is common. Repeated liquid nitrogen treatment may be painful, inconvenient, and costly. Vascular pulsed dye laser is effective and not as painful or debilitating as liquid nitrogen treatment. Home treatments with salicylic acid pads, along with judicious trimming to maintain comfort, seem to be most helpful. Glutaraldehyde, which produces a brown discoloration of treated surfaces, has also been used successfully.

14. What causes the black dots within a wart?

The small black dots, incorrectly referred to as "seeds," are actually thrombosed blood vessels.

15. Can HPV infection have a hereditary basis?

Except in the case of epidermodysplasia verruciformis, warts are not inherited. However, our immune systems are inherited, and some people seem to have inherited an immune system that places them at risk for acquiring HPV infection. For example, women with HPV involving the cervical and/or vaginal areas have given birth to babies with laryngeal warts.

16. Are some people more susceptible to warts than others?

Immunocompromised individuals, such as those with HIV infection or cancer, or transplant patients on immunosuppressive drugs are more susceptible to warts than others. Sexual intercourse at an early age is a known risk factor for acquiring genital warts. Children with atopic dermatitis may have warts that are more extensive and more difficult to eradicate.

Harwood CA, Perrett CM, Brown VL, et al: Imiquimod cream 5% for recalcitrant cutaneous warts in immunocompromised individuals, *Br J Dermatol* 152:122–129, 2005.

17. Should all warts be eradicated?

It is not possible to eradicate certain warts, and it is economically impossible to eradicate all warts in the human population. With nongenital warts, if a wart is large enough to cause discomfort, is disfiguring, or is on a body part that is constantly traumatized, treatment should be considered.

18. How should external genital warts (EGWs) be treated?

Clinical examination is sufficient for evaluation. Treatment goals should be to eliminate symptomatic warts. Sexual partners of patients with EGWs should be evaluated for warts or other sexually transmitted diseases. Women with EGWs should have cervical cytologic screening. HPV detection and EGW typing are not currently required for diagnosis or management. In minors, the presence of EGWs should prompt a consideration of sexual abuse.

Lacey CJ: Therapy for genital human papillomavirus-related disease, *J Clin Virol* 32:S82–S90, 2005.

19. What methods are available for the treatment of warts?

Over-the-counter methods for eliminating warts include topical applications of acids such as salicylic or lactic acid. These may be in a liquid form or may be incorporated into plasters (Table 26-2). When choosing a treatment plan for warts, the physician's primary concern should be to not make the treatment worse than the warts. For example, a treatment worse than the disease would be to excise and suture a wart on the weight-bearing surface of the foot and then have the wart recur in the middle of a painful scar. Sometimes, the best treatment is benign neglect. Resistance and recurrence are common with all treatments.

20. What are common side effects of treatment methods?

- Scarring (liquid nitrogen, laser, acids, cantharidin)
- Blistering (liquid nitrogen, cantharidin, topical 5-fluorouracil, bleomycin) (Fig. 26-3A)
- Allergy (cantharidin, chemotherapeutic agents, tretinoin, acids, glutaraldehyde)
- Persistent hyper- or hypopigmentation (liquid nitrogen)

21. What are "fairy ring" warts?

Fairy ring warts, or satellite warts, are annular warts that may develop following any treatment that produces blisters (Fig. 26-3B).

22. Should any treatments be avoided?

- During pregnancy, chemotherapeutic agents, interferon, and retinoids should be avoided, and careful consideration should be given to use of acids and cantharidin. Liquid nitrogen and laser are safe for use during pregnancy.
- Bleomycin should be avoided around fingernails, as permanent nail dystrophy, Raynaud's phenomenon, and sclerotic changes in the distal finger have been reported.
- X-irradiation is not indicated for treatment of warts. Increased invasiveness of lesions following radiation has been reported.

Table 26-2. Treatments for Warts

TREATMENT	WART TYPE	COMMENTS
Destructive Methods		
Cryotherapy	All	Dyschromia, pain
Electrosurgery	Resistant	Scar, recurrence
Surgery	Resistant	Scar, recurrence
Carbon dioxide laser	Resistant	Scar, recurrence
Pulsed dye laser	Resistant	Not readily available
Caustic Acids		
Monochloroacetic, dichloroacetic, and trichloroacetic acid	Common	Irritation, blisters, scar
Cantharidin	Small, common	Irritation, blisters, hyperpigmentation, fairy ring warts
Chemotherapeutic Agents		
Podophyllotoxin*	External genital	Erythema, erosions, ulcers, pain
Imiquimod*	External genital	Erythema, burning, erosion
Bleomycin (intralesional)*	Common	Pain, nail loss, nail dystrophy, Raynaud's phenomenon
5-Fluorouracil (topical)*	Flat	Irritation
Miscellaneous		
Interferon*	Anogenital	Inject intralesional or intramuscular
Contact hypersensitivity	Resistant	Squaric acid
Tretinoin (topical)*	Flat	Irritation
Glutaraldehyde	Plantar	Brown discoloration, allergy
Cimetidine (oral)*	Resistant	Best in children
Salicylic acid	Common, plantar	Available over the counter
Retinoids*	Immunosuppression	Relapse when drug is discontinued
Formalin*	Plantar	Contact sensitivity

*Avoid during pregnancy.

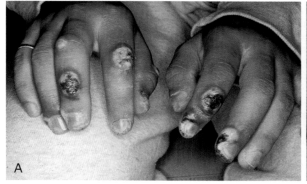 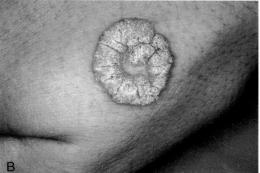

Figure 26-3. Side effects of wart treatment. **A,** Painful blisters produced by cantharidin. **B,** Fairy ring formation of warts on the wrist, at the periphery of a blister produced by previous liquid nitrogen therapy. (Panel A courtesy of Brenda Kokomo, MD; panel B courtesy of James E. Fitzpatrick, MD.)

23. Is there a best way to treat warts?

No single treatment method may be relied upon to eliminate warts permanently. Treatment choice must depend on the age of the patient, location, appearance, and symptoms of the wart:

- **Facial:** These warts are usually flat and can respond to treatment with topical tretinoin cream or imiquimod. Liquid nitrogen or pulsed dye laser may be used cautiously, but persistent hypopigmentation is an undesired side effect.

- **Weight-bearing (plantar):** These warts are treated with combinations of acid plaster or liquid acid preparations and/or pulsed dye laser. Glutaraldehyde or intralesional bleomycin may be used in refractory cases.
- **Nails:** Periungual warts may be treated with topical acids or cantharidin. Liquid nitrogen, often helpful in the treatment of common warts, should be used cautiously here because of the intense pain it causes, as well as risk of persistent nail deformity.
- **Genital:** Genital warts may be treated with liquid nitrogen, podophyllin or derivatives, topical acids, 5-fluorouracil, imiquimod, or cidofovir. Refractory warts may be treated with interferon. Carbon dioxide laser may also be indicated in some cases.
- **Children:** Salicylic acid plasters and liquids, cantharidin, liquid nitrogen, and pulsed dye laser have been used successfully. There are recent reports of success using oral cimetidine in prepubertal children with extensive common warts. Many warts regress without treatment. It is speculated that such warts are identified as foreign by the owner's immune system, which then rejects the wart.

Smolinski KN, Yan AC: How and when to treat molluscum contagiosum and warts in children, *Pediatr Ann* 34:211–221, 2005.

24. How can you tell if a wart is gone?
Treatment success is considered the return of normal body skin lines.

25. How can you be sure that warts will never come back?
You cannot.

26. Do any warts come from toads?
No. There is no supportive scientific evidence—histologic, viral, or other—that the bumps on the skin of a toad are at all related to warts.

Key Points: Human Papillomavirus Infection

1. There are over 200 known types of HPV, and over 100 have been totally sequenced.
2. Most HPV infections are not carcinogenic, but persistent infections with some genotypes, especially HPV-16 and HPV-18, are associated with a high risk of epithelial neoplasia.
3. Immunocompromised patients have a higher risk of HPV infection that is more difficult to eradicate than those in immunocompetent individuals.
4. Although there are many treatment modalities available, there is no consistently effective antiviral treatment.

27. Are molluscum contagiosum a type of wart?
No. Molluscum contagiosum is a viral infection of the skin produced by a poxvirus that is more closely related to the virus that produces smallpox. Like warts, they are more common in children and immunocompromised individuals, and can be sexually acquired. They may occur anywhere on the skin surface and present as firm, skin-colored umbilicated papules with a central core of keratin (Fig. 26-4A). Some lesions may demonstrate an intense host response (Fig. 26-4B). Many of the same treatments effective in treating warts are effective in treating molluscum contagiosum.

Scheinfeld N: Treatment of molluscum contagiosum: a brief review and discussion of a case successfully treated with adapelene, *Dermatol Online J* 13:15, 2007.

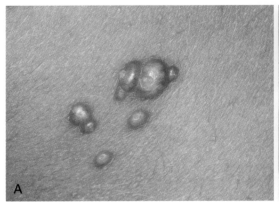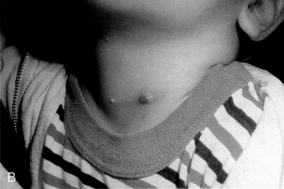

Figure 26-4. A, Multiple papules of molluscum contagiosum demonstrating a characteristic central keratotic core. **B,** Inflammatory molluscum contagiosum in a young child demonstrating both small, waxy, umbilicated papules and an inflammatory lesion simulating a furuncle. (Panel A courtesy of James E. Fitzpatrick MD; panel B courtesy of the Fitzsimons Army Medical Center teaching files.)

CHAPTER 27

BACTERIAL INFECTIONS

James E. Fitzpatrick, MD

STAPHYLOCOCCAL INFECTIONS

1. Which bacterium is the most common cause of skin infections?
Staphylococcus aureus.

2. What kinds of skin infections does *Staphylococcus aureus* produce?
- Impetigo (bullous impetigo)
- Furuncles (boils)
- Carbuncles
- Superficial folliculitis (impetigo of Bockhart)
- Staphylococcal septicemia
- Staphylococcal scalded skin syndrome
- Staphylococcal cellulitis
- Toxic shock syndrome
- Staphylococcal scarlet fever
- Wound infections
- Secondary infections of dermatitis

The most common primary infections are impetigo and furuncles.

3. Is *Staphylococcus aureus* the only bacterium that causes impetigo?
Older textbooks state that the most common cause of impetigo (impetigo contagiosum) is group A β-hemolytic *Streptococcus*. In recent years, most infections in the United States have been due to *S. aureus*, but the prevalence varies geographically. Although impetigo may be due to either organism, in many cases, both can be cultured. In these cases, it is thought that the streptococci are the primary infection and the staphylococci are secondary invaders after the infection has damaged the skin.

4. What does staphylococcal impetigo look like?
Early lesions of staphylococcal impetigo appear as thin, flaccid blisters that may demonstrate cloudy contents or layering of pus (Fig. 27-1). The base of the blister may demonstrate variable erythema. Histologically, the blisters are very superficial; the split occurs beneath the stratum corneum. For this reason, the blisters quickly collapse and may demonstrate a shiny lacquered appearance. Older lesions demonstrate a yellowish crust.

5. Why is staphylococcal impetigo frequently bullous?
Bullous impetigo is caused by staphylococci that produce toxins (exfoliative toxins A and B) capable of causing the split in the epidermis by targeting the epidermal adhesion molecule, desmoglein 1 (Dsg-1). Group II staphylococci are most commonly implicated.

Hanawaka Y, Stanley JR: Mechanisms of blister formation by staphylococcal toxins, *J Biochem* 136:747–750, 2004.

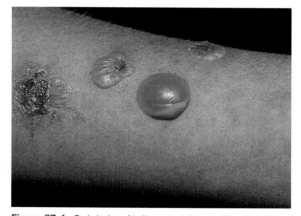

Figure 27-1. Early lesion of bullous staphylococcal impetigo demonstrating fragile bullae with layering of the pus. Collapse blister with lacquered appearance is also present. (Courtesy of the Fitzsimons Army Medical Center teaching files.)

6. How is bullous impetigo diagnosed?
The clinical appearance is usually suggestive but not diagnostic, and other superficial blistering or pustular disorders need to be considered, such as pemphigus, some bullous drug eruptions, and subcorneal pustular dermatosis. A Gram stain of the blister contents should demonstrate abundant Gram-positive cocci, but the definitive test is a culture that not only establishes the cause but also provides sensitivities to different antibiotics. The diagnosis can also be established by doing a biopsy, which demonstrates a subcorneal blister with neutrophils and cocci in the blister cavity.

7. How is bullous impetigo treated?

Oral dicloxacillin or cephalexin is the antibiotic of choice for severe infections. Oral erythromycin is frequently used in penicillin-allergic patients, although up to 20% or more of all staphylococci are resistant. Topical mupirocin is also effective and can be used if the patient cannot take oral antibiotics or if the infection is localized to a small area.

8. What is the difference between a furuncle and a carbuncle?

A furuncle (boil) is a deep follicular abscess, and a carbuncle is a more serious subtype in which there is involvement of several adjoining follicles. A furuncle may develop into a carbuncle. Carbuncles are more likely to develop complications, such as cellulitis or septicemia.

9. How do furuncles present?

Furuncles may be solitary or multiple and present as painful, erythematous, deep-seated follicular abscesses (Fig. 27-2). Patients may demonstrate mild constitutional symptoms in severe cases, or lesions may progress into carbuncles or staphylococcal cellulitis.

10. What is the best way to treat furuncles?

Nonsuppurative solitary lesions are best treated with local heat until they become fluctuant. Fluctuant furuncles should be opened and drained. Smaller

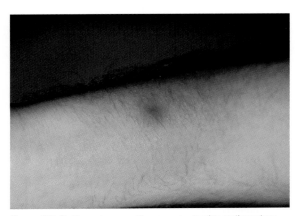

Figure 27-2. Furuncle presenting as a very tender, erythematous follicular-based abscess.

lesions may be punctured with a no. 11 blade and the contents drained, while large abscesses may require a larger incision, drainage, and a wick. Patients with many lesions, evidence of surrounding cellulitis or with systemic symptoms should be considered for oral antibiotics.

As always, the diagnosis should be confirmed with a culture and antibiotic sensitivities performed at the initial visit, since not all follicular-based abscesses are due to staphylococci. The initial antibiotic choice before the culture and antibiogram results is usually oral dicloxacillin, oral cephalexin, or oral amoxicillin/clavulanate. Oral erythromycin, azithromycin, or clarithromycin can be used if the patient is allergic to penicillin. However, if MRSA infection is clinically suspected then the initial antibiotic choice is different (see question 16).

11. Why do some patients develop recurrent staphylococcal impetigo or recurrent furunculosis?

Recurrent infections occur when *Staphylococcus aureus* establishes itself as a part of the resident microbial flora. This occurs in up to 20% of individuals. The most common sites of carriage are the anterior nasal vestibule, axilla, groin, and feet. Patients who have virulent strains are prone to the development of recurrent impetigo or furunculosis, depending on the strain. A variety of host factors, such as abnormal neutrophil chemotaxis (e.g., hypergammaglobulinemia IgE syndrome), deficient intracellular killing (e.g., chronic granulomatous disease), and immunodeficiency states (e.g., AIDS), are important in a minority of patients. Diabetes mellitus is listed in many references as being associated with recurrent furunculosis, but this is controversial.

El-Gilany AH, Fathy H: Risk factors of recurrrent furunculosis, *Dermatol Online J* 15:16, 2009.

12. How is staphylococcal carriage eliminated?

Standard treatment regimens, such as oral dicloxacillin, oral cephalexin, oral erythromycin, or even intravenous vancomycin, eliminate active infection but not staphylococcal carriage. The most commonly used regimen to eliminate staphylococcal carriage is rifampin in combination with dicloxacillin. Less common regimens utilize oral clindamycin, topical mupirocin ointment, or replacement of the microflora with a less pathogenic strain of *S. aureus* (strain 502A). The success of these regimens varies from 50% to 70%; however, recolonization is common.

13. What is staphylococcal scalded-skin syndrome?

Staphylococcal scalded-skin syndrome typically occurs in neonates, infants, or immunocompromised adults. Like bullous impetigo, it is due to group II staphylococci that produce an exfoliatoxin; however, it differs in that the infection occurs at a distant site, such as a conjunctivitis or abscess. In neonates and infants, the kidneys are not able to excrete the exfoliatoxin adequately. The high level of exfoliatoxin produces diffuse, tender erythema associated with fever that rapidly progress to flaccid bullae; the bullae wrinkle and exfoliate, leaving an oozing erythematous base (Fig. 27-3). Mortality in neonates is usually not due to the infection but is secondary to impaired temperature regulation or fluid balance.

Yamasaki O, Yamaguchi T, Sugai M, et al: Clinical manifestations of staphylococcal scalded-skin syndrome depend on serotypes of exfoliative toxins, *J Clin Microbiol* 43:1893–1899, 2005.

14. Describe the presentation of toxic shock syndrome.

Toxic shock syndrome is an acute febrile illness due to *Staphylococcus aureus* strains that produce pyrogenic exotoxins. These toxin-producing strains have been isolated classically from superabsorbent tampons in menstruating women but are also found in abscesses, wound infections, or the vaginas of nonmenstruating women.

Clinically, the hallmarks are fever, hypotension, and a diffuse erythema that resembles scarlet fever. Other manifestations include pharyngeal erythema, strawberry tongue, conjunctival infection, and gastrointestinal symptoms. Desquamation of the palms and soles occurs 1 to 2 weeks following resolution of the erythema.

15. Why is *S. aureus* frequently found in secondary infections of dermatitis and wounds?

S. aureus has receptors that allow it to bind to fibrin that is found in abundance on wound surfaces and in dermatitic skin.

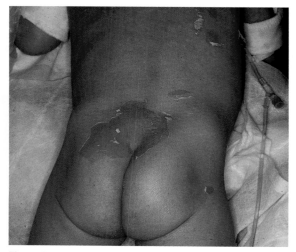

Figure 27-3. Early staphylococcal scalded-skin syndrome demonstrating diffuse erythema and early desquamation.

Key Points: Staphylococcal Skin Infections

1. *Staphylococcus aureus* is the most common cause of skin infection.
2. *Staphylococcus aureus* has replaced *Streptococcus pyogenes* as the most common cause of impetigo.
3. Bullous impetigo is always caused by *S. aureus* strains, usually phage II, type 71, that produce exfoliative toxins.
4. Approximately 20% of the population is colonized by *S. aureus*.
5. The anterior nares is the most common site of *S. aureus* colonization, but other moist sites including the axillae, groin, and toe webs can also be colonized

---

16. What is MRSA?

MRSA stands for methicillin-resistant *S. aureus*. MRSA strains have developed resistance to β-lactam antibiotics. MRSA strains are often resistant to other antibiotics as well, especially erythromycin.

17. What is the difference between HA-MRSA and CA-MRSA?

In the past, most cases of MRSA were hospital acquired but, in recent years, a distinct subtype of MRSA has emerged in the community setting. The two MRSA types are known as hospital acquired and community acquired (HA and CA-MRSA). HA-MRSA tends to cause invasive and disseminated infections in hospitalized patients, hemodialysis patients, long-term care facility patients, and patients with implanted medical devices. These strains tend to exhibit resistance to a greater number of antibiotic classes than CA-MRSA. CA-MRSA causes the same spectrum of skin infections as methicillin-sensitive (MSSA) *S. aureus*, most commonly furuncles, boils, and abscesses; however, severe, invasive infections with CA-MRSA have been reported. Additionally, CA-MRSA tends to display a narrower spectrum of antibiotic resistance than HA-MRSA. Trimethoprim-sulfamethoxazole, tetracycline, and clindamycin are antibiotics that will often cover CA-MRSA, although inducible clindamycin resistance is fairly common in CA-MRSA isolates. Therapy is dependent on the severity of infection and the strain susceptibility, with empiric antibiotic coverage determined by prevalence of CA-MRSA in a given community. More serious and hospital-acquired cases are usually treated with vancomycin or linezolid.

Elston DM: Status update: hospital-acquired and community-acquired methicillin-resistant *Staphylococcus aureus*, *Cutis* 79(Suppl 6):37–42, 2007.

STREPTOCOCCAL INFECTIONS

18. What types of cutaneous infections are produced by β-hemolytic streptococci?

Beta-hemolytic streptococci are responsible for impetigo, blistering distal dactylitis, ecthyma, erysipelas, necrotizing fasciitis, and septicemia.

19. How does streptococcal impetigo present?

Streptococcal impetigo presents as superficial, stuck-on, honey-colored crusts overlying an erosion (Fig. 27-4). The most common location is the face, but any area may be involved. In contrast to staphylococcal impetigo, blisters are absent.

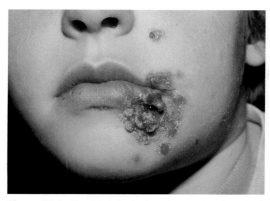

Figure 27-4. Characteristic stuck-on, honey-colored crusts of streptococcal impetigo.

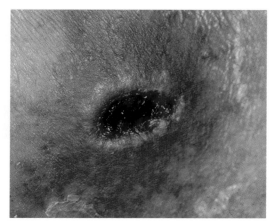

Figure 27-5. Streptococcal ecthyma demonstrating punched-out ulceration surrounded by erythema.

20. What is ecthyma?

Ecthyma is a severe form of streptococcal impetigo in which there is a thick crust overlying a punched-out ulceration of the epidermis (Fig. 27-5). Typically, it is surrounded by a zone of erythema. In contrast to streptococcal impetigo, which is usually found on the face and does not produce scarring, ecthyma is more commonly located on lower extremities and may heal with scarring.

21. What is blistering distal dactylitis?

Blistering distal dactylitis is an uncommon infection typically caused by *Streptococcus pyogenes* but occasionally caused by *Staphylococcus aureus*. It typically presents in young children as one or more tender superficial bullae on an erythematous base on the volar fat pad of a finger (Fig. 27-6). In rare instances, toes may be affected.

22. What is erysipelas?

Erysipelas, or St. Anthony's fire, is a form of cellulitis usually caused by β-hemolytic streptococci, rarely by *Staphylococcus aureus*. Patients often have a prodrome of malaise, fever, and headache. Typically, erysipelas presents on the face as an erythematous indurated plaque with a sharply demarcated border and a "cliff-drop" edge (Fig. 27-7). In severe cases, the epidermis may become bullous, pustular, or necrotic. Untreated erysipelas can be fatal due to vascular thrombosis, bacteremia, or toxin release. Streptococcal cellulitis is a more generic term that includes erysipelas but also cellulitis that lacks the characteristic cliff-drop border. Known commonly as "blood poisoning," it is most often found on extremities and is associated with lymphangitis (Fig. 27-8).

23. How do you diagnose erysipelas?

The diagnosis usually is made clinically because the organism is difficult to recover in culture. Aspiration of the advancing edge following the injection of nonbacteriostatic saline produces positive cultures in about 20% of cases.

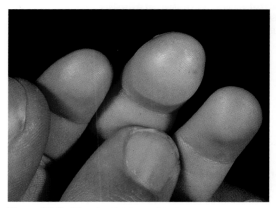

Figure 27-6. Blistering distal dactylitis demonstrating a characteristic tender superficial blister on the volar fat pad.

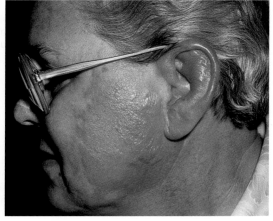

Figure 27-7. Characteristic lesion of erysipelas demonstrating indurated, erythematous plaque with sharply demarcated border.

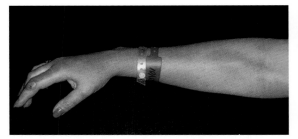

Figure 27-8. Streptococcal cellulitis that started with an injury to the index finger. Note associated lymphangitis extending up the arm.

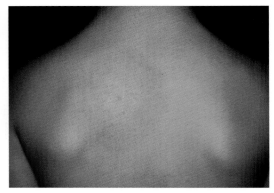

Figure 27-9. Typical lesion of erythema chronicum migrans manifesting as central papule at the tick bite site surrounded by annular erythema.

24. How is erysipelas treated?

Mild or early cases may be treated with an oral penicillin or oral erythromycin. Oral dicloxacillin is the best choice because it provides better antistaphylococcal coverage for the rare case of staphylococcal erysipelas. Severe cases or cases with central facial involvement should be hospitalized and treated with intravenous antibiotics, such as vancomycin. Erysipelas usually improves within 48 hours after institution of antibiotic therapy.

OTHER BACTERIAL INFECTIONS

25. Describe the cutaneous manifestations of Lyme disease.

Lyme disease is a multisystem disease caused by *Borrelia burgdorferi* that is transmitted to humans by ticks of the genus *Ixodes*. One to 30 days after the tick bite, patients present with variable constitutional symptoms, including fever, malaise, headache, and arthralgias. Approximately three fourths of patients develop erythema chronicum migrans that begins as an erythematous papule at the bite site and progresses to an annular erythema that may reach 20 cm or more in size (Fig. 27-9).

Müllegger RR, Glatz M: Skin manifestations of Lyme borreliosis: diagnosis and management, *Am J Clin Dermatol* 9:355–368, 2008.

26. A patient living in an endemic area for Lyme disease reports a history of a tick bite. Should that patient receive antibiotic prophylaxis?

The question of whether or not patients with tick bites in endemic areas should receive antibiotic prophylaxis is controversial. Randomized controlled trials only support the use of a 200 mg oral dose of doxycycline in a child >8 years of age when all of the following criteria are met: 1) The attached tick can be identified as a nymphal or adult form of *Ixodes scapularis* that has been attached for >36 hours, estimated by exposure or degree of tick engorgement; 2) prophylaxis can be started within 72 hours of when tick was removed; 3) ecologic information shows that local prevalence of infection of ticks with *Borellia burgdorferi* is greater than 20%; and 4) doxycycline is not contraindicated.

Wormser GP, Dattwyler RJ, Shapiro ED, et al: The clinical assessment, treatment, and prevention of Lyme disease, human granulocytic anaplasmosis, and babesiosis: clinical practice guidelines by the Infectious Diseases Society of America, *Clin Infect Dis* 43:1089–1134, 2006.

27. What types of skin infections does *Pseudomonas aeruginosa* produce?

P. aeruginosa is one of the most feared bacterial pathogens in medicine. Cutaneous infections include:

- Ecthyma gangrenosum
- Septic vasculitis
- Pseudomonal folliculitis
- External otitis media
- Toe web infection
- Wound infections (burn wounds)
- Cellulitis
- Necrotizing fasciitis
- Onycholysis (green nail syndrome)
- Paronychia

28. How does ecthyma gangrenosum differ from ecthyma?

- Ecthyma is caused by β-hemolytic streptococci, while ecthyma gangrenosum is most commonly caused by *P. aeruginosa*.
- Ecthyma is a localized infection that normally occurs in healthy young adults. Ecthyma gangrenosum usually follows septicemia in a neutropenic patient. Less commonly, it follows primary inoculation into the skin.

- Ecthyma responds rapidly to antibiotics, whereas ecthyma gangrenosum has a high mortality.
- Clinically, ecthyma gangrenosum presents as one or more red macules that become edematous and rapidly progress to hemorrhagic bullae. In the late stages, it may ulcerate (Fig. 27-10) or form an eschar surrounded by erythema.

29. Where do you usually acquire *Pseudomonas* folliculitis?

In your hot tub. *Pseudomonas* folliculitis is typically associated with hot tub use (hot tub folliculitis). Less commonly, it is associated with whirlpools or swimming pools. It is usually associated with *P. aeruginosa* serotype 0:11, although other serotypes have also been reported. *Pseudomonas* folliculitis has also been reported as a complication of depilatories used for the removal of leg hair.

Yu Y, Chang AS, Wang L, et al: Hot tub folliculitis or hot hand-foot syndrome caused by *Pseudomonas aeruginosa*, *J Am Acad Dermatol* 57:596–600, 2007.

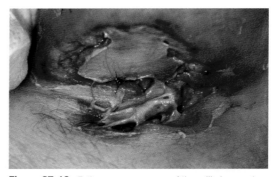

Figure 27-10. Ecthyma gangrenosum of the axilla in a neutropenic patient demonstrating massive ulceration. (Courtesy of the Fitzsimons Army Medical Center teaching files.)

30. How does *Pseudomonas* folliculitis present?

Clinically, it occurs 1 to 3 days after exposure, presenting as a diffuse truncal eruption (Fig. 27-11). The primary lesion is a follicular-based erythematous papule that frequently demonstrates a follicular pustule. Less commonly, patients may also demonstrate mastitis, abscesses, lymphangitis, and fever. Another variation is those patients that present with painful indurated lesions of the feet and/or hand that may become pustular ("*Pseudomonas* hot hand-foot syndrome"). The disease is usually self-limited, although rare patients may continue to develop recurrent folliculitis or abscesses for up to 2 months.

31. What is the best treatment for *Pseudomonas* folliculitis?

Most cases are self-limited and do not require treatment. Severe or recurrent cases can be treated with oral ciprofloxacin. Ultimately, the best treatment is prevention of infection. The most effective measures are frequent drainage of the hot tub or whirlpool to remove the buildup of desquamated skin cells that serve as the prime source of nutrients. Adequate chlorination and bromination are also necessary.

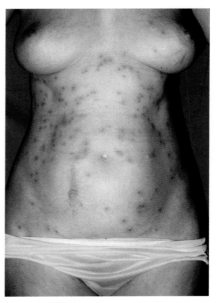

Figure 27-11. Pseudomonas folliculitis. Patient with history of recent hot tub exposure and development of numerous truncal follicular-based papules and pustules. (Courtesy of the Fitzsimons Army Medical Center teaching files.)

32. How is Wood's light used in diagnosing *Pseudomonas* infections?

P. aeruginosa produces a pigment called pyoverdin that fluoresces yellow-green on Wood's light. The Wood's light is useful in detecting pseudomonads in burn wounds, surgical infections, ulcerated ecthyma gangrenosum, and Gram-negative toe web infections.

33. What causes tularemia? Where did the name tularemia come from?

Tularemia is caused by *Francisella* (formerly *Pasteurella*) *tularensis*, a Gram-negative coccobacillus. The infection is acquired through handling of infected animals (squirrels and rabbits), tick bites, and deerfly bites. Tularemia gets its name from Tulare County in California, the site where researchers isolated the organism from ground squirrels in 1911. The term was first used by Dr. Francis, who was subsequently honored by having the genus named after him.

34. Describe the skin lesions of tularemia.

Tularemia has six presentations: ulceroglandular, glandular, oculoglandular, oropharyngeal, typhoidal, and pneumonic forms. The ulceroglandular form is the most common presentation and the one that typically demonstrates skin lesions. The primary skin lesion begins as a small papule at the inoculation site that rapidly necroses. The papule may be surrounded by an area of cellulitis and is characteristically associated with painful regional lymphadenopathy (Fig. 27-12). Systemic symptoms include fever, chills, headache, and malaise.

35. How should tularemia be treated?

The treatment of choice is streptomycin. Alternate therapies include gentamicin, chloramphenicol, and tetracycline.

36. What is trichomycosis axillaris?

Trichomycosis axillaris is a superficial infection of the hair shaft that most commonly affects the axillary hair and, less commonly, the pubic hair. It is most commonly produced by *Corynebacterium tenuis* although other *Corynebacterium* species are also frequently implicated. It is an asymptomatic infection characterized by tan or, less commonly, yellow, red, or black concretions of tightly packed bacteria that grow on and within the hair (Fig. 27-13). Treatment options include cutting the affected hair, topical aluminum chloride, topical erythromycin, or topical clindamycin.

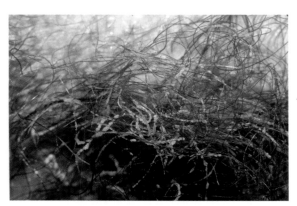

Figure 27-13. Trichomycosis axillaris. Adherent tan-white concretions on axillary hair. (Courtesy of the Fitzsimons Army Medical Center teaching files.)

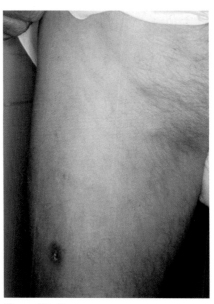

Figure 27-12. Tularemia. Patient with history of deerfly bite on thigh while fishing in New Mexico. The patient has an eschar at the bite site and a suppurative lymph node in the groin. (Courtesy of the Fitzsimons Army Medical Center teaching files.)

SYPHILIS

Clayton B. Green, MD, PhD, and James E. Fitzpatrick, MD

CHAPTER 28

"Know syphilis in all of its manifestations and relations, and all other things clinical will be added unto you."

—Sir William Osler, 1897

1. What causes syphilis?

Syphilis is caused by the spirochete *Treponema pallidum*, ssp. *pallidum*, which belongs to the order Spirochaetales. *T. pallidum* ssp. *endemicum* is a subspecies that causes bejel, or endemic syphilis. Other pathogenic treponemes for humans include *T. pallidum* ssp. *pertenue,* the cause of yaws, and *T. carateum*, the cause of pinta. There are other *Treponema* species that infect other animals or are free-living. Since 2000, there has been an increase in the number of reported cases in the United States, with 11,466 cases of primary and secondary syphilis being reported in 2007, which is a 15.7% increase when compared to the figures from 2006.

Centers for Disease Control and Prevention: *Sexually transmitted disease surveillance 2007 supplement: syphilis surveillance report*, Atlanta, March 2009, US Department of Health and Human Services, Centers for Disease Control and Prevention.

2. Describe the morphologic appearance of *T. pallidum*.

T. pallidum is a delicate spiral bacterium that measures 6 to 20 mm in length and 0.10 to 0.18 mm in width (Fig. 28-1). Because of the narrow width, it is not visible by normal light microscopy and must be visualized by darkfield microscopy, by silver stains (i.e., Warthin-Starry or modified Steiner stains), or by immunoperoxidase stains *(Treponema)*. The spiral coils are regularly spaced at a distance of about 1 mm. The typical spirochete has 6 to 14 coils. The organism reproduces by transverse fission.

3. Where did syphilis originate?

The origin of syphilis had been a point of great debate among experts, with some authorities favoring a New World origin because of an epidemic of syphilis that ravaged Europe in the last decade of the 15th century, when it was referred to as the "Great Pox" (as opposed to smallpox). Because this epidemic coincided with the return of Columbus from America in 1493, this suggested that it was imported from the West Indies. Of interest, Columbus himself is thought to have died from syphilitic aortitis. Other authorities maintained that it had always been present in the Old World. Studies on skeletal remains clearly demonstrate that while treponemal disease was present in the Old World, epidemic syphilis was imported from the New World.

Tognotti E: The rise and fall of syphilis in Renaissance Europe, *J Med Humanit* 30:99–113, 2009.

4. How is syphilis transmitted?

Syphilis is most commonly acquired as a sexually transmitted disease but also may be acquired congenitally (see Chapter 57) or, rarely, by blood transfusions. The organism is very fragile and easily killed by heat, cold, drying, soap, and disinfectants. Since the spirochete is so fragile, the possibility that an infection could be acquired from a toilet seat is statistically very remote.

5. What are the chances of getting syphilis from having sexual intercourse with an infected individual?

The definitive study has obviously never been done, but epidemiologic studies show that the chances are about one in three. It is believed that the treponemes cannot penetrate intact epidermis or mucosa and that most infections are acquired through microscopic or macroscopic breaks in the skin.

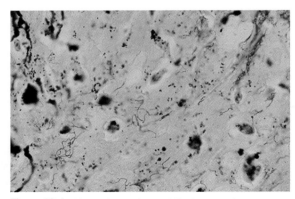

Figure 28-1. Biopsy of secondary syphilis demonstrating numerous spirochetes in the epidermis (Warthin-Starry stain, ×1000).

6. Following inoculation, how long does it take for the primary chancre to appear?

Experimental study on both rabbits and human volunteers has shown that the appearance of the primary chancre is related to the size of the inoculum. The primary chancre normally appears in 10 to 90 days, with the average time being about 3 weeks. The organism reaches the regional lymph nodes within hours.

7. Describe the typical Hunterian chancre.

The classic Hunterian chancre develops at the site of inoculation as a painless ulcer with a firm, indurated border (Fig. 28-2). The size may vary from a few millimeters to several centimeters in diameter. Associated unilateral or bilateral, painless, regional, nonsuppurative lymphadenopathy develops in 50% to 85% of patients approximately 1 week after the appearance of the primary ulcer. It is important to realize that up to 50% of all chancres are atypical. Painful ulcers, multiple ulcers (Fig. 28-3), secondarily infected ulcers, and nonindurated ulcers are variations on the classic chancre.

Lee V, Kinghorn G: Syphilis: an update, *Clin Med* 8:330–333, 2008.

8. Do syphilitic chancres occur on sites other than the genitalia?

Extragenital chancres occur in 5% of all cases of primary syphilis, although the incidence may be as high as 10%. The most common extragenital sites are the lip, which is associated with oral sex, and anus, which is associated with anal intercourse. Anal intercourse may also produce rectal or colonic chancres as high as 20 cm into the bowel. Other reported sites include the tongue, tonsil, finger, thumb (Fig. 28-4), eyelid, chin, nipple, umbilicus, axilla, and even the lower limb. A high index of suspicion is required to diagnose extragenital chancres.

Scott CM, Flint SR: Oral syphilis—reemergence of an old disease with oral manifestations, *Int J Oral Maxillofac Surg* 34:58–63, 2005.

9. What is the best way to diagnose primary syphilis?

Diagnosis cannot be based on clinical presentation alone, and, unfortunately, *T. pallidum* cannot be cultured. The most specific and rapid method of diagnosing primary syphilis is the demonstration of the spirochete utilizing darkfield examination by a trained observer. This test is not readily available to most community physicians and usually requires sending the patient to a sexually transmitted disease (STD) clinic or medical center. The material for examination can be obtained from either the ulcer or an aspirate from an enlarged lymph node. A single negative darkfield examination does not rule out the possibility of syphilis, and it should not be regarded as negative until there are negative examinations on 3 consecutive days. Primary syphilis can also be diagnosed by biopsying the primary ulcer and demonstrating the organism by special stain.

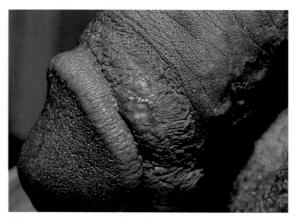

Figure 28-2. Typical Hunterian chancre of syphilis demonstrating characteristic indurated border.

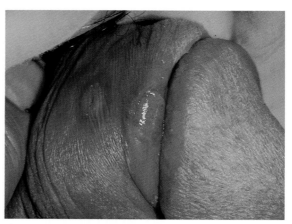

Figure 28-3. A typical presentation of primary syphilis demonstrating two chancres. (Courtesy of William James, MD.)

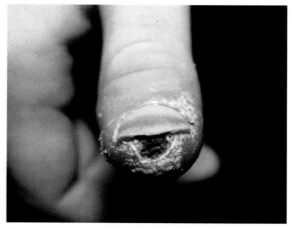

Figure 28-4. Extragenital chancre of syphilis on the thumb. (Courtesy of the teaching files of Fitzsimons Army Medical Center.)

In lieu of these procedures, a presumptive diagnosis can be made by serologic tests (see Chapter 3). The Venereal Disease Research Laboratory (VDRL) test and rapid plasma reagin (RPR) test are negative in early primary syphilis and should be repeated weekly for 1 month to be considered as negative. The diagnosis is more likely if a rising titer can be demonstrated. The fluorescent treponemal antibody-absorption (FTA-ABS) test turns positive earlier and is more sensitive.

10. How is primary syphilis treated?

The recommended treatment for primary syphilis is benzathine penicillin G, 2.4 million units in a single intramuscular (IM) dose or procaine penicillin, 600,000 units IM daily for 10 to 14 days. Nonpregnant patients who are allergic to penicillin can be treated with either doxycycline (100 mg orally two times per day for 14 days), tetracycline (500 mg orally four times per day for 14 days), or ceftriaxone (125 mg IM every day for 10 days, 250 mg IM every other day, or 1000 mg IM for 8 to 10 days).

Treatment failures have been reported with all regimens, and patients should have follow-up serologic titers at 3, 6, 12, and 24 months to ensure a fourfold decline in titers. Failure of non-treponemal antibody titers to fall fourfold within 6 months of treatment can be considered a probable treatment failure. Patients need to be reported to the proper public health agency to ensure tracking of known sexual partners.

Centers for Disease Control and Prevention: Sexually transmitted disease guidelines 2006, *MMWR* 55:22–33, 2006.

11. What is the Jarisch-Herxheimer reaction?

This acute febrile reaction, associated with shaking chills, malaise, sore throat, myalgia, headache, and localized inflammation of infected mucocutaneous sites, usually occurs 6 to 8 hours following penicillin treatment. Tetracycline, doxycycline, and ceftriaxone are less commonly associated with this reaction. It develops in 50% of patients with primary syphilis, 75% with secondary syphilis, and 30% with neurosyphilis. There is indirect evidence that this reaction is due to the release of a treponemal lipopolysaccharide that acts like a bacterial endotoxin. Similar reactions have been reported with other infectious diseases, including leptospirosis and louse-borne relapsing fever.

12. What is the natural history of the untreated syphilitic chancre?

The untreated syphilitic chancre lasts for about 2 to 8 weeks and then disappears. The primary chancre may relapse, in which case it is referred to as chancre redux.

13. When does secondary syphilis begin?

Secondary syphilis usually begins about 6 weeks after the onset of the primary chancre. In approximately 25% of cases, the primary ulcer will still be present. In one study, 25% of patients with secondary syphilis did not recall a primary chancre.

Baughn RE, Musher DM: Secondary syphilitic lesions, *Clin Microbiol Rev* 18:205–216, 2005.

14. Do patients with secondary syphilis have any symptoms?

The most common reported symptoms include malaise (23% to 46%), headache (9% to 46%), fever (5% to 39%), pruritus (42%), and loss of appetite (25%). Less common symptoms include painful eyes, joint or bone pain, meningismus, iritis, and hoarseness. Some textbooks incorrectly state that pruritus is uncommon in secondary syphilis.

15. List the common physical findings in secondary syphilis.

- Syphiloderm (rash): 88% to 100%
- Lymphadenopathy: 85% to 89%
- Residual primary chancre: 25% to 43%
- Condylomata lata: 9% to 44%
- Hepatosplenomegaly: 23%
- Mucous patches: 7% to 12%
- Alopecia: 3% to 11%

16. Describe the syphiloderm of secondary syphilis.

The syphiloderm of secondary syphilis is most commonly a maculopapular dermatitis (Fig. 28-5A, B) with variable scaly (70%), papular (12%), or macular (10%) lesions. Less common morphologic appearances include annular (Fig. 28-5C, D), pustular, and psoriasiform lesions. The rash typically demonstrates a widespread symmetrical distribution, although in some patients, lesions may be localized to a single anatomic region, such as the palms and soles. In a large study done in the United States, the most common sites of involvement, in descending order, were the soles, trunk, arms, genitals, palms, legs, face, neck, and scalp.

Dave S, Gopinath DV, Thappa DM: Nodular secondary syphilis, *Dermatol Online J* 9:9, 2003. (Readers can go to this journal online and see clinical photographs.)

17. What are condylomata lata? How do they differ from condylomata acuminata?

Condylomata lata are whitish or grayish, elevated, broad, flat papular lesions of secondary syphilis that primarily occur in moist areas, such as the penis (Fig. 28-6A), labia, inner thighs, and anal region. These papular lesions may coalesce

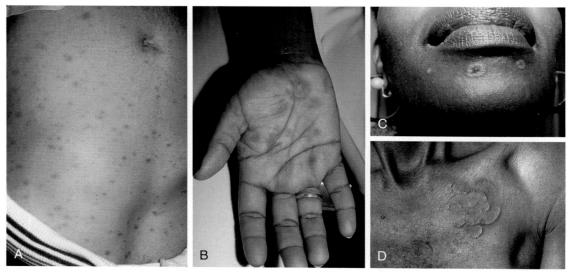

Figure 28-5. Secondary syphilis. **A,** Hyperpigmented macules of secondary syphilis in a patient who was initially treated for chancroid. Note the strong similarity of these lesions to pityriasis rosea. **B,** Characteristic papulosquamous lesions of secondary syphilis on the palm of a nurse. Macular or papulosquamous lesions on the palms are not diagnostic but are suggestive of secondary syphilis. **C,** Annular lesions of secondary syphilis on the face. **D,** Striking annular lesions of the chest in a patient with secondary syphilis. (Panel B courtesy of the Fitzsimons Army Medical Center teaching files; panel D courtesy of the Walter Reed Army Medical Center teaching files.)

Figure 28-6. A, Exophytic condylomata lata of the penis in a patient referred to the author for treatment of "venereal warts." **B,** Discrete, white, focally eroded mucous patches of secondary syphilis.

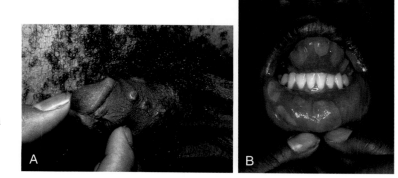

to form verrucous plaques that are easily confused with condylomata acuminata, which are genital warts caused by human papillomavirus. Condylomata lata are more common in women than men.

Begovac J, Lukas D: Images in clinical medicine. Condylomata lata of secondary syphilis, *N Engl J Med* 352:708, 2005.

18. What are mucous patches?

Shallow, usually painless erosions of the mucous membranes (Fig. 28-6B). Some mucous patches demonstrate linear shapes and have been described as resembling "snail tracks."

19. Is there anything characteristic about the alopecia of secondary syphilis?

The hair loss primarily affects the scalp but may also involve the eyebrows and eyelashes. It presents as a nonscarring, patchy alopecia that is described as a "moth-eaten" pattern (see Figure 20-8). This classic pattern appears to be uncommon in the 20th century. The most common pattern of hair loss in secondary syphilis today is a nonspecific diffuse hair loss due to a telogen effluvium (see Chapter 20).

20. How good are physicians at recognizing the signs and symptoms of secondary syphilis?

In a retrospective study of 34 patients with secondary syphilis who had been seen previously by community physicians, only 40% of physicians listed secondary syphilis as the primary diagnosis. Another 14% included secondary syphilis in their differential diagnosis. In sum, almost one half of physicians did not consider the diagnosis.

21. What is the best way to diagnose secondary syphilis?

The diagnosis of secondary syphilis requires a health care provider with a strong index of suspicion. The cutaneous manifestations of secondary syphilis may mimic other skin diseases, including pityriasis rosea, psoriasis, erythema multiforme, pityriasis lichenoides et varioliformis acuta, and some drug reactions. It is a good rule of thumb to consider secondary syphilis in any patient having a generalized dermatitis with associated lymphadenopathy.

As with primary syphilis, the most specific tests are the demonstration of the spirochete either in a skin biopsy or on darkfield examination, which can be performed on either the secondary skin lesions or on aspirates from lymph nodes. In contrast to primary syphilis, serologic tests are almost invariably positive. The only exception is when there is a false-negative reaction due to a prozone phenomenon, which occurs in 1% to 2% of patients with secondary syphilis. The prozone phenomenon occurs when the titers are very high and can be eliminated by diluting the serum.

Hoang MP, High WA, Molberg KH: Secondary syphilis: a histologic and immunohistochemical evaluation, *J Cutan Pathol* 31:595–599, 2004.

Key Points: Syphilis

1. Syphilis is a sexually transmitted disease that can also be transmitted from the mother to the fetus.
2. Syphilis is produced by the spirochete *Treponema pallidum*, ssp. *pallidum*.
3. Secondary syphilis is protean in its clinical appearance and can be difficult to recognize, with studies showing that up to one half of community physicians will not clinically suspect secondary syphilis.
4. The most specific and rapid method of diagnosing primary syphilis is the demonstration of the spirochete utilizing darkfield examination by a trained observer.
5. Patients with syphilis have an increased incidence of other sexually transmitted infections such as gonorrhea, HIV infection, and venereal warts.

---

22. How should secondary syphilis be treated?

The treatment should be the same as for primary syphilis.

23. What stage follows untreated secondary syphilis?

The mucocutaneous lesions of secondary syphilis usually heal without scarring in 2 to 10 weeks, although hyperpigmentation or hypopigmentation may persist. Following the resolution of secondary syphilis, patients enter the latent stage of infection. During this stage, approximately one fourth of patients experience relapsing secondary lesions. Most relapses occur in the first year, but these may occur for up to 5 years.

24. How is latent syphilis treated?

For the purpose of treatment, the Centers for Disease Control and Prevention defines infections of <1 year as early latent syphilis and infections of >1 year as late latent. The World Health Organization considers early latent syphilis to extend up to 2 years.

Like primary and secondary syphilis, early latent syphilis is treated with 2.4 million units (mu) of benzathine penicillin G intramuscularly in a single dose. Late latent syphilis or latent syphilis of unknown duration is treated with a total of 7.2 mu of benzathine penicillin G administered as three doses of 2.4 mu intramuscularly at 1-week intervals. Penicillin-allergic patients are treated with doxycycline or tetracycline for 2 weeks in early latent syphilis and for 4 weeks in late latent syphilis.

25. When should lumbar punctures be done in patients with syphilis?

Lumbar punctures to rule out neurosyphilis are recommended for patients with late latent syphilis of more than 1-year duration or unknown duration who demonstrate neurologic symptoms, treatment failure, serum nontreponemal antibody titer equal to or greater than 1:32, other evidence of active syphilis (iritis, aortitis, gumma), nonpenicillin treatment, or positive HIV test. Syphilis frequently attacks the central nervous system, as demonstrated by the fact that 40% of patients with primary or secondary syphilis demonstrate cerebrospinal fluid pleocytosis, and 24% of patients with secondary syphilis demonstrate a reactive VDRL. In patients with syphilis/HIV coinfection there is evidence to suggest that lumbar puncture may be indicated in all coinfected patients since the disease is more aggressive; however, this is also controversial.

Chan DJ: Syphilis and HIV co-infection: when is lumbar puncture indicated? *Curr HIV Res* 3:95–98, 2005.

26. What happens to patients with untreated latent syphilis?

Approximately one third of patients with untreated latent syphilis develop tertiary syphilis. The other two thirds of patients will not develop later effects of the disease.

27. Name the three major presentations of tertiary syphilis.

- Late benign syphilis
- Cardiovascular disease
- Neurosyphilis (general paresis or tabes dorsalis)

Marra CM: Update on neurosyphilis, *Curr Infect Dis Rep* 11:127–134, 2009.

28. What are the mucocutaneous features of late benign syphilis?

Late benign syphilis usually occurs 1 to 46 years after resolution of the secondary skin lesions. Although almost any organ may be involved, the most common organ is the skin (70%) followed by the mucous membranes (10%) and bones (10%). The primary lesion of late benign syphilis is the *gumma*. A gumma is a granulomatous lesion that contains treponemes only rarely; it probably represents a hypersensitivity reaction.

The skin lesions of late benign syphilis present as nodules and plaques that demonstrate a tendency for central healing and peripheral extension. The central healed areas characteristically demonstrate scarring and atrophy (Fig. 28-7). The mucosal lesions may involve any mucosal surface but demonstrate a tendency to extend to and destroy the nasal cartilage, producing a "saddle nose" deformity. Involvement of the mucosa over the hard palate may produce a perforation.

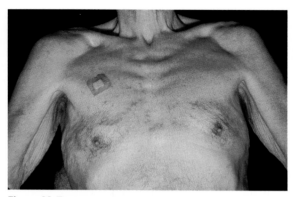

Figure 28-7. Tertiary cutaneous syphilis demonstrating characteristic annular appearance with mild central atrophy. (Courtesy of Richard Gentry, MD.)

Rocha N, Horta M, Sanches M, et al: Syphilitic gumma—cutaneous tertiary syphilis, *J Eur Acad Dermatol Venereol* 18:517–518, 2004.

29. What was the Tuskegee Study?

The Tuskegee Study is one of the most iniquitous prospective medical studies ever done in the United States. Untreated black men with syphilis, without their knowledge or consent, were randomized into treated and untreated groups and then followed so that the complications and mortality of untreated syphilis could be monitored. This study was part of the impetus to establish strict guidelines for biomedical research. In 1997, President Clinton formally apologized to the survivors for this United States Public Health Service (USPHS) study.

HANSEN'S DISEASE (LEPROSY)

Kehua Li, MD, and Loren E. Golitz, MD

CHAPTER 29

1. What causes leprosy?

Leprosy is a chronic granulomatous infection caused by *Mycobacterium leprae*, affecting primarily skin and peripheral nerves. *M. leprae* is a noncultivable, gram-positive, obligate intracellular, acid-fast bacillus. There is an apparent genetic susceptibility to acquiring infection.

Moschella SL: An update on the diagnosis and treatment of leprosy, *J Am Acad Dermatol* 51:417–426, 2004.

2. Why is leprosy called Hansen's disease?

Leprosy is referred to as Hansen's disease to honor Gerhard Armauer Hansen, a Norwegian physician, who discovered the leprosy bacterium in 1873. *Mycobacterium leprae* was the first bacillus to be associated with a human disease. In addition, as with acquired immune deficiency syndrome, there are considerable social stigmata associated with having leprosy. Therefore, rather than referring to patients as lepers and the disease as leprosy, it is often preferable to use the term Hansen's disease.

Gelber RM: Hansen's disease, *West J Med* 158:583–590, 1993.

3. How is leprosy transmitted?

Although the mode of transmission is still uncertain, current evidence favors respiratory transmission. Average incubation times are 2 to 5 years for tuberculoid leprosy and 8 to 12 years for lepromatous cases. Evidence for congenital and percutaneous transmission has been presented, but these are probably rare.

4. Are children and adults equally susceptible to acquiring leprosy?

Children and young adults seem to be most susceptible to acquiring leprosy. Only about 5% of adults at risk, such as marriage partners, develop leprosy. As many as 60% of children who have a parent with leprosy develop the disease. *M. leprae* may be present in breast milk; there is some evidence to suggest that the infection can be transmitted via the placenta.

5. Are humans the only host for *M. leprae*?

It was once believed that humans were the only natural reservoir for *M. leprae*. More recently, four other animals have been shown to carry the infection: the nine-banded armadillo, chimpanzee, sooty mangabey monkey, and cynomolgus macaque. Up to 10% of wild armadillos in Louisiana and eastern Texas have naturally acquired leprosy.

Bruce S, Schroeder TL, Ellner K, et al: Armadillo exposure and Hansen's disease: an epidemiologic survey in southern Texas, *J Am Acad Dermatol* 43:223–228, 2000.

6. Is leprosy a systemic disease?

Yes. Although the peripheral nerves and skin are most notably affected, leprosy has involved every organ except for the central nervous system (CNS) and lung.

7. How common is leprosy?

There were about 2.7 million persons with leprosy worldwide in 1994, with 600,000 new cases yearly. Leprosy is endemic in 53 countries, including India, Bangladesh, and Brazil. There are approximately 6,500 cases of leprosy in the United States. Around 200 to 250 new cases are reported each year in the United States, with about 175 of these being new cases diagnosed for the first time; 166 new cases were reported in the U.S. in 2005.

8. Are there endemic areas for leprosy in the United States?

Southern Texas and Louisiana are considered endemic for leprosy. Southern California and Florida also have many cases. Large cities such as New York and San Francisco have many leprosy cases from other countries.

9. How is leprosy recognized clinically?

The three most useful features are skin lesions, areas of cutaneous anesthesia, and thickened nerves. Other features are nasal stuffiness, inflammatory eye changes, and loss of eyebrows. A reactional state in lepromatous leprosy causes multiple tender red nodules resembling erythema nodosum (erythema nodosum leprosum).

10. Is there more than one kind of leprosy?

Four major variants of leprosy represent a spectrum of disease: indeterminate leprosy, tuberculoid leprosy, lepromatous leprosy, and dimorphous (or borderline) leprosy (Fig. 29-1). The lepromatous form is seen twice as frequently in men as

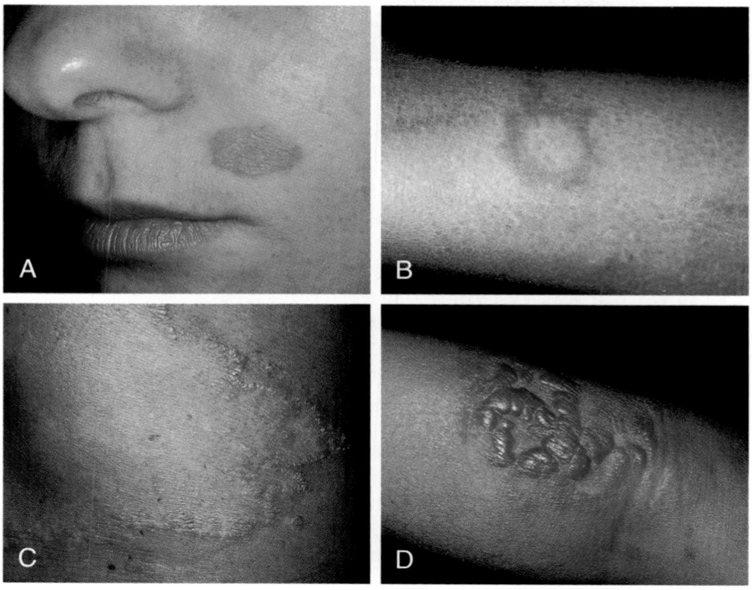

Figure 29-1. Skin lesions in four variants of leprosy. **A,** Indeterminate leprosy. A solitary erythematous macule on the face of a young family member of a patient with lepromatous leprosy. **B,** Tuberculoid leprosy. A solitary, well-circumscribed, annular anesthetic patch on the leg. **C,** Dimorphous leprosy. A solitary anesthetic annular patch with a scaly border on the trunk. **D,** Lepromatous leprosy. Coalescent brown, firm nodules on an extremity.

in women. Although it varies from country to country, about 90% of the leprosy cases in the United States are of the lepromatous type.

11. Does indeterminate leprosy mean that you do not know what type it is?

No. Indeterminate leprosy is believed to be the very first sign of infection with the leprosy bacillus. It usually manifests as a solitary macular skin lesion that is vaguely defined and either erythematous or hypopigmented. Patients with indeterminate leprosy may clear spontaneously or progress to one of the other three types of leprosy.

12. What are the two "polar" forms of leprosy? How do they differ?

Tuberculoid leprosy and lepromatous leprosy are considered the two polar forms, and they tend to remain stable clinically. Patients with tuberculoid leprosy have a high degree of immunity against *M. leprae* and have few skin lesions and few organisms in their skin. Patients with lepromatous leprosy have low immunity against *M. leprae* and have many skin lesions and millions of organisms in their skin (Table 29-1).

13. Describe dimorphous leprosy.

Dimorphous leprosy, also known as borderline leprosy, shows features intermediate between tuberculoid and lepromatous leprosy. It is a less stable form of leprosy, and its clinical features and immune status may change over time. If dimorphous leprosy develops more features of lepromatous leprosy, it is referred to as dimorphous-lepromatous. If it develops features of tuberculoid leprosy, it is called dimorphous-tuberculoid.

14. What is the unusual feature of the cell-mediated immunity in lepromatous leprosy?

Patients with lepromatous leprosy have a specific anergy to *M. leprae*. This is in contrast to diseases such as sarcoidosis and Hodgkin's lymphoma, in which there is loss of immunity to a wide variety of antigens. The clinical spectrum of leprosy appears to depend mainly on an individual's ability to develop effective cell-mediated immunity against *M. leprae*. In endemic areas, most individuals appear to be completely resistant to infection with the leprosy bacillus.

Table 29-1. Clinical Features of Leprosy Skin Lesions

CUTANEOUS LESIONS	TUBERCULOID	DIMORPHOUS	LEPROMATOUS
Number	Few	Many	Numerous
Size	Large	Large and small	Small
Symmetry	Asymmetrical	Symmetrical	Symmetrical
Sensation	Anesthetic	Variable	Variable
Surface	Rough, scaly	Rough, scaly	Smooth
Edge	Sharp	Sharp	Vague

15. Define the cytokine response to *M. leprae* in tuberculoid versus lepromatous patients.

Studies of circulating cytokines in leprosy patients and cytokine production in skin show those tuberculoid patients have a helper T cell type I (Th1) response to *M. leprae* with predominant interleukin-2 (IL-2) and interferon (IFN)-? production, while lepromatous cases have a response of Th2-type cytokines.

16. How is the diagnosis of leprosy usually made?

The diagnosis of leprosy is usually made by demonstrating cutaneous anesthesia, by finding enlarged superficial nerves, and by demonstrating leprosy bacilli in the skin.

- Cutaneous anesthesia is best diagnosed by using a wisp of cotton to demonstrate loss of light touch. In tuberculoid and dimorphous leprosy, sensation is lost within the center of skin lesions, which are often annular. In lepromatous leprosy, the loss of light touch sensation typically occurs first in fingers and toes, while anesthesia in individual skin lesions may be variable.
- Nerve enlargement in tuberculoid and dimorphous leprosy occurs within or adjacent to specific skin lesions. In lepromatous leprosy, large peripheral nerves can be palpated. The easiest nerves to palpate are the posterior auricular nerve behind the ear and the ulnar nerve at the elbow (Fig. 29-2).
- The demonstration of *M. leprae* in the skin may be accomplished by a "slit skin smear" by experienced personnel. For those not experienced with the technique, it is easier and more reliable to simply perform a skin biopsy and request a special stain for the leprosy bacillus.

Hartzell JD, Zapor M, Peng S, Straight T: Leprosy: a case series and review, *South Med J* 97:1252–1256, 2004.

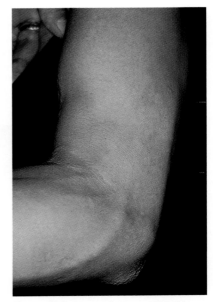

Figure 29-2. Nerve enlargement. Palpable or visually enlarged nerves may be a sign of leprosy.

17. What area should be biopsied to detect *M. leprae*?

The raised, active margin of tuberculoid and dimorphous skin lesions. For lepromatous leprosy, the biopsy specimen should be taken from a cutaneous papule or nodule.

18. Can the same acid-fast stain used for *Mycobacterium tuberculosis* be used for the leprosy bacillus?

M. leprae is less acid-fast than *M. tuberculosis*, and a modified acid-fast stain known as the Fite stain should be used to demonstrate organisms in tissue (Fig. 29-3).

19. What are Virchow cells?

Lepromatous leprosy exhibits an extensive cellular infiltrate separated from the epidermis by a narrow grenz zone of collagen. In florid early lesions, macrophages contain abundant live bacilli. In time, and with therapy, degenerate bacilli accumulate in macrophages, and these cells are called lepra cells or Virchow cells; they have foamy cytoplasms and are Fite stain–positive.

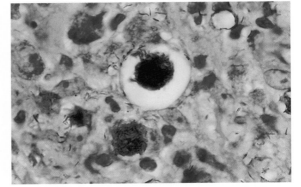

Figure 29-3. Fite stain for *Mycobacterium leprae*. This skin biopsy shows clusters of acid-fast leprosy bacilli. The clusters are called globi. (Courtesy of James E. Fitzpatrick, MD.)

20. Is the lepromin skin test helpful in making a diagnosis of leprosy?

No, but it is useful in classifying leprosy into the various subtypes. Lepromin is a crude preparation of killed bacteria from a lepromatous nodule or from infected armadillo liver. An intradermal injection of 0.1 mL of lepromin is read at 48 hours for erythema (Fernandez reaction) or at 3 to 4 weeks for a papule or nodule (Mitsuda reaction). Patients with tuberculoid leprosy have strongly positive reactions, while dimorphous and lepromatous patients are usually negative. The reaction in indeterminate leprosy is variable.

21. Is the neuropathy in lepromatous leprosy the same as that in diabetic neuropathy?

No. Although the neuropathy is similar in the two diseases, it is a true "stocking-glove" anesthesia in diabetes mellitus. In leprosy, the cooler parts of the skin and nerves are affected, which gives the peripheral neuropathy a spotty and variable expression. For example, the dorsal aspects of the hands may be anesthetic, while the palms are partially spared. This has led some neurologists to misdiagnose leprosy patients as malingerers or neurotics.

22. Describe a patient with advanced lepromatous leprosy.

The skin shows widespread, hyperpigmented papules and nodules with a predilection for cool parts of the body, such as the earlobes, nose, fingers, and toes. There may be loss of the lateral eyebrows (madarosis) (Fig. 29-4), redness of the conjunctiva, a stuffy nose, flattening of the nasal bridge (Fig. 29-5A), and a palpable postauricular nerve. There is marked anesthesia of the extremities with some atrophy of the thenar and hypothenar muscles (Fig. 29-5B). Contraction of the fourth and fifth fingers may be seen, resulting in difficulty in extending the fingers fully. Ulcers or sores of the hands and feet may be present secondary to minor trauma or burns (Fig. 29-5C). A plantar ulcer

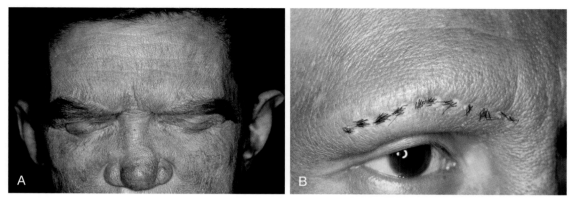

Figure 29-4. Madarosis (loss of eyebrows) is an important sign in leprosy. **A,** This patient has heavy eyebrows due to hair transplants and dark skin color due to the drug clofazimine. **B,** This patient has just received eyebrow transplants.

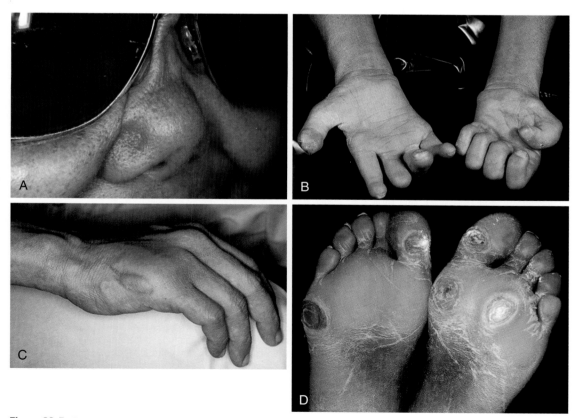

Figure 29-5. Features of advanced lepromatous leprosy. **A,** Destruction of the cartilage of the nose producing a "saddle nose" deformity. **B,** The hands often show contractures, and muscle atrophy of the thenar and hypothenar eminences. **C,** Accidental burn. Because of anesthetic extremities, patients with leprosy are subject to burns and other minor trauma. **D,** Mal perforans ulcers. Patients with lepromatous leprosy develop foot ulcers surrounded by thick keratin as a result of peripheral anesthesia. (Panel A courtesy of the Fitzsimons Army Medical Center teaching files.)

surrounded by hyperkeratotic skin (mal perforans ulcer) may be present over a pressure area (Fig. 29-5D). The physician should inquire whether the patient is from an endemic area for leprosy.

23. What are the most common complications in leprosy?
1. Traumatic ulcers in anesthetic extremities
2. Reactional states that follow successful drug therapy

24. What are the reactional states of leprosy?
There are two types of reactions that may occur spontaneously but often follow the initiation of antibacterial therapy by months to years. Approximately half of all leprosy patients experience one of these acute inflammatory episodes at some point in their disease course.

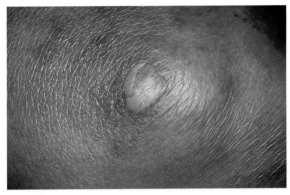

Figure 29-6. Erythema nodosum leprosum. The reactive state in lepromatous leprosy resembles erythema nodosum but may be bullous, as seen in this patient.

Type I reactions (reversal reactions) complicate unstable dimorphous leprosy and represent alterations in the patient's cell-mediated immunity. The immunity may be either upgraded or downgraded. Typically, in type I reactions, existing lesions become acutely inflamed.

Type II reactions (most commonly erythema nodosum leprosum [ENL]) occur in lepromatous leprosy (Fig. 29-6). ENL reactions are believed to represent immune complex precipitation in blood vessels due to released antigens from *M. leprae* organisms that have been damaged by antibiotic therapy. The patients develop red, tender nodules mainly on their extremities, associated with constitutional symptoms including fever, arthralgias, lymphadenitis, and neuritis.

Burdick AE: Leprosy including reactions. In Lebwohl M, Heymann WR, Berth-Johnes J, Coulson I, editors: *Treatment of skin disease*, New York, 2002, Mosby, pp 336–339.

25. What drugs are used in multidrug therapy for leprosy?
Because of the resistance to dapsone, multidrug therapy is currently used for leprosy and has resulted in a dramatic improvement in prognosis and a decrease in reported new cases worldwide. Only four drugs are readily available in the United States to treat leprosy: dapsone, rifampin, clofazimine, and ethionamide. Of these agents, only rifampin is bactericidal.

Recommended therapy for lepromatous leprosy in the United States is dapsone, 100 mg/day for life, and rifampin, 600 mg/day for 3 years. For tuberculoid leprosy, the recommended treatment is dapsone, 100 mg/day for 5 years, and rifampin, 600 mg/day for 6 months.

26. Do the recommendations of the World Health Organization (WHO) differ from those of the U.S.?
Due to economic and other factors, the WHO treatment recommendations are different from those of the U.S. The WHO multidrug therapy (MDT) recommends for multibacillary leprosy rifampin, 600 mg, and clofazimine, 300 mg once a month, and daily dapsone 100 mg and clofazimine 50 mg for 12 months. Paucibacillary leprosy is treated with dapsone, 100 mg/day, and rifampin, 600 mg/month for 6 months. Since 1995, WHO has provided free MDT for all leprosy patients worldwide.

Key Points: Hansen's Disease (Leprosy)

1. Leprosy is a chronic granulomatous infection caused by *Mycobacterium leprae*, affecting primarily skin and peripheral nerves.
2. The mode of transmission of leprosy is still not proven, but current evidence favors respiratory transmission.
3. The diagnosis of leprosy is usually made based on skin lesions, cutaneous anesthesia, and enlarged superficial nerves and by demonstrating leprosy bacilli in the skin.
4. Patients with tuberculoid leprosy have a high degree of immunity against *M. leprae* and have few skin lesions and few organisms in their skin.
5. Patients with lepromatous leprosy have low immunity against *M. leprae* and have many skin lesions and millions of organisms in their skin.

---

27. What are the side effects of the drugs for leprosy treatment?
Overall, dapsone is a safe drug, and it is safe to use during pregnancy. All patients on dapsone experience hemolysis of older red blood cells with a mild drop in hematocrit. Patients who are glucose-6-phosphatase dehydrogenase deficient may develop severe hemolysis. Methemoglobinemia is also regularly observed but is usually not a significant problem, because the level usually does not exceed 12% of the total hemoglobin. Idiosyncratic reactions such as pancytopenia, peripheral neuropathies, acute psychosis, and a potentially fatal

infectious mononucleosis-like condition may also develop. Rifampin, as a P450 inducer, may decrease the effect of other drugs. Hepatotoxicity and red urine are banal.

28. What is the most bothersome cutaneous side effect of clofazimine?

The most bothersome side effect of clofazimine is a red to brown to purple discoloration of the skin (see Fig. 29-4A). Some patients may also demonstrate acquired ichthyosis.

29. How are the reactional states of leprosy treated?

For type I reactions, because of the risk of permanent nerve damage, prednisone, 40 to 80 mg/day, is recommended. Mild type II reactions may be controlled with aspirin, nonsteroidal antiinflammatory agents, and rest. More severe type II reactions may be controlled with thalidomide, 400 mg at night. Thalidomide should not be given to women of childbearing age because of its severe teratogenic effects. If thalidomide is not available, type II reactions can usually be controlled with prednisone, 40 to 80 mg/day.

30. Should family members of leprosy patients be treated?

Dapsone prophylaxis of all family members is not currently recommended. However, children and spouses should be examined at least once a year by experienced medical personnel.

31. Can leprosy be eliminated as a worldwide disease, as smallpox has been?

The worldwide prevalence of leprosy has been reduced from 10 to 12 million in 1988 to 2.7 million in 1994, but the disease is far from being eliminated. Leprosy vaccines are being studied. The sequencing of the entire genome of *M. leprae* was completed in 2001.

Lockwood DNJ, Bryceson ADM: Leprosy. In Champion RH, Burton JL, Burns DA, Breathnach SM, editors: *Rook/Wilkinson/Ebling textbook of dermatology*, Oxford, 1998, Blackwell Scientific Publications, pp 1215–1235.

MYCOBACTERIAL INFECTIONS

Genevieve L. Egnatios, MD, and Karen E. Warschaw, MD

1. What is the classification system of mycobacteria?

Extensive taxonomic work has been done to classify the more than 60 species of organisms belonging to the genus *Mycobacterium*. In the 1950s, Runyon classified the atypical mycobacteria based on their rate of growth, ability to form pigment, and colony characteristics (Fig. 30-1). The **Runyon classification** may also include distinctions among obligate human pathogens requiring direct person-to-person transmission, facultative human pathogens found in the environment that are rarely responsible for direct person-to-person spread, and nonpathogens (Table 30-1).

2. What are the staining characteristics of mycobacteria?

Mycobacteria are aerobic, non–spore-forming, nonmotile bacilli. They do not stain readily, but their most useful staining characteristic is acid fastness. Acid fastness refers to the ability to retain carbol fuchsin dye after washing with acid or alcohol as a result of a high content of cell wall mycolic acids, fatty acids, and other lipids. The acid-fast stain is also called the Ziehl-Neelsen stain. Other staining methods include the Dieterle, Fite, hematoxylin-eosin, auramine-rhodamine, and phenolic acridine orange stains. Acid fastness is also shared by *Nocardia*, *Rhodococcus*, *Legionella micdadei*, *Isospora*, and *Cryptosporidium*.

TUBERCULOSIS

3. How many species of *Mycobacterium* cause infection in human beings?

There are approximately 30 species of *Mycobacterium* that cause disease in humans. The primary culprits include *M. tuberculosis* complex, *M. leprae*, and atypical mycobacteria.

4. Name three mycobacteria in the tuberculosis complex responsible for tuberculosis.

The three species most significant to human disease in the *M. tuberculosis* complex include *M. tuberculosis*, *M. bovis*, and *M. africanum*. Under certain conditions, the attenuated strain of *M. bovis*, bacillus Calmette-Guérin (BCG), may also cause disease.

5. What is tuberculosis?

Tuberculosis is a systemic infectious disease that can affect any organ system, including the skin. Only approximately 5% to 10% of infections lead to clinical disease. The lungs, however, are the most commonly involved organ. Cutaneous tuberculosis has a broad clinical spectrum depending on the route of infection, virulence of the organism, and immune status of the host (Table 30-2). Lupus vulgaris and scrofuloderma, although rare, are the two most common forms of cutaneous tuberculosis.

6. What is the difference between a primary and secondary infection?

Primary-inoculation tuberculosis occurs in a host not previously infected. A secondary infection occurs in a previously infected host either as a reactivation years later from a primary focus, endogenous spread to new areas, or exogenous reinfection.

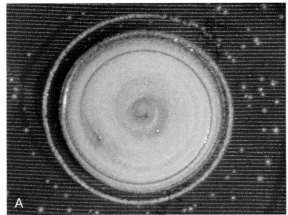
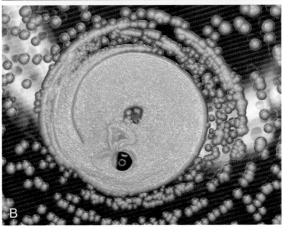

Figure 30-1. A, *M. scrofulaceum.* The slow-growing colonies that are forming yellowish-orange pigment without light (scotochromogen). **B,** *M. chelonei.* Rapid-growing colonies (within 7 days) without evidence of pigment production (rapid grower). (Courtesy of the Fitzsimons Army Medical Center teaching files.)

Table 30-1. Classification of Pathogenic Mycobacteria

CLASSIFICATION	OBLIGATE HUMAN PATHOGEN	FACULTATIVE HUMAN PATHOGEN
Slow Growers		
M. tuberculosis complex		
M. tuberculosis	x	
M. bovis	x	
M. africanum	x	
M. mycoti	x	
Photochromogens (Runyon Group 1) **Form Yellow-Orange or Rust Pigment with Light**		
M. kansasii		x
M. marinum		x
M. simiae complex (*M. simiae, M. triplex, M. genavense,* *M. heidelbergense,* and *M. lentiflavum*)		x
Others include *M. intermedium,* and *M. asiaticum*		x
Scotochromogens (Runyon Group 2) **Form Light Yellow to Orange Pigment with and without Light**		
M. scrofulaceum		x
M. szulgai		x
Others include *M. injectum, M. lentiflavum,* *M. gordonae*		x
Nonchromogens (Runyon Group 3) **Unable to Form Pigment**		
M. avium-intracellulare complex (*M. avium,* *M. intracellulare,* and other unidentified species)		x
M. haemophilum		x
M. xenopi		x
M. ulcerans		x
Others include *M. celatum, M. genavense,* *M. gastri,* and *M. malmoense*		x
Rapid Growers (Runyon Group 4) **Growth within 7 Days**		
M. fortuitum		x
M. abscessus		x
M. chelonei ssp. *chelonei, abscessus,* unnamed subspecies		x
Others include *M. phlei, M. smegmatis,* *M. fredericksbergense*		x
Noncultivable **Unable to Cultivate in Media**		
M. leprae	x	

Data from Bhambri S, Bhambri A, Del Rosso JQ: Atypical mycobacterial cutaneous infections, *Dermatol Clin* 27(1):63–73, 2009.

7. Explain the route of infection in cutaneous tuberculosis.

Cutaneous tuberculosis may be acquired by three possible routes. The first route is exogenous infection acquired from an outside source (primary-inoculation tuberculosis and tuberculosis verrucosa cutis). The second route of infection is endogenous spread. This can occur by contiguous spread (scrofuloderma) or by autoinoculation (periorificial tuberculosis) as organisms are passed from internal organ involvement. The final route is through hematogenous or lymphatic dissemination (lupus vulgaris, miliary tuberculosis, and gummas).

Semaan R, Traboulsi R, Kanj S: Primary mycobacterium tuberculosis complex cutaneous infection: report of two cases and literature review, *Int J Infect Dis* 12(5):472–477, 2008.

Table 30-2. Classification of Cutaneous Tuberculosis

CLASSIFICATION	PRIMARY INFECTION (NONIMMUNE HOST)	SECONDARY INFECTION (IMMUNE HOST)
Exogenous		
Primary inoculation tuberculosis	x	
Tuberculosis verrucosa cutis		x
Endogenous		
Scrofuloderma		x
Periorificial tuberculosis		x
Hematogenous/lymphatic		
Lupus vulgaris		x
Acute miliary tuberculosis	x	
Gummas	x	

Data from Semaan R, Traboulsi R, Kanj S: Primary mycobacterium tuberculosis complex cutaneous infection: report of two cases and literature review, *Int J Infect Dis* 12(5):472–477, 2008.

8. Who is at risk of acquiring tuberculosis?

In the United States, the incidence of tuberculosis was decreasing until 1985 when it reached its nadir. Since 1985, the incidence of tuberculosis has markedly increased. Crowded urban environments, immigration, poverty, homelessness, intravenous drug abuse, loss of tuberculosis control programs, increased use of immunosuppressive medications (e.g., TNF-α inhibitors), and, most importantly, the HIV epidemic account for the rising incidence. High-risk groups include the elderly, urban homeless, alcoholics, intravenous drug abusers, prison inmates, migrant farm workers, minorities, and immunosuppressed patients (with HIV or from iatrogenic causes).

9. Describe the histopathologic hallmark of tuberculosis.

The caseation granuloma (also known as tubercle) is the histopathologic hallmark of tuberculosis. This consists of giant cells and epithelioid cells and usually has varying amounts of caseation necrosis. This pattern can also be seen in other infections and is not pathognomonic. Acid-fast bacilli are usually easy to find in the early lesions, but there are very few bacilli once granulomas develop.

10. How can one acquire primary cutaneous tuberculosis?

Primary-inoculation tuberculosis occurs from direct inoculation of *M. tuberculosis* into the skin and includes the chancre at the site and affected regional lymph nodes. The organism cannot penetrate intact skin and requires a break in the skin, such as a minor cut or abrasion. Reports have also implicated tattooing, ear piercing, circumcision, mouth-to-mouth resuscitation, and needle-sticks. In some cases, there is no documented injury.

Semaan R, Traboulsi R, Kanj S: Primary mycobacterium tuberculosis complex cutaneous infection: report of two cases and literature review, *Int J Infect Dis* 12(5):472–477, 2008.

11. Describe the clinical manifestation of primary-inoculation cutaneous tuberculosis.

Primary tuberculosis may occur in any age group, but is most common in children up to 4 years of age and young adults. The face, mucous membranes (conjunctiva and oral mucosa), and lower extremity are the usual sites of infection. A tuberculous chancre develops 2 to 4 weeks after inoculation and presents as a painless, firm, red-brown papule/nodule, which slowly enlarges, eventually eroding to form a sharply demarcated ulcer (Fig. 30-2). Regional, hard, nonpainful lymphadenopathy occurs 3 to 8 weeks after infection. The combination of the tuberculous chancre and lymphadenopathy is analogous to the Ghon complex in the lungs. The purified protein derivative (PPD) may initially be negative and diagnosis is confirmed by culture.

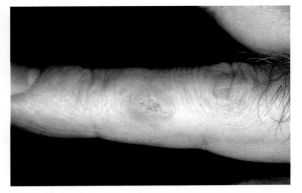

Figure 30-2. Primary-inoculation tuberculosis presenting as an eroded papule. The patient was a microbiologist in a hospital laboratory, and this was probably an accidental inoculation. (Courtesy of James E. Fitzpatrick, MD.)

12. What are the different types of cutaneous tuberculosis?

Tuberculosis of the skin can be divided into two categories: true cutaneous tuberculosis infections and tuberculid reactions. True cutaneous tuberculosis includes lupus vulgaris, tuberculosis verrucosa cutis, cutaneous miliary tuberculosis, cutaneous primary tuberculosis, and tuberculosis cutis orificialis (Fig. 30-3). A tuberculid refers to a cutaneous or mucosal lesion that represents an immunologic response to a previous infection of tuberculosis at a remote site. Special stains and culture of a tuberculid lesion are negative. Tuberculid reactions include lichen scrofulosorum, papulonecrotic tuberculid, and erythema induratum.

13. What laboratory tests are used to diagnose *Mycobacterium tuberculosis*?

Mycobacterium tuberculosis can be diagnosed using acid-fast bacilli (AFB) stains, culture, polymerase chain reaction (PCR), or interferon-gamma release assay (IGRA). Diagnosis of cutaneous tuberculosis is challenging and requires the correlation of clinical findings with diagnostic testing.

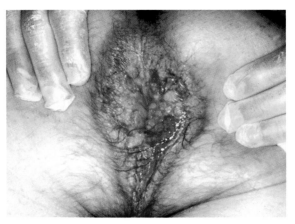

Figure 30-3. Tuberculosis cutis orificialis. Erythematous eroded plaque of perianal area. (Courtesy of James E. Fitzpatrick, MD.)

14. Is lupus vulgaris related to lupus erythematosus or lupus pernio?

No. Lupus erythematosus is an autoimmune connective tissue disease. Lupus pernio is a cutaneous manifestation of sarcoidosis that presents as a violaceous patch on the face. Lupus vulgaris is a form of cutaneous tuberculosis. The term lupus is used to depict erosion as if "gnawed by a wolf." Vulgaris means common or ordinary. Both of these terms are used in a variety of unrelated diseases.

15. Describe the clinical manifestations of lupus vulgaris.

Lupus vulgaris is a chronic progressive form of cutaneous tuberculosis that originates from another site and involves the skin or mucous membranes via contiguous, lymphatic, or hematogenous spread. In 40% of patients, there is underlying lymphadenitis, and 10% to 20% have underlying pulmonary involvement. The primary skin lesion is an asymptomatic macule or papule that is brown-red in color and has a soft gelatinous consistency (Fig. 30-4A). Diascopy, a test where a glass slide is gently pressed against the skin lesion, may be helpful in diagnosing lupus vulgaris. Lupus vulgaris lesions have a characteristic "apple jelly" color with this technique. Squamous cell carcinoma arising in a longstanding lesion is the most serious complication (Fig. 30-4B).

16. Where and when does lupus vulgaris develop?

Lupus vulgaris most often affects patients in their second or third decade of life. The most common site of involvement is the head and neck and, in particular, the nose, cheek, and earlobe. There may be extension to involve the oral, nasal, or conjunctival mucosa. In the tropics, the buttocks and lower extremities are more often involved.

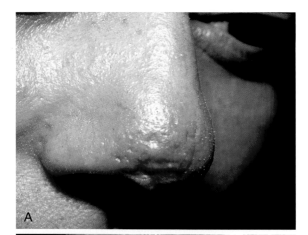

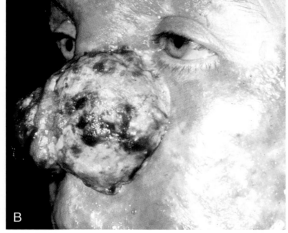

Figure 30-4. Lupus vulgaris. **A,** Red-brown plaque on nasal tip. **B,** Lupus vulgaris with squamous cell carcinoma.

17. What is scrofuloderma?

Scrofuloderma is a form of cutaneous tuberculosis that originates in tuberculous lymph nodes, bones, joints, or epididymis and spreads directly to the overlying skin. The most common locations include the lateral neck and the parotid, submandibular, and supraclavicular areas. The skin lesion presents as a firm subcutaneous nodule. As the lesion matures, there is extensive necrosis leading to a soft, doughy consistency, ulceration with bluish margins, and formation of a sinus tract. Necrotic cheesy material may drain from sinus tracts (Fig. 30-5).

18. Name the vaccination against tuberculosis. What type of vaccination is it?

Bacillus Calmette-Guérin (BCG) is a live attenuated strain of *Mycobacterium bovis*. It was discovered in 1921, but has not been widely used in the United States, with the exception of a very small number of at-risk infants who cannot receive chemoprophylaxis. In third-world countries, the BCG vaccine is widely used. This vaccination is contraindicated in immunosuppressed individuals who are at risk of disseminated *M. bovis* infection. Intravesical BCG is also commonly used as treatment for bladder cancer, and there have been reports of cutaneous tuberculous lesions following this therapy.

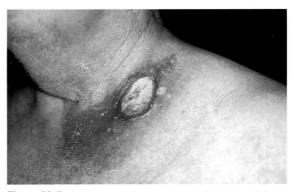

Figure 30-5. Scrofuloderma. Erythematous to violaceous nodule with ulceration. The lesion is an extension from an underlying lymph node.

Hillyer S, Gulmi FA: Cutaneous BCG of the penis after intravesical therapy for bladder cancer: a case report in a 66-year-old male, *Can J Urol* 16(5):4866–4869, 2009.

Gontero P, Bohle A, Malmstrom PU, et al: The role of Bacillus Calmette-Guérin in the treatment of non–muscle-invasive bladder cancer, *Eur Urol* 57:410–429, 2010. [Epub ahead of print.]

Ng YH, Bramwell SP, Palmer TJ, Woo WK: Cutaneous mycobacterial infection postintravesical BCG installation, *Surgeon* 4(1):57–58, 2006.

19. What drugs are used in the treatment of tuberculosis?

Drugs used in the treatment of tuberculosis can be classified into first-line essential, first-line supplemental, and second-line antituberculous drugs. First-line essential chemotherapeutic agents include isoniazid, rifampin, and rifabutin. First-line supplemental chemotherapeutic agents include pyrazinamide and ethambutol. Second-line drugs include cycloserine, ethionamide, levofloxacin, moxifloxacin, gatifloxacin, p-aminosalicylic acid, streptomycin, amikacin/kanamycin, and capreomycin. Isoniazid is the cornerstone of therapy, and rifampin is the second major antituberculous drug. Currently, the Center for Disease Control (CDC) endorses a number of 6-month and 9-month protocols. The 6-month regimens include an intensive 2-month therapy with three to four agents followed by a 4-month therapy with isoniazid plus rifampin or rifapentine.

Available at http://www.cdc.gov/mmwr/preview/mmwrhtml/rr5211a1.htm. Treatment of Tuberculosis Accessed December 13, 2009.

20. What are the major side effects of antituberculous agents?

See Table 30-3.

21. What factors have led to multidrug-resistant tuberculosis?

Multidrug-resistant tuberculosis (MDRTB) is defined as combined resistance to isoniazid and rifampin, and can be either primary or acquired. Primary MDRTB occurs in a person who has not previously been treated, whereas acquired

Table 30-3. First-Line Antituberculous Agents and Major Side Effects		
DRUG	**SIDE EFFECT**	**SPECIAL COMMENT**
Isoniazid	Peripheral neuritis Hepatitis	From pyridoxine deficiency Occurs with 1%–2%, increased risk with age >35
Rifampin	Hepatitis Orange stain of secretions	More common when given with isoniazid May permanently stain contact lenses
Rifabutin	Neutropenia Hepatitis Orange stain of secretions	Occurs in HIV patients More common when given with isoniazid May permanently stain contact lenses
Rifapentine	Hepatitis Orange stain of secretions	More common when give with isoniazid May permanently stain contact lenses
Pyrazinamide	Hyperuricemia	May precipitate gout
Ethambutol	Optic neuritis	Avoid in children under age 13

Data available at http://www.cdc.gov/mmwr/preview/mmwrhtml/rr5211a1.htm. Accessed December 13, 2009.

MDRTB is a result of treatment failure. The main factors leading to MDRTB include patient noncompliance in drug therapy, inability or unwillingness to find adequate health care, and inappropriate treatment regimens. Homelessness, intravenous drug use, and HIV infection favor the spread of drug-resistant tuberculosis. Resistance is prevalent in Asia, South America, and Africa. In the United States, miniepidemics of drug resistance are centered in New York City, Miami, and Michigan. Spread to health care workers is a major concern. Treatment cure rates of up to 96% have been published in the medical literature, but this requires aggressive and often very complicated management of the disease.

22. Are there any special treatment considerations for cutaneous tuberculosis?

Treatment of cutaneous tuberculosis is the same as for systemic tuberculosis and consists of effective chemotherapeutic agents. Small lesions of lupus vulgaris or tuberculosis verrucosa cutis may be excised, but the treatment must also include standard antituberculous therapy. Surgical drainage of scrofuloderma may shorten the treatment course, and surgical intervention is necessary in any draining lesion.

Key Points: Mycobacterial Infections

1. Cutaneous tuberculosis has a broad clinical spectrum, depending on the route of infection, virulence of the organism, and immune status of the host. Lupus vulgaris and scrofuloderma, although rare, are the two most common forms of cutaneous tuberculosis.
2. Caseation granuloma (also known as tubercle) is the histopathologic hallmark of tuberculosis, although it can also be seen in other infections and is not pathognomonic.
3. *Mycobacterium tuberculosis* can be diagnosed using acid-fast bacilli (AFB) stains, culture, polymerase chain reaction (PCR), or interferon-gamma release assay (IGRA).
4. Atypical mycobacteria are ubiquitous and are found in soil, water, and domestic and wild animals. The presentation of these infections is quite variable, leading to frequently missed diagnoses.
5. Rapidly growing mycobacteria are a cause of cutaneous infections associated with immunosuppression and cutaneous surgical and cosmetic procedures (e.g., mesotherapy and tattoos). Tap water is an important reservoir for these pathogens.

23. What is the mechanism of action of TNF-α in tuberculosis?

TNF-α mediates host defense against infection. It is a key player in granuloma formation and containment of *M. tuberculosis* organisms. TNF-α inhibitors (etanercept, adalimumab, and infliximab) have been associated with reactivation of tuberculosis. Because of this risk, patients must be screened for tuberculosis prior to beginning treatment with a TNF-α inhibitor. If the PPD is positive, but the chest x-ray is negative, the patient may still receive the TNF-α inhibitor after starting antitubercular treatment for latent tuberculosis. The preferred regimen is 6 to 9 months of isoniazid. However, the risk of developing active tuberculosis is not obviated, and there have been reports of this despite an adequate course of isoniazid.

Saraceno R, Chimenti S: How to manage infections in the era of biologics? *Dermatol Ther* 21(3):180–186, 2008.

ATYPICAL MYCOBACTERIA

24. Describe the pathogenesis of the atypical mycobacteria.

Atypical mycobacteria (also known as nontuberculous mycobacteria, or NTM) are ubiquitous and are found in soil, water, and domestic and wild animals. Tap water is the major reservoir for the atypical mycobacteria that cause human disease. Because they are found everywhere, isolation of these organisms does not necessarily constitute proof of disease. In contrast to *M. tuberculosis*, they are not transmitted from person to person. Immunosuppression, organ damage, Mohs micrographic surgery, cutaneous surgery, punch biopsy, acupuncture, mesotherapy, injections, cardiothoracic surgery, breast reconstruction, facial plastic surgery, laser resurfacing, liposuction, body piercing, pedicures, tattoos, or minor cuts and abrasions are some of the clinical settings in which these organisms can cause disease. The presentation of these infections is quite variable, leading to frequently missed diagnoses. Depending on geographic location, atypical mycobacteria may account for 0.5% to 30% of all mycobacterial infections.

Drage LA, Ecker PM, Orenstein R, et al: An outbreak of *Mycobacterium chelonae* infections in tattoos, *J Am Acad Dermatol* 62:501–506, 2010. [Epub ahead of print.]

25. How is the diagnosis of atypical mycobacteria made?

Often the diagnosis is delayed because of the varied clinical and histopathologic findings. After inoculation, there is an incubation period of 1 to 29 weeks. Classically, this is followed by an eruption of painful nodules that increase to 2 to 5 cm in size, and which then drain purulent fluid for 7 to 14 days before forming a scar over 1-month period. Other skin lesions have been reported including folliculitis, furuncles, abscesses, cellulitis, nodules, draining lesions, ulcers, and fistulae. Granulomatous infiltrate, diffuse lymphohistiocytic infiltrate, mixed inflammatory infiltrate, granulomas rheumatoid nodules, abscesses, panniculitis, and folliculitis have been observed in biopsy specimens. Staining for acid-fast bacteria with Fite or auramine-rhodamine is often unrevealing. Thus the current gold standard is skin biopsy for tissue culture followed DNA sequencing.

Regnier S, Cambau E, Meningaud JP, et al: Clinical management of rapidly growing mycobacterial cutaneous infections in patients after mesotherapy, *Clin Infect Dis* 49(9):1358–1364, 2009.

Drage LA, Ecker PM, Orenstein R, et al: An outbreak of *Mycobacterium chelonae* infections in tattoos, *J Am Acad Dermatol* 62:501–506, 2010. [Epub ahead of print.]

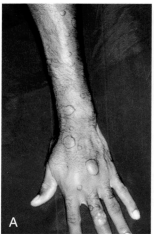
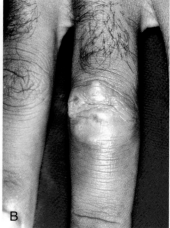
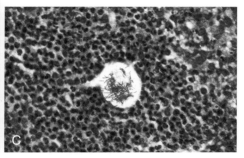

Figure 30-6. Swimming pool granuloma caused by *M. marinum*. **A,** Erythematous nodule on middle finger with sporotrichoid spread along the afferent lymphatics. **B,** Close-up of finger nodule. **C,** Ziehl-Neelsen staining demonstrating numerous acid-fast mycobacteria in a patient with swimming pool granuloma. (Courtesy of James E. Fitzpatrick, MD.)

26. What is a "swimming pool granuloma"?

It is an inoculation caused by *Mycobacterium marinum*, although, very rarely, it can be caused by *Mycobacterium gordonae*. *M. marinum* is ubiquitous in aquatic environments, including both fresh and salt water. The organism is inoculated into the skin through small cuts or abrasions while swimming or cleaning aquariums. Following an incubation period of 2 to 3 weeks (1 week to 2 months in some instances), a small violaceous papule develops at the site of inoculation. The lesion gradually enlarges into a dark red to violaceous plaque. A sporotrichoid pattern may be seen with violaceous nodules along the afferent lymphatics (Fig. 30-6A,B). The most common sites include hands, feet, elbows, and knees (sites prone to trauma). The diagnosis of cutaneous *M. marinum* infection is mainly clinical, with supporting evidence from histologic features and the response to therapy (Fig. 30-6C). The lesions typically heal spontaneously but may disseminate. This infection may respond to multiple single and combination antibiotic regimens.

27. What is a Buruli ulcer?

Buruli ulcer, caused by *Mycobacterium ulcerans*, is another of the inoculation mycobacterioses and is the third most common mycobacterial disease in immunocompetent individuals. It occurs in warm tropical climates, most notably Africa, Australia, and Mexico. The organism is inoculated into the skin through minor cuts, most commonly on the extensor surface of the extremities. Over a period of 4 to 6 weeks, a painless subcutaneous swelling develops; it may or may not be pruritic. The swelling then ulcerates and has a necrotic center, undermined borders, and can attain the size of an entire limb. Treatment is primarily surgical.

28. Describe the clinical manifestations of *Mycobacterium avium-intracellulare* complex (MAC) in both non-AIDS and AIDS patients.

Mycobacterium avium complex (MAC) includes *M. avium*, *M. intracellulare,* and other unidentified species, although it has recently become clear that *M. avium* is the most common cause. These organisms have gained importance with the epidemic of HIV infection. HIV-negative persons most commonly present with pulmonary involvement. Cutaneous disease is rare but may occur as a manifestation of primary intracutaneous inoculation or disseminated disease. The cutaneous lesions are quite variable and include ulcers, abscesses, deep nodules, or inflammatory plaques (Fig. 30-7). Eighty percent to 90% of childhood lymphadenitis is caused by MAC. AIDS patients with MAC generally present with widely disseminated disease (pulmonary, lymph node, gastrointestinal tract, bone). Isolated cutaneous disease is unusual but reported.

Bhambri S, Bhambri A, Del Rosso JQ: Atypical mycobacterial cutaneous infections, *Dermatol Clin* 27(1):63–73, 2009.

29. Which atypical mycobacteria are associated with mesotherapy?

Mesotherapy is the microinjection of drugs into the dermis. It has a variety of applications and despite the dearth of scientific data, is popular in Europe and

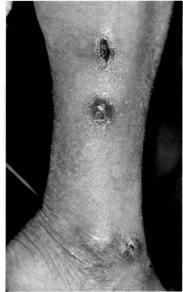

Figure 30-7. *Mycobacterium avium-intracellulare* infection presenting as nodules and ulcerations in an HIV-infected patient. (Courtesy of Margaret Muldrow, MD.)

South America as a procedure to reduce fat and cellulite and to perform body contouring. It is also offered in the United States. Most often the service is delivered in nonmedical settings under nonsterile conditions. A number of cases have been reported in the literature describing infection with rapidly growing mycobacteria following mesotherapy. The organisms include *M. chelonae, M. fredericksbergensis, M. abscessus,* and *M. fortuitum.*

Difonzo EM, Campanile GL, Vanzi L, Lotti L: Mesotherapy and cutaneous *Mycobacterium fortuitum* infection, *Int J Dermatol* 48(6):645–647, 2009.

Regnier S, Cambau E, Meningaud JP, et al: Clinical management of rapidly growing mycobacterial cutaneous infections in patients after mesotherapy, *Clin Infect Dis* 49(9):1358–1364, 2009.

30. Which atypical mycobacteria are associated with tattoos?

Tattoo-associated infections have been described secondary to *M. chelonae.* Numerous patients have been reported in the literature with pruritic papules and pustules restricted to the gray parts of their tattoos. The gray wash was prepared by dilution of black pigment with tap water. Treatment with clarithromycin, azithromycin, tobramycin, or macrolide antibiotics resulted in a favorable outcome. Similarly, outbreaks of furunculosis from contaminated tap water whirlpool baths in nail salons have also been associated with *M. chelonae* and *M. fortuitum* (Fig. 30-8). Thirty-four patients with cutaneous abscesses following liposuction performed by a single physician were found to be infections of *M. chelonae.* The tap water in the office was the source.

Drage LA, Ecker PM, Orenstein R, et al: An outbreak of *Mycobacterium chelonae* infections in tattoos, *J Am Acad Dermatol* 62:501–506, 2010. [Epub ahead of print.]

31. Which atypical mycobacteria have been associated with soft tissue fillers?

In 2002 there were two cases of *M. abscessus* infection following the injection of soft tissue filler. Both patients were injected with Hyacell, a product not approved by the FDA but available in South America. It had been brought illegally into the United States and was administered by an individual posing as a physician. Hyacell is a mixture of hyaluronic acid, zinc, selenium, vanadium, and unspecified "embryonic extracts." The patients developed tender nodules and were treated with resolution using clarithromycin and prednisone.

Cohen JL: Understanding, avoiding, and managing dermal filler complications, *Dermatol Surg* 34(Suppl 1):S92–S99, 2008.

32. How are infections with rapidly growing mycobacteria managed?

Surgical removal can be used in patients with a limited number of lesions. Antibiotics are added in immunocompromised patients or those with numerous lesions. *M. chelonae* has the greatest antibiotic resistance but is usually susceptible to tobramycin, clarithromycin, and linezolid. In vitro testing has also shown the efficacy of tigecycline and amikacin. Two to four months of antibiotics is recommended in localized disease and 6 months in disseminated cutaneous disease, but the optimal length of therapy is not clear. Testing for susceptibilities is advised before treatment begins in clinically significant isolates, and if treatment fails or there is a relapse. While waiting for susceptibilities results, clarithryomycin and azithromycin are useful oral agents for *M. chelonae.*

Regnier S, Cambau E, Meningaud JP, et al: Clinical management of rapidly growing mycobacterial cutaneous infections in patients after mesotherapy, *Clin Infect Dis* 49(9):1358–1364, 2009.

33. What are some of the key features of *Mycobacterium kansasii?*

M. kansasii is a photochromogenic acid-fast bacillus. It is found worldwide, including in the U.S.—particularly in the Southwest and the Midwest. The most common presentation is a pulmonary infection resembling tuberculosis, typically

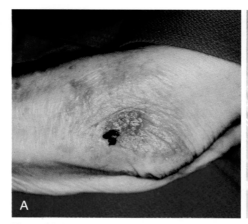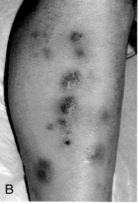

Figure 30-8. Infections with atypical mycobacteria. **A,** Infection caused by *M. fortuitum.* Erythematous plaque with ulceration and necrosis following a puncture wound. **B,** Numerous abscesses and nodules caused by *M. chelonei* infection. (Courtesy of James E. Fitzpatrick, MD.)

in older men with chronic obstructive pulmonary disease. Cutaneous presentation is heterogenous and includes an ulcer with sporotrichoid spread or cellulitis. It has a predilection for HIV-infected individuals (Fig. 30-9). In HIV-infected individuals, almost all colonized patients have disease and require treatment with ethambutol or rifampin.

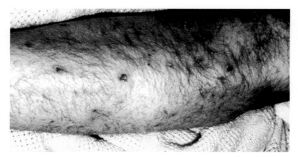

Figure 30-9. Disseminated ulcerated lesions caused by *M. kansasii* in an HIV-infected patient.

SUPERFICIAL FUNGAL INFECTIONS

Richard A. Keller, MD, and Deborah B. Henderson, MD, MPH

1. What is a dermatophyte?

A dermatophyte is a fungus that has developed the ability to live on the keratin (hair, nails, or skin scale) of animals. Dermatophytes are classed into three genera: *Microsporum, Trichophyton,* and *Epidermophyton.*

2. How are superficial fungal infections diagnosed?

Superficial fungal infections can usually be suspected clinically, but definitive diagnosis requires the demonstration of fungal pathogens by microscopic examination or culture of skin, nail, or hair scrapings from the suspected lesion. During microscopic examination, hyphae are sought in the material. The material is first placed on a glass slide, and then 1 or 2 drops of 10% to 20% potassium hydroxide (KOH) are added. A fungal stain such as chlorazol black E may be added to the preparation to aid visualization of the fungal elements. The hyphae of dermatophytes will be septate and typically demonstrate branching (see Figure 3-1). Skin scrapings can also be placed on culture media. Culturing the organism, in addition to being a diagnostic aid, permits speciation of the organism.

3. On a KOH examination, hyphal-like structures arranged in a mosaic pattern are noted. Does this indicate the presence of a dermatophyte?

"Mosaic hyphae" are not really hyphae and do not indicate the presence of a dermatophyte. If you vary the microscope's focus, the pattern can be observed to conform to the cell walls. Mosaic hyphae actually represent thickened stratum corneum cell walls. True hyphae cross the cell walls of keratinocytes and do not conform to the contour of keratinocytes.

4. What are the three most commonly used culture media for the growth of dermatophytes?

- **Sabouraud's dextrose agar:** A nonselective culture medium consisting of peptone, dextrose, agar, and distilled water. It allows the growth of bacteria as well as pathogenic and nonpathogenic yeast and molds.
- **Mycosel or mycobiotic agar:** A selective growth medium for dermatophytes. It consists of Sabouraud's agar with cycloheximide (suppresses saprophytic fungi) and chloramphenicol (suppresses bacteria). Dermatophytes and *Candida albicans* grow readily on this media, while the growth of contaminant bacteria, some yeast, and many opportunistic fungi is inhibited.
- **Dermatophyte Test Media (DTM):** Sabouraud's agar with cycloheximide, gentamicin, and chlortetracycline hydrochloride. It also has a phenol red indicator. If a dermatophyte is present, the color of the media changes from yellow to red. False-positives do occur.

5. Describe some of the presentations of superficial fungal infections caused by dermatophytes.

The superficial dermatophyte infections are classified according to their location on the affected person. This location does not necessarily reveal the identity of the offending organism. The infection will cause the production of scale. The scale may or may not be associated with erythema, vesicles, or annular plaques (Table 31-1, Fig. 31-1).

6. Which dermatophyte causes the most fungal infections of skin?

Trichophyton rubrum.

Foster KW, Ghannoum MA, Elewski BE: Epidemiologic surveillance of cutaneous fungal infections in the United States from 1999 to 2002, *J Am Acad Dermatol* 50:748–752, 2004.

7. What is the most common cause of tinea capitis in the United States?

Until the mid-1950s, *Microsporum audouinii* was the most common cause of endemic tinea capitis in the U.S., but it has since been replaced by *Trichophyton tonsurans.* Several theories have been proposed to explain the almost total disappearance of *M. audouinii* from the U.S., but the most plausible theory is that it was eradicated by the widespread use of griseofulvin. At the same time that *M. audouinii* disappeared, *T. tonsurans,* formerly an uncommon cause of tinea capitis, quickly spread. This species was probably introduced into the U.S. from Central or South America.

Foster KW, Ghannoum MA, Elewski BE: Epidemiologic surveillance of cutaneous fungal infections in the United States from 1999 to 2002, *J Am Acad Dermatol* 50:748–752, 2004.

Table 31-1. Clinical Presentations of Dermatophyte Infections

INFECTION	LOCATION
Tinea capitis	Scalp
Tinea faciei (see Fig. 31-1A)	Face
Tinea barbae	Beard
Tinea corporis (see Fig. 31-1B)	Trunk, extremities
Tinea cruris (see Fig. 31-1C)	Groin
Tinea manuum (manus)	Hands
Tinea pedis	Feet
Tinea unguium	Nails

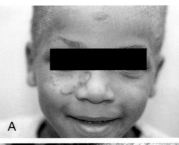

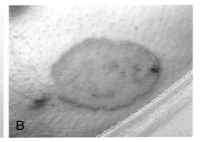

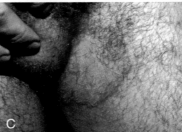

Figure 31-1. Dermatophyte infections. **A,** Tinea faciei in a child demonstrating multiple annular scaly lesions of the face. **B,** Tinea corporis. Annular lesion with scale at the edge and clearing in the central portion of the lesion. **C,** Tinea cruris. Annular scaly lesion of the groin, note the characteristic sparing of the scrotum. (Panel A courtesy of the William L. Weston, M.D. collection; panel B courtesy of the Fitzsimons Army Medical Center teaching files; panel C courtesy of the Fitzsimons Army Medical Center teaching files.)

8. Name the four clinical patterns of tinea capitis.

1. The seborrheic pattern has a dandruff-like scaling of the scalp and should be considered in prepubertal children with suspected seborrheic dermatitis (Fig. 31-2A).
2. In the black-dot pattern, hairs are broken off at the skin line, and black dots are seen within the areas of alopecia (Fig. 31-2B). In the U.S., this pattern is primarily associated with *T. tonsurans* infections.
3. A kerion is an inflammatory fungal infection that may mimic a bacterial folliculitis or an abscess of the scalp (Fig. 31-2C). The scalp is tender to the touch, and the patient usually has posterior cervical lymphadenopathy.
4. Favus is a rare form of inflammatory tinea of the scalp presenting with sites of alopecia that have cup-shaped, honey-colored crusts, which are called *scutula* and are composed of fungal mats.

   Tinea capitis is one of the most commonly misdiagnosed skin infections. Any prepubertal child who presents with a scaly scalp dermatitis or carries a diagnosis of seborrheic dermatitis should be presumed to have a dermatophyte infection of the scalp until proven otherwise. Similarly, any child who presents with one or more scalp abscesses most likely has a kerion. Kerions are frequently secondarily infected with *Staphylococcus aureus*, and unsuspecting health care providers often mistakenly treat kerions as bacterial abscesses.

Sobera JO, Elewski BE : Fungal infections. In Bolognia JL, Jorizzo, JL, Rapini RP, et al, editors: *Dermatology*, New York, 2008, Mosby, pp 1135–1163.

9. What are the types of hair invasion in tinea capitis? What dermatophytes are associated with each type?

Dermatophytes can cause three types of hair invasion:

1. **Endothrix** infections are produced by fungi that invade the inside of the hair shaft and are composed of fungal arthroconidia and hyphae (Fig. 31-3). A helpful mnemonic to remember the organisms that cause endothrix invasion is: "TVs are in houses."—T is *Trichophyton tonsurans*, V is *violaceum*, and S is *soudanense*.

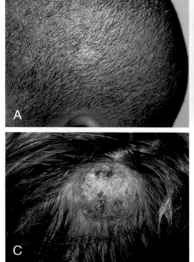
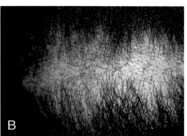

Figure 31-2. Tinea capitis. **A,** Seborrheic pattern. **B,** Black-dot pattern. **C,** Kerion presenting as a tender boggy mass in the scalp.

2. **Ectothrix** infections are produced by fungi that primarily invade the outside of the hair shaft. Some agents of small-spore ectothrix cause a fluorescent tinea capitis.
3. **Favus** infections are characterized by invasion of hair by hyphae that do not produce conidia and by the presence of linear air spaces. *T. schoenleinii* is associated with this type of invasion.

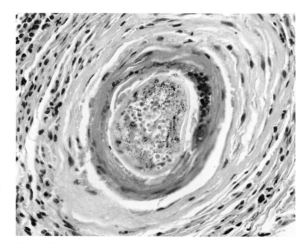

Figure 31-3. Endothrix. Cross section of a hair shaft filled with hyphae and arthrospores (hematoxylin and eosin, [H&E]).

10. What is a Wood's light? What organisms are detected by this exam?

A Wood's light is an ultraviolet light source that emits in the spectrum of 325 to 400 nm. This light was used extensively for the diagnosis of tinea capitis when *Microsporum audouinii* was the major cause of this disorder. However, it is of limited usefulness today because most cases are now produced by *Trichophyton tonsurans*, which is not fluorescent. The fluorescence is caused by pteridine. The fungi responsible for fluorescent tinea capitis can be remembered by the mnemonic **"See Cats and Dogs Fight."**

- **See:** *T. schoenleinii*
- **Cats:** *M. canis*
- **And:** *M. audouinii*
- **Dogs:** *M. distortum*
- **Fight:** *T. ferrugineum*

    Except for *T. schoenleinii*, all of these organisms produce a small-spore ectothrix pattern of hair invasion.

Wolf F, Jones E, Nathan H: Fluorescent pigment of *Microsporum*, *Nature* 182:475–476, 1958.

11. How is tinea capitis treated?

After the presence of a fungal infection is demonstrated by either culture or a positive KOH smear, treatment with an oral antifungal agent should be instituted. Most patients are placed on griseofulvin. Microsized griseofulvin at a dose of 20 to 25 mg/kg/day should be taken with meals to improve absorption. The medication is continued for 4 to 6 weeks, after which the site is recultured. Using antifungal shampoo may reduce shedding of the organism. Members of the patient's family also should be evaluated for infection or a carrier state, and treated if needed. Patients who fail to respond to griseofulvin or are intolerant should be treated with an alternative treatment regimen:

- **Fluconazole:** 6 mg/kg/day for 6 weeks
- **Itraconazole:** 3–5 mg/kg/day for 6 weeks

- **Terbinafine:** 62.5 mg/day (<20 kg), 125 mg/day (20–40 kg), 250 mg/day (>40 kg) for 2 to 6 weeks (infections by *M. canis* may require double the dose)

Sobera JO, Elewski BE: Fungal infections. In Bolognia JL, Jorizzo JL, Rapini RP, et al, editors: *Dermatology*, New York, 2008, Mosby, pp 1135–1163.

12. What is meant by a carrier state in tinea capitis?

A carrier is a person who does not have clinical signs of tinea capitis but has a positive fungal culture from the scalp. In families in whom tinea capitis is identified, the carrier rate in adults is around 30%. The presence of these carriers will reduce the cure rate for tinea capitis if they are not treated concomitantly. Treatment can include shampooing with selenium sulfide or other antifungal shampoo.

Babel D, Baughman S: Evaluation of the adult carrier state in juvenile tinea capitis caused by *Trichophyton tonsurans*, *J Am Acad Dermatol* 21:1209–1212, 1989.

Neil G, Hanslo D, Buccimazza S, Kibel M: Control of the carrier state of scalp dermatophytes, *Pediatr Infect Dis J* 9:57–58, 1990.

13. Name the three types of tinea pedis. Which dermatophyte is most commonly associated with each?

The three types of tinea pedis are interdigital infection, moccasin-type infection, and vesiculobullous or inflammatory infection. Interdigital infections present as scaling, maceration, fissuring, or erythema of the webspaces between the toes. This infection is usually associated with *Trichophyton rubrum* or *T. mentagrophytes*. Moccasin-type tinea pedis presents as generalized scaling and hyperkeratosis of the plantar surface of the foot. This form of infection is frequently associated with nail involvement. Moccasin-type tinea pedis is typically caused by *T. rubrum*. The inflammatory or vesiculobullous type will cause a vesicular eruption on the arch or side of the foot and is most often caused by *T. mentagrophytes*.

14. What nondermatophyte mold can cause mycotic infections that mimic moccasin-type tinea pedis?

Scytalidium dimidiatum has been isolated from cases of moccasin-type pedis that are resistant to standard therapy. The organism will not grow on selective dermatophyte media, such as Mycosel, Mycobiotic, or DTM, but it does grow readily on Sabouraud's agar.

Hay RJ, Moore MK: Mycology. In Burns T, Breathnach S, Cox N, Griffiths C, editors: *Rook's textbook of dermatology*, ed 8, vol 2, Malden, MA, 2010, Blackwell Publishing, pp 31.10–31.14.

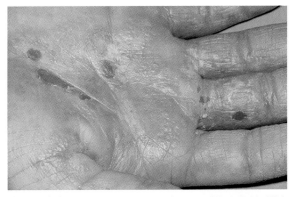

Figure 31-4. Dermatophytid reaction. (Courtesy of Mark Welch, MD.)

15. What is a dermatophytid reaction?

Dermatophytid reactions are inflammatory reactions at sites distant from the site of the associated dermatophyte infection. Types of dermatophytid reactions from tinea pedis include urticaria, hand dermatitis (Fig. 31-4), or erythema nodosum. The pathogenesis of dermatophytid reactions is not fully understood, but evidence suggests that they are secondary to a strong host immunologic response against fungal antigens.

16. Name and describe the four clinical presentations of onychomycosis.

1. Distal subungual onychomycosis presents as onycholysis, subungual debris, and discoloration beginning at the hyponychium that spreads proximally. The most common organism is *Trichophyton rubrum* (Fig. 31-5).
2. Proximal subungual onychomycosis begins underneath the proximal nail fold and is typically caused by *T. rubrum*. The patient's immune status should be investigated, because it is strongly associated with immunosuppressed conditions.
3. Superficial white onychomycosis produces a white, crumbly nail surface due to invasion of the top of the nail plate. It is usually caused by

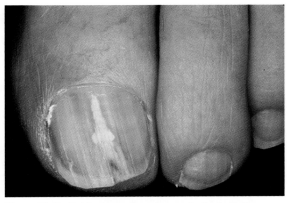

Figure 31-5. Distal subungual onychomycosis demonstrating a spikelike pattern of infection. (Courtesy of the Fitzsimons Army Medical Center teaching files.)

T. mentagrophytes; however, nondermatophytes such as *Fusarium, Acremonium,* and *Aspergillus* have been associated with this type of infection.

4. Candidal onychomycosis is seen in patients with chronic mucocutaneous candidiasis.

17. Can other diseases mimic onychomycosis?

Yes. Psoriasis, Reiter's disease, lichen planus, pachyonychia congenita, Darier's disease, and Norwegian scabies are some of the diseases that can resemble onychomycosis. For this reason, the diagnosis should be established by either a KOH examination or culture before beginning prolonged and often expensive therapies to eradicate the infection.

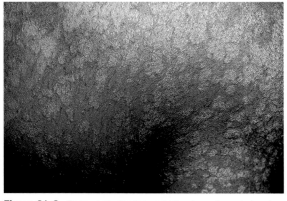

Figure 31-6. Tinea versicolor demonstrating hypopigmented scaly patches.

18. What is tinea versicolor?

Tinea versicolor (pityriasis versicolor) is a hypopigmented, hyperpigmented, or erythematous macular eruption. Macules may coalesce into large patches with an adherent fine scale (Fig. 31-6). Lesions are located predominantly on the trunk but may extend to the extremities. The proper taxonomic nomenclature of the lipophilic yeast that produces this infection is debatable. Studies indicate *Malassezia globosa* is the organism most frequently associated with tinea versicolor, although most older references list *M. furfur* as the most common organism. This eruption begins during adolescence, when the sebaceous glands become active. The eruption tends to flare when the temperatures and humidity are high. Immunosuppression, systemic corticosteroids, and sweaty or greasy skin will also cause this disease to flare.

Erchiga VC, Florencio VD: *Malassezia* species in skin diseases, *Curr Opin Infect Dis* 15:133–142, 2002.

Gupta KA, Batra R, Bluhm R, Faergemann J: Pityriasis versicolor, *Dermatol Clin* 21: 413–429, 2003.

Prohic A, Ozegovic L: *Malassezia* species isolated from lesional and non-lesional skin in patients with pityriasis versicolor, *Mycoses* 50:58–63, 2007.

19. How does *Malassezia* induce both hyperpigmentation and hypopigmentation in the skin?

In the past, *Malassezi* has been suggested to induce hypopigmentation by production of dicarboxylic acid. These compounds do not have a direct effect on melanocytes in tissue culture. The dark lesions of tinea versicolor may be due to a variation in the inflammatory response to the infection. There is not any strong evidence that influences current thought on this question (Fig. 31-7).

Hay RJ, Moore MK: Mycology. In Burns T, Breathnach S, Cox N, Griffiths C, editors: *Rook's textbook of dermatology*, ed 8, vol 2, Malden, MA, 2010, Blackwell Publishing, pp 31.10–31.14.

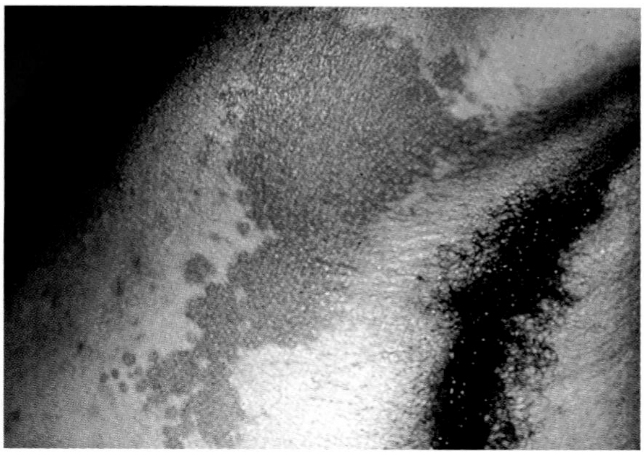

Figure 31-7. Hyperpigmented variant of tinea versicolor. (Courtesy of the Walter Reed Army Medical Center teaching files.)

20. How is tinea versicolor diagnosed? Why is it difficult to culture this organism?

Tinea versicolor is diagnosed by scraping some of the scale from a lesion and looking for the characteristic "spaghetti and meatball" under the microscope. The meatball is the yeast forms, and the spaghetti is the short hyphae. This organism is a lipophilic yeast and will grow only after a source of lipid is added to the culture media. A yellow fluorescence may be seen by Wood's light examination of affected areas.

21. Does *Malassezia* cause any other skin disease?

This organism can also produce a folliculitis of the trunk, arms, and neck area. *Malassezia* folliculitis presents as pruritic follicular papules and pustules that do not respond to antibiotic therapy. The yeast can be demonstrated by skin biopsies or direct examination of purulent material. The severity of seborrheic dermatitis has been reported to be associated with an increase in *Malassezia* microflora.

Hay RJ, Moore MK: Mycology. In Burns T, Breathnach S, Cox N, Griffiths C, editors: *Rook's textbook of dermatology*, ed 8, vol 2, Malden, MA, 2010, Blackwell Publishing, pp 31.10–31.14.

Table 31-2. Clinical Presentations of Cutaneous Candidiasis

DISEASE	CLINICAL DESCRIPTION
Intertrigo	Superficial pustules, erythema, edema, creamy exudates within skin folds
Thrush	White, adherent, cottage cheeselike plaques on oral mucosa
Perlèche	Erythema, fissuring, creamy exudate at the angles of the mouth
Paronychia	Tender, erythematous, indurated proximal nail fold, with or without a purulent discharge
Erosio interdigitalis blastomycetica	Erythema, fissuring, maceration of the webspaces between the fingers

22. What is tinea nigra?

A superficial dermatomycosis caused by *Phaeoanellomyces (Exophiala) werneckii*. This is a dematiaceous (pigment-producing) fungus. It causes an asymptomatic tan, brown, or black patch on the palms or soles. The diagnosis is made by demonstrating pigmented hyphae on a KOH examination of the lesion. Tinea nigra has been confused with acral lentiginous melanoma.

23. What is a Majocchi's granuloma?

Majocchi's granuloma is a follicular abscess produced when a dermatophyte infection penetrates the follicular wall into the surrounding dermis. Patients usually present with one or more tender boggy papules or plaques on the legs or, less commonly, arms. Pus may be seen draining from the hair follicle. *Trichophyton rubrum* or *T. mentagrophytes* are the species most commonly isolated from these lesions. Treatment should consist of an oral antifungal agent.

24. What is piedra?

Piedra refers to adherent deposits on the hair shaft caused by superficial fungal infections. Black piedra, which is caused by *Piedraia hortae*, presents as firm black nodules on the hair shaft. *Trichosporon beigelii* is the etiologic agent that produces white piedra, which results in the formation of less-adherent white concretions on the hair shaft. This organism has been reclassified into over six pathologic species, with the *T. inkin* and *T. ovoides* being the most common causes of white piedra in pubic hair.

Fitzpatrick JE: Superficial fungal skin diseases. In James WD, editor: *Textbook of military medicine*. Part III. *Disease and the environment*, Washington, DC, 1994, Office of the Surgeon General at Textbook of Military Medicine Publication, Borden Institute, Walter Reed Medical Center, pp 423–451.

Sobera JO, Elewski BE : Fungal infections. In Bolognia JL, Jorizzo JL, Rapini RP, et al, editors: *Dermatology*, New York, 2008, Mosby, pp 1135–1163.

25. Name the organism most commonly isolated from cutaneous candidiasis.

Candida albicans is the most common organism isolated from lesions of candidiasis. It is normally part of the microflora of the gastrointestinal tract.

26. How do candidal infections present clinically?

The clinical presentations vary with the sites involved, duration of infection, and immune status of the host (Table 31-2). Most sites show erythema, edema, and a thin purulent discharge (Fig. 31-8).

27. What factors predispose to candidiasis?

The factors that predispose to the development of candidiasis are both endogenous and exogenous. Exogenous factors include occlusion, moisture, and warm temperature. Endogenous factors can include immunosuppression,

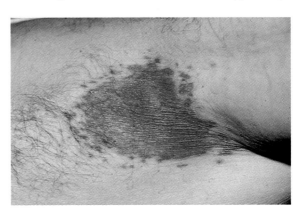

Figure 31-8. Cutanaeous candidiasis showing an erythematous plaque with characteristic satellite lesions in a body fold areas. (Courtesy of Larry Becker, MD.)

Table 31-3. Oral Antifungal Agents

CLASS	EXAMPLES	MECHANISMS OF ACTION
Antibiotic	Griseofulvin	Arrest of cellular division, dysfunction of spindle microtubules
Polyenes	Nyastatin	Binds irreversibly with ergosterol, altering membrane permeability
Azoles	Fluconazole Itraconazole Ketoconazole	Inhibits ergosterol production by inhibiting the cytochrome P-450 lanosterol 14-demethylase
Allyamines	Terbinafine	Blocks ergosterol production by inhibiting squalene epoxidase

Data from Gupta A, Sauder D, Shear N: Antifungal agents: part II, *J Am Acad Dermatol* 30:911–933, 1993.

diabetes mellitus, other endocrinopathies, antibiotics, oral contraceptives, Down syndrome, malnutrition, and pregnancy.

Wagner D, Sohnle P: Cutaneous defenses against dermatophyte and yeasts, *Clin Microbiol Rev* 8:317–335, 1995.

28. Which diseases are associated with adult-onset chronic mucocutaneous candidiasis?

Thymoma, myasthenia gravis, myositis, and aplastic anemia have been associated with the development of chronic mucocutaneous candidiasis after the third decade of life.

Hay RJ, Moore MK: Mycology. In Burns T, Breathnach S, Cox N, Griffiths C, editors: *Rook's textbook of dermatology*, ed 8, vol 2, Malden, MA, 2010, Blackwell Publishing, pp 31.10–31.14.

29. Name the different classes of oral antifungal agents and their mechanisms of action.

See Table 31-3.

Gupta A, Sauder D, Shear N: Antifungal agents: part II, *J Am Acad Dermatol* 30:911–933, 1993.

30. Which hepatic cytochrome is affected by itraconazole, ketoconazole, and fluconazole?

Cytochrome P-450 3A4. Fluconazole inhibits this enzyme at doses greater than 200 mg/day. Fluconazole is also a cytochrome 2C9 inhibitor, and it can affect the metabolism of angiotension II inhibitors, oral hypoglycemic agents, and oral anticoagulants.

Gupta AK: Systemic antifungal agents. In Wolverton SE: *Comprehensive dermatologic drug therapy*, ed 2, Phildelphia, 2007, Saunders Elsevier, pp 75–99.

Katz I, Gupta AK: Oral antifungal drug interactions: a mechanistic approach to understanding their cause, *Dematol Clin* 21:543–563, 2003.

Venkatakrishnan K, von Moltke LL, Greenblatt DJ: Effects of the antifungal agents on oxidative drug metabolism: clinical relevance, *Clin Pharmacokinet* 38:111–180, 2003.

31. Which drugs should be used with caution when using ketoconazole, itraconazole, or fluconazole? Why?

Warfarin, quinidine, digoxin, calcium channel blockers, bulsufan, HIV protease inhibitors, cyclosporine, angiotensin II inhibitors, tacrolimus, oral hypoglycemic agents, hydantoin anticonvulsants, and alcohol. These drugs should be used with caution, because the primary effect of azole antifungal drugs on hepatic enzyme metabolism is inhibition. This results in an elevation of the serum level of any drug that requires hepatic metabolism by the cytochrome P-450 3A4 enzyme in order to be removed.

Gupta AK, Ryder JE: The use of oral antifungal agents to treat onychomycosis, *Dermatol Clin* 21:469–479, 2003.

Key Points: Superficial Fungal Infections

1. *Trichophyton tonsurans* is the most common agent of tinea capitis in the United States and cannot be detected by Wood's light examination.
2. Asymptomatic dermatophyte carriers in households of children with tinea capitis are a source of treatment failures.
3. *Malassezia globosa* is the organism most commonly isolated from lesions of tinea versicolor.
4. Azole antifungal agents block the cytochrome P-450 enzyme lanosterol 14-α demethylase, which depletes ergosterol from cell membranes, whereas allylamine antifungals block ergosterol production through inhibition of squalene epoxidase.

32. Which drugs are contraindicated when using azole antifungal agents and why?

Contraindicated drugs are cisapride (pulled off the U.S. market in 2000), astemizole (pulled off the U.S. market in 1999), terfenadine (pulled off the U.S. market in 1998), lovastatin, midazolam, and triazolam. When combined with azole antifungal agents, these drugs can cause severe or life-threatening reactions. Elevated levels of cisapride, astemizole, and terfenadine are associated with cardiac arrhythmias, especially torsades de pointes. The metabolism of lovastatin is markedly reduced and can result in rhabdomyolysis. Simvastatin, atorvastatin, and cerivastatin are metabolized by the same hepatic cytochrome and also should be avoided.

33. Which oral antifungal agents can lower cyclosporine levels?

Griseofulvin and terbinafine.

34. Which drugs can affect antifungal drug levels?

Any drug that raises the gastric pH reduces the absorption of itraconazole and ketoconazole. Rifampin reduces the levels of oral azole and allylamines by induction of hepatic cytochromes. Isoniazid and phenytoin can induce the metabolism of azole antifungal agents. Cimetidine can raise terbinafine levels.

35. Which antifungal drugs have a limited spectrum of activity in the treatment of superficial fungal infections?

Griseofulvin is not effective against tinea versicolor or cutaneous candidiasis. Oral nystatin is not absorbed from the gastrointestinal tract. Topical nystatin and amphotericin are both ineffective against dermatophyte infections. Allylamines have limited effectiveness against tinea versicolor and candidiasis.

Lesher J: Therapeutic agents for dermatologic fungal diseases, In Elewski B, editor: *Cutaneous fungal infection*, ed 2, Malden, MA, 1998, Blackwell Science, pp 321–346.

32 CHAPTER

DEEP FUNGAL INFECTIONS

Larisa S. Speetzen, MD, and Karen E. Warschaw, MD

1. What is a deep fungal infection?

In contrast to the superficial dermatophytes, which are typically confined to dead keratinous tissue, certain mycotic infections have the capacity for deep invasion of the skin or production of skin lesions secondary to systemic visceral infection. They are typically acquired through direct inoculation, ingestion, and/or inhalation of spores from soil or matter. In this chapter, the deep fungal diseases are organized into three categories based on clinical presentation (Table 32-1).

SUBCUTANEOUS FUNGAL INFECTIONS

2. Discuss the characteristics of subcutaneous mycotic infections.

Subcutaneous mycotic infections are caused by a heterogeneous group of fungi and are infections of implantation (inoculated directly into the skin through local trauma). The four most important infections are sporotrichosis, chromomycosis, phaeohyphomycosis, and mycetoma. Lobomycosis and rhinosporidiosis are significantly less common. As a group, these infections involve primarily the skin and subcutaneous tissues and rarely disseminate to produce systemic disease in the immunocompetent host. These organisms are ubiquitous in soil, plants, and trees.

Queiroz-Telles F, McGinnis MR, Salkin R, Graybill JR: Subcutaneous mycoses, *Infect Dis Clin North Am* 17:59–85, 2003.

3. What is a dimorphic fungus?

Dimorphic fungi are capable of growing in both the mold and yeast forms. Examples of diseases caused by dimorphic fungi include sporotrichosis, histoplasmosis, blastomycosis, paracoccidioidomycosis, and penicilliosis.

4. What occupations are at increased risk of sporotrichosis?

Sporotrichosis is caused by a dimorphic fungus, *Sporothrix schenckii*. This organism is found worldwide, except in polar regions, and is most common in subtropical and tropical climates. It is endemic in Africa and Central and South America. In the United States, infection is most common in the Midwest. The normal habitat includes soil, thorny plants (especially roses), hay, sphagnum moss, and animals. Cats may carry *Sporothrix* on their paws and can cause infection by scratching their owners or animal handlers. A cat-transmitted epidemic was reported in Rio de Janeiro, Brazil. Occupations at risk of cutaneous inoculation include farmers, gardeners (especially rose), florists, masonry workers, Christmas tree farmers, veterinarians, and animal handlers (especially cats, rodents, and armadillos).

5. Describe the clinical manifestations of sporotrichosis.

Cutaneous sporotrichosis is more common than systemic sporotrichosis. Cutaneous sporotrichosis can be further divided into two forms: lymphangitic or lymphocutaneous disease, and fixed infection. The lymphocutaneous form accounts for approximately 80% of the cases. This classic form of sporotrichosis begins at the site of inoculation (most commonly, upper extremity) as a painless pink papule, pustule, or dermal nodule, which rapidly enlarges and ulcerates (Fig. 32-1A). Without treatment, the infection ascends along the lymphatics, producing secondary nodules and regional lymphadenopathy that may ulcerate (Fig. 32-1B). The fixed cutaneous variant (20%) is confined to the site of inoculation. The organism may rarely disseminate hematogenously to the joints, bone, meninges, or eye. Disseminated disease is most common in immunosuppressed patients, especially those with impaired cellular immunity (acquired immune deficiency syndrome [AIDS] patients). Pulmonary disease is usually due to inhalation and generally occurs in

Table 32-1. The Deep Fungal Infections		
SUBCUTANEOUS FUNGAL INFECTIONS	**SYSTEMIC OR RESPIRATORY FUNGAL INFECTIONS**	**OPPORTUNISTIC FUNGAL INFECTIONS**
Sporotrichosis	Blastomycosis	Cryptococcosis
Phaeohyphomycosis	Histoplasmosis	Aspergillosis
Chromomycosis (chromoblastomycosis)	Coccidioidomycosis	Fusariosis
Mycetoma (Madura foot)	Paracoccidioidomycosis	Mucormycosis
Lobomycosis		Penicilliosis
Rhinosporidiosis		
Zygomycosis		

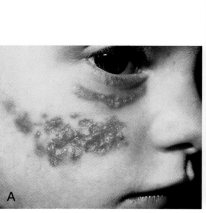
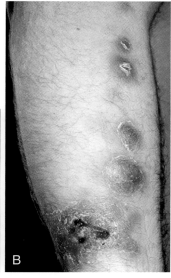

Figure 32-1. Sporotrichosis. **A,** Linear lesions secondary to a cat scratch. **B,** Erythematous, crusted, ulcerated nodule in a lymphocutaneous pattern. (Courtesy of James E. Fitzpatrick, MD.)

alcoholics, immunocompromised or debilitated patients. Both erythema nodosum and erythema multiforme have been reported as reactive eruptions to sporotrichosis.

Ramos-e-Silva M, Vasconcelos C, Carneiro S, Cestari T: Sporotrichosis, *Clin Dermatol* 25(2):181–187, 2007.

6. How is the diagnosis of cutaneous sporotrichosis made?
A strong clinical suspicion is most important. Skin biopsy shows granulomatous inflammation with neutrophilic microabscess formation. In the immunocompetent patient, fungal elements are typically not found even with special fungal stains: periodic acid–Schiff (PAS) and Gomori methenamine silver (GMS) stains. Therefore, when suspecting sporotrichosis, cultures on Sabouraud's medium are confirmatory. Colonies grow rapidly in 3 to 5 days.

7. How do you treat cutaneous sporotrichosis?
Itraconazole (100 to 200 mg/day) for 4 weeks after clinical cure is the treatment of choice for lymphocutaneous, fixed cutaneous, and disseminated cutaneous sporotrichosis, with a success rate of 90% to 100%. Terbinafine (1000 mg/day) is second-line treatment, and because potassium iodide (SSKI) is less costly than other agents, it is still recommended, especially in developing-world epidemics. Fluconazole (200 mg/day) and local hyperthermia have also been shown to be effective. Children may be safely treated with itraconazole.

Bustamante B, Campos PE: Sporotrichosis: a forgotten disease in the drug research agenda, *Expert Rev Anti Infect Ther* 2(1):85–94, 2004.

8. What other organisms may present with lymphocutaneous disease?
Several other diseases may present with a distal ulcer, proximal secondary nodules along the lymphatics, and regional lymphadenopathy. The most important organisms include nontuberculous *Mycobacterium* (*Mycobacterium marinum*, *Mycobacterium kansasii*, *Mycobacterium fortuitum* complex), *Nocardia*, leishmaniasis, cat scratch disease, and tularemia. A patient with this clinical presentation should have tissue biopsies for routine histology and cultures to include bacteria, mycobacteria, and fungi. This pattern of disease is also called *sporotrichoid*.

9. What are dematiaceous fungi?
Dematiaceous fungi are black pigmented fungi. They are slow growing and can be found in the soil, decaying vegetation, rotting wood, and the forest carpet. Subcutaneous-cutaneous disease is caused by traumatic inoculation into the skin. There are three broad categories of dematiaceous fungal infections including chromomycosis, phaeohyphomycosis, and eumycotic mycetoma (Madura foot).

10. How do you differentiate chromomycosis from phaeohyphomycosis?
Chromomycosis is a chronic subcutaneous infection characterized by the appearance in tissue biopsies of an intermediate, vegetative, pigmented fungal form with a yeastlike appearance that is arrested between yeast and hyphal formation. These pigmented, thick-walled fungal elements are called Medlar bodies (Fig. 32-2). Medlar bodies, also called copper pennies or sclerotic bodies, are diagnostic of chromomycosis, differentiating it from phaeohyphomycosis. Tissue biopsies of phaeohyphomycosis are characterized by lightly pigmented filamentous hyphae.

11. Which organisms may cause chromoblastomycosis?

Five fungal species account for most infections. The most frequent organism worldwide is *Fonsecaea pedrosoi*. Others organisms include *Phialophora verrucosa, Fonsecaea compactum, Rhinocladiella aquaspersa*, and *Cladophialophora carrionii*.

Minotto R, Bernardi CDV, Mallmann LF, et al: Chromoblasto-mycosis: a review of 100 cases in the state of Rio Grande do Sul, Brazil, *J Am Acad Dermatol* 44: 585–592, 2001.

12. Which organisms cause phaeohyphomycosis?

Phaeohyphomycosis may occur in both immunocompetent and immunocompromised patients. Due to the increasing immunocompromised patient population, there has been an increased number of fungi in this class that cause disease. Phaeohyphomycosis has been attributed to >60 genera and >100 species. The most important genera include *Scedosporium (Pseudallescheria), Alternaria, Bipolaris, Curvularia, Exophiala, Phialophora*, and *Wangiella*.

Revankar SG, Patterson JE, Sutton DA, et al: Disseminated phaeohyphomycosis: review of an emerging mycosis, *CID* 34:467–476, 2002.

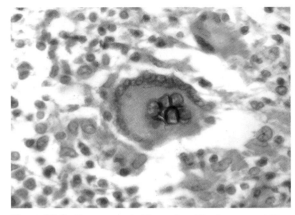

Figure 32-2. Chromomycosis. Diagnostic golden-brown, yeast-like fungi (Medlar bodies) within a multinucleated foreign body giant cell. (Courtesy of James E. Fitzpatrick, MD.)

13. How does chromomycosis present?

Chromomycosis is a chronic cutaneous and subcutaneous infection that is usually present for years with minimal discomfort. The inciting injury is often not remembered. The infection is most common on the lower extremity and 95% of cases occur in males. The typical patient is a barefoot, rural agricultural worker in the tropics. At the site of inoculation, red papules develop that eventually coalesce into a plaque. The plaque slowly enlarges and acquires a verrucous or warty surface. Satellite lesions can develop from extension of the infection through scratching. There may also be secondary bacterial infections of the lesion. If the lesion is not treated, it can evolve into a cauliflower-like mass, leading to lymphatic obstruction and elephantiasis-like edema of the lower extremity (Fig. 32-3). Neoplastic transformation to squamous cell carcinoma can occur. Diagnosis is made through potassium hydroxide (KOH) mounts from scrapings, biopsies of the lesions showing the organism and suppurative and granulomatous inflammation, and culture. Rare reports of hematogenous dissemination to the brain have been made. Chromomycosis is typically resistant to treatment. The treatment of choice for small lesions is surgical excision with a wide margin of normal skin. Chronic or extensive lesions should be treated with a combination of itraconazole therapy and surgical excision. Combination therapy with terbinafine, posaconazole, cryotherapy and local heat therapy also appear to be effective. Treatment is continued for months.

14. Describe the clinical features of phaeohyphomycosis.

The spectrum of clinical infections is broad. The most typical presentation is a subcutaneous cyst or abscess at the site of trauma and *Exophiala jeanselmei* is the most common organism. The primary lesion is a painless nodule. The nodule evolves into a fluctuant abscess. Immunocompromised patients present with multiple nodules. Dissemination is rare; however, the incidence has increased over the past 10 years. *Scedosporium proliferans* (42% cases), *Bipolaris spicifera* (8%), and *Wangiella dermatitidis* (7%) are the most common causes of disseminated disease. The primary risk factor is decreased host immunity, especially prolonged neutropenia. The outcome is poor, despite antifungal therapy, with an overall mortality rate of 79%. Cerebral phaeohyphomycosis acquired through inhalation and hematogenous dissemination is most commonly seen in immunocompetent persons with no obvious risk factors.

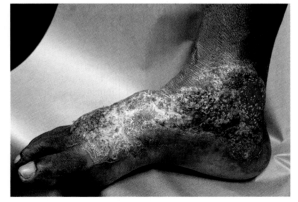

Figure 32-3. Chromomycosis. Cauliflower-like nodules and tumors on the foot and ankle with edema. (Courtesy of James E. Fitzpatrick, MD.)

15. What is Madura foot?

Madura foot, a type of mycetoma, is a localized, destructive infection of the skin and subcutaneous tissue that eventually involves deeper structures, such as muscle and bone. It may be caused by both filamentous bacteria and aerobic actinomycetes (actinomycetomas) and true fungi (eumycetoma). The most common causative fungi are *Madurella mycetomatis* and *Madurella grisea*. Less frequent causes are *Acremonium kiliense*, *E. jeanselmei*, and *Scedosporium apiospermum* (also called *Pseudallescheria boydii*).

16. What are the clinical features of Madura foot?
Madura foot is an indolent localized painless infection with three characteristic features. The first is the formation of nodules in the skin at the site of inoculation, usually a penetrating injury. The second feature is purulent drainage and fistula formation. The third and most characteristic feature is the presence of grains or granules that are visible in the purulent drainage. Seventy percent of cases involve the lower extremity, the foot in particular. Other sites of infection include the hand, head, back, and chest. Madura foot is a progressive infection leading to marked swelling and deformity in its latter stages (Fig. 32-4). Additionally, the lesions have a tendency to become painful in the latter stages, when bone involvement and deformity ravage the site. Eumycetomas are extremely difficult to manage and include medical, surgical, or a combination of both. Itraconazole and terbinafine are the most commonly used antifungal agents and are more effective than ketoconazole.

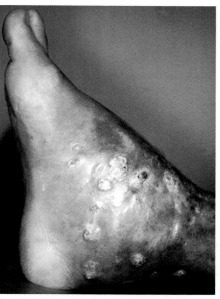

Figure 32-4. Madura foot. Swelling and deformity of the foot and ankle with purulent drainage and fistula formation.

SYSTEMIC FUNGAL INFECTIONS

17. Discuss the pathogenesis of the systemic respiratory deep fungi.
The systemic respiratory endemic fungal infections include blastomycosis, histoplasmosis, coccidioidomycosis, paracoccidioidomycosis, and penicilliosis. These infections are all due to species that show dimorphism. As a group, they cause disease in both healthy immunocompetent individuals and the immunosuppressed. These diseases are similar in pathophysiology, but each has distinct clinical characteristics. The causative organisms are found in the soil, and infection occurs with inhalation of the organism into the lung. The primary infection is pulmonary. Dissemination occurs via the lymphohematogenous route, and each fungus has a predilection for particular organ systems.

18. Where is blastomycosis endemic?
Blastomycosis, caused by the soil saprophyte *Blastomyces dermatitidis*, is endemic in North America, especially the southeastern and south central states bordering the Mississippi, Ohio, and St. Lawrence rivers (Kentucky, Arkansas, Mississippi, North Carolina, Tennessee, Louisiana, Illinois, and Wisconsin), and the Great Lakes region (Fig. 32-5). Sporadic cases have been reported in Colorado, Texas, Kansas, and Nebraska. The typical patient is a middle-aged male with occupational or recreational exposure to the soil.

McKinnell JA, Pappas PG: Blastomycosis: new insights into diagnosis, prevention, and treatment, *Clin Chest Med* 30(2):227–239, 2009.

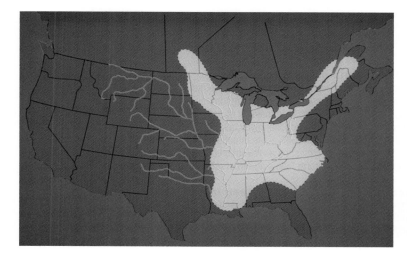

Figure 32-5. Blastomycosis. Areas depicted in yellow represent the areas reporting the most cases of blastomycosis. (Courtesy of the Fitzsimons Army Medical Center teaching files.)

19. What are the clinical manifestations of blastomycosis?

An important concept of blastomycosis is that it can mimic many other disease processes and has been called "The Great Pretender." The pulmonary manifestations range from a community-acquired pneumonia on one end of the spectrum to malignancy. Patients may have no pulmonary symptoms. Pulmonary disease is seen in 87% of patients, skin lesions in 20%, bone involvement in 15%, central nervous system in 5% to 10%, and less commonly the genitourinary system (prostate).

20. Describe the cutaneous findings in disseminated blastomycosis.

The most characteristic cutaneous presentation is a single (or multiple) crusted, verrucous plaque on exposed skin (face, hands, arms) with color variation from gray to violet (Fig. 32-6). Microabscesses can form, and pus exudes when the crust is lifted off. As the plaque progresses, there is central clearing. Ulcerative lesions are a less common cutaneous presentation. Cutaneous involvement leads to the correct diagnosis in most cases.

21. Are immunosuppressed patients at increased risk of disseminated disease with blastomycosis?

Blastomycosis, unlike other deep fungal infections (cryptococcosis, histoplasmosis, coccidioidomycosis, mucormycosis, penicilliosis, and aspergillosis), behaves, less commonly, as an opportunistic infection in the immunosuppressed host. There are, however, several reports of disseminated blastomycosis in AIDS patients, organ transplant recipients, diabetics, and patients receiving glucocorticosteroids and chemotherapy.

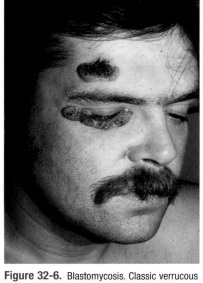

Figure 32-6. Blastomycosis. Classic verrucous plaques located on the forehead and eyelid. (Courtesy of the teaching files of Fitzsimons Army Medical Center.)

Lemos LB, Baliga M, Guo M: Blastomycosis: the great pretender can also be an opportunist. Initial clinical diagnosis and underlying diseases in 123 patients, *Ann Diagn Pathol* 6:194–203, 2002.

22. What is the treatment of blastomycosis?

Itraconazole is the treatment of choice for mild to moderate pulmonary, disseminated, or central nervous system disease. Amphotericin B is the preferred treatment of life-threatening disease and immunocompromised patients.

23. Where is histoplasmosis endemic?

Histoplasmosis is caused by *Histoplasma capsulatum*, an environmental saprophyte. It is endemic in the midwestern and south central United States, where 80% of the population is skin test–positive. It does occur in other parts of the world, but it is not found in Europe. Soil infected with excreta from chickens, pigeons, blackbirds, and bats is inhaled, leading to a pulmonary infection. Rarely, primary cutaneous disease is contracted from traumatic inoculation.

Wheat LJ, Kauffman CA: Histoplasmosis, *Infect Dis Clin North Am* 17:1–19, 2003.

24. What factors are necessary for production of the disease histoplasmosis?

The two most important factors are the number of organisms inhaled and immune status of the host. Cellular immunity is particularly important to host defense, as indicated by severe disseminated disease in human immunodeficiency virus (HIV)–infected patients.

25. Discuss the clinical manifestations of histoplasmosis.

As already mentioned, the clinical manifestations depend on the quantity of organisms inhaled and immune status of the host. Only 1% of patients exposed to a small inoculum develop symptomatic disease; in contrast, 50% to 100% of persons exposed to a heavy inoculum develop symptoms. The majority of patients with symptoms develop a flulike acute pulmonary illness characterized by fever, chills, headache, myalgias, chest pain, and nonproductive cough. Progressive disseminated histoplasmosis occurs in 1 of 2000 acute infections. High-risk groups for disseminated disease include patients with impaired cellular immunity such as HIV infection, lymphoma, or leukemia, and also infants and the elderly. Rarely, there is a primary cutaneous form following direct inoculation into the skin.

26. How common are mucocutaneous findings in disseminated histoplasmosis?

Three different patterns of disseminated histoplasmosis are described: acute, subacute, and chronic. The acute syndrome generally occurs in immunosuppressed patients and is characterized by fever, hepatosplenomegaly, and pancytopenia, with 18% developing mucocutaneous ulcers. Chronic disseminated histoplasmosis is characterized by involvement of the bone marrow, gastrointestinal tract, spleen, adrenals, and central nervous system (CNS); 67% have painful ulcerations on the tongue, buccal mucosa, gingiva, or larynx (Fig. 32-7). The treatment of choice is itraconazole and, for severe diseases and immunosuppressed patients, amphotericin.

27. Are there any other cutaneous manifestations of histoplasmosis?

Erythema nodosum and, less commonly, erythema multiforme may be seen in histoplasmosis, coccidioidomycosis, and, rarely, blastomycosis. These cutaneous hypersensitivity reactions are generally associated with a good prognosis.

28. Where is coccidioidomycosis endemic?

Coccidioidomycosis, also called San Joaquin Valley fever, is caused by *Coccidioides immitis*. It is a dimorphic fungus found in the soil of arid and semiarid regions. This organism is endemic in southern California, Arizona, New Mexico,

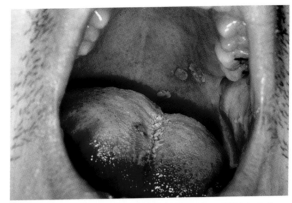

Figure 32-7. Histoplasmosis. Oral ulcerations in an HIV-infected patient. Histoplasmosis more commonly affects the oral mucosa than the skin. (Courtesy of James E. Fitzpatrick, MD.)

southwestern Texas, northern Mexico, and Central and South America (Fig. 32-8). Over 100,000 people in the U.S. are infected annually, and the number of reported cases increased by as much as 144% throughout the 1990s. Incidence is affected by annual temperature, precipitation and natural events like earthquakes.

Crum NF, Lederman ER, Stafford CM, et al: Coccidioidomycosis: a descriptive survey of a reemerging disease. Clinical characteristics and current controversies, *Medicine* 83:149–175, 2004.

29. What are the clinical manifestations of coccidioidomycosis?

Primary pulmonary infection is asymptomatic in 50% of patients. In 40%, patients present with a mild flulike illness or pneumonia. Erythema nodosum is present in 5% of patients with acute coccidioidomycosis. Hematogenous dissemination occurs in 1% to 5% of patients. Risk factors for dissemination and fatal disease include male sex, pregnancy, immunocompromised status, and race (in order of decreasing risk by race: Filipino, black, and white). Among immunosuppressed patients, lymphocytopenia correlates closely with dissemination. Coccidioidomycosis is considered an AIDS-defining illness. The most common sites of extrapulmonary disease include the skin, lymph nodes, bones/joints, and central nervous system (meninges). Cutaneous lesions of disseminated coccidioidomycosis are protean. Warty papules, plaques, or nodules are the most characteristic (Fig. 32-9). Cellulitis, abscesses, and draining sinus tracts also may occur. Rarely, cutaneous lesions can be from primary cutaneous inoculation. Erythema nodosum is the most common reactive manifestation of coccidioidomycosis and indicates a robust cell-mediated immune response. Other reactive patterns include generalized morbilliform, papular, targetoid or urticarial exanthem, interstitial granulomatous dermatitis, and Sweet syndrome.

DiCaudo DJ: Coccidioidomycosis: a review and update, *J Am Acad Dermatol* 55(6):929–942, 2009.

30. Where is paracoccidioidomycosis endemic?

Paracoccidioidomycosis (South American blastomycosis) previously has been thought to be restricted to Latin America, especially Brazil. There have been reports of cases outside this area. The disease is confined to humid tropical and subtropical forests. *Paracoccidioides brasiliensis* is the causative dimorphic fungus.

31. Why is paracoccidioidomycosis more common in men?

Paracoccidioidomycosis is most common in adult men between the ages of 30 and 60 years. Skin testing indicates that the rate of infection is equal among the sexes. However, clinical disease is more common in men, with a

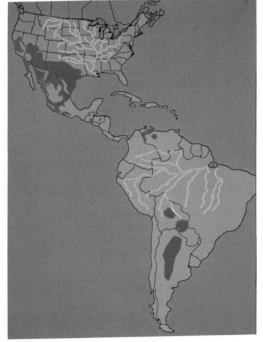

Figure 32-8. Coccidioidomycosis. Areas depicted in red represent the regions reporting the most cases of coccidioidomycosis. (Courtesy of the Fitzsimons Army Medical Center teaching files.)

male:female ratio of 15:1. It has been shown that this sex difference is due to the inhibitory action of estrogens on the mycelium to yeast transformation necessary for infectivity. Only 3% of cases occur in children and 10% in adolescents.

32. What is the most common presenting complaint of paracoccidioidomycosis?

The lung is the primary site of infection. However, respiratory complaints are the least common presenting symptom. Painful mucosal ulcerations involving the mouth and nose are the most common findings. Patients may also have enlarged cervical lymph nodes and verrucous, crusted, edematous facial lesions. Hematogenous dissemination may also cause disease in the adrenals, spleen, liver, gastrointestinal tract, and central nervous system (CNS).

Almeida OP, Jacks J: Paracoccidioidomycosis of the mouth: an emerging deep mycosis, *Crit Rev Oral Biol Med* 14:377–383, 2003.

33. Which organism is responsible for penicilliosis?

Penicilliosis is caused by the dimorphic fungus *Penicillium marneffei*. It is inhaled into the lungs and causes disease in both immunocompetent and immunocompromised patients, with a predilection to the latter.

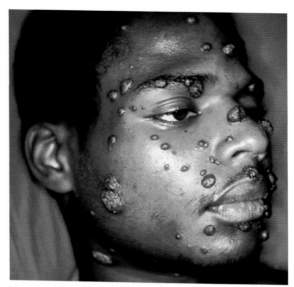

Figure 32-9. Disseminated coccidioidomycosis. Discrete verrucous papules, plaques, and nodules. (Courtesy of James E. Fitzpatrick, MD.)

34. Where is penicilliosis endemic?

Penicilliosis is endemic in southeast Asia and southern China, although there have been a few case reports in other Asian countries. The increase in HIV-infected individuals in these areas has led to the emergence of this organism as a cause of infection. Bamboo rats may serve as a reservoir.

Kullavanijaya P: Penicilliosis in AIDS, *J Dermatol* 28:667–670, 2001.

35. How does penicilliosis present clinically?

Clinical manifestations are similar between immunocompromised and immunocompetent patients. The most common clinical presentation is subacute with weeks of intermittent fevers, headache, marked weight loss, and anemia. The AIDS patients have an increased frequency of septicemia and mucocutaneous lesions. Skin lesions are a common manifestation of disseminated disease. Abscesses are common in non-HIV infected individuals. Cutaneous lesions are more diversified in the HIV patients and include molluscum contagiosum–like papules, pustules, acneiform, and morbilliform eruptions. Skin lesions are most common on the upper body. Delay in treatment is associated with 100% mortality in all patients. Biopsy and culture are used for diagnosis. Treatment options include itraconazole or amphotericin B in severe cases.

36. What is a parasitized histocyte?

Several species of bacteria and fungi infect and proliferate and actually thrive within the cytoplasm of macrophages rather than being killed by the macrophage (Table 32-2).

OPPORTUNISTIC FUNGAL INFECTIONS

37. Define opportunistic infection.

Opportunistic infections are caused by organisms that typically produce disease in a host with lowered resistance. Many opportunistic infections involve the skin. The four discussed in this chapter are cryptococcosis, aspergillosis, fusariosis, and mucormycosis.

Table 32-2. Organisms That Parasitize Histiocytes	
RARE	**RHINOSCLEROMA**
Lesions try to grow in parasitized histiocytes	Leishmaniasis Trypanosomiasis Toxoplasmosis Granuloma inguinale Peniciliosis Histoplasmosis

Table 32-3. Fungal Pathogens in HIV Infection

ORGANISM	CLINICAL FEATURES
Candida albicans	Thrush, vaginal, and esophageal candidiasis
Cryptococcus neoformans	Pulmonary and disseminated disease, meningitis, skin, eye, prostate
Histoplasma capsulatum	Disseminated disease with fever, weight loss, and predilection for reticuloen-dothelial system, adrenal glands, and CNS
Coccidioides immitis	Disseminated and pulmonary disease. Predilection for skin, lymph nodes, bones/joints, and CNS
Blastomyces dermatitidis	Disseminated and pulmonary disease. Predilection for lung, skin, bone, CNS, and prostate
Aspergillus fumigatus	Disseminated and pulmonary disease
Penicillium marneffei	Disseminated disease with fever, anemia, weight loss Mucocutaneous lesions are common
Sporotrichosis schenckii	Disseminated disease. Sites of predilection: joints/bones, eyes, and meninges

38. What are the common fungal pathogens in HIV infection?

Candida and *Cryptococcus* species are the most common fungal infections in HIV-infected patients. See Table 32-3 for other fungal pathogens and their most frequent clinical presentation.

Ampel NM: Emerging disease issues and fungal pathogens associated with HIV infection, *Emerg Infect Dis* 2:109–116, 1996.

39. Discuss the fungal infections seen in organ transplant recipients.

Organ transplant recipients are at increased risk of localized and disseminated disease from dermatophytes, yeast (candidiasis, *Malassezia*, cryptococcosis, *Trichosporon*), dimorphic organisms, and nondermatophyte molds (aspergillosis, fusariosis, mucormycosis). Skin manifestations due to *Candida* spp., *Aspergillus* spp., dematiaceous fungi, and *Pityrosporum* typically occur shortly after transplantation. Cryptococcosis occurs 6 months or later after transplantation, and the endemic dimorphic fungi can cause disease any time following transplantation. Emerging mold pathogens in the transplant patients have included *Aspergillus fumigatus* species, *Fusarium*, *Scedosporium*, and Zygomycetes.

Virgili A, Zampino MR, Mantovani L: Fungal skin infections in organ transplant recipients, *Am J Clin Dermatol* 3:19–35, 2002.
Wingard JR: The changing face of invasive fungal infections in hematopoietic cell transplant recipients, *Curr Opin Oncol* 17:89–92, 2005.

40. Discuss the important epidemiologic factors of cryptococcosis.

Cryptococcosis is caused by *Cryptococcus neoformans*, a ubiquitous encapsulated yeast found worldwide in the soil. Several strains are associated with pigeon and other avian excreta, and another strain is associated with eucalyptus trees. During the pre-AIDS era (prior to 1980), cryptococcal infections were rare and about 50% occurred in patients with lymphoreticular malignancies. Cryptococcosis is rare in immunocompetent patients, and patients at risk are those with impaired cellular immunity (advanced HIV patients, organ transplants, lymphoreticular malignancies, patients receiving corticosteroid therapy). The incidence of cryptococcosis is inversely proportional to the CD4 lymphocyte count. The prevalence of cryptococcosis in patients infected with HIV has declined with aggressive antiretroviral therapy. The mortality rate of untreated disseminated disease is 70% to 80%.

Perfect JR, Casadevall A: Cryptococcosis, *Infect Dis Clin North Am* 16:837–874, 2002.

Key Points: Deep Fungal Infections

1. Deep fungal infections can be divided into subcutaneous (localized), systemic, and opportunistic categories.
2. Neutropenic patients are particularly at risk for systemic phaeohyphomycosis, aspergillosis, fusariosis, and mucormycosis.
3. Patients with impaired cellular immunity are particularly at risk for disseminated sporotrichosis, histoplasmosis, coccidioidomycosis, penicilliosis, *Cryptococcus*, and *Candida*.
4. The differential diagnosis of lymphocutaneous (sporotricoid) spread includes sporotrichosis, atypical mycobacteria, leishmaniasis, *Nocardia*, tularemia, and cat scratch disease.

41. How is an infection with cryptococcosis acquired?

Infection occurs primarily from inhalation of the organism leading to a primary lung infection. Immunocompetent patients generally present with a mild pulmonary infection. Disseminated disease via the hematogenous route occurs in 10% to 15% of immunosuppressed patients, with a predilection for the meninges. It is the leading cause of fungal meningitis. Other organs involved include the skin (10% to 20%), eye, bone, and prostate. There are a few rare reports of primary inoculation cutaneous disease, which manifests itself as a solitary papule/nodule. However, cutaneous disease is generally indicative of disseminated disease and a poor prognosis.

Neuville S, Dromer F, Morin O, et al, for the French Cryptococcosis Study Group: Primary cutaneous cryptococcosis: a distinct clinical entity, *CID* 36:337–347, 2003.

42. What are the cutaneous manifestations of disseminated cryptococcosis?

Cryptococcosis is a great imitator of a wide variety of cutaneous diseases. These include molluscum contagiosum–like lesions (Fig. 32-10), Kaposi sarcoma–like lesions, pyoderma gangrenosum–like lesions, herpetiform lesions, cellulitis, ulcers, subcutaneous nodules, and palpable purpura. Lesions are most commonly found on the head, neck, and genitals, but can be found anywhere. Cutaneous lesions are found in 10% to 20% of HIV-infected patients. Histologic features are characteristic with periodic acid–Schiff stain with diastase demonstrating budding yeast surrounded by a clear space representing the capsule (Fig. 32-11).

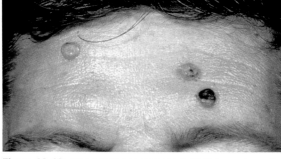

Figure 32-10. Disseminated cryptococcosis. Multiple papules and nodules that resemble molluscum contagiosum. (Courtesy of James E. Fitzpatrick, MD.)

43. What patient population is at increased risk of aspergillosis?

Neutropenia and corticosteroid therapy, especially when combined, are the two most important risk factors for aspergillosis. Solid organ transplant patients, bone marrow transplant recipients, and leukemic patients, in particular, are at high risk. Other at-risk patients include HIV-infected individuals, patients on broad-spectrum antibiotics, and patients on immunosuppression therapy.

44. How common are cutaneous lesions in aspergillosis?

Aspergillus species are ubiquitous saprophytes in the air, soil, and decaying vegetation. It is primarily a respiratory pathogen, with the lungs and sinuses as the major sites of infection. Disseminated disease occurs in 30% of aspergillosis cases, and cutaneous lesions develop in fewer than 11%. There are several documented reports of primary invasive skin infections occurring in neutropenic patients associated with intravenous catheters and adhesive tape contaminated with spores.

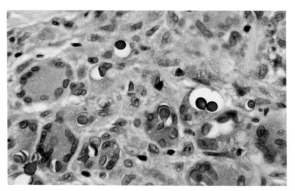

Figure 32-11. Cryptococcosis. Periodic acid–Schiff stain with diastase demonstrating budding yeast surrounded by a clear space representing the capsule. (Courtesy of the Fitzsimons Army Medical Center teaching files.)

45. Describe the cutaneous lesions in aspergillosis.

Patients may have single or multiple lesions that begin as a well-circumscribed papule, which over several days enlarges into an ulcer with a necrotic base and surrounding erythematous halo (Fig. 32-12). The organism has a propensity to invade blood vessels, causing thrombosis and infarction. The skin lesions can be very destructive and extend into cartilage, bone, and fascial planes. Aspergillosis should be considered in the differential diagnosis of necrotizing lesions.

46. What opportunistic fungus is clinically and histologically similar to *Aspergillus*?

Patients with prolonged neutropenia, especially leukemia patients, are susceptible to infections with *Fusarium*. In this patient population, *Fusarium*

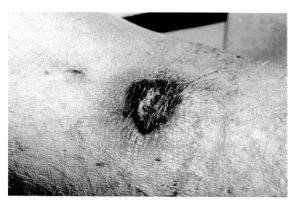

Figure 32-12. Aspergillosis cellulitis at the site of adhesive tape demonstrating erythematous plaques with pustules.

species are the second most common pathogenic mold. *Fusarium* is a filamentous mold found in soil and plants. Inhalation into the lungs is the primary route of infection; however, primary cutaneous infection from indwelling catheters may occur. The lung is the usual site of infection; however, 75% of patients have hematogenous spread with a predilection for the skin and sinuses. The cutaneous lesions caused by *Fusarium* are similar to aspergillosis. The typical presentation is a painful erythematous nodule with central ulceration and necrosis. Cellulitis and onychomycosis have also been reported. Histologically, the two are identical (septate hyphae with acute angle branching). The treatment of choice is amphotericin B and the mortality rate is 50% to 80%.

Dignani MC, Anaissie E: Human fusariosis, *Clin Microbiol Infect* 10:67–75, 2004.

47. What are the most important predisposing factors for acquiring mucormycosis?

Mucormycosis is caused by rapidly growing molds from several genera, including *Apophysomyces*, *Mucor*, *Rhizopus*, *Absidia*, and *Rhizomucor*. These organisms are ubiquitous in decaying vegetation, fruit, and bread. Approximately one third of patients have diabetes, and diabetics in ketoacidosis are at especially high risk. Other reported associations include malnutrition, uremia, neutropenia, corticosteroid therapy, burns, antibiotic therapy, neonatal prematurity, deferoxamine therapy, and HIV-infected individuals with a history of intravenous drug use. The neutrophil is the predominant component of host defense.

Gonzalez CE, Rinaldi MG, Sugar AM: Zygomycosis, *Infect Dis Clin North Am* 16:895–914, 2002.

48. Discuss the clinical manifestations of rhinocerebral mucormycosis.

Rhino-orbital-cerebral mucormycosis is the most common form of mucormycosis. Other clinical variants include pulmonary, cutaneous, gastrointestinal, and disseminated. Most commonly, the organism is deposited in the nasal turbinates or lung through inhalation. The majority of patients with Rhino-orbital-cerebral mucormycosis are diabetics (often in ketoacidosis) or have leukemia. Patients present with fever, headache, facial edema, proptosis, facial pain, orbital cellulitis, and cranial nerve dysfunction. The patients may have loss of vision from retinal artery thrombosis. This form is often fatal. Treatment consists of rapid diagnosis with aggressive debridement and antifungal therapy.

Eucker J, Sezer O, Graf B, Possinger K: Mucormycoses, *Mycoses* 44:253–260, 2001.

49. Can mucormycosis be acquired from contaminated dressings?

Yes. Primary cutaneous mucormycosis can occur when the spores are directly inoculated into abraded skin. In the 1970s, there was a nationwide epidemic associated with contaminated elastic dressings. Patients presented with a cellulitis under the covered areas. Primary cutaneous mucormycosis has also been reported from gardening, intramuscular injections, intravenous lines, arthropod bites, automobile accidents, and burns. Cutaneous disease accounts for approximately 10% of reported cases and can also be from hematological spread.

50. What is the treatment of mucormycosis?

The treatment of mucormycosis includes rapid diagnosis in conjunction with correction of any underlying diseases. Biopsy sample of necrotic tissue demonstrates thick, nonseptate hyphae branching at right angles. Culture is only positive in 30% of cases. Also indicated is administration of amphotericin B, and aggressive surgical debridement of necrotic tissue in order to minimize mortality. Emerging treatments include posaconazole, and adjuvant treatment with interferon gamma and granulocyte-macrophage– or granulocyte colony–stimulating factors.

Tarrand JJ, Lichterfeld M, Warraich I, et al: Diagnosis of invasive septate mold infections. A correlation of microbiological culture and histologic or cytologic examination, *Am J Clin Pathol* 119(6):854–858, 2003.

51. For what fungal infections might patients on biologic therapies be at risk?

Patients on TNF-α agonists most commonly are at risk for histoplasmosis, candidiasis, and aspergillosis. There may be a different degree of risk with each of the agents—infliximab creating a higher risk than etanercept or adalimumab. In endemic areas, patients are also at risk for primary or reactivation of latent coccidioidomycosis. One recent series reported 13 cases of coccidiomycosis, with two patients dying of disseminated disease. Close monitoring of current and past residents of endemic areas in the form of baseline and serial chest x-ray and serology is indicated.

Tsiodras S, Samonis G, Boumpas DT, Kontoyiannis DP: Fungal infections complicating tumor necrosis factor alpha blockade therapy, *Mayo Clin Proc* 83(2):181–194, 2008.

52. What fungal species are considered potential agents of bioterrorism?

Also known as the "lid lifter," coccidioidomycosis sporulates easily in culture and is highly infectious. It is the only fungus on the Select Agent List of the Department of Health and Human Services.

Centers for Disease Control and Prevention: National Select Agent Registry, Available at: http://www.selectagents.gov/. Accessed July 25, 2010.

CHAPTER 33

PARASITIC INFESTATIONS

Jeffrey J. Meffert, MD

1. Where and how does one acquire cutaneous parasitic diseases?

Parasitic skin diseases may arise from systemic spread or direct penetration of the skin. Cutaneous parasitic infestations are a major source of morbidity, affecting millions worldwide. Tropical climates, crowding, poor nutrition, sanitation problems, and limited medical resources are all associated with increased variety and severity of parasitoses. Ecologically temperate climates and industrialized societies are also afflicted by significant parasitic infestations because of local vectors, distant vacations, and widespread travel to and from areas of endemic infection for business, political, humanitarian, or military purposes. Immunosuppression due to drugs or disease leads to cutaneous manifestations of parasitic diseases that may be caused by unusual organisms.

2. What is "creeping eruption"?

Properly known as cutaneous larva migrans, and popularly known as "sandworms," creeping eruption occurs when the larva of dog and cat hookworms (*Ancylostoma caninum* and *A. braziliense*, respectively) penetrate intact, exposed skin and begin migrating through the epidermis. The most common location for the eruption is the sole of the foot, although other sites such as the buttocks, back, and thighs, which may have rested on contaminated sand, are susceptible. Lacking the enzymes necessary to penetrate and survive in the deeper dermis, the larvae wander a serpiginous route at a speed up to 3 cm/day. Clinically, the primary lesion is a pruritic, erythematous, serpiginous burrow (Fig. 33-1). Although the larvae usually die in 2 to 8 weeks, survival up to 22 months has been reported. Several cases of cutaneous larva migrans–related erythema multiforme have been reported.

A variety of other animal hookworm species may also cause creeping eruption. Human hookworms may briefly cause a similar eruption, but the better-adapted parasites soon find their way into the circulation.

Richey TK, Gentry RH, Fitzpatrick JE, et al: Persistent larva cutaneous migrans due to *Ancylostoma*, *South Med J* 89:609–611, 1996.

Vaughan TK, English JC 3rd: Cutaneous larva migrans complicated by erythema multiforme, *Cutis* 62:33–35, 1998.

3. How do you treat creeping eruption?

An older method was to freeze the leading point of the burrow. This sometimes produced significant tissue destruction and often missed the larva, which may be up to 2 cm ahead of the visible burrow. A classic treatment is 10% topical thiabendazole suspension applied four times a day for at least 2 days after the last sign of burrow activity; however, this medication is not always readily available. This regimen has a high cure rate and minimal toxicity. Rare cases may require oral thiabendazole. Oral ivermectin, indicated for the treatment of larval currens, may have a role in the treatment of this disease as an off-label use.

4. What is different about larva currens?

Larva currens, or "racing larva," is caused by *Strongyloides stercoralis*, a nematode with a normal life cycle similar to the hookworm. *Strongyloides*, however, is unique in that it can complete its life cycle within the human host and bypass the obligate soil phase of the hookworms. Autoinfection may occur to a point of overwhelming infestation and host death, especially in immunocompromised victims. The serpentine eruption of larva currens appears much the same as creeping eruption but is more likely to occur on the thighs, buttocks, or perineum due to larval penetration from the nearby colon. The eruption is more fleeting and lasts no more than a few days, during which the larva's migratory speed through the dermis may be clocked at up to 10 cm/hr (Fig. 33-2). A nonspecific rash or hives may also occur because of hypersensitivity to the parasite.

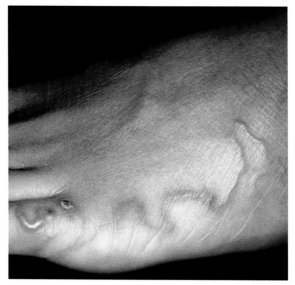

Figure 33-1. Creeping eruption. Cutaneous larva migrans due to canine hookworm. (Courtesy of the Fitzsimons Army Medical Center teaching files.)

5. Are there other nematode infestations that cause skin disease?

Enterobius vermicularis (pinworms) may cause a noisome perianal itch, but secondary complications including dermatitis, bacterial infections, and local abscesses can develop. Treatment is a single dose of mebendazole. *Trichinella spiralis*, which is acquired by eating undercooked pork, may cause a diffuse rash, nail bed splinter hemorrhages, and a subtle but persistent periorbital edema (trichinosis).

6. How do filarial infections differ from other nematode infections?

All the filariae have an insect vector integral to their life cycle and live in pairs within their mammalian host. The microfilarial offspring of this couple are the primary source of morbidity. The most important filarial diseases are filariasis, loiasis, and onchocerciasis (Table 33-1).

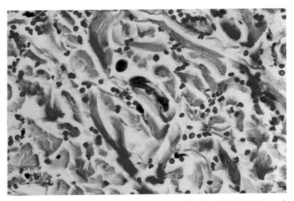

Figure 33-2. Larva currens. Biopsy demonstrates migrating larva of *Strongyloides stercoralis* in the dermis. (Courtesy of the Fitzsimons Army Medical Center teaching files.)

7. Where is onchocerciasis most prevalent? How is it transmitted?

Onchocerciasis, a disease produced by the tissue nematode *Onchocerca volvulus,* affects millions of people in Africa and Central and South America. The infective larval forms are transmitted to humans through the bite of the black fly *(Simulium)* (Fig. 33-3). The common term for onchocerciasis, *river blindness,* takes its name from its feared complication and the fast-flowing rivers where the parasite and vectors are found.

Nguyen JC, Murphy ME, Nutman TB, et al: Cutaneous onchocerciasis in an American traveler, *Int J Dermatol* 44:125–128, 2005.

8. Does river blindness cause cutaneous manifestations?

As the larval forms of *Onchocerca* develop into adult worms at the site of the bite, they produce subcutaneous nodules called onchocercomas, where numerous microfilariae are produced. They migrate into the skin, inducing a secondary dermatitis, skin pigmentation changes, skin thickening, frank elephantiasis, and an often disabling itching. The microfilariae also may migrate into the tissue of the eye and produce blindness due to severe uveal and corneal inflammation.

9. What are some of the problems with onchocerciasis treatment?

Diethylcarbamazine is effective treatment for the microfilarial stage, but a hypersensitivity reaction to large numbers of dying parasites in the anterior chamber of the eye may cause irreversible blindness and, in some cases, death. A safer course, in otherwise asymptomatic victims, is periodic "nodulectomy," which removes the adult worms and significantly lowers the morbidity of onchocerciasis.

10. What is loiasis?

Loiasis, an infection endemic in the jungles of west and central Africa, is produced by the adult form of the tissue nematode, *Loa loa,* which is transmitted through the bite of various flies including deer flies (*Chrysops* species). Usually

Table 33-1. Parasitic Infestations of the Skin	
PARASITIC INFESTATION	**VECTOR OR MODE OF TRANSMISSION**
Filariasis	Mosquito
Onchocerciasis	Black fly
Creeping eruption	Soil contact and larval penetration
African trypanosomiasis	Tsetse fly
American trypanosomiasis	Kissing bug
Leishmaniasis	Sand fly
Schistosomiasis	Water contact and cercarial penetration
Dracunculiasis, sparganosis	Ingestion of larva
Echinococcosis, cysticercosis	Ingestion of cysts
Amebiasis	Direct contact or ingestion of cysts
Loiasis	Horse and deer flies
Demodex	Person-to-person contact in childhood

asymptomatic, this filarial disease may cause large areas of transient edema (Calabar swelling) as the worm migrates, and it may even migrate visibly across the conjunctiva. Subcutaneous nodules may also be seen in this disease, but the worm's unique migration habits lead to the common name "eyeworm."

11. What causes elephantiasis?

The term *elephantiasis* is applied to many dermatologic conditions that ultimately result in severe lymphatic obstruction and stasis. The affected limb may become massively enlarged, initially with pitting edema but later with a woodlike induration. The skin becomes discolored, and patches of warty growths may eventually cover the entire affected area. Lymphangitis and mechanical obstruction from lymphatic filariasis is but one way of causing elephantiasis. Offending organisms include *Wuchereria bancrofti*, *Brugia malayi*, and *B. timori*. The *Brugia* species cause elephantiasis of the extremities most commonly, while *Wuchereria* is notorious for genital disease that may eventuate in massive scrotal enlargement (Fig. 33-4).

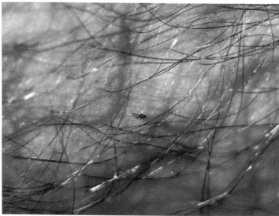

Figure 33-3. *Simulium* species. Black fly caught in the act of biting one of the editors (JEF). Note the small size compared with the hair shafts. (Courtesy of James E. Fitzpatrick, MD.)

12. Can other filarial diseases affect the skin?

Dirofilaria tenuis, the raccoon heartworm, can cause subcutaneous nodules. *Dracunculus medinensis*, or guinea worm, wanders through the subcutaneous tissue as part of its life cycle and eventually settles down where it may cause nodules and ulceration. Ivermectin, with or without coadministration of albendazole, has been used in many of the filarial diseases described previously. Dosages range from 200 to 400 mg/kg. The native treatment for *Dracunculus* is to snare the worm (up to 120 cm long in the female worm) through the skin and roll it up on a stick (the matchstick technique). Some medical historians believe that the caduceus (Fig. 33-5A), the symbol for a physician, has its origins from the ancient method of extracting the *Dracuncula* worm with a stick (Fig. 33-5B).

13. What is myiasis?

Myiasis is a disease in which various species of flies lay their eggs on or in human skin. When laid in an open wound, such as a chronic leg or decubitus ulcer, the eggs hatch into larvae (maggots) that feed on damaged skin and complete their life cycle. This is called "wound myiasis" and causes mild to severe inflammation, depending upon the fly species and wound location. In other cases, maggot nibbling of ulcer debris may actually dramatically improve the wound, and wound myiasis has been intentionally induced for this purpose.

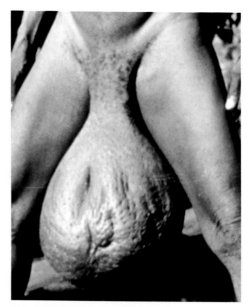

Figure 33-4. Marked scrotal enlargement in elephantiasis. (From Zaiman H, Jong EC: Parasitic diseases of the skin and soft tissue. In Stevens DL, editor: *Atlas of infectious diseases*, vol II, New York, 1995, Churchill Livingstone.)

14. What is a warble?

More properly called *furuncular myiasis* in humans, a warble occurs when fly eggs or larvae are introduced into intact skin. A large larva, more than 1 cm in length in some species, grows over time. Careful examination usually reveals a "snorkel" protruding through the skin of a boil that moves when the abscess is manipulated. Surgical extirpation is the treatment of choice, although other therapies, including occlusion of the furuncle opening with petrolatum or a piece of meat, have been reported to be successful (Fig. 33-6).

15. What is Congo floor maggot?

Unlike other forms of myiasis in which the larva feeds and pupates within the host tissue, the Congo floor maggot (*Auchmeromyia luteola*) lives in the soil or in the earthen floors of huts and crawls upon the host in the night for a blood meal. The larva, which may grow up to 18 mm long, requires 6 to 20 feedings before it pupates in the dirt. They carry no disease and may be avoided by sleeping on a raised bed.

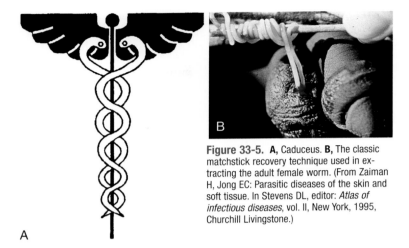

Figure 33-5. **A,** Caduceus. **B,** The classic matchstick recovery technique used in extracting the adult female worm. (From Zaiman H, Jong EC: Parasitic diseases of the skin and soft tissue. In Stevens DL, editor: *Atlas of infectious diseases*, vol. II, New York, 1995, Churchill Livingstone.)

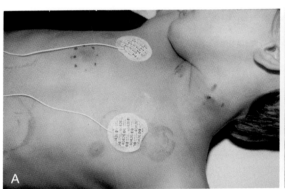

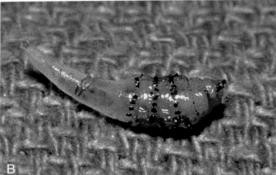

Figure 33-6. Cutaneous myiasis. **A,** Two lesions of furuncular myiasis in a young child. The lesions were acquired in Panama. **B,** Furuncular larva after removal from patient. (Panel A courtesy of the Fitzsimons Army Medical Center teaching files.)

16. What is tungiasis?

The sand flea, *Tunga penetrans*, can burrow into the foot where the female lays eggs, causing painful abscesses. Treatment is best accomplished by killing the female with chloroform or surgical excision. While late lesions will spontaneously ulcerate, potential complications include secondary infection and tetanus.

17. What is the difference between a chigoe and a chigger?

Chigoe is another name for *Tunga penetrans*. The chigger is a trombiculid mite.

18. Do chiggers burrow into the skin to lay eggs like the sand flea?

They usually do not burrow beneath the skin, but the larval forms attach via their mouth parts (adults do not bite) and feed on tissue juices and lymph. They may feed for a few days if not removed, although the intense itching usually starts within a few hours after attachment. They prefer to feed in areas where the clothing is found in close contact with the skin, such as under socks and belts (Fig. 33-7). In some parts of Asia, they are a vector of scrub typhus and may be discouraged from attachment by wearing proper clothing, permethrin repellents, and by washing in hot, soapy water.

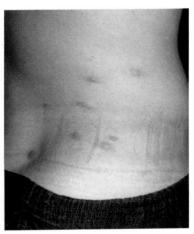

Figure 33-7. Chigger bites. Note that they tend to accentuate under areas of pressure by clothing. (Courtesy of the Fitzsimons Army Medical Center teaching files.)

19. What is leishmaniasis?

Leishmaniasis, also known as Baghdad boil, kala-azar, espundia, oriental sore, and a variety of other colorful terms, is caused by *Leishmania* species, a protozoan parasite with a multicontinental distribution. Biting sand flies (*Phlebotomus* species) spread the disease between humans and a large variety of wild and domestic animal reservoirs. Several species and subspecies of *Leishmania* may produce infection, and the clinical manifestations and disease severity are generally species specific. Most forms cause nodules and chronic ulcerations of the skin that can spread lymphatically and lead to widespread cutaneous disease (Fig. 33-8).

Markle WH, Makhoul K: Cutaneous leishmaniasis: recognition and treatment, *Am Fam Physician* 69:1455–1460, 2004.

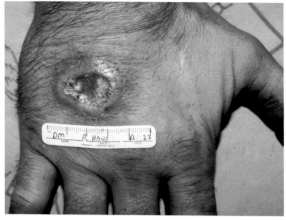

Figure 33-8. Cutaneous leishmaniasis.

20. Name the different types of leishmaniasis.

See Table 33-2.

21. Can leishmaniasis be contracted in the United States?

While most cases of leishmaniasis seen in the U.S. are acquired elsewhere, a form of cutaneous disease caused by *L. mexicana* may be acquired in central Texas and has been nicknamed "Highway 90 disease" by those familiar with its distribution. The standard treatment for leishmaniasis includes antimonial medications, but other medications such as ketoconazole, fluconazole, and physical modalities such as hyperthermia have anecdotally been shown to improve the lesions.

Davis AJ, Kedzierski L: Recent advances in antileishmanial drug development, *Curr Opin Investig Drugs* 6:163–169, 2005.
Furner BB: Cutaneous leishmaniasis in Texas: report of a case and review of the literature, *J Am Acad Dermatol* 23:368–371, 1990.

22. How does cutaneous amebiasis, due to *Entamoeba histolytica*, present?

Usually the result of direct extension from hepatic or colorectal disease, cutaneous amebiasis presents with serpiginous, warty ulcers of the anogenital area called *amebomas*. These ulcers may produce extensive tissue loss and predispose to severe secondary bacterial infections. Less common presentations include infection by direct inoculation of the perineum in dysenteric infants wearing diapers and on the penis following anal intercourse with an infected person.

23. What are the skin findings in American trypanosomiasis?

American trypanosomiasis, or Chagas' disease, is caused by the parasite *Trypanosoma cruzi*, which is introduced through the conjunctiva or skin following the bite of blood-sucking reduviid bugs (kissing bugs). This insect has the disgusting habit of defecating on the skin following its human blood meal, and the infected feces are inoculated into the conjunctiva or wound. A unilateral conjunctivitis and lid edema (Romana's sign) are usually the first clinical signs. Later, the patient may become systemically ill with various rashes and subcutaneous nodules, as well as cardiac and gastrointestinal lesions that may be fatal.

24. What are the skin findings in African trypanosomiasis?

African trypanosomiasis, also called *sleeping sickness*, is due to *Trypanosoma gambiense* or *T. rhodesiense*. It may present with a trypanosomal chancre (primary cutaneous African trypanosomiasis) at the site of the bite, followed by nodules and dermatitis (secondary cutaneous African trypanosomiasis) (Fig. 33-9). The cardiac and neurologic complications of both forms of trypanosomiasis are the most serious clinical concerns.

McGovern TW, Williams W, Fitzpatrick JE, et al: Cutaneous manifestations of African trypanosomiasis, *Arch Dermatol* 131:1178–1182, 1995.

Table 33-2. Types of Leishmaniasis		
SPECIES	**DISEASE**	**DISTRIBUTION**
L. donovani group	Visceral leishmaniasis, kala-azar	India, Asia, Middle East, Africa
L. tropica group	Old World cutaneous leishmaniasis, oriental sore, newly discovered viscerotropic disease	India, Middle East
L. viannia group (*L. braziliensis* group)	New World mucocutaneous leishmaniasis, espundia	Latin America
L. mexicana group	American cutaneous leishmaniasis	Mexico, Central America, Texas, South America

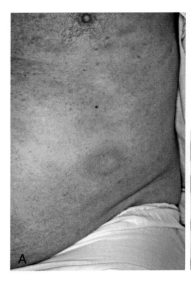
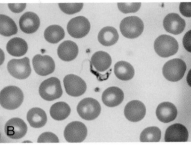

Figure 33-9. **A,** A big game hunter returning from Africa with oval secondary lesion of African trypanosomiasis. **B,** Peripheral smear from the patient demonstrating a circulating trypanosome. (Courtesy of the Fitzsimons Army Medical Center teaching files.)

25. Describe the cutaneous manifestations of schistosomiasis as they relate to the parasite's life cycle.

Schistosomiasis is a trematode (fluke) infection produced by one of three species of the genus *Schistosoma*. Schistosomes have a complex life cycle that involves development in freshwater snails (intermediate host) and the release of free-swimming cercariae that penetrate the human skin. Penetration produces a transient pruritus and burning followed by blisters, bruising, and crusted papules over the next few days. As the worm reaches maturity in the portal or caval venous system, the ova are released by the adult female and passed into the feces or urine. Some ova are deposited in the skin and may produce nodules, ulcers, and warty tumors. The anogenital region is most often involved through direct extension from the bladder or rectum, but spread through the bloodstream and lymphatics may produce lesions at other sites.

26. Are swimmer's itch and sea bather's eruption the same thing?

No. **Swimmer's itch**, also called *clam digger's itch* and *bather's itch*, is caused by the penetration of the skin by schistosome cercariae that normally infest birds. When first exposed, the victim will have a prickly eruption within a few minutes of cercarial penetration that rapidly resolves. Repeated exposure with an allergic response leads to larger, longer-lasting, and more pruritic papules that may cause pustules, blisters, and dermatitis. As with creeping eruption, the parasite cannot complete its life cycle because it cannot penetrate the epidermis.

Sea bather's eruption is caused by contact with larval forms of a marine jellyfish. In contrast to swimmer's itch, which presents with lesions in exposed areas, sea bather's eruption typically presents with pruritic macules and papules in areas covered by clothing. It is felt that the clothing holds the larvae close to the skin long enough to cause a small sting.

27. What is sparganosis?

Sparganosis is an infection produced by various species of the tapeworm *Spirometra*, which is seen most commonly in Asia and Southeast Asia. Sparganosis is typically acquired by drinking water containing infected copepods or the ingestion of inadequately cooked snake or frog meat. Clinically, it presents as pruritic or painful nodules that contain the encysted tapeworm. "Application sparganosis" occurs when an eye or ulcer is contaminated by a poultice made from these same animals and is characterized by similar nodules at the site of inoculation (Fig. 33-10). Sparganosis is best treated by surgical removal of the tapeworm.

Kimura S, Kashima M, Kawa Y, et al: A case of subcutaneous sparganosis: therapeutic assessment by an indirect immunofluorescence antibody titration using sections of the worm body obtained from the patient, *Br J Dermatol* 148:369–371, 2003.

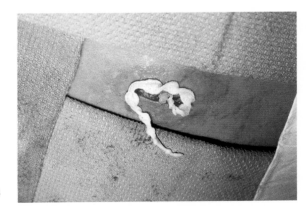

Figure 33-10. Sparganosis. Spirometra species due to a poultice made from a frog. (Courtesy of the Fitzsimons Army Medical Center teaching files.)

28. Can other tapeworms affect the skin?

Taenia solium (pork tapeworm) may produce cysticercosis cutis, which is acquired from the oral ingestion of eggs, usually due to poor sanitary habits. Clinically, it presents as painless subcutaneous nodules containing the larval stage of the tapeworm. *Echinococcus granulosus*, a dog tapeworm, produces fluctuant, cystic tumors in the skin (hydatid disease) as well as generalized hives and itching. It is acquired from the ingestion of contaminated food or water.

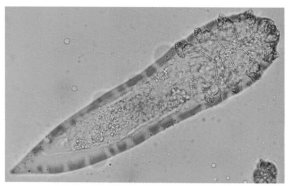

Figure 33-11. *Demodex folliculorum* (mineral oil preparation, original magnification ×500).

29. What is *Demodex*?

These microscopic mites reside by the thousands in the hair follicles *(D. folliculorum)* and sebaceous glands *(D. brevis)* of adult humans. They resemble carrots with legs and live off sebum and squamous debris (Fig. 33-11).

30. Does *Demodex* cause skin disease?

The role of *Demodex* in facial eruptions, particularly rosacea, has been a topic of debate for decades. Many convincing reports describe a recalcitrant folliculitis, often seen in immunosuppressed patients, which responds to mite-killing topical therapy. The contribution of *Demodex* to garden-variety rosacea is less certain, although patients with refractory rosacea pattern erythema and nodules have responded to miticidal therapy.

Forton F, Germaux MA, Brasseur T, et al: Demodicosis and rosacea: epidemiology and significance in daily dermatologic practice, *J Am Acad Dermatol* 52:74–87, 2005.

Key Points: Parasitic Infestations

1. A variety of parasitic diseases may have cutaneous manifestations.
2. Because of international travel and global conflict, what were once considered exclusively tropical diseases may show up in a North American clinic.
3. Cutaneous eruptions may be common minor nuisances, such as larval migrans and swimmer's itch, or more serious systemic infections, such as onchocerciasis and trypanosomiasis.
4. Many parasitic skin diseases are arthropod vector-borne, providing opportunities to interrupt the organisms' life cycle for both prevention and treatment.

31. What are morgellons?

There are those who believe that many, if not most, patients diagnosed with delusions of parasitosis actually have infestations with small parasites known as *morgellons*. Complaining of stinging or biting sensations, patients will present with fibers and serum crusts, claiming that these are the creatures that exited the skin. Most reported victims live in California, central Texas, and Florida. Those who believe that morgellons are an unrecognized and underdiagnosed health threat have at various times linked them with latent Lyme disease, biologic contamination from meteorites, and clandestine bioweapons gone awry. Treatment is difficult but usually involves prolonged courses of antibiotics and homeopathic therapies. Health care providers should be aware there are Websites showing images of plant and clothing fibers, mixed with scale crust, that are positively identified as "morgellons." In addition, there are weblogs describing how ignorant physicians are ignoring their patients' needs and suggesting where they can go for a sympathetic ear and what products they may buy to get a cure.

Centers for Disease Control (CDC): Unexplained dermopathy: http://www.cdc.gov/unexplaineddermopathy/. Accessed July 25, 2010.

CHAPTER 34

ARTHROPOD BITES AND STINGS

C. Paul Sayers, MD

1. What are arthropods? Are most arthropods harmful to humans?

Arthropods compose the largest number and most diverse group of animals on earth. They are invertebrates that arise from eggs and share these three anatomic features:

- Segmented bodies (head, thorax, abdomen)
- Hard outer exoskeleton derived from cutis
- Symmetrically paired and jointed appendages (legs, antennae, mouth parts)

  Less than 0.5% of the 1 million named species are injurious to humans. Most are harmless, while others are even beneficial to humans.

  Arthropods may be classified as follows:
- Arachnids (spiders, ticks, mites, scorpions): Medically important
- Insects (e.g., bees, lice, fleas, beetles, mosquitos, butterflies, moths): Medically important
- Millipedes
- Centipedes
- Crustaceans

2. Describe various ways arthropods injure humans. What insect or arachnid would cause the injury?

- Vesication/blister: Blister beetle
- Envenomation: Bees, ants, spiders
- Allergic sensitization (salivary proteins and enzymes in bee venom): Bed bugs, mosquitos, bees, and ants
- Invasion: Human botfly; tungiasis: penetrating fleas
- Contact urticaria: Setae from butterflies and moths
- Necrosis: Brown recluse spider
- Secondary infection: Any bite or sting, usually staphylococci
- Vector of disease: Mosquito, tick
  - Tick
- Bacterial: Lyme disease
- Rickettsial: Rocky Mountain spotted fever
- Viral: Colorado tick fever
  - Mosquito: West Nile, malaria, yellow fever, filariasis
  - Deer fly, tick: Tularemia
  - Human body lice: Epidemic typhus
  - Tsetse fly: African sleeping sickness
  - Black fly: Onchocerciasis

Alexander JOD: *Arthropods and the human skin*, Berlin, 1984, Springer-Verlag.

BITES AND STINGS

3. How do you diagnose a bite or sting?

The annoyance of the mosquito or the immediate pain of the bee sting rarely poses a problem of recognition. Diagnostic problems arise when the arthropod is not seen or felt but leaves a nonspecific papular rash with redness, pain, itching, or swelling. A careful history, common knowledge of local arthropod populations, and a physical examination with a high index of suspicion is necessary. Arthropod bites may present with itchy, red papules in a particular distribution or pattern that suggests an area of potential arthropod exposure. For example, grouped bites around an exposed ankle suggest a nonflying arthropod such as a flea, mite, chigger mite, or bedbug. Mysterious bites are often secondary to a zoonotic source, which includes exposures to pets, pests such as rats and mice, and nesting birds or bats near the home or workplace. Consultation with a veterinarian or entomologist is extremely beneficial in unusual cases. A biopsy of the skin lesion often will show perivascular dermatitis with eosinophils.

4. Why are some bites and stings extremely painful or dangerous while others are simply itchy, red, irritating papules?

The host reaction largely depends on whether the bite or the sting is defensive, toxic, or for feeding purposes. The highly visible, buzzing yellow bee or wasp stings primarily in defense of the hive. The venom causes rapid onset of severe pain for immediate negative feedback and defense.

The bite of spiders, on the other hand, contains toxins and proteolytic, digestive enzymes; thus spiders subjugate and then liquify their prey for food. Unfortunately, these venoms are often quite painful and destructive when injected into humans.

The bites of ectoparasites that require blood for nutrition or reproduction, such as the mosquito, are almost always painless and asymptomatic until allergic or irritant reactions take place. The salivary products are often allergenic and cause itching and redness.

5. One person on a hike is "eaten alive" by mosquitos while his companions are not bothered at all. Do ectoparasites such as mosquitos, ticks, fleas, and mites bite randomly?

No. Most arthropods are attracted to their hosts by a number of physical and chemical stimuli such as warmth, composition of sweat, carbon dioxide, vibrations, and odor. On the other hand, lipids derived from the degenerative epidermal cells often have a repellent quality to them. Thus, to arthropods, some human hosts are far more attractive than others.

6. Why are bite reactions to ectoparasites so much different in different people?

The severity of bug bite reactions depends most on the immunologic status of the patient. In general, a severely symptomatic eruption may result from only a few bites in an immunologically sensitized person, while many bites may produce no symptoms at all in a person with an acquired immunologic tolerance.

In clinical settings and in experimental models, continuous exposure to biting arthropods will produce five stages of reactivity. Confusing clinical reactions may emerge because the immunologic reaction may range from nonreactive to severe and even tolerant, depending on the patient's immune status.

- **Stage 1:** Bite is nonreactive in persons never exposed before.
- **Stage 2:** After a 2-week period of exposure, a delayed red papule begins within 24 hours after a bite and subsides within a week.
- **Stage 3:** An immediate wheal after a bite, followed by a delayed papule 24 hours later, becomes the clinical presentation.
- **Stage 4:** Immediate wheal develops as usual but the delayed hypersensitivity is lost.
- **Stage 5:** With continual exposure, immunologic tolerance begins, and there is no reaction after even prolonged exposure to insect bites; that is, with the immediate as well as the delayed response is lost.

Dahl MV: Cutaneous reactions to arthropod bites and stings, *Clin Cases Dermatol* 3:11–16, 1991.

7. How do you treat bee stings?

The best treatment for stings is prevention. Exposure to areas of wildflowers, dandelions, or clover fields should be avoided. Always wear shoes. Brightly colored clothing, flowery designs, and the use of colognes, perfumes, and scented soaps should be minimized. When confronted by agitated bees or wasps, avoid rapid movements and either stand still or withdraw very slowly to prevent further aggravation.

The venom-containing barbed stinger, if still present at the site of the sting, should be removed by gently scraping the skin horizontally with a dull knife or credit card (Fig. 34-1). Stinger removal with forceps compresses the venom

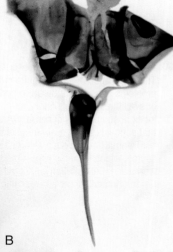

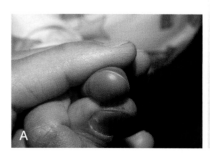

Figure 34-1. A, Bee sting on the thumb of a young child demonstrating painful, indurated erythema. **B,** Stinger that was removed from the thumb by scraping laterally with a index card. (Courtesy of the Fitzsimons Army Medical teaching files.)

gland, forcing more venom into the skin, and should be avoided. Symptomatic care with rest, elevation, and ice to the area are helpful. Antihistamines may also be useful. Early signs of systemic toxicity or allergic reactions should be noted.

8. What are the signs of serious systemic reactions to bee, wasp, or ant stings?
Profound anaphylactic reaction is the most serious and may occur with bronchospasm, urticaria, angioedema, and finally, vascular collapse and even death.

9. How do you treat anaphylactic syndrome from a bee sting?
If a reaction begins, treatment includes subcutaneous injection of epinephrine, 1:1000 in aqueous solution. This may be repeated in 15 to 20 minutes. In addition, intravenous diphenhydramine and cortisone as well as oxygen, fluids, vasopressors, and bronchodilators may also be used as needed. Since most fatalities occur within the first hour, early intervention by the allergic patient with a self-administered epinephrine injection may prevent a reaction from developing. Emergency treatment kits may be prescribed and carried at all times (Ana-Kit by Hollister-Stier [Spokane, WA], or EpiPen/EpiPen Jr by Dey Pharma [Basking Ridge, NJ]). Education and sting avoidance and evaluation for venom immunotherapy should be considered.

10. What are the unique characteristics of fire ants and their sting?
The fire ant, accidentally introduced into the United States in the 1930s from Brazil, now occupies most of the Southeast, limited only by cold winter weather in the north and the deserts of the Southwest. When the ants are provoked, they may attack en masse, administering up to several thousand stings to a victim. The sting is actually initiated by the ant biting the flesh and then pivoting slightly and repeatedly stinging the victim to form an annular eruption of sterile pustules and sting reaction sites. The sting site develops a large wheal and flare punctuated by a small sterile pustule, which ulcerates and potentially scars. The large erythematous wheal will then gradually desquamate over the next couple of days, and the sting site resolves normally. The unusual fire ant venom, a piperidine alkaloid, has become a leading cause of anaphylactic reaction to venomous animals in the United States. Treatment of the ant stings is symptomatic. Select patients with severe local or generalized sting reactions may be considered for immunotherapy.

Nguyen SA, Napoli DC: Natural history of large local and generalized cutaneous reactions to imported fire ant stings in children, *Ann Allergy Asthma Immunol* 94:387–390, 2005.

11. What species of spiders are medically important?
The brown recluse (*Loxosceles reclusa*) and the female black widow (*Latrodectus mactans*) (Fig. 34-2) are the most serious spiders in the United States. The hobo spider (*Tegenaria agrestis*) in the Pacific Northwest has been reported to produce dermonecrotic arachnidism, a serious necrotic reaction in the skin induced by the venom. However, whether or not this spider produces dermonecrotic arachnidism is controversial; some authorities believe that the reported bites have come from other causes. As many as 16 other species may bite humans, causing a small amount of pain or even necrosis at the site, but these reactions are transient, self-limiting, and require little attention. Most species are either too small or the biting mouthparts will not penetrate the human skin and, therefore, inject an insignificant amount of venom.

12. How do you diagnose and treat the black widow spider bite?
The female black widow spider is 10 to 15 mm long and has a black, globose abdomen, often with a red hourglass figure on the ventral surface. This spider is found in all 48 contiguous states. The venom is a potent neurotoxin.

Initially, the bite may sting slightly and then begins to burn. The skin changes are usually minimal, but the systemic symptoms of pain and muscle cramping may become intense. Diaphoresis, dizziness, anxiety, salivation, and other neurotoxic symptoms may ensue. Treatment of this neurotoxin should be prompt. Antisera are available and afford prompt relief, especially in the very young, old, or those with a history of heart disease or hypertension. Calcium gluconate, muscle relaxants, and pain medications are also used.

Elston DM: What's eating you? *Latrodectus mactans* (the black widow spider), *Cutis* 69:257–258, 2002.

13. How do brown recluse spider bites present?
Unlike the black widow, the brown recluse produces a dermonecrotic toxin that can cause severe necrosis of the skin as well as a hemolytic toxin that

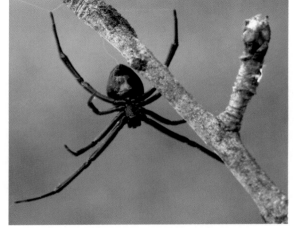

Figure 34-2. Female black widow spider demonstrating the characteristic hour glass on the ventral surface. (iStock_6222259)

causes severe, even life-threatening, hemolysis. The brown recluse is a shy, reclusive, brown spider with a dark brown violin-like marking on the dorsum of the cephalothorax, hence the name fiddleback spider. The spider is located largely in the Midwest but has been reported along the East Coast, in Texas, and in California. The bite commonly occurs when a person is cleaning old storage rooms or woodpiles outdoors, where the spider resides. Often, the spider is not seen or recovered at the time of the bite. The initial bite may be painless but is usually sharp and stinging for 6 to 8 hours and then is replaced by dull, aching pain that gradually increases in intensity and is accompanied by itching. The bite then begins to show a central blue color (impending necrosis), a surrounding white area (a vasospasm and ischemia), and a peripheral red halo (inflammation). Extension of this reaction demonstrates a remarkable gravitational spread to dependent areas. Over the next 2 to 4 days, the extent of the necrosis will be known. If a larger area of necrosis develops after a few days, a rare but serious and life-threatening systemic reaction to the hemolytic toxin may occur. Therefore, observation for hematologic changes such as red blood cell hemolysis or disseminated intravascular coagulopathy (DIC) should be observed.

14. How should brown recluse spider bites be treated?

First aid measures are important and can be remembered by the mnemonic **RICE. R**est, **i**ce, **c**ompression, and **e**levation of the bite site decrease blood flow, temperature, and enzymatic activity of the dermonecrotic toxin. General wound care, tetanus toxoid, antibiotics such as erythromycin or cephalexin for secondary infection, and observation for systemic hematologic problems may be necessary until the wound heals. Although dapsone and corticosteroids have been used to treat brown recluse spider bites, the use is controversial because some animal studies and nonrandomized human series have not demonstrated a beneficial effect. As serious as these bites can be, it is important to remember that most bites are inconsequential and heal without any problem. In those rare patients with hemolytic anemia, blood transfusions and intravenous fluid replacement is indicated.

Elston DM, Miller SD, Young RJ 3rd, et al: Comparison of colchicine, dapsone, triamcinolone, and diphenhydramine therapy for the treatment of brown recluse spider envenomation: a double-blind, controlled study in a rabbit model, *Arch Dermatol* 141:595–597, 2005.

Mold JW, Thompson DM: Management of brown recluse spider bites in primary care, *J Am Board Fam Pract* 17:347–352, 2004.

Key Points: Dermonecrotic Arachnidism

1. The brown recluse spider (*Loxosceles reclusa*) is the most common cause of dermonecrotic arachnidism.
2. The hobo spider (*Tegenaria agrestis*) in the Pacific Northwest has been reported to produce dermonecrotic arachnidism, although this is controversial.
3. In a small percentage of cases, brown recluse spider bites may progress to large ulcers that may spread along gravitational lines.
4. The use of systemic corticosteroids and dapsone for the treatment of brown recluse spider bites is controversial, with the most recent evidence suggesting that they are not effective.

INFESTATIONS

15. What is scabies?

Scabies is a contagious infestation caused by a mite that affects humans and other mammals, such as dogs, cats, horses, cows, pigs, and others. There are approximately 40 known species of scabies. *Sarcoptes scabiei* var. *hominis* is the etiologic agent of human scabies and is a full-time ectoparasite living, eating, and breeding on the human host. The female mates, burrows into the upper epidermis, lays her eggs, and eventually dies after 1 month. The mite and its feces cause severe pruritus.

16. How is scabies characterized clinically?

- There is an insidious onset of red to flesh-colored, pruritic papules.
- The itch is almost always worse at night.
- Secondary cases are almost always present—person-to-person transmission.
- The rash has a distinctive distribution involving the interdigital webs of the hands, the volar wrists, extensor elbows, axillary areas, central abdomen, genitalia, buttocks, and anterior thighs. The papular lesions affecting the shaft and glans penis as well as the scrotum are almost diagnostic. Facial lesions in adults are absent. Difficult cases include the very young, who may have pustules on the face or scalp.
- The rash consists of pruritic papules, but a diagnostic linear burrow consisting of a very fine scale is often seen in the interdigital web area or on the volar wrists (Fig. 34-3A). Nodular lesions commonly occur on male genitalia (Fig. 34-3B).
- The diagnosis is confirmed by scraping a small linear scaly burrow to reveal the female mite, her eggs, or fecal material under the microscope. Recovery of the diagnostic mite on scraping is often difficult in the excessively clean patient or patients that have been partially treated. Less commonly the diagnosis is established by visualizing the mite on a skin biopsy (Fig. 34-4).

17. What is Norwegian scabies?

Norwegian (crusted) scabies is a massive infestation with inordinate numbers of scabies mites due to inadequate host response. The large numbers of organisms cause a hyperplastic growth of the epithelium. Scratching may be absent

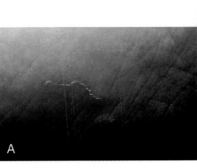

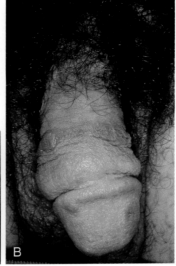

Figure 34-3. Scabies. **A,** Characteristic linear burrow. **B,** Nodular scabies most commonly presents in male genitalia as markedly pruritic papules. The lesion is almost diagnostic. (Courtesy of the Fitzsimons Army Medical Center teaching files.)

because itching is variable. The condition is seen in debilitated patients, those with mental illness, sensory neuropathy, paresis, and immunosuppressed patients such as those with acquired immune deficiency syndrome, post-transplantation, or undergoing topical or systemic corticosteroid therapy. Topical treatment with permethrin and keratolytics is difficult, so oral ivermectin (200 μg/kg) has been used with good success.

Tran L, Siedenberg E, Corbett S: Crusted (Norwegian) scabies, *J Emerg Med* 22:285–287, 2002.

18. What agents are used to treat scabies?

Sixty grams of 5% permethrin cream should be applied at night from the neck down with special attention to the subungual areas on the fingernails and the genitalia as well as the waistline. The cream

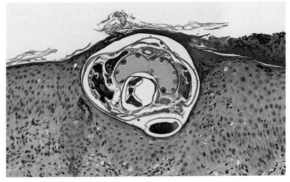

Figure 34-4. Biopsy of scabies demonstrating mite in burrow. (Courtesy of James E. Fitzpatrick, MD.)

should be removed in the morning and the clothes and linen from the night before should be thoroughly washed in hot water and dried. This entire procedure should be repeated in 4 to 5 days. All members of the family should be treated to eliminate asymptomatic, incubating cases. A shortened two-hour application may be used in pregnancy, if indicated.

Between 5% and 10% sulfur ointment may be applied every day for 3 days after a tepid or lukewarm bath. This method is particularly attractive to use in pregnant or lactating women and infants under the age of 2 months. Ivermectin 200 to 400 μg/kg may be administered twice, two weeks apart (not FDA approved). Until further data becomes available, this therapy should not be used in young children or pregnant/breast-feeding women.

Karthikeyan K: Treatment of scabies: newer perspectives, *Postgrad Med J* 81:7–11, 2005.
Bolognia JL, Jorizzo JL, Rapini R Petal: *Dermatology*, Spain, 2008, Mosby-Elsevier.

19. Discuss the three varieties of lice that affect humans.

The head louse (*Pediculus humanus* var. *capitus*) is 2 to 4 mm long with three pairs of legs that are of equal length. The body is dorsoventrally flattened. The entire life cycle is spent in the scalp hair. The visible eggs or nits are deposited on the hair shaft, singly and close to the scalp. Pruritus of the scalp with secondary infection is common. Associated cervical and occipital lymphadenopathy is common. Head lice are more common in school-aged children, especially young females with longer hair (Fig. 34-5).

The large **body louse** (*Pediculus humanus* var. *corporis*) resembles the head louse in configuration, only being larger. It lives and reproduces in the lining of the clothes and leaves the clothing only for feeding, being rarely found on the skin. The patient presents with pruritic papules and areas of hyperpigmentation from healing. This problem occurs in the setting of poverty, overcrowding, and poor hygiene in individuals who rarely change or clean their clothes.

The **pubic louse** (*Phthirus pubis*), or crabs, is smaller, broad-shouldered, and has a narrow head. The major crablike body is dorsoventrally flattened and has three pairs of legs. Eggs are found on the hair shaft. The pubic louse may also be found on short occipital scalp, body, eyebrow, eyelash, and axillary hair. One third of sexually active patients with pediculosis pubis have other sexually transmitted diseases.

20. How should lice infestations be treated?

Head and pubic lice infestations are treated similarly. Due to resistance and safety, a 5% permethrin cream is applied 8 to 12 hours overnight, the treatment is repeated in one week (with occlusion), and the scalp (within ¼ inch) is observed for viable nits. Ovide (malathion 0.5%) is applied 8 to 12 hours (approved for individuals over 6 years of age) and the treatment is repeated in 7 days. Finally, oral ivermectin 200 to 250 mg/kg is given on day 1 and day 8. As with scabies, children should get less than 15 kg, and pregnant/lactating women should probably not get oral ivermectin. Removal of the nits with a specially designed, fine-toothed comb ensures that the infestation is clear. All close contacts should also be treated. Body lice are eliminated by thorough cleaning of the clothes or changing them for new ones. The patient needs symptomatic relief only and a fresh change of clothes.

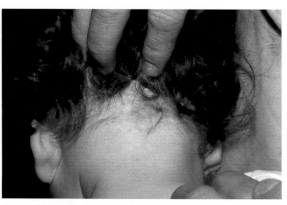

Figure 34-5. Pediculosis. Young girl with pruritic papules on posterior scalp and lower neck. The diagnosis was established by finding nits attached to hair shafts. (Courtesy of the Fitzsimons Army Medical Center teaching files.)

Elston DM: Drugs used in the treatment of pediculosis, *J Drugs Dermatol* 4:207–211, 2005.

ZOONOTIC INFESTATIONS

21. How do flea infestations typically present?

Only the adult flea is a parasitic bloodsucker, while the immature, wormlike, legless, eyeless larvae scavenge for food for the next 1 to 6 months before pupating. The adult fleas are small, approximately 3 mm in size, and streamlined with no neck or waist. They are laterally compressed, taller than broad. Bristles, combs, and claws are used to cling to their host and move briskly through the hair. They are wingless but have powerful rear legs to reach the ankles of their prospective hosts (Fig. 34-6).

Clinical symptoms in pets often vary tremendously, according to their immunologic status. The asymptomatic pet without pruritus often is immunologically tolerant of fleas and, therefore, will have a large number of fleas and flea dirt (flea feces with blood) easily found on the coat. On the other hand, on the severely affected pet with severe pruritus, the organisms may be sparse to absent.

Steen CJ, Carbonaro PA, Schwarz RA: Arthropods in dermatology, *J Am Acad Dermatol* 50:819–842, 2004.

22. How do you treat a flea infestation?

Treatment of the patient is symptomatic. The pet should be treated with insecticidal powders, shampoos, and dips. For each adult flea found on the animal, there are perhaps hundreds of adults, eggs, larvae, and pupae in the bedding material of the pet. Apply strict environmental controls: Vacuum the pet's sleeping areas throughout, wash or destroy the bedding, and apply an insecticide containing a residual pyrethroid and a growth regulator hormone to the area.

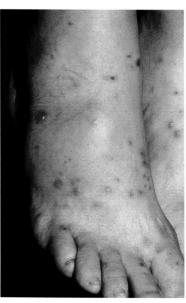

Figure 34-6. Flea bites. Papulovesicular lesions commonly found near the exposed ankles of women.

23. How is *Cheyletiella* infestation recognized in humans? In animals? How does it compare to canine scabies?

Cheyletiella species are free-living, nonburrowing, ectoparasitic mites of dogs, cats, and rabbits. The mite is about the same size as the scabies mite but can be easily differentiated by the presence of pincher-like palps tipped with strong claws used for grasping fur (Fig. 34-7). The eggs are attached to the hair shaft of the animal. The most common sources of the infestation are long-haired cats and new puppies. Animals are often asymptomatic, but a white dandruff-like scale on their backs and necks is often seen on close examination. Small, yellow-white scales which are the mites themselves, are also seen, and hence the disease is called "walking dandruff."

Infested patients complain of pruritic eruptions, which occur most commonly in the sites that correspond to a dog sitting on the patient's lap, volar forearms, abdomen, and anterior thighs. The red papules may develop vesicles, pustules, and even necrosis, and the severity and the extent of the rash depends on the duration of contact with the pet. Diagnosis is made by microscopic examination of the pet. Treatment is directed toward the pet, the pet contacts, and the environment. The patient requires symptomatic care with antiitch medications. *Cheyletiella* is common, and the infestation often goes undiagnosed or unrecognized.

Canine scabies is rarely asymptomatic. Usually the symptoms are severe: redness, scaling, pruritic on the face, margins of the ears and distal extremities. Puppies are always symptomatic. In man, the mite can penetrate clothing and symptoms are severe and onset may occur within an hour. The rash resembles the distribution of *Cheyletiella*—chest, anterior arms, and thighs—but the inverse distribution of human scabies. The face is frequently affected, but hands and genitalia are not affected. The itch is nocturnal and increases with warmth. No burrows are seen. Lindane does not work for pets, so ivermectin and dips are used on all the animals.

Other animals with mite infestations that affect humans include the following:

- *Ornithonyssus sylviarum* (northern fowl mite): Chickens
- *Ornithonyssus bacoti* (tropical rat mite): Rats
- *Ornithonyssus bursa* (tropical fowl mite): Sparrows
- *Dermanyssus gallinae* (poultry mite): Chickens
- Feline scabies: Cats

Lee B: *Cheyletiella*: report of 14 cases, *Cutis* 47:11, 1992.

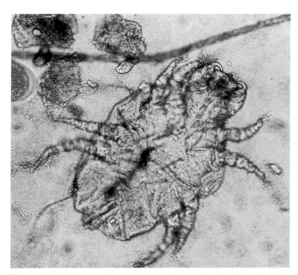

Figure 34-7. *Cheyletiella* mite resembles scabies in size but is identified by the hooklike palps anteriorly.

24. Where do bedbugs live? What do their bites look like?

The human bedbug, *Cimex lectularius,* is a reddish-brown, wingless insect resembling the size and shape of a ladybug that has been stepped on (Fig. 34-8A). They dine alone at night—rapidly and painlessly—but live gregariously during the day in dark closets, behind wallpaper, or under furniture and are not usually seen. Once thought to be associated only with unclean housing, bedbugs can be found in the most pristine homes and may be passively brought in on luggage, clothing, or secondhand furniture. Relatives of the human bedbug may be associated with bats or birds that live in or nearby the home.

The pruritic bites are often multiple and grouped into a "breakfast, lunch, and dinner" pattern (Fig. 34-8B). Treatment of the patient is symptomatic, but fumigation of the home is necessary to get rid of the pest. With a good description of the bug, patients are often able to recover one to confirm the diagnosis.

Thomas I, Kihiczak GG, Schwartz RA: Bedbug bites: a review, *Int J Dermatol* 43:430–433, 2004.
Kolb A, Needham GR, Neyman KM, et al: Bedbugs dermatologic therapy 22:347–352, 2009.

25. Do species of bedbugs that parasitize other animals bite humans?

Yes. Close relatives of the human bedbug often inhabit the nests of birds or bats (Fig. 34-9) that are located in the attic or eaves of homes. They may bite humans, particularly if the natural host leaves the nest. In fact, bird or bat bugs are much more common than human bugs.

Eads RB, Fancy DB, Smith DB: The swallow bug, *O. vicarius* Horvath (Hemiptera: Cimicidae), a human household pest, *Proc Entomtol Soc Wash* 82:81, 1980.

26. What are zoonotic dermatoses?

Zoonotic dermatoses, also called "cryptic bites," are caused by arthropods that infest animals. These include:

- Pets: Dogs, cats, rabbits, gerbils
- Fleas: Only adult fleas bite for blood; immature fleas are scavengers

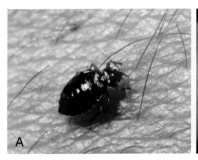

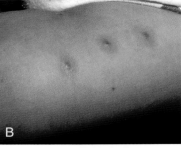

Figure 34-8. A, Human bedbug feeding of human skin. **B,** The bedbug bite typically occurs on the trunk and extremities in a generalized asymmetrical papular eruption that may be grouped into a "breakfast, lunch, and dinner" pattern.

- *Cheyletiella*: Common mite of dogs, cats, rabbits
- Scabies: Canine
- Nesting birds: Swallows, sparrows, pigeons, starlings on or near the house; bites begin when the birds have fledged. Swallow bugs (*Oeciacus vicarus, C. adjunctus*) are not rare
- Bats in attics: *C. pilosellus*
- Pests: Rats, mice

These bites are chronic, recurrent, painless, and very itchy; the organisms are too small to see. Treatment is to disinfect the pet, get rid of any pests, including nearby bats and birds, then spray the area for insects and mites. This should be tightly coordinated. If the natural host of the swallow/bat bug is gone, the bugs will seek new sources of blood, and the bites may increase in number.

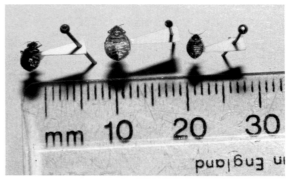

Figure 34-9. Comparison of the bat bug (*left*), human bed bug (*center*), and swallow bug (*right*). Note that all species are elliptically shaped and dorsoventrally flattened.

INSECT VECTORS

27. What are the kissing, or assassin, bugs?

Assassin bugs are triatomids, a subfamily of the reduviids, of the order Hemiptera, or "true bugs," and are generally adapted to nocturnal, rapid (3 to 5 minutes), painless feedings on blood. They live in rural settings, finding refuge in animal burrows, poorly constructed buildings, and occasionally drawn toward lighted homes at night in the southwest United States, Central America, and South America. The bites form red papules that can lead to allergic sensitization and moderately severe itching that last for weeks. Later, large patches of urticaria may develop, as well as systemic anaphylactic reaction.

Vetter R: Kissing bugs (*Triatoma*) and the skin, *Dermatol Online J* 7:6, 2001. (This is a free online journal that includes photographs.)

28. Why are kissing bugs important?

In Central and South America, many triatomids, particularly the kissing bug, or *binchugas*, are infected with the etiologic agent of Chagas' disease (American trypanosomiasis), which is spread to humans from contamination of broken skin with the bug's feces. This triatomid has the unusual feature of defecating immediately after a blood meal so that the itch-induced scratching will contaminate the bite wound with the fecal material containing infectious organisms. It is a leading cause of heart disease in Central and South America and accounts for the death of a large number of young adults in South America. The organism, *T. cruzi*, also affects the esophagus, colon, and nervous system.

29. What diseases are transmitted by ticks?

- **Viruses:** Colorado tick fever, tick-borne encephalitis
- **Rickettsia:** Rocky Mountain spotted fever, ehrlichiosis, typhus
- **Bacteria:** Lyme disease, relapsing fever, tularemia, babesiosis

Shapiro ED: Tick-borne diseases, *Adv Pediatr Infect Dis* 13:187–218, 1997.

30. What is the most common tick-borne infectious disease in the United States?

Lyme disease. It is caused by the *Borrelia burgdorferi*, a spirochete, and transmitted by the hard ticks: *Ixodes scapularis* (deer tick), in the Northeast and the upper Midwest (Minnesota and Wisconsin), and *I. pacificus* in the Pacific states.

31. How does Lyme disease present?

The classic presentation is that of a person—in spring or early summer, living in an endemic area—with a history of a tick bite associated with fever and an annular, spreading rash called *erythema chronicum migrans*. Unfortunately, not all components are always present. As many as 50% of people with Lyme disease never develop the important sign of erythema chronicum migrans, and another 50% of the people do not recall a tick bite.

In addition to constitutional symptoms of general malaise, aches and pains, and fever, the disease may be complicated by cardiac, neurologic, and arthritic symptoms. Treatment in the early phase consists of antibiotics such as amoxicillin, erythromycin, or, most likely, doxycycline for a 3-week period of time. If Lyme disease progresses on to a more chronic problem, or there is evidence of neurologic symptoms, it is often necessary to use ceftriaxone in order to cross the blood–brain barrier.

32. Why do the tick bites often go unnoticed?

The nymphal form of the tick is the most common type to bite humans and is roughly the size of the dot on the letter *i* on this page. In addition to the small size, the bite is painless, due to the tick's salivary secretion of anesthetic, anticoagulant, and cement.

33. How do tick bites affect humans? How are ticks removed once they are attached to the skin?

The tick bite may cause a foreign body reaction, allergic reaction to salivary proteins, reaction to a toxin (e.g., tick paralysis), or, more importantly, infectious disease carried by the tick (Fig. 34-10). Prompt removal of an attached tick may prevent transmission of potential tick-borne infectious disease. Suffocation techniques with petrolatum, heating with matches, or application of irritants should be avoided. Removal of the attached tick should be done by gentle, steady traction by blunt forceps or glove-protected fingers that grip the tick near the head's attachment. Direct contact with the tick should be avoided to prevent contact with infectious organisms. The site and date of the tick removal should be recorded for future observations. The tick can be saved for identification and possible analysis for infectious disease.

Gammons M, Salam G: Tick removal, *Am Fam Physician* 15:643–645, 2002.

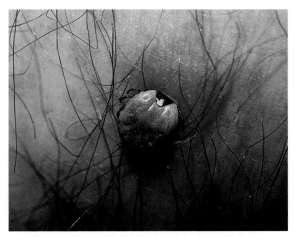

Figure 34-10. Attached feeding tick with an allergic host response manifesting as erythema and induration. (Courtesy of the Fitzsimons Army Medical Center teaching files.)

34. How do you prevent tick bites?
- Wear protective clothing, including long-sleeved shirts and pants tucked into the socks. The clothing should be white or light-colored to facilitate close and frequent inspection for ticks.
- Permethrin-containing spray may be applied to the clothing, where it remains through several washings. This spray serves as a repellent as well as an insecticide.
- Apply repellent containing N,N-diethyl-m-toluamide (DEET) on exposed areas on hands and face. The concentration of deet in the newer preparations is in the 30% to 35% range to lessen concerns about systemic absorption and toxicity.

35. Name some important arthropod-borne diseases.
See Table 34-1.

Table 34-1. Selected Diseases Transmitted by Arthropods	
INFECTIOUS DISEASE	**VECTOR**
Anaplasmosis (human granulocytotropic)	Hard ticks
Arboviruses (including yellow fever, dengue, encephalitis)	Mosquitos, ticks
Babesiosis	Hard ticks
Boutonneuse fever (tick-bite fever) (*Rickettsia conorii*)	Rabbit flea
Chagas disease	Triatomid (kissing) bugs
Colorado tick fever	Hard ticks
Ehrlichiosis, monocytotropic (*Ehrlichia ewingii*)	Hard ticks
Endemic relapsing fever (*Borrelia duttoni*)	Soft ticks
Epidemic relapsing fever (*Borrelia recurrentis*)	Human body lice
Epidemic typhus (*R. prowazekii*)	Human body lice
Filariasis (*Wuchereria bancrofti, Brugia malayi*)	Mosquitos
Leishmaniasis (*Leishmania* spp.)	Phlebotomid flies
Loiasis (*Loa loa*)	Tabanid flies
Lyme disease (*Borrelia burgdorferi*)	Hard ticks
Malaria (*Plasmodium* spp.)	Mosquitos
Murine typhus (*R. mooseri*)	Rat fleas, lice
Onchocerciasis (*Onchocerca volvulus*)	Black flies
Plague (*Yersinia pestis*)	Rat fleas

Continued

Table 34-1. Selected Diseases Transmitted by Arthropods—cont'd

INFECTIOUS DISEASE	VECTOR
Q fever (*Coxiella burnetii*)	Hard ticks, fleas
Rickettsial pox (*R. akari*)	Mouse mites
Rocky Mountain spotted fever (*R. rickettsii*)	Hard ticks
Scrub typhus (*R. tsutsugamushi*)	Mites (chiggers)
Trypanosomiasis, African sleeping sickness	*Glossina* (tsetse) flies
West Nile fever	Mosquitos

Adapted from Braunstein, WB: Ectoparasites. In Mandell GL, Bennett JE, Dolin R, editors: *Principles and practice of infectious diseases*, ed 6, Philadelphia, 2005, Elsevier, pp 3301–3302.

36. What are the most effective insect repellents?

The most effective repellent for the prevention of bites of mosquitos, chiggers, blackflies, midges, and fleas is DEET. An 8% to 10% concentration is adequate for children and a 20% to 50% concentration for adults. A new preparation, extended-duration topical arthropod repellent (Editar), provides a slow release and is marketed by 3M as Ultrathon and by Amway as Hour Guard. Permethrin aerosol (Permanone) applied to clothing is the best tick repellent.

Elston DM: Insect repellents: an overview, *J Am Acad Dermatol* 38:644–645, 1998.

CUTANEOUS MANIFESTATIONS OF INTERNAL MALIGNANCY

Simone A. Ince, MD, and John L. Aeling, MD

1. List the five criteria that establish an association between a skin disease and internal malignancy.

In the late 1950s, Helen Curth, while evaluating acanthosis nigricans, established five criteria necessary to make this association. These five criteria are called Curth's postulates:

1. Concurrent onset of the cutaneous disease and internal malignancy—or at the onset of the cutaneous disease, the internal malignancy is recognizable
2. Parallel course of the skin disease and internal malignancy
3. A specific type or site of malignancy associated with the skin disease
4. Sound statistical evidence that the malignancy is more frequent in patients with the skin disease than in age- and sex-matched controls
5. A genetic link between a syndrome with skin manifestations and an internal malignancy

2. What is Sweet's syndrome?

Sweet's syndrome occurs mostly in women 30 to 60 years of age and consists of characteristic skin lesions, fever, malaise, and leukocytosis. Less commonly, there is involvement of the joints, eyes, lungs, kidneys, and liver. Approximately 20% of cases have an association with a hematopoietic malignancy or, more rarely, a solid tumor.

3. Describe the cutaneous lesions of Sweet's syndrome.

The clinical hallmark of Sweet's syndrome is the presence of sharply demarcated, painful plaques on the face, neck, upper trunk, and extremities (Fig. 35-1). The surface of the plaques has a mammillated (nipple-like) appearance and often shows papulovesicles and pustules. Some lesions have a target-like appearance, and lesions on the lower extremities may resemble erythema nodosum. Oral mucous membrane and eye lesions can be seen. Skin lesions may develop at the site of minor skin trauma or needle-sticks in a small subset of patients. This phenomenon is called *pathergy* and is also seen in pyoderma gangrenosum and Behçet's syndrome.

4. Are any laboratory abnormalities found in Sweet's syndrome?

Leukocytosis. Ten thousand/mm³ is present in 60% of patients. Elevated sedimentation rates, increased numbers of segmented neutrophils, lymphopenia, anemia, thrombocytopenia, and increased C-reactive protein levels can be seen. A handful of cases have been reported with antineutrophilic cytoplasmic antibodies.

5. What cancers are associated with Sweet's syndrome?

The most commonly associated malignancy is acute myelogenous leukemia, but chronic myelogenous leukemia, lymphocytic leukemia, T- and B-cell lymphomas, polycythemia, and, rarely, solid tumors also have been reported. There are no clinical or histopathologic differences between patients with and without associated cancer. Patients with persistent laboratory abnormalities, especially anemia, thrombocytosis, and thrombocytopenia, require close observation and thorough diagnostic evaluation.

Bae-Harboe Y-SC, Salter SA, Kimball A: Acute febrile neutrophilic dermatosis, *eMedicine Online* August 2009. Available at: http://www.emedicine.com.

6. Describe the clinical appearance of acanthosis nigricans.

Acanthosis nigricans appears as velvety, hyperpigmented, papillomatous, dirty-appearing skin. It is most frequently seen on the neck, axilla, groin, and dorsal hand surfaces. It is often associated with numerous skin tags and rarely affects mucosal surfaces (Fig. 35-2).

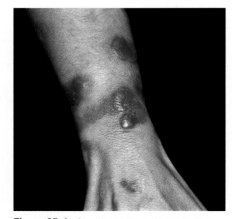

Figure 35-1. Sweet's syndrome demonstrating painful red indurated plaques on on the hand and arm. (Courtesy of James E. Fitzpatrick, MD.)

7. What clinical disease states are associated with acanthosis nigricans?

Acanthosis nigricans is a common skin finding, reported in 7.1% of children aged 11 to 16, and is frequently associated with obesity. It is commonly found in association with diabetes and other endocrinopathies with insulin resistance. Paraneoplastic acanthosis nigricans is rare and is most commonly associated with gastrointestinal cancer, especially gastric carcinoma. When associated with malignancy, it is usually abrupt in onset, severe, and may involve mucous membranes and palmar skin. Findings of tripe palms (resembling rugose bovine intestine) and the sign of Leser-Trélat, discussed later in this chapter, are often seen in patients with paraneoplastic acanthosis nigricans.

Miller J, Rapini R: Acanthosis nigricans, *eMedicine Online,* June 2002. Available at: http://www.emedicine.com/ derm/topic1.htm.

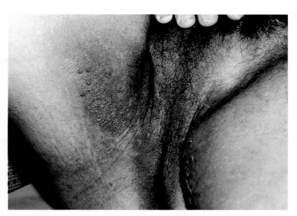

Figure 35-2. Acanthosis nigricans with hyperpigmented velvety skin lesions and small tags on the proximal thigh and groin.

8. What is necrolytic migratory erythema?

This characteristic skin eruption is associated with an α-cell tumor of the pancreas. It presents as erythema with superficial pustules and erosions, typically involving the face, intertriginous skin, and acral extremities (Fig. 35-3). Alopecia, weight loss, glossitis, stomatitis, nail dystrophy, anemia, and diabetes are frequent associations. The eruption tends to migrate and desquamate, and most patients have elevated glucagon serum levels (glucagonoma syndrome). Skin biopsy shows necrosis of the upper portion of the epidermis and is usually diagnostic. This unique skin disease is probably related to low serum amino acid levels.

Zettouni N, Harvey N: Glucagonoma syndrome, *eMedicine Online,* http://www.emedicine.com. May 2008.

9. What is hypertrichosis lanuginosa?

Hypertrichosis lanuginosa (malignant down) is an acquired excessive growth of lanugo hair. It usually begins on the face, neck, and ears and eventually can involve most hair-bearing skin. Glossitis is frequently an associated finding. If drug-related causes (such as minoxidil, diazoxide, and cyclosporine) can be excluded, there is a high association with internal malignancy. The most common associated cancers are lung, breast, gastrointestinal, and carcinoid. This rare cutaneous finding has also been reported in patients with anorexia nervosa.

10. What is Trousseau's sign?

Trousseau's sign consists of recurrent and migratory superficial thrombophlebitis, affecting both large and small cutaneous veins, which is associated with an internal cancer. Crops of oval to linear, erythematous, tender skin lesions are seen most commonly on the arms, legs, flanks, and abdomen. Thrombosis of internal veins can also occur and lead to a variety of symptoms. Men are more commonly affected. The most commonly associated cancers are lung and pancreatic carcinoma.

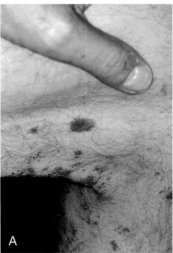

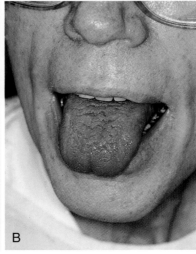

Figure 35-3. Glucagonoma syndrome. **A,** Erosive plaques on the leg. **B,** Atrophic glossitis.

Superficial migratory thrombophlebitis can also be seen in Behçet's syndrome and several coagulation factor deficiencies, including deficiencies of factor V Leiden, factor XII, antithrombin III, protein S and C, and plasminogen activating factor. Hypercoagulable states also occur in patients with anticardiolipin antibody syndrome, liver disease, nephritis, pregnancy, infection, and oral contraceptive use.

Varki A: Trousseau's syndrome: multiple definitions and multiple mechanisms, *Blood* 110:1723–1729, 2007.

11. Describe the classical skin lesions of dermatomyositis.

The classic eruption of dermatomyositis is a reddish-purple erythema involving the face, typically the eyelids (heliotrope sign). The rash may be faint or quite inflamed and edematous (Fig. 35-4A).

In addition to the facial rash, lesions on the scalp, neck, upper trunk, and extensor extremities are common. As the lesions mature, scaling and atrophy may develop. The erythema on the hands occurs over the knuckles rather than over the phalanges, as is typical of lupus erythematosus. Cuticular telangiectasias can be seen in both lupus erythematosus and dermatomyositis. Frequently, flat-topped, red-to-violaceous papules known as *Gottron's papules* develop over the knuckles of patients with dermatomyositis (Fig. 35-4B).

The skin lesions of dermatomyositis may precede clinical or laboratory evidence by weeks, months, or years. A few patients may never develop muscle dysfunction. The skin lesions are notoriously resistant to topical steroid therapy.

12. Is dermatomyositis associated with internal malignancy?

The true incidence of malignancy associated with dermatomyositis is difficult to define. In 153 patients with dermatomyositis, an associated malignancy was found in 8.5% of the total and 19.2% of the men. The cancer may occur before, during, or after the development of dermatomyositis. Most of the reported cases have been in patients over age 40, although cases in children have been reported.

The type of cancer reported to be associated with dermatomyositis parallels the incidence of cancer found in the general population, though a slight increase in ovarian carcinoma has been noted. Patients newly diagnosed with dermatomyositis should have age-appropriate cancer screening, and female patients should be screened for ovarian carcinoma.

Callen JP, Wortman RL: Dermatomyositis, *Clin Dermatol* 24:363–373, 2006.

13. What are the three components of Sézary's syndrome?

As originally described, Sézary's syndrome represents a triad of findings: (1) cutaneous erythema, (2) lymphadenopathy, and (3) 10% to 15% atypical mononuclear cells in peripheral blood.

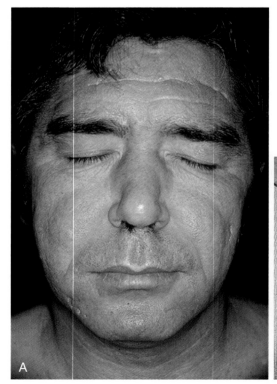
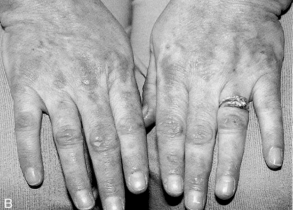

Figure 35-4. Dermatomyositis. **A,** Facial erythema and heliotrope sign. **B,** Classic hand lesions and Gottron's papules on the knuckles.

This syndrome is a subset of cutaneous T-cell lymphoma (CTCL). Erythroderma can also be associated with drug reactions, psoriasis, and other cutaneous diseases. Patients with Sézary syndrome frequently have intolerable itching, often to the point that they are suicidal. Lymphadenopathy, nail dystrophy, and hair loss are common associated features. The diagnosis is established by a skin biopsy showing CTCL, the presence of at least 15% atypical mononuclear cells in peripheral blood, and the typical clinical picture. Approximately 10% to 15% of patients with erythroderma will have an associated lymphoma or, more rarely, leukemia.

Foss F: Mycosis fungoides and the Sézary syndrome, *Curr Opin Oncol* 5:421–428, 2004.

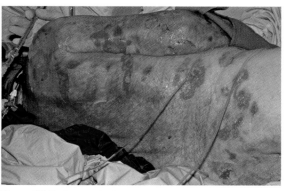

Figure 35-5. Paraneoplastic pemphigus demonstrating extensive superficial blisters and erosions. (Courtesy of James E. Fitzpatrick, MD.)

14. What is paraneoplastic pemphigus?

Paraneoplastic pemphigus is a superficial blistering skin disease with a reported association with lymphoma, although a few cases are reported with solid tumors. The clinical picture may resemble pemphigus vulgaris, bullous pemphigoid, Stevens-Johnson syndrome, with significant oral mucous membrane involvement (Fig. 35-5). The disease responds poorly to immunosuppressive therapy and frequently is fatal.

15. Discuss the laboratory findings in patients with paraneoplastic pemphigus.

Skin and oral mucous membrane biopsy specimens reveal epidermal acantholysis, epidermal spongiosis, suprabasilar clefts, basal cell vacuolar changes, and dyskeratotic keratinocytes. Direct immunofluorescent examination reveals IgG and, less commonly, IgA with or without complement in the intracellular spaces and C3, IgG, or IgM at the basement membrane zone. Antibodies have been demonstrated against desmoplakins, proteins in keratinocyte attachment plaques (desmosomes), and a 230-kDa protein in the basement membrane (bullous pemphigoid antigen). Rat bladder is a useful substrate for indirect immunofluorescent examination and shows positive staining with serum from patients with paraneoplastic pemphigus but will be negative with serum from patients with classic pemphigus vulgaris.

Zhu X, Zhang B: Paraneoplastic pemphigus, *J Dermatol* 34:503–511, 2007.

16. What is the characteristic finding in erythema gyratum repens?

This rare skin eruption is characterized by a widespread, ever-changing pattern of skin lesions resembling wood grain. The erythematous circinate lesions may have a fine scale and move up to 1 cm a day. Almost all patients with this unique dermatosis have an associated malignancy. It was first reported in conjunction with breast cancer, which remains the most common association, but has also been reported with lung, bladder, cervical, and prostate cancers. The skin lesions clear within a few weeks after removal of the malignancy and usually recur if the cancer returns.

DelRosario R, Allen K, Kaneshiro S: Erythema gyratum repens, *eMedicine Online,* http://www.emedicine.com. May 2009.

17. How do the lesions in Bazex syndrome (acrokeratosis paraneoplastica) progress?

This syndrome begins with acral violaceous erythema on the ears, nose, hands, and feet. Early lesions may show small vesicles. As the lesions progress, they become hyperkeratotic and psoriasiform, especially on the hands and feet. Paronychia and nail dystrophy are common. Later, the eruption may generalize, and lesions on the face may appear dermatitic or lupus-like. The syndrome is more common in men and is associated with squamous cell carcinoma of the upper aerodigestive tract.

There is another Bazex syndrome inherited as an autosomal dominant disease. This syndrome is characterized by acral follicular atrophoderma, early development of multiple facial basal cell carcinomas, and, in some patients, hypohidrosis.

Buxtorf K, Hubscher E, Panizzon R: Bazex syndrome, *Dermatology* 202:350–352, 2001.

18. Where does Paget's disease most commonly occur?

On the female breast, although cases have been reported in men. It begins as a small eczematous patch on the nipple that gradually spreads onto the areola and eventually to the skin of the breast. The borders of the lesion are sharply marginated, and the surface may be crusted, moist, erythematous, and/or scaly (Fig. 35-6). Paget's disease of the breast invariably has an underlying ductal carcinoma, although often there is no breast mass and mammograms can be normal. Any chronic eczematous lesion on the nipple or areola that is unresponsive to topical therapy should have an excisional biopsy, which includes nipple ducts and underlying breast tissue. The associated ductal carcinoma may be small and focal and is easily missed by small punch or shave biopsy.

Extramammary Paget's disease occurs on the axilla, groin, or anogenital skin. The disease may present with solitary or multiple lesions. It is often associated with an underlying adnexal carcinoma, and about 20% of cases have carcinoma of the rectum or genitourinary tract.

Kao GF: Paget disease, mammary, *eMedicine Online* November 2007.
Wilde JL: Extramammary Paget's disease, *eMedicine Online,* http://www.emedicine.com. November 2007.

19. Which disorder of protein metabolism is associated with skin lesions and malignancy?

Primary systemic amyloidosis. The cause of this disease is a plasma cell dyscrasia, even though bone marrow aspiration, in some cases, may be normal. The most common associated skin lesions are purpura or ecchymoses that are seen most frequently on thin skin areas, that is, eyelids, neck, groin, axilla, umbilicus, or oral mucosa. The hemorrhagic lesions may occur on areas of clinically normal skin or in skin having waxy papules, plaques, nodules, or tumors. The intracutaneous bleeding is due to infiltration of blood vessel walls with amyloid protein. Other less common skin lesions include alopecia, nail dystrophies, scleroderma-like lesions, macroglossia, cutis verticis gyrata, bullous lesions, and dyspigmentation.

Nyirady J, Schwartz RA: Primary systemic amyloidosis, *eMedicine Online*, http://www.emedicine.com. April 2009.

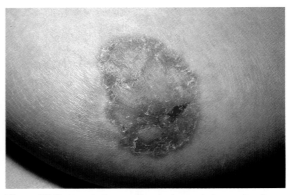

Figure 35-6. Paget's disease. Sharply demarcated area of erythema and scale crust that had been treated as a dermatitis, showing partial destruction of the nipple. The patient had an underlying ductal breast carcinoma. (Courtesy of the Fitzsimons Army Medical Center teaching files.)

20. List the autosomal dominant diseases that have prominent skin findings and internal cancer.

See Table 35-1.

21. Describe the cutaneous features of Gardner's syndrome.

The cutaneous hallmark of the syndrome is epidermoid cysts, which often appear before puberty, frequently on the extremities. These cysts may be many or few. The syndrome is also characterized by osteomas (typically on facial bones), fibrous and desmoid tumors, abnormal dentition, lipomas, hypertrophy of retinal pigmented epithelium, and leiomyomas of the gastrointestinal tract. The syndrome is characterized by the early onset of colonic polyposis and has a very high incidence of colon cancer.

22. What are the clinical findings in Cowden's syndrome (multiple hamartoma syndrome)?

This syndrome is characterized by a triad of findings: (1) small keratotic facial papules (Fig. 35-7A), (2) cobblestoning of the oral mucosa (Fig. 35-7B), and (3) acral keratotic skin lesions. These patients also have benign tumors of neural,

Table 35-1. Autosomal Dominant Diseases with Skin Findings and Malignancy

DISORDER	SKIN FINDINGS	CANCER	ASSOCIATIONS	AFFECTED GENE
Cowden's syndrome	Keratotic facial papules Acral keratosis Soft tissue tumors	Breast Thyroid	Mucosal papules Fibrocystic disease of the breast	*PTEN*
Torre's syndrome	Sebaceous tumors Keratoacanthomas	Colon	Colon polyps	*MSH2, MLH1*
Gardner's syndrome	Epidermoid cysts	Colon	Colon polyps Osteomas Desmoids Abnormal dentition	*APC*
Peutz-Jeghers syndrome	Pigmented macules on mucosa, face, acral extremities	Intestinal	Intestinal polyps	*STK11*
Multiple mucosal neuroma syndrome	Neuromas of lips, tongue, and oral mucosa	Thyroid	Pheochromocytoma Marfanoid habitus	*RET*
Neurofibromatosis	Neurofibromas Café-au-lait macules	Neurofibrosarcoma (rare)	Lisch nodules Seizures Deafness	Neurofibromin
Hereditary leiomyomatosis/renal cell cancer syndrome	Multiple leiomyomas of skin and uterus	Papillary renal cell carcinoma	Fumarate hydratase	

APC, Adenomatosis polyposis coli; MLH1, micronuclear linker histone; MSH2, melanocyte stimulating hormone; PTEN, phosphate and tension homologue deleted on chromosome 10; RET, RET protooncogene (rearranged during transfection); STK11, serine threonine kinase.

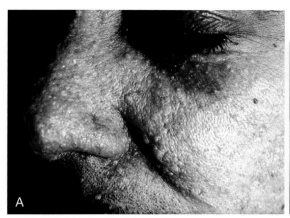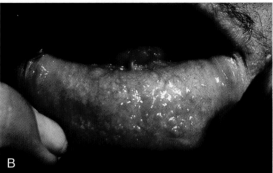

Figure 35-7. Cowden's syndrome. **A,** Typical small keratotic papules on the face. **B,** Characteristic cobblestone papules on the mucosal surface of the lower lip.

fibrous, vascular, and epithelial origin. Multiple small tumors of facial hair follicles (trichilemmomas) are pathognomonic of this syndrome. Fibrocystic disease of the breast is common, and 30% of women will develop breast cancer. Many other associated cancers have been reported, with thyroid cancer being the second most common malignancy.

23. When do the characteristic skin lesions of Peutz-Jeghers syndrome appear?
Brown to blue-black macules (lentigines) are present at birth or early infancy on the lips, oral mucosa, nasal mucosa, palms, soles, dorsal hand surfaces, central face, and elbows. Polyps of the small intestine develop in 90% of patients; polyps may also occur in the stomach, colon, and rectum. There is an increased incidence of gastrointestinal malignancy, but it is not nearly as common as in patients with Gardner's syndrome. In one series, 16 fatal malignancies were seen in 72 cases, with an average age at death of 36 years. Intussusception occurs in about 50% of cases.

24. How does multiple mucosal neuroma syndrome typically present?
As the name implies, this syndrome is characterized by the development of multiple flesh-colored papules on the tongue, lips, and, occasionally, other mucosal surfaces early in life. These patients have a characteristic appearance with thick prominent lips and a marfanoid habitus. Ninety percent of these patients develop medullary thyroid carcinoma, and half will suffer from pheochromocytoma that is often multifocal and/or bilateral.

25. What is Torre's syndrome (Muir-Torre's syndrome)?
This syndrome includes cutaneous sebaceous neoplasia and a high incidence of low-grade colon cancer. The sebaceous tumors include sebaceous adenomas, epitheliomas, and carcinomas. In addition, about one third of patients develop keratoacanthomas. The sebaceous skin tumors may be few or many, but even one sebaceous adenoma should alert the clinician that the patient may have this syndrome.

Winship IM, Dudding T: Lessons from the skin-cutaneous features of familial cancer, *Lancet Oncol* 9:462–472, 2008.

26. Is the sign of Leser-Trélat (eruptive seborrheic keratoses) associated with internal malignancy?
This association remains controversial. Seborrheic keratoses are common in older patients, and so is cancer. There have been many skin lesions and skin diseases reported to be associated with internal malignancy, but these associations are difficult to prove and probably are spurious. Examples include dermatitis herpetiformis, bullous pemphigoid, pemphigus vulgaris (excluding paraneoplastic pemphigus), persistent erythemas (excluding erythema gyratum repens), cutaneous vasculitis, pruritus, scleroderma, and ichthyosis.

Schwartz R: The sign of Leser-Trélat, *eMedicine Online* May 2009.

27. Is dry scaly skin associated with internal malignancy?
Yes. Acquired ichthyosis was first reported to be associated with Hodgkin's disease in the 1940s. In 32 patients with acquired ichthyosis, Hodgkin's disease was reported in 80% of the cases and was the presenting symptom in a few patients. This association is also reported with T-cell lymphoma, leukemia, Kaposi's sarcoma, malignant histiocytosis, leiomyosarcoma, and multiple myeloma.

Moore RL, Devere TS: Epidermal manifestations of internal malignancy, *Dermatol Clin* 26(1):17–29, vii, 2008.

28. Which recessively inherited diseases have skin findings and associated internal malignancy?
See Table 35-2.

Table 35-2. Recessively Inherited Diseases with Skin Findings and Malignancy

DISORDER	INHERITANCE	CLINICAL FINDINGS	CANCER	AFFECTED GENE
Wiskott-Aldrich syndrome	X-linked recessive	Chronic dermatitis Thrombocytopenia Recurrent infections	Lymphoma, especially non-Hodgkin's	WAS
Bloom's syndrome	Autosomal recessive	Photosensitivity Telangiectasia of sun-exposed skin Short stature Decreased serum immunoglobulins Recurrent infections Sister chromatid exchange	Lymphomas Leukemias	RecQ3
Ataxia-telangiectasia (Louis-Bar syndrome)	Autosomal recessive	Progressive cerebellar ataxia Telangiectasia Recurrent sinus and pulmonary infections Decreased/absent serum IgA	Lymphomas (increased cancer risk also seen in heterozygotes)	ATM
Dyskeratosis congenita	X-linked recessive Autosomal dominant	Skin atrophy and hyperpigmentation Nail dystrophy Oral precancerous leukokeratosis	Oral cancers Other malignancies	DKC1 TERC

WAS, Wiskott-Aldrich syndrome; RecQ3, DNA helicase Rec Q protein-like-3; ATM, ataxia telangiectasia mutated; DKC1, dyskerin; TERC, telomerase RNA component.

29. Can pyoderma gangrenosum be associated with internal malignancy?

Yes. Pyoderma gangrenosum (PG) is an ulcerative skin disease of unknown etiology. The lesions are painful, may rapidly enlarge, and are characterized by an erythematous or violaceous undermined border with a necrotic center (Fig. 35-8). The most common diseases associated with PG are inflammatory bowel disease, rheumatoid arthritis, and a small subset may have monoclonal IgA gammopathy. In a review of several studies, PG was associated with internal malignancy in 7.2% of patients. Leukemia is the most frequently reported malignancy with myelocytic and myelomonocytic leukemia accounting for the majority of cases. Other reported hematologic cancers are multiple myeloma, polycythemia vera, and lymphoma. In two thirds of the cases associated with myelocytic leukemia, the PG preceded or was concurrent with the diagnosis of the leukemia.

There are rare sporadic reports of PG associated with solid tumors.

Callen J. Jackson JM: Pyoderma gangrenosum: an update, *Rheumatol Dis Clin N Am* 33:787–802, 2007.

30. What is erythromelalgia?

Erythromelalgia is a rare skin disease characterized by erythematous, painful, burning of the feet, ankles, and lower extremities. The disease is aggravated by heat exposure and relieved by cooling. Many patients can find relief only by soaking their legs in ice water. The incidence of associated malignancy has been variably reported as between 3% and 65% of cases. Some authors subdivide the disease into two subtypes: the idiopathic type, which frequently begins in childhood, and the secondary type associated with hematologic malignancies, usually polycythemia vera or essential thrombocythemia.

Nardino RT, Silber AL: Erythromelalgia, *eMedicine Online,* http://www.emedicine.com. August 2009.

31. Can pruritus be a sign of malignancy?

Generalized pruritus without skin lesions has been reported as a symptom of internal malignancy. Pruritus is reported as an initial symptom of Hodgkin's disease in 5% to 10% of patients and in 3% of those with non–Hodgkin's lymphoma. The relationship of this symptom to visceral solid cancers is far less clear.

Lober CW: Pruritis and malignancy, *Clin Dermatol* 11:125–128, 1993.

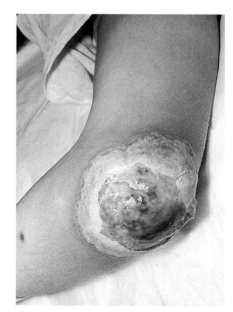

Figure 35-8. A young woman with acute-onset pyoderma gangrenosum.

Key Points: Cutaneous Manifestations of Internal Malignancy

1. Patients with biopsy-proven Sweet's syndrome should have a complete blood count to evaluate for an underlying hematologic malignancy.
2. Acanthosis nigricans is a common condition, and most cases are associated with insulin resistance. Paraneoplastic acanthosis nigricans is rare, may be of explosive onset, and associated with tripe palms and the sign of Leser-Trélat.
3. Patients with refractory oral pemphigus vulgaris should be evaluated for paraneoplastic pemphigus.
4. Patients with dermatomyositis should have age-appropriate cancer screening, and women should be screened for ovarian carcinoma.
5. Any refractory eczematous eruption on the breast should be biopsied to exclude mammary Paget's disease.

32. Is vasculitis associated with malignancy?

Vasculitis is rarely associated with internal malignancy. In one large review of 200 patients with vasculitis and cancer, 77.5% had a hematologic malignancy.

Paydas S, Zorludemir S, Sahin B: Vasculitis and leukemia, *Leuk Lymphoma* 40:105–112, 2000.

33. What is multicentric reticulohistiocytosis?

Multicentric reticulohistiocytosis is a rare disease characterized by multiple skin papules and nodules in patients with severe arthritis. Skin biopsy shows characteristic histology of a diffuse histiocytic cellular infiltrate with large multinucleate giant cells with ground-glass cytoplasm. Associated malignancy was reported in 28% of the patients in 82 cases reported in the literature. The disease preceded the development of cancer in 73% of the patients. This association is controversial, there was no consistent cancer reported, and there are no careful prospective studies.

Rapini RP: Multicentric reticulohistiocytosis, *eMedicine Online,* http://www.emedicine.com. March 2008.

34. What is carcinoid syndrome? Does it have prognostic significance?

Carcinoid syndrome is a systemic manifestation of neuroendocrine carcinoid tumors that manifest most commonly by flushing that progresses to persistent telangiectasia (Fig. 35-9) and diarrhea. Less common findings include bronchospasm, cardiac valvular dysfunction, and pellagra-like skin changes (photodistributed dermatitis). It is estimated that 10% of patients with carcinoid tumors will develop this syndrome. Development of this syndrome has prognostic significance, as liver metastases underlie most cases, and thus it signifies metastatic, unresectable disease.

Santacroce L, Diomede D, Balducci L: Malignant carcinoid syndrome, *eMedicine Online,* http://www.emedicine.com. November 2009.

35. What is FAMM syndrome?

FAMM is the **f**amilial **a**typical **m**ultiple mole **m**elanoma–pancreatic cancer syndrome, and it appears to be related to germline mutations in cyclin-dependent kinase inhibitor 2A (CDKN2A). Affected patients have numerous clinically atypical nevi, increased lifetime risk for melanoma, and a family history of melanoma and/or pancreatic cancer. Affected families benefit from screening for early detection of pancreatic cancer.

Lynch HT, Fusaro R, Lynch JF, et al: Pancreatic cancer and the FAMM syndrome, *Fam Cancer* 7:103–112, 2008.

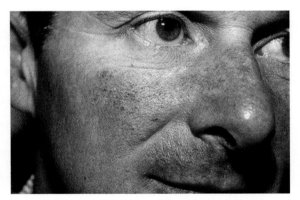

Figure 35-9. Carcinoid syndrome. Patient with long history of flushing and development of persistent telangiectasias of the face. (Courtesy of the Fitzsimons Army Medical Center teaching files.)

CUTANEOUS MANIFESTATIONS OF ENDOCRINOLOGIC DISEASE

Shayla Francis, MD, and Carl F. Bigler, MD

1. How does endocrinologic disease cause skin disorders?

There are several mechanisms by which endocrinologic diseases produce cutaneous changes:

- Hormones interact with cell surface receptors to regulate cellular function. Many cell types in the skin have hormonal receptors. Deficient or excess hormone levels can alter skin metabolism. An example is the warm and moist skin associated with hyperthyroidism due to the thyroid-stimulating hormone (thyrotropin, TSH) receptors in the skin.
- Hormone deficiency or excess may affect the skin indirectly rather than through specific receptors. An example is the hyperglycemia of diabetes that results in increased cutaneous infections from impaired immune function.

For some unusual skin disorders that are highly suggestive of endocrinologic disease, such as necrobiosis lipoidica diabeticorum, the pathogenesis is not understood.

Ciafarani F, Baldini E, Cavalli A, et al: TSH receptor and thyroid-specific gene expression in human skin, *J Invest Dermatol* 130:93–101, 2010.

2. What is necrobiosis lipoidica?

This disease is characterized by granulomatous inflammation and fibrosis with a marked predilection to occur on the pretibial areas, although it may occur at other sites. Early lesions present as nondiagnostic erythematous papules and evolve into annular lesions that have a yellowish-brown color, dilated blood vessels, and central epidermal atrophy (Fig. 36-1). Fully developed pretibial lesions can be diagnosed by clinical appearance.

3. Do all patients with necrobiosis lipoidica have diabetes?

No. In a study of 171 patients with necrobiosis lipoidica, about 60% had diabetes. Many other patients subsequently developed diabetes, had abnormal glucose tolerance tests, or had a strong family history of diabetes. Only about 10% of patients were not in a high-risk group to develop diabetes. In a more recent study with 65 patients, 22% either had or developed diabetes. Patients with necrobiosis lipoidica should be screened for diabetes.

Peyrí J, Moreno A, Marcoval J: Necrobiosis lipoidica, *Semin Cutan Med Surg* 26:87–89, 2007.

Wee SA, Possick P: Necrobiosis lipoidica, *Dermatol Online J* 10:18, 2004. (Readers can go to this article online and read case history, see clinical photographs, biopsy, read discussion, and get references.)

4. Is necrobiosis lipoidica diabeticorum common in patients with diabetes?

No. It occurs in 0.3% of patients with diabetes and may occur in both insulin-dependent and insulin-resistant diabetic patients. It is most frequently seen in adults but has rarely been reported in children with insulin dependent diabetes.

de Silva BD, Schofield OM, Walker JD: The prevalence of necrobiosis lipoidica diabeticorum in children with type 1 diabetes, *Br J Dermatol* 141(3):593–594, 1999.

5. Does glucose control affect necrobiosis lipoidica diabeticorum?

It is unclear whether tight glucose control changes the appearance or clinical course of the disease. Multiple studies have suggested that there is no effect, but Cohen et al conclude that tighter glucose control might prevent presentation of the lesions.

Cohen O, Yaniv R, Karasik A, Trau H: Necrobiosis lipoidica and diabetic control revisited, *Med Hypotheses* 46(4):348–350, 1996.

6. What other skin findings are associated with insulin resistance?

Acanthosis nigricans. Insulin-like growth factors are produced by the liver in response to high levels of circulating insulin. These growth factors bind to epidermal growth factor receptors or other receptors and produce thickening of the epidermis and hyperkeratosis. Acanthosis nigricans can be found in 30% to 50% of patients with diabetes and correlates with obesity and insulin resistance. Acanthosis nigricans may predict the future development of diabetes in high-risk populations with strong family histories for diabetes and obesity.

Hermanns-Le T, Scheen A, Pierard GE: Acanthosis nigricans associated with insulin resistance: pathophysiology and management, *Am J Clin Dermatol* 5:199–203, 2004.

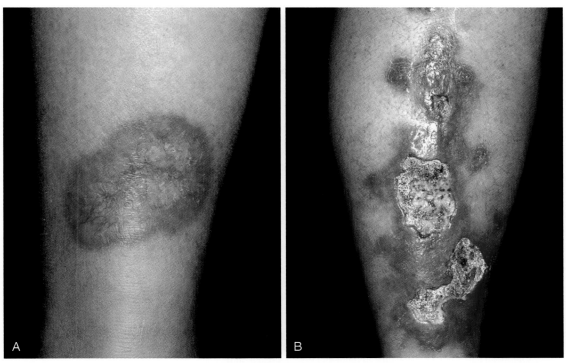

Figure 36-1. Necrobiosis lipoidica diabeticorum. **A,** Typical yellow-red plaque of a developed lesion. **B,** Late lesion with central atrophy and extensive ulceration. (Courtesy of James E. Fitzpatrick, MD.)

7. What does acanthosis nigricans look like?

Acanthosis nigricans presents as velvety, hyperpigmented plaques, most commonly in neck creases and axillae (Fig. 36-2). The patient may complain about "dirty skin" under the arms that is impossible to clean. The tops of knuckles may also demonstrate small papules.

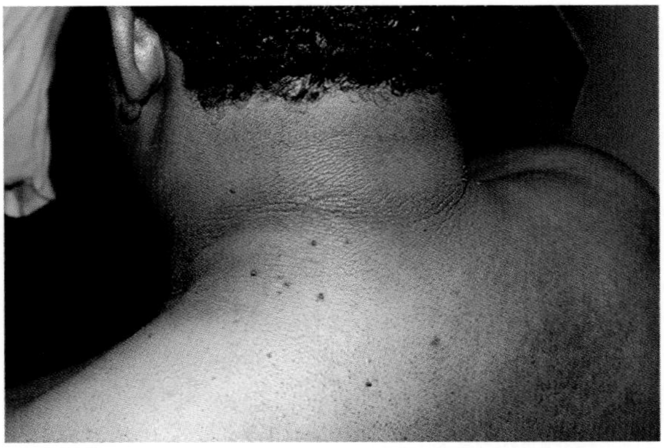

8. Is diabetes the only condition associated with acanthosis nigricans?

No. There are many causes of insulin resistance and hyperinsulinemia. Endocrine diseases, such as Cushing's syndrome with excess cortisol, acromegaly with excess growth hormone, or polycystic ovarian disease, and medications that promote hyperinsulinemia are also associated with acanthosis nigricans. Certain malignancies, most commonly gastrointestinal adenocarcinomas, may autonomously make insulin-like growth factors and thus produce acanthosis nigricans. Oral acanthosis nigricans suggests malignancy as the cause.

Figure 36-2. Velvety hyperpigmentation of the neck crease in a patient with classic acanthosis nigricans. (Courtesy of James E. Fitzpatrick, MD.)

Higgins S, Freemark M, Prose N: Acanthosis nigricans: a practical approach to evaluation and management, *Dermatol Online J* 14(9):2, 2008.

9. What bacterial infections are more common in diabetic patients?

Cutaneous bacterial infections are relatively more common and severe in patients with diabetes. Diabetic foot ulcers are a leading cause of morbidity and health care cost. Foot numbness from diabetic neuropathy prevents recognition of injury and hyperglycemia impairs white blood cell function, allowing bacterial infection. Staphylococcal folliculitis or skin abscesses are well described in diabetic patients and respond well to antibiotics and surgical drainage of abscesses. Diabetic patients may develop external necrotizing ear infections caused by *Pseudomonas aeruginosa*.

There is increasing evidence that diabetes mellitus is an important risk factor for tuberculosis. It also may affect disease presentation and treatment response. Additionally, evidence suggests that tuberculosis might induce glucose intolerance and worsen glycemic control in people with diabetes.

Dooley KE, Chaisson RE: Tuberculosis and diabetes mellitus: convergence of two epidemics, *Lancet Infect Dis* 9:737–746, 2009.

10. What are the most common fungal skin infections associated with diabetes?

Candidiasis, usually caused by *Candida albicans*. Mucocutaneous candidiasis is characterized by red plaques with adherent white exudate and satellite pustules. Candidal vulvovaginitis is extremely common. Perianal dermatitis in either men or women may be caused by *Candida*. Other mucocutaneous forms of candidiasis include thrush (infection of oral mucosa), perlèche (angular cheilitis), intertrigo (infection of skinfolds), erosio interdigitalis blastomycetica chronica (finger webspace infection), paronychia (infection of the soft tissue around the nail plate), and onychomycosis (infection of the nail). The mechanism appears to involve increased levels of glucose that serve as a substrate for *Candida* species to proliferate. Patients with recurrent cutaneous candidiasis of any form should be screened for diabetes.

Dermatophytosis is also common in the general population as well as in diabetic patients. A recent epidemiologic study found that among all dermatophyte infections, *Trichophyton rubrum* was the most frequently isolated. Tinea pedis was identified as the most frequent, followed by tinea unguium, tinea corporis, tinea cruris, tinea manuum, and tinea capitis including kerion.

Watanabe S: Dermatomycosis—classification, etiology, pathogenesis, and treatment: *Nippon Rinsho* 66:2285–2289, 2008.

11. Are there more dangerous fungal infections associated with diabetes?

Rarely, mucormycosis will complicate diabetic ketoacidosis. Mucormycosis is a severe and progressive infection of the soft tissues caused by saprophytic fungi such as *Mucor*, *Rhizopus*, and *Absidia* species. This infection is poorly responsive to systemic antifungals and is often fatal.

12. Why are diabetic patients in ketoacidosis especially prone to mucormycosis?

These fungi prefer an acid pH, grow rapidly in high-glucose media, and are some of the few fungi that utilize ketones as a growth substrate. All these growth requirements are present in patients with diabetic ketoacidosis.

13. What other skin disorders are commonly encountered in diabetic patients?

Diabetic dermopathy (atrophic, scarred, hyperpigmented papules on the anterior leg), periungual telangectasias, yellow skin and nails, skin tags, and diabetic thick skin occur commonly. Bullous disease of diabetes (tense bullae of the lower extremities), vitiligo, and scleroderma-like symptoms such as diabetic stiff hands and thickened skin on the upper back (scleredema adultorum) are less common associations.

Van Hattem S, Bootsma AH, Thio HB: Skin manifestations of diabetes, *Cleve Clin J Med* 75(11):772, 774, 776–777, 2008.

14. Describe the clinical manifestation of pretibial myxedema.

Pretibial myxedema is characterized by brawny, indurated plaques over the pretibial areas. These plaques may be skin-colored or have an unusual brownish-red color (Fig. 36-3A). On biopsy, the skin is infiltrated by mucinous ground substance (Fig. 36-3B). Pretibial myxedema is specific for Graves' disease, a frequent cause of hyperthyroidism, but occurs in only 3% to 5% of patients with the disease. Pretibial myxedema is often associated with Graves' ophthalmopathy (bulging eyes or exophthalmos) and acropachy (clubbed nails). Treatment of hyperthyroidism has no effect on pretibial myxedema.

Ai J, Leonhardt JM, Heymann WR: Autoimmune thyroid diseases: etiology, pathogenesis, and dermatologic manifestations, *J Am Acad Dermatol* 48:641–659, 2003.

15. Why does treatment of Graves' disease have no effect on pretibial myxedema?

Graves' hyperthyroidism is an autoimmune disease produced by autoantibodies that bind to thyrotropin (TSH) receptors in the thyroid gland, stimulating the thyroid to produce and release thyroid hormone. Pretibial connective tissue also has thyrotropin receptors. Stimulation of these receptors is the proposed mechanism of mucin production in pretibial connective tissue. Treatment of Graves' disease treats hyperthyroidism but not the underlying autoimmune disease.

Daumerie C, Ludgate M, Costagliola S, Many MC: Evidence for thyrotropin receptor immunoreactivity in pretibial connective tissue from patients with thyroid-associated dermopathy, *Eur J Endocrinol* 146:35–38, 2002.

16. What are the skin manifestations of hypothyroidism?

- **Mild hypothyroidism:** The skin is dry, scaly, cold, and pale. Dryness and scale may make the skin pruritic. The nails are brittle.
- **Severe and long-standing hypothyroidism:** There may be yellow and diffusely thickened skin (Fig. 36-4), loss of the outer third of the eyebrows and enlarged and thickened lips and tongue.

17. Why do hypothyroid patients have yellow skin?

The yellow skin is due to excess serum carotene that is deposited in the stratum corneum. Carotenemia results from impaired hepatic conversion of carotene to vitamin A in patients with hypothyroidism.

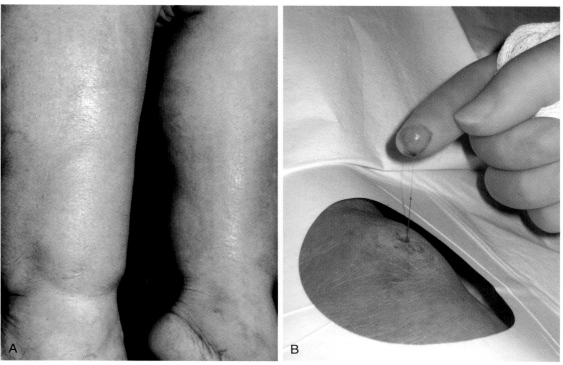

Figure 36-3. Pretibial myxedema. **A,** Large indurated skin-colored plaques. **B,** A positive "string sign" of mucin extending from the biopsy site to the surgical glove. (Panel B courtesy of Scott Freeman, MD.)

18. Why do hypothyroid patients have thickened skin?

There is increased dermal mucopolysaccharide or mucin within the skin (myxedema).

19. How does the myxedema of hypothyroidism differ from pretibial myxedema of Graves' disease?

Myxedema of hypothyroidism has smaller quantities of mucin with a generalized distribution over the entire surface area of skin. Pretibial myxedema often has dermal pools of mucin and is localized to the anterior legs.

20. Are the skin changes of hypothyroidism reversible with thyroid replacement?

Yes.

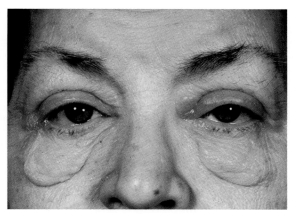

Figure 36-4. Patient with severe generalized myxedema demonstrating intensive periocular edema and very yellow skin.

21. What are the skin manifestations of hyperthyroidism?

They are the opposite of hypothyroidism. Hyperthyroid skin is moist, warm, smooth, and erythematous. The nails may separate from the nailbed (onycholysis). The skin may be pruritic. Because itchy skin may occur with either high or low thyroid hormone, patients with itchy skin of unknown cause should have thyroid disease excluded.

22. Which hormone gives the skin a darkened or tanned appearance?

Adrenocorticotropic hormone (ACTH) darkens the skin by stimulating melanocytes to produce melanin. In contrast to normal tanning, the darkening is often accentuated in palmar creases and mucous membranes. (A note of caution: dark skin creases and mucous membranes may be a normal variant in more darkly pigmented races.) The most common cause of elevated ACTH levels is Addison's disease, in which hypofunctioning adrenals and deficient serum cortisol remove the negative feedback inhibition of the pituitary gland that increases ACTH production.

Slominski A, Tobin DJ, Shibahara S, Wortsman J: Melanin pigmentation in mammalian skin and its hormonal regulation, *Physiol Rev* 84:1155–1228, 2004.

23. What skin disease is associated with insulin-dependent diabetes, hypothyroidism, and Addison's disease?

Vitiligo. This is a trick question. Vitiligo is not caused by deficient hormones but is an autoimmune disease that results in the destruction of melanocytes and is associated with the autoimmune endocrinopathies. Vitiligo presents clinically as white macules, most commonly on the face and hands. Vitiligo is present in 4% of patients with insulin-dependent diabetes, 7% of patients with Graves' disease, and 15% of patients with Addison's disease. There is also a familial predisposition to this group of diseases.

24. What skin findings are associated with glucocorticoid excess or Cushing's disease?

The skin is generally thin and atrophic. Wound repair is inhibited, and striae developed in sites such as the abdomen, upper chest, and buttocks, where the skin is normally stretched. These striae are often large and purple in color, in contrast to idiopathic or pregnancy-induced striae (Fig. 36-5). The skin has a ruddy appearance, and telangiectasias may be prominent. The skin bruises and tears easily. Other skin changes include hypertrichosis, dryness, fragility of the skin, and facial acne. These changes may also be seen in skin that has been treated with high-strength topical steroids for long periods of time. Broadened facial features (moon facies), increased subcutaneous fat on the upper back and neck (buffalo hump), and truncal obesity are also characteristic.

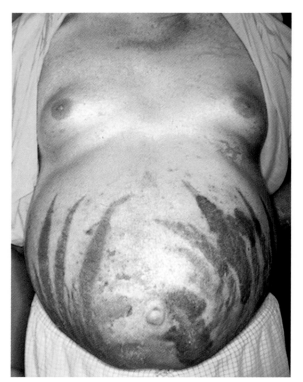

Figure 36-5. Cushing's syndrome (excess glucocorticoids), showing truncal obesity and abdominal striae. (Courtesy of James E. Fitzpatrick, MD.)

25. Are the skin changes caused by excess glucocorticoids reversible?

Partially. Striae and telangiectasias may fade but often do not disappear.

26. Which hormones have the greatest effect on sebaceous glands and hair?

The androgens. Androgens at the time of puberty induce sebaceous gland activity and the development of acne. Excess androgen in women may cause acne, hirsutism (increased facial hair), and/or alopecia. Associated signs may include hyperpigmentation of genital and areolar skin and clitoromegaly. Possible causes of hirsutism and acne in women include adrenal and ovarian tumors, prolactin-producing pituitary tumors, polycystic ovarian disease, adrenal enzyme deficiencies, and familial acne and hirsutism that may be related to increased end-organ sensitivity to normal circulating levels of androgens. Most acne and hirsutism in women is benign and familial. Screening tests for tumors include serum prolactin; dehydroepiandrosterone sulfate (DHEAS), which is an androgen produced by the adrenal glands; and free testosterone.

27. Are there medications and nutritional supplements that may cause acne?

Yes. Supplements and medications that have androgen effects and can cause acne may not appear in the patient's list of medications. New-onset acne in a recreational weightlifter, either male or female, may result from the abuse of androgens. New-onset acne in a young woman may be from birth control pills that are low in estrogen. The progesterone-like hormone in many birth control pills and in all long-acting depository forms may have androgen effects. New onset acne in a perimenopausal woman may result from small amounts of testosterone added to some estrogen supplements. High-dose glucocorticoid therapy can also cause acne. The acne that occurs from changing hormone levels takes 4 to 6 weeks to appear.

Hartgens F, Kuipers H: Effects of androgenic-anabolic steroids in athletes, *Sports Med* 34:513–554, 2004.

28. What hormonal methods are available to treat acne?

Estrogens often antagonize the effects of androgens. High-dose estrogen birth control pills that use progesterone-like hormones with few androgen effects have been approved for the treatment of acne in women. Spironolactone, an aldosterone antagonist that acts as a relatively weak antiandrogen, has been used to treat hormone related acne in women over the age of 35. Additionally, it has been used for treatment of hirsuitism, androgenic alopecia, and hydradenitis suppurativa due to its antiandrogen effects.

Shaw J: Antiandrogen and hormonal treatment of acne, *Dermatol Clin* 14:803–811, 1996.

29. What are xanthelasma?

Xanthelasma (palpebra) are distinctive yellowish plaques on the eyelids and around the eyes caused by cholesterol deposition within the skin (Fig. 36-6). Although people with xanthelasma may have normal total cholesterol and triglyceride levels, they often have more subtle lipid abnormalities associated with high cardiovascular risk and deposition of cholesterol within blood vessels. As opposed to other xanthomas, treatment of xanthelasma with surgical excision is often successful.

Elabjer B, Busic M, Sekelj S, Kristovijevic E: Operative treatment of large periocular xanthelasma, *Orbit* 28:16–19, 2009.

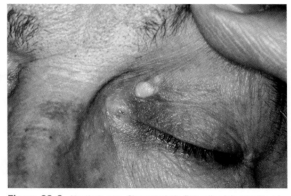

Figure 36-6. Xanthelasma. Characteristic flat yellowish papules of the upper eyelid. (Courtesy of the Fitzsimons Army Medical Center teaching files).

30. What are eruptive xanthomas?

Eruptive xanthomas are multiple, small, skin-colored to yellow-brown papules that occur in crops, most commonly on the buttocks, thighs, or elbows (Fig. 36-7A). On biopsy, there is accumulation of triglyceride within histiocytes and around blood vessels in the skin. These distinctive papules are a cutaneous sign of very high triglyceride levels. These patients are at risk to develop pancreatitis, which may be severe. Often, eruptive xanthomas are precipitated by the new onset of diabetes.

Naik NS: Eruptive xanthomas, *Dermatol Online J* 7:11, 2001. (Readers can go to this article online, read case history, see clinical photographs, biopsy, read discussion, and get references.)

31. How do eruptive xanthomas differ from tuberous xanthomas?

Tuberous xanthomas are larger and deeper than eruptive xanthomas and may be palpated as nodules similar to a large radish, a small turnip, or other vegetable tuber or root within the deep dermis or subcutaneous fat (Fig. 36-7B). These xanthoms are the result of cholesterol accumulation within these tissues, in contrast to the smaller, papular, eruptive xanthomas that contain triglyceride. Tuberous xanthomas are a marker of high cholesterol levels, and these patients

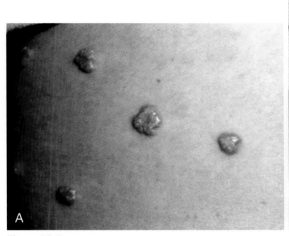

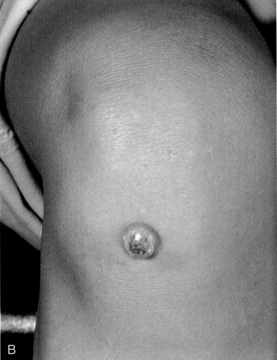

Figure 36-7. A, Eruptive xanthomas demonstrating typical yellow-brown papules. This patient's triglyceride level was 7760. **B,** Tuberous xanthoma manifesting as a large nodular xanthoma of the knee. (Courtesy of James E. Fitzpatrick, MD.)

are at risk for coronary artery disease at a young age. Tendinous xanthomas (e.g., similar lesions attached to large tendons, such as the Achilles tendon) may also be present.

32. What are the cutaneous features of acromegaly?

Acromegaly is the result of excess pituitary growth hormone present after puberty. Bone thickening is prominent and results in coarse facies and enlarged hands. The skin changes are the result of the production of insulin-like growth factors and, thus, overlap with changes due to insulin resistance. The skin is hypertrophied and thickened, and acanthosis nigricans may be present. These changes may be accentuated on the scalp as whorled furrowing (cutis vertices gyrata) in 30% of patients.

Centurión SA, Schwartz RA: Cutaneous signs of acromegaly, *Int J Dermatol* 41:631–634, 2002.

Key Points: Xanthomas

1. The presence of one or more xanthomas on the skin usually indicates the presence of an abnormality of lipid metabolism or, less commonly, a monoclonal gammopathy.
2. Xanthomas are histologically characterized by the accumulation of lipids in tissue macrophages.
3. The presence of eruptive xanthomas always indicates the presence of high levels of triglycerides.
4. Patients with eruptive xanthomas are at increased risk to develop pancreatitis.
5. Most patients with xanthelasma often have normal serum levels of triglycerides and cholesterol but often have other abnormalities of apolipoprotein metabolism.

---

33. How does panhypopituitarism affect the skin?

The skin in patients with panhypopituitarism appears pale, and there are fine wrinkles around the eyes and mouth. Body hair and genital hair are sparse. Sweat and sebum production are also diminished. The skin dryness and thickening are not as prominent as in primary hypothyroidism because there is some autonomous thyroid gland function in panhypopituitarism.

34. How do you diagnose endocrine disease from skin findings?

- Most skin findings are nonspecific but related to the specific effect of the hormone on the skin. An example is dry, thickened skin in hypothyroidism or skin infections in diabetes. Dry skin and skin infections may occur in many other diseases or, in most cases, such as dry skin in a dry climate or folliculitis, happen in otherwise normal people.
- Nonspecific skin findings are grouped with nonspecific findings from other organ systems to suggest the appropriate endocrine diagnosis. Dry, thickened skin with weight gain, fatigue, depression, and lethargy would be highly suggestive of hypothyroidism. Multiple skin or mucous membrane infections with yeast or bacteria coupled with increased urination should prompt tests for diabetes.
- More specific skin findings often occur in a minority of patients with endocrinologic disease but are highly suggestive of the diagnosis when present. Patients with acanthosis nigricans or necrobiosis lipoidica should be screened for diabetes. Pretibial myxedema is a feature of Graves' hyperthyroidism. Xanthelasma is associated with cardiovascular risk and more subtle lipid abnormalities. Eruptive xanthomas occur with marked hypertriglyceridemia and tuberous xanthomas with very high serum cholesterol.

SKIN SIGNS OF GASTROINTESTINAL DISEASE

Christina S. O'Hara, MSIII, 2LT MC, and Paul M. Benson, MD, COL (Ret), MC

1. List some of the hallmark skin signs seen with diseases of the digestive tract.

- **Cirrhosis:** Jaundice, ascites, purpura, spider angiomas
- **Peutz-Jeghers syndrome (PJS):** Lip lentigo
- **Inflammatory bowel disease:** Pyoderma gangrenosaum on legs
- **Gardner's syndrome:** Osteomas, epidermoid inclusion cysts

It is logical that many diseases of the skin also involve the oral and anal mucosa because, embryologically, the foregut (forming the oral epithelium) and the hindgut (creating the anal mucosa) share a common ectodermal component in the first few weeks of fetal development. Therefore, the skin becomes a "mirror" of underlying pathology, both obvious and occult, in the gastrointestinal (GI) system.

Fitzpatrick JE: Cutaneous manifestations of gastrointestinal disease. In McNally PR, editor: *Gastroenterology secrets*, ed 3, Philadelphia, 2006, Elsevier Mosby, pp 559–566.

2. What is jaundice (icterus) and when is it apparent in the skin?

On average, 250 to 350 mg of bilirubin is normally generated daily, with 70% to 80% arising from senescent red blood cells and the remainder coming from heme proteins in the bone marrow and liver. Jaundice is the overaccumulation of bilirubin and various bile pigments in the skin and other organs. It is first seen in the sclera of the eye, skin (especially the face), and hard palate. Jaundice may result from stone obstruction, hemolysis with overproduction of bilirubin, ineffective erythropoiesis, or intrinsic liver disease. Jaundice is best seen in bright daylight and may be overlooked indoors. Jaundice is not clinically apparent until serum bilirubin exceeds 2.0 to 2.5 mg/dL in the adult and 5 mg/dL in the neonate. Jaundice may be the first and sole sign of hepatic dysfunction.

Kliegman R, Nelson WE: *Nelson textbook of pediatrics.* ed 18. Philadelphia, 2007, Saunders Elsevier, p 3147.

3. What can a jaundice color spectrum tell me about the types of liver disease in a patient?

Yellow discoloration of the skin is caused by bilirubin, while orange shades come from xanthorubin (intrahepatic jaundice). A deep green skin color is due to marked biliverdinemia and is characteristic of obstructive jaundice, as seen with pancreatic cancer. Patients with hepatobiliary disease, especially obstructive jaundice, often have severe pruritis; constant scratching results in inflammation of the skin follow by postinflammatory hyperpigmentation. The combination of postinflammatory hyperpigmentation and bile pigments imparts a bronze color to the skin. "Bronzing" is also encountered in hemochromatosis and primary Addison's disease.

Do not forget about exogenous plant pigments, metabolic diseases, and trematode ingestion when examining a patient who appears jaundiced. The differential diagnosis of jaundice includes carotenemia (excessive ingestion of carotenoids), lycopenia (via tomato juice), *Clonorchis sinensis* (travel to Asia) or *Fasciola hepatica* (ingesting watercress) infection, and the sallow skin of myxedema.

4. List the top ten skin findings suggestive of hepatic and biliary tract disease.

Jaundice	Purpura
Pigment changes	Loss of body hair
Spider angioma	Gynecomastia
Palmar erythema	Peripheral edema
Dilated abdominal wall veins	Non-palpable gallbladder

Hepatobiliary diseases are associated with alterations of the vasculature, including spider angiomas, palmar erythema, and cutaneous varices. Spider angiomas are classically associated with chronic liver disease, yet may also be seen in pregnancy, oral contraceptive use, and in normal persons, especially children. The vascular spider consists of a coiled central arteriole with smaller vessels radiating outward like the legs of a spider. In chronic liver disease, they are numerous and are found on the face, neck, upper chest, hands, and forearms. "Liver palms" refers to the mottled erythema and increased warmth of the palms (and sometimes the soles of the feet) in chronic liver disease. Palmar erythema also may be seen in pregnancy, lupus erythematous, pulmonary disease, and hyperthyroidism.

Portal venous hypertension due to chronic liver disease leads to the development of collateral circulation, with esophageal varices as an example. In the skin, this is observed as dilation of the abdominal wall veins (Fig. 37-1). Caput medusa refers to the dilated periumbilical veins and has been known for centuries as a marker of advanced liver disease. In men with chronic liver disease, induction of a "hyperestrogen state" (due to a decreased efficacy of estrogen breakdown in the liver) leads to gynecomastia, testicular atrophy; loss of axillary, truncal, and pubic hair; and a female pattern of pubic hair. Purpura, ecchymoses, and gingival bleeding reflect impaired hepatic production of various clotting factors, especially the vitamin K–dependent factors. Peripheral edema and ascites indicate hypoalbuminemia and/or portal venous hypertension.

5. What is the most common skin symptom associated with liver disease?

Pruritis is common and it may be severe. It is particularly intense in primary biliary cirrhosis, diseases caused by biliary tract obstruction, and cholestatic jaundice. Constant scratching may lead to excoriations, pigment disturbances, and thickening of the skin (lichenification).

6. What diseases associated with intestinal bleeding may also leave clues in the skin?

See Table 37-1.

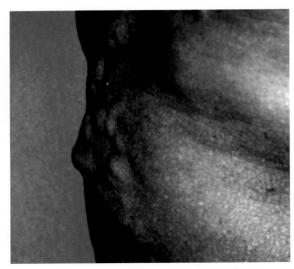

Figure 37-1. Profile view showing dilation of the umbilical vein in the epigastrium. Enlarged abdominal wall veins reflect portal venous hypertension. The patient also had esophageal varices.

7. What is pyoderma gangrenosum?

Pyoderma gangrenosum (PG) is a severe ulcerative condition that affects 1 in 100,000 United States citizens per year and, in over 70% of cases, affects the lower legs (Fig. 37-2). It is one of the skin lesions associated with the abdominal pain and bleeding of inflammatory bowel disease. PG originates as a small, tender pustule that breaks down to form a painful, rapidly expanding necrotic ulcer with a cyanotic, raised and undermined edge. Lesions may develop at sites of minor trauma, a phenomenon known as pathergy. The ulcers of PG may become quite large. They frequently heal with a thin, atrophic scar.

The exact cause of PG is unknown, but immune complex–mediated neutrophilic vascular reactions in the skin have been postulated. After the diagnosis of PG is made, the next step should be to look for an underlying cause. Important conditions to search for include chronic infectious hepatitis, inflammatory bowel disease (ulcerative colitis or Crohn's disease), rheumatoid arthritis, lupus erythematosus, HIV infection, and leukemia. About 2% of patients with ulcerative colitis have PG, and the course of both illnesses maybe parallel. Some patients may have PG for several years before developing inflammatory bowel disease. In general, firstline treatment is corticosteroids and cyclosporine. Infliximab (TNF-α antibody) is the treatment of choice for PG with underlying inflammatory bowel disease or rheumatoid arthritis.

Brooklyn T, Dunnill G, Probert C: Diagnosis and treatment of pyoderma gangrenosum, *BMJ* 333(7560):181–184, 2006.

8. A patient presents with anemia, blood in the stool, and red macules on his lips/tongue. What diagnosis should I first consider?

The most likely cause is hereditary hemorrhagic telangiectasia (HHT), also known as Olser-Weber-Rendu syndrome. This is an autosomal dominant genetic disorder with highest prevalence in the Dutch Antilles (1:1330). Two subtypes exist: HHT-1 and HHT-2, due to *ENG* (9q33-34) and *ALK-1* (2q13) TGFB-1 receptor mutations, respectively. Affected individuals develop linear, punctuate, and papular red lesions on the lips, face, mucous membranes, fingers (Fig. 37-3), and toes beginning in childhood. The entire GI tract may also be affected with similar lesions, and bleeding may be minimal

Table 37-1. Conditions Associated with GI Bleeding and Skin Lesions	
INFLAMMATORY CONDITIONS	**VASCULAR MALFORMATIONS AND TUMORS**
Ulcerative colitis	Hereditary hemorrhagic telangiectasia
Crohn's disease	(Osler-Weber-Rendu)
Henoch-Schönlein purpura	Kaposi's sarcoma
Polyarteritis nodosa	Blue rubber bleb nevus syndrome
HEREDITARY POLYPOSIS SYNDROMES	**MISCELLANEOUS**
Gardner's syndrome	Ehlers-Danlos syndrome
Peutz-Jeghers syndrome	Pseudoxanthoma elastica
Multiple hamartoma syndrome (Cowden's syndrome)	

(causing a chronic iron-deficiency anemia), or massive (leading to an acute, severe and sometimes fatal blood loss). The disease prevalence of GI manifestation is 15% to 45%. The mucous membranes, especially the nasal mucosa, are also involved. In children, an important early clue to the diagnosis is recurrent severe nosebleeds (epistaxis) prior to the presence of other more typical findings. Diagnosis results from the positive finding of three out of four Curaçao criteria (epistaxis, telangiectasias, visceral lesions, first-degree relative with HHT). Patients continue to develop new lesions throughout life. Individuals with the HHT-1 subtype have an increased risk of arteriovenous malformations of the lungs, liver (causing cirrhosis), and central nervous system.

Letteboer TG, Mager JJ, Snijder RJ, et al: Genotype-phenotype relationship in hereditary haemorrhagic telangiectasia, *J Med Genet* 43(4):371–377, 2006.

Sabba C, Pasculli G, Lenato GM, et al: Hereditary hemorrhagic telangiectasia: clinical features in ENG and ALK1 mutation carriers, *J Thromb Haemost* 5(6):1149–1157, 2007.

9. What other diagnoses should I consider when seeing a patient with macules on the lips?

A number of conditions have pigmented macules on the lips. The most important one concerning the GI tract is Peutz-Jeghers syndrome (PJS). It is one of the "classic" polyposis syndromes with intestinal polyps, an increased risk of cancer, and characteristic skin findings in 95% of cases. PJS is an autosomal dominant disorder that appears at birth or in infancy with small round to oval macules that vary from brown to blue-brown in color. They most often occur on the lips and buccal mucosa, but the nose, palms, soles, fingers, hard palate, and gingiva may also be affected. Be sure to examine the mouth. It is important to remember that the lip macules are not present at birth.

Individuals with PJS also have multiple polyps in the small intestine, most commonly in the jejunum and ileum. Polyps present around 11 to 13 years of age. When only a few polyps are present, there may be no symptoms. However, when present in large numbers, the polyps may cause intussusception with resultant abdominal pain and bleeding (most common) or obstruction. The polyps are hamartomatous polyps, which means that they are composed of benign elements normally present in the gut. There is a 2% to 3% risk, however, of intestinal malignancy in patients with PJS. It is thought that among the masses of benign polyps is the occasional adenomatous polyp that is a precursor lesion of intestinal cancer. There is a 37% chance of any type of cancer by age 65 in PJS. In addition, it has been recently discovered that patients with this syndrome have a higher risk of developing cancer of the ovary, uterus, breast, endometrium, testicles, GI, lungs, and pancreas. Recent studies have indicated that PJS arises from mutations in a tumor supressor gene (19p13.5, gene *STK11/LKB1*), which normally regulates cell cycle progression. Forty percent of gene mutations are spontaneous.

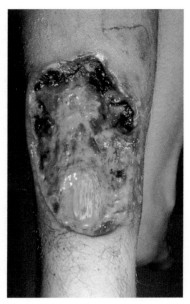

Figure 37-2. Pyoderma gangrenosum. Large necrotic undermined ulcer of the lower leg with exposed tendon in a patient with ulcerative colitis. (Courtesy of the Fitzsimons Army Medical Center teaching files.)

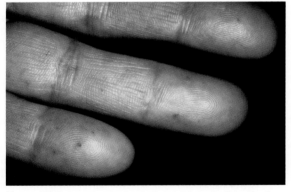

Figure 37-3. Hereditary hemorrhagic telangiectasia (Osler-Rendu-Weber disease). Punctate telangiectasias of the fingers that provide a cutaneous clue to the diagnosis of a genodermatosis with involvement of the gastrointestinal tract. (Courtesy of the Fitzsimons Army Medical Center teaching files.)

Thiers BH, Sahn RE, Callen JP: Cutaneous manifestations of internal malignancy, *CA Cancer J Clin* 59(2):73–98, 2009.

10. What is the best treatment for patients with Peutz-Jeghers syndrome?

Surgery. The gold standard is prophylaxis and polypectomy of the entire small bowel. Treatment of patients with inhibitors of cyclooxygenase-2 (COX-2 inhibitors, celecoxib) may lead to a dramatic reduction in the burden of polyps and need for surgical resection. Ongoing research indicates that Rapamycin (sirolimus) shows promise for PJS treatment by binding to FKBP12, which results in antiproliferative effects and dramatic reduction of polyp production/size.

Kopacova M, Tacheci I, Rejchrt S, Bures J: Peutz-Jeghers syndrome: diagnostic and therapeutic approach, *World J Gastroenterol* 15(43):5397–5408, 2009.

11. What is pseudoxanthoma elasticum (PXE)? How does this cause GI bleeding?

PXE is inherited in an autosomal dominant or autosomal recessive fashion, due to mutations in the *ABCC6* gene, which codes for a cellular transport protein. The basic defect is in the elastic tissue in various organs—the skin, blood vessels, eyes, and heart. Recent studies indicate that in PXE, extracellular material accumulates due to a defective MRP6 transmembrane transporter; this is thought to cause the calcification of elastic fibers and fragmentation of the tissue. As a result, a major part of the structural framework in these tissues is weakened, leading to disastrous consequences.

Changes of PXE in the skin develop in adolescence or early adulthood and typically begin on the sides of the neck. The skin lesions consist of asymptomatic, yellowish pebbly plaques on the neck, axillae, antecubital fossae, abdomen, and thighs or other large flexor surfaces. PXE has a peculiar texture and color reminiscent of "plucked chicken skin." PXE typically presents in a reticular pattern.

Internally, the yellowish papules of PXE are seen in the mouth, esophagus, and stomach. Involvement of the elastic tissue of the gastric arteries may result in sudden, massive hemorrhage. Involvement of the eye, specifically Bruch's membrane, causes angioid streaks of the retina. Sudden hemorrhage with acute loss of vision may be a presenting sign. Involvement of large vessels results in claudication, hypertension, and angina at an early age.

Finger RP, Charbel Issa P, Ladewig MS, et al: Pseudoxanthoma elasticum: genetics, clinical manifestations and therapeutic approaches, *Surv Ophthalmol* 54(2):272–285, 2009.

12. What is Gardner's syndrome?

Gardner's syndrome is another polyposis syndrome inherited in an autosomal dominant fashion. Mutations of the *APC* gene on chromosome 5c21 are responsible for the syndrome. APC is a tumor suppressor protein with a role in cell-to-cell adhesion, signal transduction, and transcriptional activation. Patients with this syndrome have numerous epidermal inclusion cysts in the skin (50% to 65%), various dental abnormalities including osteomas of the mandible, intraabdominal desmoid tumors, and innumerable premalignant adenomatous polyps throughout the colon (Fig. 37-4). Congenital retinal pigmentation may also develop. The incidence of Gardner's syndrome in the United States is 1 in a million, average age of onset is 22, and the lifetime risk of colon cancer in untreated patients is 100%. In

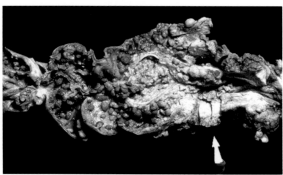

Figure 37-4. Gardner's syndrome. Segment of colon demonstrating numerous polyps and colon adenocarcinoma at the site of the *arrow*. (Courtesy of the Fitzsimons Army Medical Center teaching files.)

addition, patients have a predisposition to periampullary and thyroid cancers. Deforming osteomas may require excision although Gardner's skin manifestations do not typically require treatment. Underlying polyp excision is preferred, and second-line sulindac or tamoxifen is recommended for abdominal desmoid polyps or extraabdominal manifestations.

Schwartz R: Gardner syndrome, *eMedicine Dermatology*. Available at: http://emedicine.medscape.com/article/1093486-overview. Accessed December 7, 2009.

Nandakumar G, Morgan JA, Silverberg D, Steinhagen RM: Familial polyposis coli: clinical manifestations, evaluation, management, and treatment, *Mt Sinai J Med* 71:384–391, 2004.

13. How can cancer of the gastrointestinal tract present in the skin?

The skin may be involved with GI tract malignancy in several ways. First, the skin may be a site of metastasis from a primary GI tract cancer. This happens most frequently with adenocarcinoma of the colon (Fig. 37-5). Secondly, the skin and GI tract may be both affected by a genetic disease, such as the pancreatic cancer syndrome associated with multiple atypical nevi and melanoma (chromosme 9p21, *CDKN2A*). There is also a large group of paraneoplastic dermatoses, that is, a skin condition associated with an underlying malignancy (indirect involvement). Examples include "malignant" acanthosis nigricans, superficial migratory thrombophlebitis, and glucagonoma syndrome. In a few instances, such as excess glucagon secretion in the glucagonoma syndrome, the link between the skin and gut is clear. In other cases (such as acanthosis nigricans), the skin condition may occur in many individuals without cancer, so a thorough evaluation of the patient is necessary.

Thiers BH, Sahn RE, Callen JP: Cutaneous manifestations of internal malignancy, *CA Cancer J Clin* 59(2):73–98, 2009.

14. What is "malignant" acanthosis nigricans (AN)?

AN may be caused by endocrine disorders (insulin resistance), obesity (Fig. 37-6), medications, genetic abnormalities, or underlying cancer. However, the sudden onset of widespread AN in an adult with weight loss should suggest an underlying malignancy. Many different cancers have been reported with "malignant" AN, but almost 60% of patients have adenocarcinoma of the stomach. In most of these cases, AN develops when the tumor is

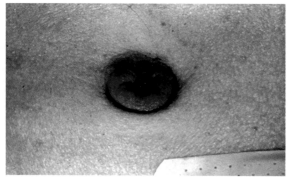

Figure 37-5. Sister Mary Joseph nodule. Metastatic lesion of colon cancer to the umbilicus.

in an advanced stage. One third of patients have AN before, one third during, and one third present after the discovery of the internal malignancy. In some cases, successful resection of the adenocarcinoma leads to regression of the AN. Gastric adenocarcinoma secrete TNF-α, which inevitably stimulates the epidermal growth factor (EGF) receptor to cause proliferation of keratinocytes.

Malignant AN initially presents abruptly as a darkening and thickening of the skin, occasionally with pruritus. This morphology progresses into symmetrical hyperpigmented, velvety plaques that occur most commonly around the posterior neck, axilla, and groin. Treatment for malignant AN is correction of the underlying pathology.

"Tripe palms" is another form of AN, and refers to AN of the palms in which there is a velvety furrowing of the palmar surfaces. It is almost always associated with internal malignancy. When Tripe palms occurs in the absence of AN, squamous cell carcinoma should be suspected. The sign of Leser-Trélat (increased numbers or the explosive onset of seborrheic keratoses) can also be associated with AN and tripe palms and it stems from the same circulating epidermal growth factors. Leser-Trélat may also be seen with tumors of the female reproductive tract and lymphoproliferative disorders.

Thiers BH, Sahn RE, Callen JP: Cutaneous manifestations of internal malignancy, *CA Cancer J Clin* 59(2):85–86, 2009. (Triple palms, Leser-Trélat)

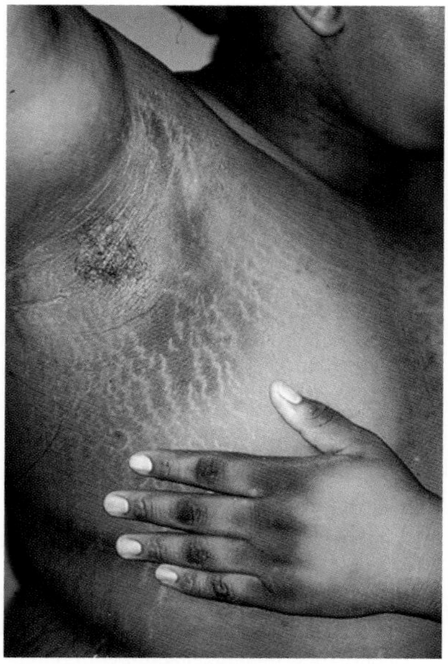

Figure 37-6. Acanthosis nigricans. Velvety hyperpigmented lesions of the neck, axilla, and knuckles in an obese individual. (Courtesy of the Fitzsimons Army Medical Center teaching files.)

15. What is superficial migratory thrombophlebitis (SMT)?

Many conditions may produce a state of increased blood coagulability, leading to venous thrombosis. One important GI-related cause is pancreatic cancer, which may be asymptomatic at the time the thrombophlebitis develops. Fifty percent of cases of SMT are associated with an underlying malignancy.

Superficial migratory thrombophlebitis presents as cropped, tender, erythematous, linear cords along the course of superficial veins of the trunk and extremities. Lesions in one area may be resolving, while new lesions are developing elsewhere. It is essential that any patient presenting with superficial migratory thrombophlebitis undergo a thorough evaluation to rule out underlying malignancy.

Recent work has focused on the association of superficial migratory thrombophlebitis and mucin-secreting abdominal adenocarcinomas. A low-grade disseminated intravascular coagulation occurs through mucin interaction with L and P selectins leading to aggregation and emboli formation, none of which requires thrombin generation. The thrombophlebitis is remarkably resistant to oral anticoagulant therapy such as warfarin, but does respond well to low-molecular-weight (LMW) heparin therapy, which is postulated to inhibit tumor growth, instead of acting in its traditional anticoagulatory role. Current research indicates that dalteparin and nadroparin may also illicit improved outcomes and survival rates. SMT is not specific for GI malignancies and has also been associated with carcinoma of the lung and breast, Hodgkin's disease, and multiple myeloma. Nonmalignant associations include Behçet's disease and rickettsial infections.

Thayalasekaran S, Liddicoat H, Wood E: Thrombophlebitis migrans in a man with pancreatic adenocarcinoma: a case report, *Cases J* 2:6610, 2009.

Key Points: Jaundice

1. Bilirubin has a strong affinity for tissues rich in elastic tissue, which is why it accumulates earliest in the sclera of the eye followed by the skin (especially the face), hard palate, and abdominal wall.
2. The yellow coloration in the skin is due to bilirubin while the orange shades come from xanthorubin and the greenish hue is due to biliverdin.
3. Patients with jaundice that has an orange hue are more likely to have intrahepatic jaundice while patients with a greenish hue are more likely to have obstructive jaundice.
4. Clinically apparent jaundice is not noticeable until the serum bilirubin exceeds 2.0 to 2.5 mg/dL in the adult.
5. Infants may have much higher levels of bilirubin in the serum (i.e., >5.0 mg/dL) before they become clinically jaundiced.

---

16. How is inflammation of the fat (panniculitis) associated with pancreatic disease?

The pancreas is a 99% exocrine- (pancreatic digestive enzyme) and a 1% endocrine- (insulin, glucagon) producing organ. Acute pancreatitis caused by viral infection, drugs, alcohol, pancreatic cancer, or trauma leads to massive outpouring of digestive enzymes. Patients with pancreatitis are often extremely ill with fever, vomiting, eosinophilia, and severe abdominal pain. About 2% to 3% develop tender red fluctuant nodules on the lower legs (Fig. 37-7) associated with joint pain and swelling. Predominantly seen with chronic pancreatitis or pancreatic cancer, these nodules rupture and discharge a thick, oily liquid. Schmid's triad, (panniculitis, polioarthritis, and eosinophilia) denotes a poor prognosis. The disease is caused by pancreatic lipase, phospholipase, trypsin, and amylase that migrate into tissue to cause the inflammation. It is felt that these pancreatic enzymes cause autodigestion of the fat in the subcutaneous tissue and periarticular fat pads. The histopathology is distinctive, demonstrating lobular liquefactive necrosis and ghostlike fat cells with neutrophils and other inflammatory cells. Administration of octreotide (inhibiting pancreatic enzyme manufacture) results in the cessation of symptoms. Steroids and nonsteroidal antiinflammatory drugs (NSAIDs) do not effectively treat skin nodules.

Garcia-Romero D, Vanaclocha F: Pancreatic panniculitis, *Dermatol Clin* 26(4): 465–470, 2008.

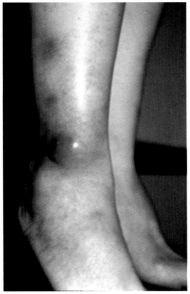

Figure 37-7. Pancreatic panniculitis. Tender, erythematous, fluctuant nodules on the lower legs of a patient with acute pancreatitis.

17. What chronic liver disease associated with photosensitivity causes blistering and scarring of the skin?

Porphyria cutanea tarda (PCT) is a metabolic disease characterized by skin fragility, chronic blistering, and scarring of the dorsal hands, forearms, ears, and face associated with photosensitivity to sunlight (Fig. 37-8). In addition to the blistering and scarring, skin findings include thickened, coarse hairs (hypertrichosis) over the temples, forehead, and cheeks; occasional shiny, thickened, scleroderma-like changes of the face, scalp, posterior neck, and torso; and hyperpigmentation or hypopigmentation.

PCT is either of autosomal dominant inheritance with incomplete penetrance or is acquired. There is a high incidence of liver disease and iron overload in patients with PCT. Factors that may trigger attacks of PCT include alcohol abuse, hepatitis C infection, estrogens (especially oral contraceptives), and HIV infection. The biochemical defect in chromosome 3q12 (*UROD* gene) leads to a deficiency of the hepatic and red blood cell enzyme uroporphyrinogen decarboxylase. This is the fifth enzyme in the metabolic pathway of the synthesis of hemoglobin. The liver's resultant overproduction of porphyrin precursors (photosensitizing compounds) causes a thickening of the dermal vascular architecture following exposure to sunlight.

A useful laboratory test that can be performed in the office is the demonstration of pink-red fluorescence of the patient's urine when exposed to ultraviolet light. A Wood's light emitting ultraviolet A

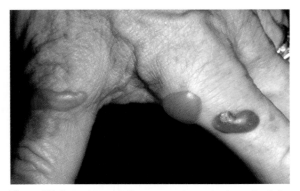

Figure 37-8. Vesicles and blisters, some hemorrhagic, on the digits of a patient with porphyria cutanea tarda.

(UVA) can be used for this test. Patients also have increased total body iron stores reflected in increased serum iron and ferritin levels. Quantitative measurement of the urine porphyrins in a 24-hour urine specimen will confirm the diagnosis.

Treatment of PCT includes elimination of alcohol and other predisposing medications, photoprotection, phlebotomy, and low-dose antimalarial therapy (chloroquine).

Kauppinene R: Porphyrias, *Lancet* 365 (9455):241–252, 2005.

18. What chronic skin disease is associated with a gluten-sensitive enteropathy?

Dermatitis herpetiformis (DH) is an immunobullous skin disease. Onset typically occurs between 20 and 40 years of age and affects men in a 2:1 ratio to women. Patients develop intensely itchy papules, papovesicles, and occasionally tense blisters in a grouped (herpetiform), symmetrical distribution over the scalp and posterior neckline, shoulders and back, elbows, knees, and the lumbosacral region (Fig. 37-9). Rarely, urticarial lesions without papulovesicles may be the only manifestation of the disease. Lesions on the palms are uncommon, and the mucous membranes are only rarely involved. Over 90% of patients will have histologic evidence of a gluten-sensitive enteropathy, ranging from increased intraepithelial lymphocytes to complete villous atrophy of the jejunum.

The disease in the skin and the intestinal tract (small intestine) is triggered by dietary gluten found in many grains (but not in rice, corn, or oats). There are usually no abdominal symptoms but an occasional patient may complain of bloating, cramping, and diarrhea. A diet completely free of gluten will clear the skin and intestinal tract lesions; however, this diet is difficult for many patients to maintain. The skin disease is characterized by the accumulation of

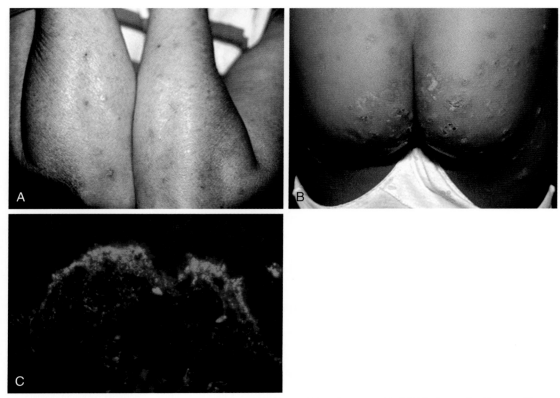

Figure 37-9. Dermatitis herpetiformis. **A,** Papules and vesicles with excoriations in a symmetrical distribution on the elbows and knees are typical of dermatitis herpetiformis. **B,** Excoriations and secondary infection due to intense itching and scratching are common. Lesions may be confused with scabies and folliculitis. **C,** Direct immunofluorescence of lesional skin in dermatitis herpetiformis showing granular deposits of IgA in the tips of dermal papillae.

polymorphonuclear neutrophils (PMNs) and granular deposits of IgA in the tips of the dermal papillae. These two findings are considered diagnostic of DH. In addition, most patients, as with celiac patients, show increased frequency of HLA-A1, HLA-B8, HLA-DR3, and HLA-DQw2 haplotypes. Current research indicates that epidermal transglutaminase 3 is the autoantigen in DH, which when coupled with gluten and a predisposition to gluten sensitivity, cross reacts with IgA antibodies.

Patricio P, Ferreira C, Gomes MM, Filipe P: Autoimmune bullous dermatoses: a review, *Ann N Y Acad Sci* 1173:203–210, 2009.
Zone JJ: Skin manifestations of celiac disease, *Gastroenterol* 128:S87–S91, 2005.

19. How is dermatitis herpetiformis treated?

Treatment includes strict adherence to a gluten-free diet and the use of either dapsone (diaminodiphenylsulfone) or sulfapyridine. Dapsone is the more effective of the two. Be sure to check G6PD levels and complete blood count prior to starting dapsone. The condition is lifelong with only rare periods of brief remission. Approximately 1% of patients will develop enteropathy-associated B-cell or less commonly T-cell lymphomas. These patients have a history of poor adherence to a gluten-free diet.

Patricio P, Ferreira C, Gomes MM, Filipe P: Autoimmune bullous dermatoses: a review, *Ann N Y Acad Sci* 1173:203–210, 2009.

CUTANEOUS MANIFESTATIONS OF RENAL DISEASE

Todd T. Kobayashi, MD, Lt Col, USAF, MC, and Kathleen M. David-Bajar, MD

1. What types of skin changes are associated with renal disease?

There are three main categories of skin disease associated with renal diseases:

- Cutaneous manifestations of renal failure; skin changes in nearly all patients
- Systemic diseases with prominent renal and cutaneous manifestations (e.g., Henoch-Schönlein purpura)
- Diseases affecting the kidney in which skin biopsy may be helpful in making the diagnosis, even when cutaneous findings are not prominent (e.g., primary systemic amyloidosis)

Pico MR, Lugo-Somolinos A, Sanchez JL, Burgos-Calderon R: Cutaneous alterations in patients with chronic renal failure, *Int J Dermatol* 31:860–863, 1992.

2. What cutaneous findings occur in renal failure?

See Table 38-1.

3. Do cutaneous signs of chronic renal failure resolve when the patient is treated with hemodialysis?

Generally, no. Many of the cutaneous changes associated with chronic renal disease persist after the patient is treated with hemodialysis. Some complaints (e.g., pruritus) may actually worsen after dialysis treatments are begun.

4. What cutaneous findings are present in patients being treated with dialysis?

Many of the skin changes described in patients with chronic renal failure are also found in patients with renal failure undergoing treatment with either peritoneal dialysis or hemodialysis. A high percentage of patients receiving dialysis complain of pruritus that may be severe. In some instances, the pruritus worsens with dialysis. Patients on renal dialysis may develop a bullous eruption similar to porphyria cutanea tarda (Fig. 38-1A). Acne has been described in association with dialysis and therapy with testosterone. Several perforating diseases are associated with chronic renal failure, with or without renal dialysis, including Kyrle's disease, reactive perforating collagenosis, and perforating folliculitis. Some authors group all of the perforating diseases seen in these patients under one term—*acquired perforating dermatosis of chronic renal failure*. The pathogenesis of these conditions is not understood. Dialysis patients may also develop

Table 38-1. Cutaneous Findings in Chronic Renal Failure

FINDING	% AFFECTED	FINDING	% AFFECTED
Changes in cutaneous pigmentation	70%	Keratotic pits of palms and soles	14%
Yellowish tinge	40%	Perforating disorder	4%
Hyperpigmentation of palms and soles	30%	Finger pebbles	86%
Hyperpigmentation, diffuse or photodistributed	22%	Calcinosis cutis	1%
Pallor	8%	Calciphylaxis	1%
Cutaneous infections	70%	Uremic frost	3%
Onychomycosis	52%	Porphyria and pseudoporphyria	1.2%–18%
Tinea pedis	25%		
Nail changes	66%		
Half-and-half nails	39%		
Pale nails	23%		
Splinter hemorrhages	11%		
Xerosis (dry skin) and/or pruritus	63%		

Data from Pico MR, Lugo-Somolinos A, Sanchez JL, Burgos-Calderon R: Cutaneous alterations in patients with chronic renal failure, *Int J Dermatol* 31:860–863, 1992.

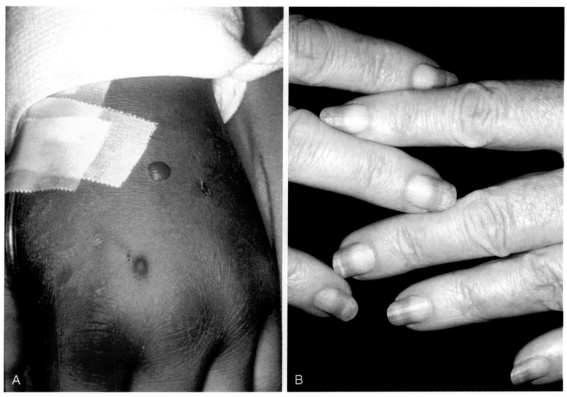

Figure 38-1. Cutaneous findings. **A,** Tense vesicle on the dorsal hand of a patient undergoing renal dialysis. **B,** Half-and-half nails in a patient with chronic renal failure.

cutaneous complications from this treatment, such as infections or contact dermatitis in the area of the peritoneal cannula or arteriovenous fistula.

Fuchs E, Lynfield Y: Dialysis acne, *J Am Acad Dermatol* 23:125, 1990.

5. Describe the nail changes in chronic renal failure.

Both half-and-half nails and Muehrcke's nails are associated with chronic renal failure. In half-and-half nails, the proximal half of the nail is white, and the distal portion retains the normal pink color (Fig. 38-1B). This is believed to be due to edema of the nail bed. Muehrcke's nails are associated with hypoalbuminemia and have two transverse parallel white bands, separated from each other and from the lunula by areas of normal pink nail.

Muehrcke RC: The fingernails in chronic hypoalbuminaemia: a new physical sign, *BMJ* 9:1327–1328, 1956.

6. What is uremic frost?

Although a rare finding today, this discoloration of the face was originally described as a classic manifestation of chronic renal failure. Whitish deposits were noted about the face and neck, believed to be due to deposition of crystallized urea from sweat. Table 38-2 summarizes the abnormalities of skin color associated with renal failure.

Walsh SR, Parada NA: Images in clinical medicine. Uremic frost, *N Engl J Med* 352:e13, 2005.

Table 38-2. Abnormalities of Skin Color Associated with Renal Failure

SKIN FINDING	COLOR	DISTRIBUTION	ETIOLOGY
Uremic frost	White	Face, nostrils, neck	Deposition of crystallized urea from sweat
Pallor	Yellowish	Generalized	Anemia, urochrome deposition
Hyperpigmentation	Brown	Photodistributed or generalized	Increased β-melanocyte stimulating hormone
Bruising	Red-purple-green-yellow-brown	Sites of trauma	Hemostatic abnormalities

7. What causes the pallor of chronic renal failure?

This pallor is due mainly to the anemia that invariably accompanies chronic renal failure. In addition, a yellowish cast may be noted and is believed to be due to urochrome deposition in the skin.

8. What causes the pigmentary changes of the skin seen in chronic renal failure?

It is the result of increased amounts of melanin present in the basal layer of the epidermis and superficial dermis. It has been proposed that such patients have decreased metabolism of β-melanocyte–stimulating hormone (β-MSH) by diseased kidneys, leading to elevated plasma levels of β-MSH, a hormone that stimulates melanocytes to produce more melanin.

9. Is pruritus a common finding in all renal failure?

No. Patients with acute renal failure do not develop pruritus. However, it is common in patients with chronic renal failure. Also, some patients with chronic renal failure treated with dialysis have exacerbation of their pruritus. The precise cause of uremic pruritus is unknown. One study suggests that uremic patients have a histamine-releasing factor in their sera that is depleted or diminished by ultraviolet B (UVB) light. Nitric oxide or pruritogenic cytokines may play a role in the pruritus of chronic renal failure. Another study found a reduction in the total number of skin nerve terminals in uremic patients and proposed that skin innervation is altered in chronic renal failure patients, possibly as a consequence of neuropathy. Secondary hyperparathyroidism, which sometimes develops in chronic renal failure, may also induce pruritus.

Goicoechea M, de Sequera P, Ochando A, et al: Uremic pruritus: an unresolved problem in hemodialysis patients, *Nephron* 82:73–74, 1999.
Urbonas A, Schwartz RA, Szepietowski JC: Uremic pruritus: an update, *Am J Nephrol* 21:343–350, 2001.

10. How is the pruritus of renal failure treated?

First of all, a specific diagnosis should be sought. Patients with renal failure may develop other skin conditions associated with pruritus, such as scabies or allergic contact dermatitis. Also, reactions to medications may be associated with pruritus. Xerosis is often present and can be treated with avoidance of irritants, use of mild or no soap for cleansing the skin, and the frequent use of emollients. When pruritus is believed to be due to secondary hyperparathyroidism, surgical therapy may be indicated. When no specific cause for pruritus is found, treatment with ultraviolet B light may be beneficial.

11. Are there skin changes associated with renal transplants?

Skin signs of chronic renal failure may resolve following successful renal transplantation (in contrast to hemodialysis). Cutaneous infections (viral, bacterial, atypical mycobacterial, and fungal) may develop, secondary to immunosuppressive therapy given following transplantation. After years of immunosuppression, benign (verrucae, premalignant keratoses, porokeratosis) and malignant cutaneous tumors (squamous cell carcinoma, malignant melanoma, Kaposi's sarcoma) may develop. Sometimes numerous tumors may arise simultaneously or at increasingly alarming rates, often demonstrating aggressive histology and a propensity to metastasize. Lowering immunosuppressive therapy, aggressive treatment of skin tumors, and potentially adding a systemic retinoid such as acitretin may help control this serious problem.

12. What is transepidermal elimination? What is its relationship to kidney disease?

These are a group of diseases in which altered components of skin are eliminated via the epidermis, a process termed *transepidermal elimination*. Several different perforating diseases have been associated with chronic renal failure, including Kyrle's disease, reactive perforating collagenosis, and perforating folliculitis. Because features of more than one type of perforating disorder have been noted in skin biopsies from patients with chronic renal failure, it has been suggested that this condition be referred to as the *acquired perforating dermatosis of chronic renal failure*. This eruption occurs in up to 10% of patients on dialysis but has also developed in patients with renal failure even without dialysis treatment. The lesions consist of keratotic papules and nodules on the trunk and extremities (Fig. 38-2). They occur more commonly in black patients. Skin biopsy confirms the diagnosis. Recently, treatment with narrow band ultraviolet B radiation has been reported to be effective in the treatment of this condition. This eruption may resolve spontaneously over a period of months.

Ohe S, Danno K, Sasaki H, et al: Treatment of acquired perforating dermatosis with narrowband UVB, *J Am Acad Dermatol* 50:892–894, 2004.
Patterson JW: The perforating disorders, *J Am Acad Dermatol* 10:561–581, 1984.

13. What are the differences between Kyrle's disease, reactive perforating collagenosis, and perforating folliculitis?

All three disorders are classified as perforating diseases; however, as originally defined, *Kyrle's disease* is due to an abnormal clone of keratinocytes that perforates through the epidermis down into the dermis. In contrast, *reactive perforating collagenosis* is a disease in which presumably abnormal collagen is being extruded from the dermis through the epidermis. *Perforating folliculitis* is a disease characterized by follicular plugs and curled-up hairs that perforate through the follicle into the dermis. Kyrle's disease is a controversial entity, with some authorities doubting its existence.

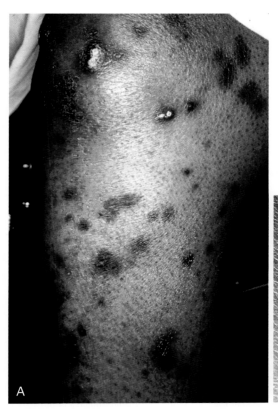
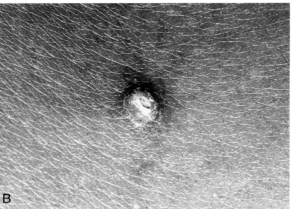

Figure 38-2. Perforating disease of chronic renal failure. **A,** Small erythematous papules with central crusts or scales are seen on the lower legs. Central umbilication of the papules can be seen, the area of "perforation." The hyperpigmented macules are areas of prior involvement. **B,** Close-up of hyperkeratotic papule demonstrating cell area of perforation. (Courtesy of James E. Fitzpatrick, MD.)

14. Describe the porphyria-like eruption of dialysis.

Patients with chronic renal failure on dialysis sometimes develop skin fragility, blisters, hyperpigmentation, and hypertrichosis that is indistinguishable from the cutaneous lesions seen in porphyria cutanea tard (PCT). Although most of these patients do not have elevated levels of porphyrins (pseudoporphyria), some do. When these patients are anuric, plasma and fecal specimens are submitted for porphyrin studies. Elevated porphyrin levels are due to decreased elimination, poor erythropoiesis, decreased activity of uroporphyrinogen decarboxylase (enzyme responsible for PCT), and failure of hemodialysis to remove porphyrins. Hepatitis C infection, iron overload, and medications are exacerbating factors.

Green JJ, Manders SM: Pseudoporphyria, *J Am Acad Dermatol* 44:100–108, 2001.

Poh-Fitzpatrick MB, Masullo AS, Grossman ME: Porphyria cutanea tarda associated with chronic renal disease and hemodialysis, *Arch Dermatol* 116:191–195, 1980.

Key Points: Cutaneous Manifestations of Renal Disease

1. Uremic frost is the presence of white deposits in the head and neck area seen in patients with severe renal failure.
2. The pruritus of renal failure often responds to ultraviolet light B (UVB) therapy.
3. Small vascular lesions called angiokeratoma corporis diffusum are most commonly found in a bathing suit distribution area. These angiokeratomas are characteristic of Fabry's disease, a genetic disorder that affects the kidney.
4. Nephrogenic systemic fibrosis is a recently described disease characterized by papules, plaques, and thickened skin of the trunk and extremities. It is associated with impaired renal function and deposition of gadolinium in tissues from gadolinium-based contrast media.

---

15. What is Fabry's disease?

Fabry's disease (angiokeratoma corporis diffusum universale) is the result of defective activity of a lysosomal enzyme, α-galactosidase A, which leads to deposition of neutral glycosphingo-lipids, particularly trihexosyl ceramides, in many cells and tissues of the body. It is inherited in an X-linked recessive pattern, with nearly all patients being male. Heterozygous females are generally asymptomatic, although they often have characteristic corneal opacities.

Desnick RJ, Brady RO: Fabry disease in childhood, *J Pediatrics* 144:S20–S26, 2004.

16. Describe the skin lesions in Fabry's disease.

Angiokeratomas are the skin lesions seen in Fabry's disease. They begin as pinpoint erythematous to purplish macules or flat papules with slight scaling and often start in early childhood with progressive increase in size and number. They are typically distributed in the "bathing suit area," the area between the waist and the knees. These lesions may be quite subtle. A skin biopsy may aid in establishing the diagnosis because special stains such as Sudan black B, scarlet red, or periodic acid–Schiff may demonstrate glycolipid deposition in the skin. Electron microscopy is frequently used to help establish the diagnosis because it demonstrates characteristic cytoplasmic glycolipid deposits (typically, within endothelial cells). Other findings in patients with Fabry's disease include acroparesthesias and acute attacks of severe pain, particularly in the palms and soles, often beginning in childhood. In adult life, cardiac ischemia and infarcts, transient ischemic attacks, stroke, and progressive kidney failure may develop. Recently, treatment with enzyme replacement therapy has become available in Europe (α Gal A) and the United States (agalsidase β [Fabrazyme]).

17. What are the five vasculitic diseases that frequently involve both the kidneys and skin?

- Leukocytoclastic vasculitis
- Henoch-Schönlein purpura
- Polyarteritis nodosa
- Microscopic polyarteritis
- Wegener's granulomatosis

When skin lesions suggestive of vasculitis occur, a skin biopsy should be done to confirm the diagnosis and determine the type of vessel and inflammation involved (see also Chapter 15). Vessel involvement may vary from small postcapillary venules (leukocytoclastic vasculitis) to medium-sized arteries (polyarteritis nodosa). If vasculitis is confirmed, testing should be done to determine if the kidneys are also involved.

18. How should skin biopsy be used for the diagnosis of systemic amyloidosis?

In primary systemic amyloidosis, immunoglobulin light-chain proteins and serum amyloid P (SAP) are deposited in skin, tongue, heart, spleen, joints, peripheral nerves, and carpal ligaments due to an underlying plasma cell dyscrasia or multiple myeloma. Cutaneous changes may be present, including purpura of the upper trunk, face, and neck and eyelid purpura, which is very characteristic of primary systemic amyloidosis (Fig. 38-3). Waxy papules, particularly on the palms and fingertips, have also been reported. Secondary systemic amyloidosis is due to chronic inflammatory diseases such as tuberculosis and other infections, connective tissue diseases, hidradenitis suppurativa, and familial periodic fever syndromes, and is due to deposition of a distinctive nonimmunoglobulin protein designated AA (amyloid A protein), of which the precursor is an acute-phase reactant produced by the liver. Cutaneous lesions due to amyloid deposits are rarely seen in this type of amyloidosis. Even when there are no cutaneous changes present, skin biopsy may help make a diagnosis of primary or secondary systemic amyloidosis. Clinically, normal skin, abdominal fat, tongue, rectal, and minor salivary gland biopsies have been used to confirm the diagnosis, thus avoiding the need for more invasive biopsies of internal organs.

Wong CK, Wang WJ: Systemic amyloidosis. A report of 19 cases, *Dermatology* 189:47–51, 1994.

19. What is nephrogenic systemic fibrosis (nephrogenic fibrosing dermopathy)?

Nephrogenic systemic fibrosis is a recently described systemic disorder with prominent cutaneous findings seen in patients with impaired renal function who have received gadolinium-based contrast media. Many, but not all, of the patients have been on hemodialysis. It presents as thickened or edematous skin that primarily affects the extremities and trunk. Some patients may also demonstrate discrete papules or plaques. In severe cases, there may be restriction of movement or disabling contracture of the joints. Fibrosis may also involve extracutaneous sites including the sclera (yellow scleral plaques), the heart, lungs, and the skeletal muscle. Histologically, biopsies demonstrate increased numbers of CD34-positive and procollagen-positive fibroblasts and increased mucin in early lesions with marked fibrosis in later lesions, often involving the subcutaneous fatty septae. By energy dispersive spectroscopy, particles of gadolinium can be detected within involved tissues. Treatment has been disappointing as the condition is often refractory to all treatments.

High WA, Ayers RA, Chandler J, et al: Gadolinium is detectable within the tissue of patients with nephrogenic systemic fibrosis, *J Am Acad Dermatol* 56:21–26, 2007.

20. What are some diseases that have both skin and renal manifestations?

See Table 38-3.

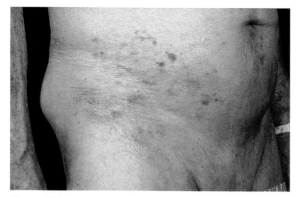

Figure 38-3. Systemic amyloidosis. Extensive purpura in a patient with diffuse, cutaneous systemic amyloidosis. A skin biopsy demonstrated amyloid deposited in the dermis and subcutaneous tissue. (Courtesy of the Fitzsimons Army Medical Center teaching files.)

Table 38-3. Diseases with Both Skin and Renal Manifestations

DISEASE	PATHOGENESIS	CUTANEOUS FINDINGS	ASSOCIATED SYSTEMIC FINDINGS
Systemic sclerosis	Autoimmune disease involving anti–Scl-70, anticentromere, and other antinuclear antibodies resulting in progressive sclerosis of skin and internal organs	Scleroderma, morphea, sclerodactyly, telangiectatic mats, calcinosis cutis, Raynaud's syndrome	Internal organ involvement is frequent and may affect the esophagus, heart and kidneys; lung involvement is the leading cause of death
Primary systemic amyloidosis (accumulation of amyloid fibrils within vital organs leads to atrophy of normal tissue and interferes with the normal functioning of the organ)	Deposits of immunoglobulin light chain (AL), or, less often, heavy chain (HL), around vessels and functional units of skin and internal organs	Pinch purpura; petechiae and ecchymosis around eyelids, neck, axilla, and anus; waxy or purpuric papules, nodules, or plaques on face, neck, scalp, and digits; hemorrhagic blisters Mucosa: macroglossia	Renal proteinuria and failure, hypoalbuminemia, edema, cardiac failure (congestive heart failure), neurologic deficits (peripheral and autonomic neuropathy), gastrointestinal (motility problems)
Secondary systemic amyloidosis (accumulation of amyloid fibrils within vital organs leads to atrophy of normal tissue and interferes with the normal functioning of the organ)	Deposits of amyloid A protein (AA) (chronic inflammatory diseases and hereditary periodic fever syndromes); deposits of β2 microglobulin (patients with chronic renal failure receiving hemodialysis)	No, or rare, cutaneous findings, but skin often biopsied for diagnosis (abdominal fat pad, minor salivary gland, rectal mucosa, buccal mucosa, tongue)	AA amyloidosis usually affects the kidneys, liver, spleen, adrenals and heart; synovial deposits of β2 microglobulin: carpal tunnel syndrome, bone cysts and destructive spondyloarthropathy
Tuberous sclerosis (Bourneville disease) Epiloia (*epi*lepsy, *lo*w *i*ntelligence, angiofibroma)	*TSC1* (chromosome 9q34) and *TSC2* (chromosome 16p13); their protein products are hamartin and tuberin, respectively, which are integral to cell cycle and growth regulation	Skin: congenital hypopigmented macules (ash leaf macules), confetti-like hypopigmentation, facial angiofibromas, collagenomas (Shagreen patch), periungual fibromas, café-au-lait macules; mucosa: gingival fibromas and dental enamel pits	Hamartomas can be found in the eye, brain, kidneys, liver, heart, lungs, and bones, sometimes progressing to malignancy; seizures, mental deficits and neuropsychiatric disturbances are common
Nail-patella syndrome (hereditary osteoonychodysplasia)	*LMX1B* gene: regulates collagen synthesis Dysregulation of the synthesis of collagen in the glomerular basement membrane may contribute to the nephrosis	Hypoplasia of radial side of thumbnails, triangular lunula, absent or hypoplastic nails	Absent or hypoplastic patella, radial head dysplasia, iliac crest exostosis (iliac horns); nephropathy and renal insufficiency
Birt-Hogg-Dube Syndrome	*FLCN* (*BHD*) gene encodes the tumor suppressor protein folliculin	Fibrofolliculomas, trichodiscomas, and acrochordons	Lung cysts, spontaneous pneumothorax, and renal tumors (oncocytomas and chromophobe renal cell carcinoma); colon polyps; neural tumors
Hereditary leiomyomatosis and renal cell cancer (HLRCC)	*FH* gene: fumarate hydratase enzyme activity decreased	Multiple cutaneous leiomyomata or single leiomyoma with positive family history	Uterine leiomyomata (fibroids) and renal tumors

1. How significant is the occurrence of skin disease in the setting of HIV infection?

Dermatologic diseases are frequently encountered in HIV-infected patients. In one study of 100 serial outpatients, a 92% prevalence of skin disease was noted. Skin disease may also be the first manifestation of HIV disease and may suggest HIV infection because of increased severity of presentation, atypical clinical appearance, or increased resistance to treatment. In addition, mucocutaneous disease, such as an infection or neoplasm, may be the initial sign of a systemic process in an HIV-infected patient. Highly active antiretroviral therapy (HAART) was introduced in 1997 and has significantly decreased the occurrence and severity of many skin conditions associated with HIV infection, such as Kaposi's sarcoma, eosinophilic folliculitis, oral hairy leukoplakia, and molluscum contagiosum.

2. Outline the clinical spectrum of cutaneous disease associated with HIV infection.

See Table 39-1.

3. What are the most common dermatoses associated with HIV infection?

Papulosquamous dermatoses are among the most commonly seen cutaneous manifestations of HIV infection, and these include seborrheic dermatitis (Fig. 39-1) and xerosis. Other common dermatologic conditions include bacterial infections, such as *Staphylococcus aureus* skin infections. Fungal infections, such as mucocutaneous candidiasis (oropharyngeal and vulvovaginal) and dermatophytosis (tinea pedis, tinea cruris, tinea manuum, and onychomycosis), are also commonly encountered. Frequently seen viral infections include human papilloma virus infections (condyloma acuminata, common and plantar warts), as well as infections with herpes simplex virus, varicella-zoster virus, molluscum contagiosum, and Epstein-Barr virus (oral hairy leukoplakia).

4. Can mucocutaneous changes occur as a result of primary HIV infection?

Yes. The earliest cutaneous sign of HIV infection is an exanthem consisting of discrete, erythematous macules and papules that usually measure 10 mm or less. They are located primarily over the trunk but also are seen on the palms and soles. These lesions may become hemorrhagic. The exanthem of acute HIV infection is not clinically or histologically specific. Mucosal changes described include oral, genital, and anal ulcers. These changes are associated with an acute febrile illness.

5. What is the most common bacterial pathogen in HIV disease? How does it manifest itself?

Staphylococcus aureus is the most common cutaneous bacterial pathogen in HIV disease. Cutaneous infections due to *S. aureus* most commonly present as a superficial folliculitis. Less common manifestations include impetigo, ecthyma, furunculosis, cellulitis, abscesses, and botryomycosis. In addition, *S. aureus* can secondarily infect underlying primary dermatoses such as eczema, scabies, herpetic ulcers, and Kaposi's sarcoma, or can colonize intravenous catheter sites. Staphylococcal colonization (carriage) of the nose and flexures (perineal, toe webspaces) is known to increase in HIV disease and may account for the increased incidence of cutaneous infections. As in the general population, infections with community-acquired methicillin-resistant *S. aureus* (MRSA) are becoming increasingly common.

Ahuja D, Albrecht H: HIV and community-acquired MRSA, *AIDS Clin Care* 21:21–23, 2009.

6. What is the most common cutaneous malignancy in HIV disease?

Kaposi's sarcoma (KS) or, more specifically, epidemic Kaposi's sarcoma. In the Swiss HIV Cohort Study, the risk for KS and non–Hodgkin's lymphoma continued to be at least 20-fold higher among HAART-treated individuals compared with that of the general population. Most cases occurred in homosexual or bisexual men with HIV disease. However, KS has also been reported in HIV-negative homosexual males. Human herpesvirus–8 is associated with epidemic as well as other types of KS.

Chang Y, Cesarman E, Pessin MS, et al: Identification of herpesvirus-like DNA sequences in AIDS-associated Kaposi's sarcoma, *Science* 266:1865–1869, 1994.

Clifford GM, Polesel J, Richenbach M, et al: Cancer risk in the Swiss HIV Cohort Study: associations with immunodeficiency, smoking, and highly active antiretroviral therapy, *J Natl Cancer Inst* 97:425–432, 2005.

Schwartz RA, Micali G, Nasca MR, et al: Kaposi sarcoma: a continuing conundrum, *J Am Acad Dermatol* 59:179–206, 2008.

Table 39-1. Mucocutaneous Diseases Seen in HIV Infection*

NEOPLASTIC DISEASES	INFECTIOUS DISEASES
Kaposi's sarcoma	**Bacterial**
Lymphoma	*Staphylococcus aureus* infections
Squamous cell carcinoma	Syphilis
Basal cell carcinoma	Bacillary angiomatosis
PAPULOSQUAMOUS DISEASES	**Fungal**
	Candida, *Penicillium marneffei*
Seborrheic dermatitis	Dermatophytosis
Xerosis/acquired ichthyosis	Cryptococcosis
Psoriasis	Histoplasmosis
Reiter's syndrome	**Viral**
MISCELLANEOUS DISEASES	Human papillomavirus (HPV)
	Molluscum contagiosum
Eosinophilic folliculitis	Herpes simplex virus (HSV)
Drug eruptions	Varicella-zoster virus (VZV)
Hyperpigmentations	Cytomegalovirus (CMV)
Photoeruptions	Epstein-Barr virus
Pruritus	**Arthropods**
Lipodystrophy	Scabies
Granuloma annulare	
Aphthosis	

*Costner M, Cockerell CJ: The changing spectrum of the cutaneous manifestations of HIV disease, *Arch Dermatol* 134:1290–1292, 1998.
Dover JS, Johnson RA: Cutaneous manifestations of human immunodeficiency virus infection: parts 1 and 2, *Arch Dermatol* 127:1383–1391, 1549–1558, 1991.
James W, editor: AIDS: a ten-year perspective, *Dermatol Clin* 9:391–615, 1991.

7. What are the cutaneous clinical features of epidemic Kaposi's sarcoma?

Epidemic Kaposi's sarcoma has a widespread, symmetrical distribution of rapidly progressive macules, patches, nodules, plaques, and tumors. Common areas of involvement include the trunk, extremities, face, and oral cavity. Early lesions consist of erythematous macules, patches, or papules that may have a bruiselike halo. They enlarge at different rates and tend to be oval or elongated in shape, following the lines of skin cleavage. The color varies from pink to red, purple, or brown and can easily mimic purpura, hemangiomas, nevi, sarcoidosis, pityriasis rosea, secondary syphilis, lichen planus, basal cell carcinoma, and melanoma. The surface may become scaly, hyperkeratotic, ulcerated, or hemorrhagic.

Disfigurement and pain secondary to edema can occur, especially on the face, genitals, and lower extremities. *Koebnerization*, or formation of new lesions at sites of trauma, can be seen. Secondary bacterial infection can also occur. Lesions can be arranged in several known patterns, such as a follicular (clustered) pattern (Fig. 39-2), pityriasis rosea–like pattern, or dermatomal pattern.

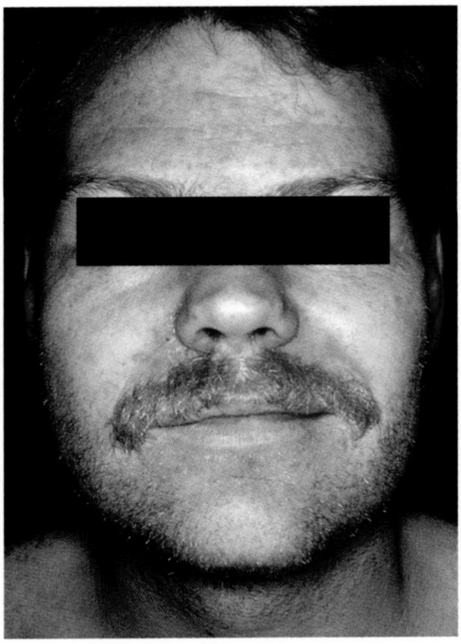

8. How is Kaposi's sarcoma treated?

Therapy of localized disease may be with intralesional vinblastine, radiotherapy, liquid nitrogen cryotherapy, surgical excision, and topical alitretinoin. Treatment of more extensive disease includes α-interferon as well as single- or multiple-agent chemotherapy with vinblastine, vincristine, bleomycin, or liposomal doxorubicin.

Conant M, The International and North American Panretin Gel KS Study Groups: topical alitretinoin gel as treatment for cutaneous lesions of AIDS-related Kaposi's sarcoma: results of multicenter, double-blind, vehicle-controlled trials, Presented at the 6th Conference on Retroviruses and Opportunistic Infections, Chicago, 1999.

Walmsley S, Northfelt DW, Melosky B, et al: Treatment of AIDS-related cutaneous Kaposi's sarcoma with topical alitretinoin (9-cis-retinoic acid) gel. Panretin Gel North American Study Group, *J Acquir Immune Defic Syndr* 22:235–246, 1999.

Figure 39-1. Seborrheic dermatitis. Erythematous patches with yellow scale are present on the forehead, nose, and paranasal areas of an HIV-positive patient. (Courtesy of James E. Fitzpatrick, MD.)

9. Is the course of syphilis altered in HIV-infected individuals?

Although the course of syphilis in most HIV-infected patients is not different from that in a normal host, it may differ in several ways.

- Altered clinical manifestations of syphilis, including the usual painless chancre becoming painful secondary to bacterial infection. Lues maligna, a rare manifestation of secondary syphilis, can occur and consists of pleomorphic skin lesions with pustules, nodules, and ulcers with necrotizing vasculitis.

- Altered serologic tests for syphilis, with limited or absent antibody tests for syphilis, including repeatedly negative reagin and treponemal antibody tests. Seronegative secondary syphilis, as well as exaggerated antibody responses, has been reported. Loss of treponemal antibody positivity has also been noted.
- There may be concurrent coinfection with another sexually transmitted disease.
- There may be a decreased latency period with accelerated development of tertiary syphilis within months to years.
- There may be a lack of response to antibiotic therapy with relapses.

Gregory N, Sanchez M, Buchness MR: The spectrum of syphilis in patients with human immunodeficiency virus infection, *J Am Acad Dermatol* 22:1061–1067, 1990.

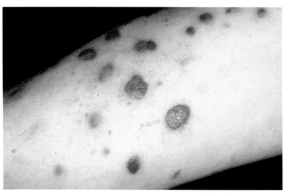

Figure 39-2. Kaposi's sarcoma. Multiple violaceous papules and plaques. (Courtesy of James E. Fitzpatrick, MD.)

10. How does syphilis increase the risk for HIV infection?

The syphilitic chancre can itself serve as a source of HIV transmission in the HIV-infected person. An HIV-negative patient with a genital ulcer, such as in primary syphilis, can be at increased risk for acquiring HIV if exposed to an HIV-positive sexual partner.

11. What is oral hairy leukoplakia?

Oral hairy leukoplakia, which is predictive for development of AIDS, is primarily seen in HIV-infected patients but also has been described rarely in HIV-negative immunosuppressed organ transplant recipients. It is due to Epstein-Barr virus replication within clinical lesions. Oral hairy leukoplakia occurs primarily on the lateral edges of the tongue as parallel, vertically oriented, white plaques, producing a corrugated appearance (Fig. 39-3A). It can infrequently also involve the dorsal and ventral aspects of the tongue, the buccal or labial mucosa, and the soft palate. The plaque in this condition does not rub off with scraping (unlike candidal thrush) and is usually asymptomatic. Histologically, parakeratosis, acanthosis, and ballooning cells (koilocytes) are seen. In situ Epstein-Barr virus DNA hybridization of lesional scrapings or tissue sections shows positive nuclear staining within epithelial cells. Lesions may respond to acyclovir, zidovudine, podophyllin, tretinoin, or excision but do not respond to anticandidal treatment.

Resnick L, Herbst JS, Raab-Traub N: Oral hairy leukoplakia, *J Am Acad Dermatol* 22:1278–1282, 1990.

12. Name the four types of oropharyngeal candidiasis that can be seen in HIV disease.

Pseudomembranous candidiasis appears as whitish, cottage-cheese–like or creamy plaques at any site in the oropharynx. These are removable when scraped and may leave a reddish surface. *Erythematous candidiasis* appears as well-demarcated patches of erythema on the palate or dorsal tongue. Lesions of erythematous candidiasis on the tongue can look smooth and depapillated. *Hyperplastic candidiasis* appears as a white coating on the dorsum of the tongue that persists with scraping (Fig. 39-3B). *Angular cheilitis* consists of erythema, cracking, and fissuring of the mouth corners. More than one type of oropharyngeal candidiasis can coexist.

Figure 39-3. Oral changes. **A,** Oral hairy leukoplakia. Vertically oriented white plaques with a corrugated appearance are seen on the lateral edge of the tongue. **B,** Hyperplastic candidiasis. A white coating that does not scrape off is present on the dorsal surface of the tongue in this HIV-positive patient.

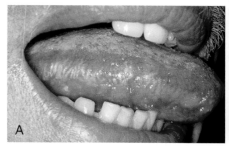
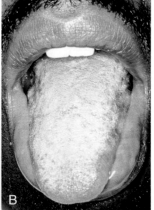

13. What is HIV-associated eosinophilic folliculitis?

HIV-associated eosinophilic folliculitis is a chronic, pruritic dermatosis of unknown etiology characterized by discrete, erythematous, follicular, urticarial papules on the head and neck, trunk, and proximal extremities (Fig. 39-4). Most cases occur in males, but the disease has been reported in females. Bacterial cultures are negative, and the eruption does not resolve with antistaphylococcal treatment. It is associated with peripheral eosinophilia, an elevated serum IgE level, and advanced HIV infection (CD4 counts lower than 250 cells/mm^3). Eosinophilic folliculitis is not specific for HIV infection, as it has rarely been described in association with hematologic malignancies.

Transverse histologic sections are superior to vertical sections in the diagnosis of this disease. Histopathologic findings include a perivascular and perifollicular mixed infiltrate with variable numbers of eosinophils and spongiosis of the follicular infundibulum or sebaceous gland with a mixed infiltrate. Treatment options include potent topical corticosteroids, antihistamines, ultraviolet B phototherapy, itraconazole, oral metronidazole, permethrin cream, and isotretinoin.

Piantanida EW, Turiansky GW, Kenner JR, et al: HIV-associated eosinophilic folliculitis: diagnosis by transverse histologic sections, *J Am Acad Dermatol* 38:124–126, 1998.

Simpson-Dent SL, Fearfield LA, Staughton RCD: HIV-associated eosinophilic folliculitis: differential diagnosis and management, *Sex Transm Infect* 75:291–293, 1999.

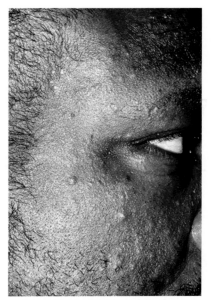

Figure 39-4. Eosinophilic folliculitis. Multiple pruritic, firm, urticaria-like pink papules are present on the face of this HIV-positive patient.

14. Is the incidence of drug eruptions increased in HIV disease?

Definitely, and especially with sulfonamides and amoxicillin clavulanate. About half of HIV-infected patients with *Pneumocystis carinii* pneumonia treated with intravenous trimethoprim-sulfamethoxazole develop a widespread macular or papular erythematous eruption within weeks of initiating treatment. In HIV disease, sulfonamides are commonly used in the prophylaxis and treatment of *P. carinii* pneumonia and central nervous system (CNS) toxoplasmosis. More severe drug reactions, such as Stevens-Johnson syndrome and toxic epidermal necrolysis, have also been reported in HIV patients.

15. Describe clinical features of molluscum contagiosum infection in the HIV-infected host.

Molluscum contagiosum, a poxvirus infection, is seen in approximately 8% to 18% of patients with symptomatic HIV disease and AIDS. Although molluscum lesions often appear as dome-shaped, flesh-colored umbilicated papules, they can have an unusual appearance, involve atypical sites, and be widespread.

In HIV disease, molluscum lesions tend to occur on the face, trunk, intertriginous areas, and buttocks as well as in the genital area. Beard area lesions are commonly seen, and these are probably spread by shaving. Lesions can be large (>1 cm, giant molluscum) or hyperkeratotic; can simulate skin cancers, common and genital warts, and keratoacanthomas; and can become confluent. Lesions can also involve the follicular epithelium with sparing of the interfollicular epithelium. Molluscum lesions can be associated with a localized chronic dermatitis surrounding a centrally located lesion (molluscum dermatitis). With progressive immune dysfunction, lesions increase in number and become diffuse. Disseminated cryptococcosis, histoplasmosis, and *Penicillium marneffei* infection can mimic facial molluscum contagiosum.

Mastrolorenzo A, Urbano FG, Salimbeni L, et al: Atypical molluscum contagiosum infection in an HIV-infected patient, *Int J Dermatol* 37:378–380, 1998.

16. How is molluscum contagiosum treated?

Treatment options include liquid nitrogen cryotherapy, curettage, electrodesiccation, trichloroacetic acid, topical wart preparations, laser ablation, tretinoin, topical fluorouracil and imiquimod, and topical or intravenous cidofovir. However, treatment of widespread lesions in advanced HIV disease is problematic, as lesions are numerous and tend to recur.

Buckley R, Smith K: Topical imiquimod therapy for chronic giant molluscum contagiosum in a patient with advanced human immunodeficiency virus I disease, *Arch Dermatol* 135:1167–1169, 1999.

17. Is the prevalence of common and genital warts increased in HIV infection?

The prevalence of human papillomavirus (HPV) infections is increased in HIV disease, including verruca vulgaris (common warts) and condyloma acuminata (genital warts). Lesions can be numerous, large, confluent, and resistant to standard treatment with increasing immunodeficiency. Condyloma acuminata occur in the genital and perianal areas, where it is associated with receptive anal intercourse. In HIV disease, the incidence of HPV-associated intraepithelial neoplasia of the cervix and of the anus in homosexual men is increased. Resolution of recalcitrant hand warts temporally related to protease inhibitor–containing antiretroviral therapy has been reported.

Spach DH, Colven R: Resolution of recalcitrant hand warts in an HIV-infected patient treated with potent antiretroviral therapy, *J Am Acad Dermatol* 40:818–821, 1999.

18. What causes bacillary angiomatosis?

Bacillary angiomatosis is a gram-negative bacillary disease caused by *Bartonella henselae* and *B. quintana*. The disease can involve the skin, as well as the liver, spleen, lymph nodes, and bone. Cutaneous lesions consist of solitary or multiple red-to-violaceous, vascular-appearing papules and nodules that can simulate hemangiomas, pyogenic granulomas, and Kaposi's sarcoma. Organisms can be demonstrated in lesional biopsies by Warthin-Starry stain. An association between bacillary angiomatosis in humans and traumatic exposure to cats having *B. henselae* blood infection has been shown. Treatment is with erythromycin or doxycycline, but clarithromycin and azithromycin have also been used.

19. How does varicella-zoster virus infection present in the HIV-positive patient?

Primary infection with the varicella-zoster virus (VZV, chickenpox) in HIV disease may be associated with complications such as pneumonia, encephalitis, hepatitis, profuse eruptions, and even death. Reactivation of latent VZV infection is increased in HIV disease. Reactivation usually manifests itself as a typical unidermatomal eruption, but with advanced immunodeficiency, multidermatomal and disseminated eruptions can occur. These eruptions may be vesiculobullous, hemorrhagic, necrotic, or poxlike and may be very painful. Chronic, painful verrucous and ecthymatous (poxlike) lesions can occur and appear as hyperkeratotic warty nodules and necrotic ulcerations, respectively.

Weinburg JM, Mysliwiec A, Turiansky GW, et al: Viral folliculitis: atypical presentations of herpes simplex, herpes zoster, and molluscum contagiosum, *Arch Dermatol* 133:983–986, 1997.

Key Points: Cutaneous Manifestations of HIV-infection

1. *Staphylococcus aureus* is the most common cause of bacterial infection in the HIV-infected population.
2. Atypical molluscum contagiosum manifestations in the HIV-infected population include giant molluscum, disseminated lesions, confluent lesions, lesions distributed in atypical sites such as the perianal area, and lesions mimicking warts, skin cancers, and keratoacanthomas.
3. Chronic varicella-zoster infection can manifest as verrucous, hyperkeratotic nodules and as ecthymatous, poxlike ulcerations.
4. Bacillary angiomatosis is caused by *Bartonella henselae* and *B. quintana*.
5. Side effects of HAART include the lipodystrophy syndrome, painful periungual inflammation (paronychia), and injection site reactions (enfuvirtide).

20. Do any photosensitive dermatoses occur in HIV disease?

Various photosensitive dermatoses have been described in HIV disease, and these include porphyria cutanea tarda (PCT), lichenoid photoeruptions, and chronic actinic dermatitis. Photosensitivity may, in fact, be the presenting sign of HIV infection.

Most cases of PCT in HIV infection are acquired and many are associated with historical or serologic evidence of hepatitis B or C infection, as well as with elevated transaminase levels and history of alcohol abuse. Patients present with blisters, erosions, crusting, scarring, and increased skin fragility on the face and dorsal hands. In one study, urinary and stool porphyrin excretion patterns classic for PCT occurred in hepatitis C–positive AIDS patients without any clinical evidence of porphyria.

Lichenoid photoeruptions in HIV infection occur most often in black individuals with advanced HIV disease and may be associated with photosensitizing drug use. Patients present with pruritic, violaceous plaques that begin on the face, neck, dorsal hands, and arms. The plaques may become hyperpigmented, hypopigmented, or depigmented and may extend to non–sun-exposed sites. Histopathologic features are primarily those of lichenoid drug eruption or hypertrophic lichen planus, but some patients have findings of lichen nitidus. Patients may improve or clear with discontinuation of a photosensitizing drug, sun avoidance, and sunscreen use.

Chronic actinic dermatitis has been described in markedly immunosuppressed patients and presents as a chronic pruritic and idiopathic eczematous dermatitis in a photodistribution. Phototesting shows increased sensitivity to ultraviolet B. Histologic findings demonstrate eczematous, lymphoma-like, and psoriasiform changes.

O'Connor WJ, Murphy GM, Darby C, et al: Porphyrin abnormalities in acquired immunodeficiency syndrome, *Arch Dermatol* 132:1443–1447, 1996.

21. What is known about granuloma annulare in the setting of HIV infection?

A recent study of 34 consecutive HIV-positive patients with a clinical and histologic diagnosis of granuloma annulare revealed that the generalized form of granuloma annulare was a more common clinical pattern than the localized form of granuloma annulare. In this study, two patients with localized granuloma annulare had perforating lesions, both clinically and histologically. Although granuloma annulare can occur in all stages of HIV infection, it is slightly more common in patients with AIDS. Generalized granuloma annulare lesions appear as multiple, discrete, skin-colored dermal papules distributed on the trunk and extremities. Localized granuloma annulare lesions present as solitary or few discrete papules or annular plaques on one area of the body. The histologic findings of HIV-associated granuloma annulare are similar to those of non–HIV-infected individuals. There are no known cases of diabetes mellitus reported in association with HIV and granuloma annulare.

Toro JR, Chu P, Yen T-S B, et al: Granuloma annulare and human immunodeficiency virus infection, *Arch Dermatol* 135:1341–1346, 1999.

22. Describe some of the potential cutaneous side effects of antiretroviral therapy.

A syndrome of lipodystrophic changes is temporally associated mainly with use of protease inhibitors, and possibly with nucleoside reverse transcriptase inhibitors. It is characterized by enlargement of the dorsocervical fat pad ("buffalo hump"), breast hypertrophy, visceral abdominal fat accumulation ("crix belly," "protease paunch") (Fig. 39-5), peripheral fat wasting with prominence of the superficial veins, and loss of fat in the buccal, temporal, and buttocks areas. Lipodystrophic changes have been associated with hypertriglyceridemia, hypercholesterolemia, hyperglycemia, insulin resistance, and hyperinsulinemia. Evidence of associated Cushing's syndrome or disease is lacking. Lipodystrophic changes have occasionally been reported in patients not taking protease inhibitors. Histologic findings in patients with lipoatrophy include atrophy of the subcutaneous fat, fat lobules with variably sized and often large adipocytes, prominent capillary vascular proliferation, and focal lymphocytic infiltrate and lipogranuloma formation. The exact mechanism involved in these changes is not clear. In addition, antiretroviral therapy has recently been temporally associated with

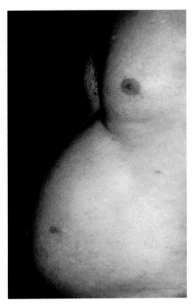

Figure 39-5. Lipodystrophy. Visceral abdominal fat accumulation is seen in this HIV-positive patient who had been taking indinavir for 3 years.

symptomatic angiolipomatosis. Also, painful periungual inflammation (paronychia) of the fingernails and toenails has been reported with use of indinavir and lamivudine. Cutaneous side effects have been described with enfuvirtide (Fuzeon, T-20) use. This drug is a member of a new class of HAART known as fusion inhibitors and is administered subcutaneously. Reported skin side effects are very common and include erythema, induration, nodules, and cysts at the injection sites (Fig. 39-6A,B).

Dank JP, Colven R: Protease inhibitor-associated angiolipomatosis, *J Am Acad Dermatol* 42:129–131, 2000.
James J, Carruthers A, Carruthers J: HIV-associated facial lipoatrophy, *Dermatol Surg* 28:979–986, 2002.
Lalezari JP, Henry K, O'Hearn M, et al: Enfuvirtide, an HIV-1 fusion inhibitor, for drug-resistant HIV infection in North and South America, *N Engl J Med* 348:2175–2185, 2003.
Ward HA, Russo GG, Shrum J: Cutaneous manifestations of antiretroviral therapy, *J Am Acad Dermatol* 46:284–293, 2002.

23. What is the immune restoration syndrome?

Immune restoration syndrome (IRS) is also known as immune reconstitution syndrome, immune reactivation syndrome, and immune reconstitution inflammatory syndrome. It consists of the paradoxical recrudescence of quiescent disease or the appearance of new internal and cutaneous diseases that are temporally associated within weeks to months of HAART initiation. New or recurrent skin disease may consist of initial or recurrent herpes zoster, eosinophilic folliculitis,

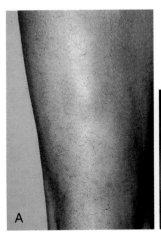

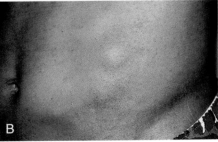

Figure 39-6. A and **B,** Enfuvirtide injection site reactions manifesting as erythematous subcutaneous nodules. (Courtesy of the Walter Reed Army Medical Center teaching files.)

erythema nodosum with pulmonary sarcoidosis with or without cutaneous sarcoidosis, extensive cytomegalovirus ulceration, reactions to prior tattoos, disseminated cutaneous *M. avium* complex infection, alopecia universalis and Graves' disease, and leprosy complicated by type 1 reactional state. The IRS is attributed to the immunologic recovery produced by HAART, with restoration of pathogen-specific immunity.

Hirsch HH, Kaufmann G, Sendi P, et al: Immune reconstitution in HIV-infected patients, *CID* 38:1159–1166, 2004.

DISCLAIMER

The views expressed in this article are those of the authors and do not reflect the official policy of the Department of the Army, the Department of Defense, or the U.S. government.

CUTANEOUS SIGNS OF NUTRITIONAL DISTURBANCES

CHAPTER 40

Carl W. Demidovich, MD

1. When do skin abnormalities occur in association with nutritional disturbances?

Skin manifestations occur when structural or enzymatic processes are affected by a deficiency or excess of a particular nutrient. This can be seen with dietary insufficiency or excess, malabsorption, drug interference, catabolic states, and metabolic, renal, hepatic, and inherited disorders. Nutrients include protein, carbohydrate, fat, vitamins, minerals, and trace elements.

Heath ML, Sidbury R: Cutaneous manifestations of nutritional deficiency, *Curr Opin Pediatr* 18:417–422, 2006.

2. Do nutritional disturbances involve the skin exclusively?

Absolutely not. Nutritional disorders are generalized conditions that cause multisystem disorders. Inadequate diet usually causes multiple nutrient deficiencies, with the resulting clinical picture a combination of these deficiencies. Clinical history, review of systems, and physical examination are of utmost importance when attempting to determine the underlying etiology of skin findings suggestive of a nutritional disorder.

3. Which skin changes are seen with protein and calorie deprivation in adults?

In clinical observations and prospective experiments, adults with starvation demonstrate rough, inelastic, pallid, gray skin with pigmentary changes in the malar and periorificial areas. Hair is thinned and growth of nails is slow. Nails may also demonstrate fissuring. There is decreased subcutaneous fat and, with time, muscle wasting.

4. What is marasmus?

Marasmus (from the Greek meaning *wasting*), or childhood caloric malnutrition, is a combined or proportional energy and protein deficiency with resultant catabolism and utilization of muscle and fat. There are no specific or significant skin findings. Infants often demonstrate a "monkey facies" due to loss of buccal fat that normally gives the face a rounded appearance.

Oumeish OY, Oumiesh I: Nutritional skin problems in children, *Clin Dermatol* 21:260–263, 2003.

5. What is kwashiorkor?

Kwashiorkor (from the Ga language of Ghana, meaning "sickness of the weanling"), or childhood protein malnutrition, is a result of protein deficiency with concurrent normal to excessive carbohydrate intake. It is a common affliction worldwide, and is seen in developed countries in association with poverty, neurologic disease, and malabsorption. There is muscle wasting with preservation of normal fat stores. The low ratio of protein to energy is felt to disrupt the body's usual hypometabolic response to caloric deficiency and is biochemically manifest as markedly increased lipid peroxidation. Clinically, edema, hypoalbuminemia, growth retardation, fatty liver, psychomotor changes, and prominent skin findings are seen.

Lenhartz H, Ndasi R, Anninos A, et al: The clinical manifestation of the kwashiorkor syndrome is related to increased lipid peroxidation, *J Pediatr* 132:879–881, 1998.

6. Describe the skin findings in kwashiorkor.

In black children, initial circumoral pallor progresses to diffuse depigmentation. In white children, there is diffuse blanching erythema that rapidly progresses to dusky nonblanching purple macules and papules. Classic findings include mosaic skin (dry, fine areas of desquamation with cracking along skin lines) and enamel paint dermatosis (Fig. 40-1), which evolves into large areas of erosion and desquamation. Hair in affected patients is sparse, thin, fragile, and depigmented. This hair depigmentation may produce the flag sign, which is alternating pigmented and depigmented bands seen along the hair shafts corresponding to periods of normal and inadequate nutrition.

Buno IJ, Morelli JG, Weston WL: The enamel paint sign in the dermatologic diagnosis of early-onset Kwashiorkor, *Arch Dermatol* 134:107–108, 1998.

7. How can I remember the differences in skin findings associated with kwashiorkor and marasmus?

Kwashiorkor, or protein malnutrition, may be memorized by thinking of "KP," the military term for "kitchen patrol." Kwashiorkor is associated with peeling skin, as are hands of dishwashers.

8. Do skin abnormalities occur with fat deficiency?

Essential fatty acid deficiency occurs with deficiency of linoleic acid, a precursor of arachidonic acid. It is seen primarily with malabsorption syndromes and with prolonged total parenteral nutrition. Skin findings consist of a periorificial or generalized dermatitis caused by increased transepidermal water loss due to loss of the barrier function of the skin. Periorificial dermatitis cannot be clinically differentiated from lesions seen in acrodermatitis enteropathica (see question 18). Dietary or intravenous linoleic acid supplementation is curative, although adults often respond to only topical application.

Smit EN, Muskiet FA, Boersma ER: The possible role of essential fatty acids in the pathophysiology of malnutrition: a review, *Prostaglandins Leukot Essent Fatty Acids* 71:241–250, 2004.

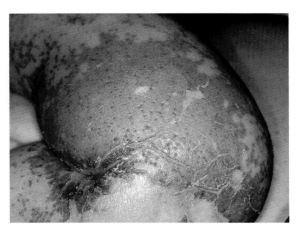

Figure 40-1. Enamel paint dermatosis in a child with kwashiorkor. (Courtesy of William Weston, MD.)

9. Are any skin findings associated with fat excess?

Yes. Obesity researchers have documented an increased incidence of plantar hyperkeratosis (thickened soles), acanthosis nigricans, striae, and skin tags in patients overweight by more than 100%. Excess fat deposition predisposes to intertrigo, a dermatitis occurring between skinfolds, sometimes associated with secondary bacterial or candidal infection.

Yosipovitch G, DeVore A, Dawn A: Obesity and the skin: skin physiology and skin manifestations of obesity, *J Am Acad Dermatol* 56:901–916, 2007.

10. Which water-soluble vitamin abnormalities have skin findings?

Nearly all of the water-soluble vitamins demonstrate skin findings in deficiency states. There is considerable overlap in the skin findings, especially among the B-complex deficiencies, which is expected because they all function as coenzymes or cofactors in redox, carboxylation, or transamination reactions. Common clinical findings in riboflavin (B2), pyridoxine (B6), cobalamin (B12), and biotin deficiencies include angular cheilitis, periorificial dermatitis, and glossitis.

Barthelemy H, Chouvet B, Cambazard F: Skin and mucosal manifestations in vitamin deficiency, *J Am Acad Dermatol* 15:1263–1274, 1986.

11. What is beriberi?

Beriberi is the name applied to severe vitamin B1 (thiamine) deficiency. Vitamin B1 deficiency is most commonly seen in alcoholism, imbalanced diets (e.g., polished rice diet), gastrointestinal disease, gastrointestinal surgery (e.g., gastric bypass surgery for obesity), and pregnancy. The mucocutaneous manifestations consist of limb edema and glossitis. The most important extracutaneous manifestations include mental confusion, peripheral neuropathies, confabulation, Wernicke encephalopathy, and congestive heart failure.

Towbin A, Inge TH, Garcia VF, et al: Beriberi after gastric bypass surgery in adolescence, *J Pediatr* 145:263–267, 2004.

12. Name the four "Ds" of pellagra.

- Diarrhea
- Dermatitis
- Dementia
- Death

Pellagra (Italian, *pelle-*, meaning skin, and *agra-*, meaning sharp, burning, or rough) is a deficiency of niacin that manifests classically as the "four Ds." Great variability is seen in the extent and type of gastrointestinal, neurologic, and skin manifestations. Niacin is available in animal products, enriched wheat flour, and is synthesized from tryptophan. Pellagra is most commonly seen in alcoholics and in patients on isoniazid therapy, which interferes with tryptophan metabolism.

Hegyi J, Schwartz RA, Hegyi V: Pellagra: dermatitis, dementia, and diarrhea, *Int J Dermatol* 43:1–5, 2004.

13. Describe the dermatitis in pellagra.

The dermatitis is characteristically, but not invariably, photodistributed. Acutely, it is erythematous and may be associated with either pruritus or burning. Within 2 to 3 weeks, it becomes dry, scaly, and thickened. Casal's necklace is a term used to describe sharply demarcated dermatitic lesions that develop around the neck and clinically resemble a necklace (Fig. 40-2). Dermatitic lesions also occur in the perineal and genital areas, over bony prominences, and on the face. The skin abnormalities in pellagra respond rapidly to niacin supplementation and heal in a centrifugal fashion.

14. Does scurvy still exist?

Yes, but it is rare. Vitamin C present in fresh fruits and vegetables is a necessary cofactor in collagen synthesis. Deficiency states initially demonstrate enlargement and keratosis of hair follicles with development of corkscrew hairs in adults. Within weeks, there is a proliferation of blood vessels around hair follicles (Fig. 40-3) and in the interdental papillae of gingiva with hemorrhage. Impaired collagen synthesis results in poor wound healing. Recent reports also describe clinical findings of purpura mimicking vasculitis and extensive ecchymoses on the lower extremities. Infantile scurvy is often associated with lower extremity fractures and subperiosteal hemorrhage and demonstrates a characteristic radiographic ground-glass osteopenia. It occurs most commonly between six and twenty four months and is associated with dietary deficiency of medical, social or economic cause.

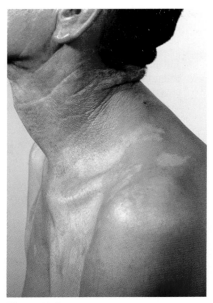

Gonzalez-Gay MA, Garcia-Porrua C, Lueiro M, et al: Scurvy can mimic cutaneous vasculitis: three case reports, *Rev Rheum Engl Ed* 66:360–361, 1999.

Pimentel L: Scurvy: historical review and current diagnostic approach, *Am J Emerg Med* 21:328–332, 2003.

Jenny C: Evaluating infants and young children with multiple fractures, *Pediatrics* 118(3):1299–1303, 2006.

15. Do deficiencies of the fat-soluble vitamins occur?

Yes, but less commonly because these vitamins have significant storage depots. Vitamin K deficiency is seen with malabsorption syndromes and in the newborn period prior to bacterial colonization of the intestine. Clinical lesions range from petechiae to massive hemorrhages. Vitamin D and E deficiencies are not associated with skin findings.

Figure 40-2. Pellagra, showing the typical photodistributed dermatitis on the neck and chest known as "Casal's necklace." (Courtesy of Richard Gentry, MD.)

16. What abnormalities occur with vitamin A deficiency?

This disorder primarily involves the skin and eyes. Phrynoderma, the name applied to the cutaneous eruption of vitamin A deficiency, is a keratotic follicular eruption that initially appears on the proximal extremities. It eventually extends to the trunk, back, abdomen, buttocks, and neck. Although phrynoderma is widely accepted as being specific for vitamin A deficiency, it has recently been suggested that it may be a manifestation of severe malnutrition associated with deficiencies of multiple critical vitamins and essential fatty acids. Facial lesions may resemble large comedones of acne. Eye symptoms include nyctalopia (delayed dark adaptation, the earliest finding), night blindness, and xerophthalmia. Objective findings are Bitot's spots, which are areas of shed corneal epithelium, and in severe disease, keratomalacia. Vitamin A deficiency is most commonly caused by malabsorption disorders.

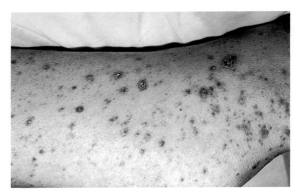

Figure 40-3. Scurvy. Characteristic perifollicular hemorrhage and follicular hyperkeratosis.

Maronn M, Allen DM, Esterly NB: Phrynoderma: a manifestation of vitamin A deficiency?...The rest of the story, *Pediatr Dermatol* 22:60–63, 2005.

Sommer A: Vitamin A deficiency and clinical disease: an historical overview, *J Nutr* 138:1835–1839, 2008.

17. Is vitamin A excess toxic?

Yes. Hypervitaminosis A may develop either acutely or chronically. Acute toxicity is rare but is most commonly due to vitamin A overdose. It has also been documented in Arctic explorers consuming polar bear livers, which are rich in vitamin A. Clinically, it presents as large areas of desquamation associated with headache and vomiting. Chronic toxicity is more common and displays features associated with side effects of retinoid therapy: alopecia, exfoliation, and skin dryness. Pseudotumor cerebri with papilledema may occur early before any other signs. All symptoms and signs resolve in days to weeks following cessation of supplementation.

18. What is acrodermatitis enteropathica?

Acrodermatitis enteropathica is a rare autosomal recessive disorder of intestinal zinc absorption. Zinc is normally incorporated into multiple types of enzymes present in all body tissues but is concentrated five- to sixfold in the epidermis. Deficiency of this trace element results in dramatic findings. The classic triad consists of acral dermatitis, alopecia, and diarrhea. Growth failure, anemia, impaired wound healing, and mental and emotional disturbances are also seen. The periorificial and acral dermatitis (Fig. 40-4) was considered to be pathognomonic in the past, but more recent reports have described similar cutaneous eruptions in essential fatty acid deficiency, biotin deficiency, and infants treated for organic acidurias. Acrodermatitis enteropathica develops in days to weeks after birth in bottle-fed infants and shortly after weaning in breastfed infants. Uncommonly, signs and symptoms are first noted at puberty.

Maverakis E, Fung MA, Lynch PJ, et al: Acrodermatitis enteropathica and an overview of zinc metabolism, *J Am Acad Dermatol* 56:116–124, 2007.

19. Has the gene responsible for inherited acrodermatitis enteropathica been identified?

Yes. The responsible gene is the *SLC39A4* gene, which has been localized to the chromosomal region 8q24.3. A number of different mutations of this gene, which is responsible for encoding for an intestinal zinc transporter of the ZIP family, have been identified.

Nakano A, Nakano H, Nomura K, et al: Novel SLC39A4 mutations in acrodermatitis enteropathica, *J Invest Dermatol* 120:963–966, 2003.

20. How is acrodermatitis enteropathica diagnosed and treated?

Diagnosis is made by demonstrating low plasma or serum zinc levels. Hair zinc levels reflect only long-term status and may not reflect early deficiency. Oral or intravenous zinc supplementation promotes rapid improvement, with reversal of most clinical manifestations in hours to days. Untreated infants develop failure to thrive, with progressive deterioration and death.

Key Points: Pellagra

1. Pellagra is due to deficiency of niacin and/or nicotinic acid.
2. Pellagra is most common in patients with corn-rich diets, alcoholism, gastrointestinal disease, carcinoid, and some drugs.
3. The classic tetrad of pellagra all start with the letter D: diarrhea, dermatitis, dementia, death.
4. Casal's necklace is the distinctive photosensitive eruption seen in pellagra that presents as a "necklace" around the neck.

21. Can zinc deficiency be acquired?

Yes, in association with diabetes mellitus, collagen vascular disease, pregnancy, Crohn's disease, nephrotic syndrome, dialysis, renal tubular disease, burns, antimetabolite drugs, alcoholism, malabsorption syndromes, and HIV infection. Clinical findings are similar to those of the inherited form of acrodermatitis enteropathica.

22. What is carotenoderma?

Carotenoderma is a yellow or orange skin discoloration most prominent on the palms, soles, and central face. It is more common in children and is associated with ingestion of carotene found in carrots, oranges, squash, spinach, yellow corn, butter, eggs, pumpkin, yellow turnips, sweet potatoes, and dried seaweeds. It is clinically apparent when serum carotene levels are three to four times normal. The discoloration spares the sclera and mucosal surfaces, which can be used to differentiate this benign condition from jaundice (Fig. 40-5). Elimination of the offending food results in normalization of skin color in 2 to 6 weeks. Carotenemia also occurs in diabetes mellitus and hypothyroidism due to impaired hepatic conversion of carotene to vitamin A. It has been reported in anorexia nervosa with undetermined etiology.

Maharshak N, Shapiro J, Trau HZ: Carotenoderma: a review of the current literature, *Int J Dermatol* 42:178–181, 2003.

23. Has supplementation with micronutrients or homeopathic remedies been associated with any cutaneous disorders?

Yes. Ginkgo, garlic and ginseng inhibit platelet activation and aggregation and may increase intraoperative bleeding and cause postoperative hematoma and ecchymosis. It is recommended to stop these supplements one week before surgery. Certain Chinese herbal supplements and proprietary medicines have been reported to contain inorganic arsenic. This has caused chronic arsenicism, clinically manifested as Bowen's disease (squamous cell carcinoma in situ) and arsenical keratoses on the palms and soles.

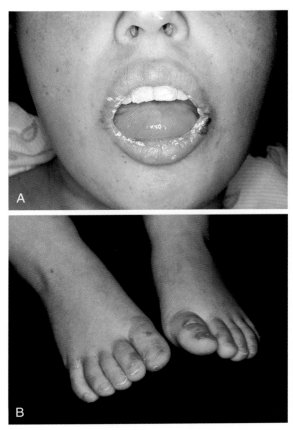

Figure 40-4. Acrodermatitis enteropathica. **A,** Periorificial dermatitis in a young patient with acrodermatitis enteropathica. **B,** Acral dermatitis in a young patient with characteristic involvement around the nails. (Courtesy of James E. Fitzpatrick, MD.)

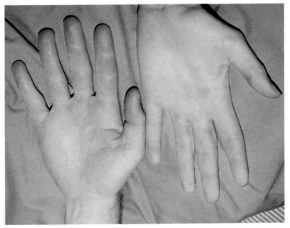

Figure 40-5. Characteristic yellow discoloration of skin in a patient with carotenoderma contrasted with normal skin color. The patient was eating up to one bunch of carrots per day. (Courtesy of James E. Fitzpatrick, MD.)

BENIGN MELANOCYTIC TUMORS

Michael R. Campoli, MD, PhD, and Patrick Walsh, MD

1. What is a mole?

A mole is a small burrowing mammal belonging to the family *Talpidae*. It is also a term commonly used to describe a melanocytic nevus.

2. What is a nevus?

Derived from the Latin term meaning "spot" or "blemish," nevus was originally used to describe a congenital lesion or birthmark (mother's mark). In modern usage, the term describes a cutaneous hamartoma, or benign proliferation of cells. However, when the term is used without a descriptive adjective, it usually refers to a melanocytic nevus. Examples of nevi used in the context of a birthmark are epidermal nevus and nevus sebaceous.

3. Are there different types of melanocytic nevi?

Yes. Melanocytic nevi can be classified according to their histology based on 1) location of the nevus cells (e.g., junctional, compound, or intradermal nevi), 2) cytologic atypia (e.g., atypical [dysplastic] nevi, and 3) morphology and architectural arrangement of nevus cells (e.g., Spitz and spindle cell nevi). Melanocytic nevi can also be classified based on their appearance (e.g., halo nevi or blue nevi). In addition, there are congenital melanocytic and acquired nevi.

4. How do melanocytes get to the skin?

Melanocytes arise from the cranial and truncal neural crest cells in embryonic life. The development of melanocytes from neural crest cells, as well as their ability to migrate, is dependent upon interactions between specific receptors and extracellular ligands, including endothelin 3 and the endothelin B receptors, α–melanocyte stimulating hormone and the melanocortin-1 receptor stem cell factor and its receptor KIT, each of which induce expression of the microphthalmia-associated transcription factor (MITF). MITF is the most critical regulator of pigment cell development and survival. Bone morphogenic protein (BMP) is a negative regulator of this process.

Melanocytes migrate via the mesenchyme and reach their final location in the skin, uveal tract of the eye (choroid, ciliary body, and iris), leptomeninges, inner ear (cochlea), and sympathetic chain lining the colon early during embryogenesis. The melanocytes that migrate to the skin take up residence on the epidermal side of the dermal–epidermal junction, the basal layer of the hair matrix, as well as the outer root sheath of the bulge region of the hair follicle. The latter region is where melanocyte stem cells are thought to reside.

5. Explain the natural developmental history of melanocytic nevi.

Melanocytic nevus cells are derived from melanocytes and differ from normal epidermal melanocytes in a number of ways. They are no longer dendritic; they do not distribute melanin to surrounding keratinocytes; and they are less metabolically active. Melanocytic nevi are benign clonal proliferations of cells expressing the melanocytic phenotype, and are thought to be derived from precursor cells that acquire genetic mutations. These mutations are thought to activate proliferative pathways and/or or suppress apoptosis, allowing for the accumulation of melanocytic cells in the skin. The type of nevus that is formed is thought to be dependent upon the specific mutation, as well as local environmental factors. *B-Raf* mutations are commonly seen in acquired melanocytic nevi. Acquired melanocytic nevi are thought to begin as a proliferation of nevus cells along the dermal–epidermal junction (forming a junctional nevus; Fig. 41-1A). With continued proliferation of nevus cells, they extend from the dermal–epidermal junction into the dermis (forming a compound nevus). The junctional component of the melanocytic nevus may resolve, leaving only an intradermal component (intradermal nevus; Fig. 41-1B). However, it should be stressed that there is debate regarding the direction of nevus growth.

Melanocytic nevi form naturally, possibly due to ultraviolet light exposure, from the ages of 6 months to 40 years and later. They may also resolve spontaneously. However, the appearance or disappearance of any melanocytic lesion should be brought to the attention of a physician.

Cane JF, Trainor PA: Neural crest stem and progenitor cells, *Annu Rev Cell Dev Biol* 22:267–286, 2006.
Grichnik J: Melanoma, nevogenesis, and stem cell biology, *J Invest Dermatol* 128:2365–2380, 2008.

6. What is a halo nevus?

A halo nevus, also known as a Sutton's nevus or leukoderma acquisitum centrifugum, is a melanocytic nevus with a surrounding well-circumscribed annulus of hypo- or depigmented skin (Fig. 41-1C). Halo nevi can be solitary or multiple and generally affect individuals under the age of 20 years. In general, those patients with halo nevi have an overall increased number of melanocytic nevi. Halo nevi are commonly associated with vitiligo, with ~20% to 50% of vitiligo patients demonstrating halo nevi. Conversely, ~15% to 25% of patients with halo nevi have vitiligo. Although both halo nevi and vitiligo may look similar clinically, recent studies strongly suggest that halo nevi and vitiligo have separate pathogenetic mechanisms. Although not completely understood, the pathogenesis of halo nevi is thought to be related to 1) an immune response against antigenically altered nevus cells or 2) a cell-mediated or humoral immune response against nonspecifically altered nevus cells. It is not completely understood whether this represents an abnormal immunologic response or whether the immune system is recognizing an atypical clone of nevomelanocytes.

Although most pigmented lesions with halos are benign, malignant melanoma can rarely be seen with an associated halo. If a pigmented lesion has an irregular border and halo or shows other atypical features, it should be biopsied.

De Vijlder HC, Westerhof W, Schreuder GM, et al: Difference in pathogenesis between vitiligo vulgaris and halo nevi associated with vitiligo is supported by an HLA study, *Pigment Cell Res* 17:270–274, 2004.

7. What is a congenital nevus?

A melanocytic nevus that is present at birth. For the purpose of management, any melanocytic nevus that arises during the first year of life is considered "congenital." Congenital melanocytic nevi (CMN) are usually characterized as small, large, or giant, although there is no universally accepted definition of these categories. Small CMN are usually defined as being up to 1.5 cm in diameter, large CMN as being between 1.5 and 20 cm in diameter, and giant CMN as being more than 20 cm in diameter. Another scheme for classifying small, large, and giant CMN considers the percentage of the body surface area the lesion covers, or the ease of surgical removal and repair of the resulting surgical defect. Still another classification scheme describes giant CMN as being as large as two of the patient's palms for lesions on the trunk and extremities, or the size of one palm for lesions on the face or neck (Fig. 41-1D).

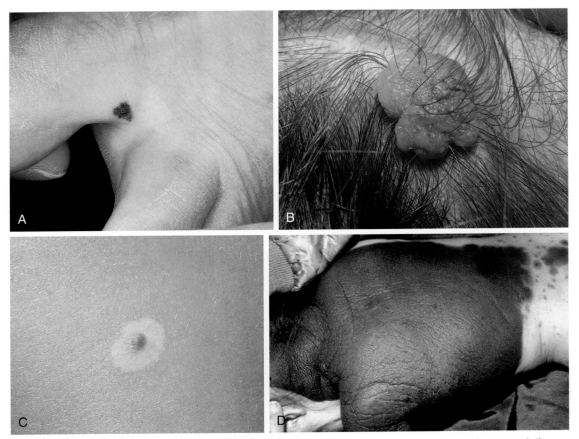

Figure 41-1. A, Junctional nevi are typically small, flat, and dark brown in color. **B,** An intradermal nevus also may be very exophytic or papillomatous, as shown here. **C,** Typical halo nevus of the back demonstrating a central brownish-red papule. **D,** Large congenital nevus with multiple smaller congenital nevi. These lesions present a surgical challenge and a significant cosmetic problem.

8. **What is the risk of developing a malignant melanoma in a congenital nevus?**

Although there is little agreement about the risk of developing melanoma within a CMN, some general guidelines can be stated. The risk appears to relate to the size of the CMN. A small or medium CMN does not appear to have any significantly greater risk for melanoma than an acquired melanocytic nevus. The best evidence suggests that there is about a 1% to 4% chance of developing melanoma in CMN > 60 cm. The need for removal of congenital nevi is one of the most controversial issues in pediatric dermatology. It should be stressed that surgical removal of the CMN does not decrease their risk for melanoma.

Kinsler VA, Birley J, Atherton DJ: Great Ormond Street Hospital for Children Registry for Congenital Melanocytic Naevi: prospective study 1988–2007. Part 1— epidemiology, phenotype, and outcomes, *Br J Dermatol* 160:143–150, 2009.
Kinsler VA, Birley J, Atherton DJ: Great Ormond Street Hospital for Children Registry for Congenital Melanocytic Naevi: prospective study 1988–2007. Part 2—evaluation of treatments, *Br J Dermatol* 160:387–392, 2009.

9. **What is a blue nevus?**

Blue nevi and related melanocytic proliferations (i.e., congenital dermal melanocytoses including Mongolian spot, nevus of Ito and nevus of Ota) are a heterogenous group of congenital and acquired melanocytic lesions that have in common several clinical, histologic, and immunochemical features. They have been termed dermal dendritic melanocytic proliferations, because they are usually composed, at least in part, of dendritic melanocytes within the dermis. The deep dermal location of the pigment-producing cells, and therefore the pigment, causes the lesion to have its blue, black, or gray appearance due to the Tyndall effect (Fig. 41-2).

Blue nevi are usually acquired and have their onset most commonly in childhood and adolescence, but ~25% are congenital. In general, melanocytes disappear from the dermis during embryonic migration, but some cells do remain in the scalp, sacral region and dorsal aspect of the distal extremities. These sites correlate to the most common locations for blue nevi to occur. The three commonly identified varieties of blue nevi are the common blue nevus, cellular blue nevus, and combined blue nevus–melanocytic nevus.

10. **Can blue nevi become malignant?**

Yes. Malignant blue nevi can develop de novo in existing cellular blue nevi, or in a nevus of Ota (see below). Most commonly, the lesion presents as an expanding dermal nodule that may ulcerate. As with other forms of cutaneous melanoma, metastases may develop. Malignant blue nevi are tumors of older individuals. It is more frequent in males then females. The scalp and extremities are the most common sites of occurrence. The prognosis in malignant blue nevi is poor. However, malignant blue nevi are rare, and often there is controversy regarding their histopathologic diagnosis.

Zembowicz A, Mihm MC: Dermal dendritic melanocytic proliferations: an update. *Histopathology* 45:433–451, 2004.

11. **What is a combined melanocytic nevus?**

A combined melanocytic nevus is a blue nevus with an overlying melanocytic nevus. The blue nevus may be a common or cellular blue nevus. The overlying melanocytic nevus can be junctional, compound, or intradermal. This is found in 1% of all excised melanocytic nevi.

12. **How does a nevus of Ota differ from a nevus of Ito?**

The nevus of Ota (also called nevus fuscoceruleus ophthalmomaxillaris) is characterized clinically as a blue to gray hyperpigmentation of the skin, mucosa, and conjunctiva in the distribution of the trigeminal nerve. Less commonly, it may also involve the meninges (meningeal melanocytoma), where it may develop a hemorrhage or, rarely, a malignant melanoma. Histologically, it is composed of heavily melanized dendritic dermal melanocytes in the upper dermis. The nevus of Ito is similar in histology to the nevus of Ota but is distributed along the neck and shoulder in the distribution of the posterior supraclavicular and lateral cutaneous brachial nerves. Both lesions are considered congenital dermal melanocytoses and are more common in Asians and African-Americans. About 80% of all reported cases have been woman.

13. **What is the best way to treat nevus of Ota?**

Most lesions are a cosmetic issue only and treatment is not necessary unless it starts to affect the patient's self-esteem. In the past, scarring treatment modalities such as excision and cryotherapy were utilized. In the last 10 years, the use of Q-switched ruby, alexandrite, and Nd:YAG lasers has markedly improved the cosmetic appearance of these lesions, and they have become the treatment of choice. Although malignant changes are extremely rare, nevus of Ota patients with eye

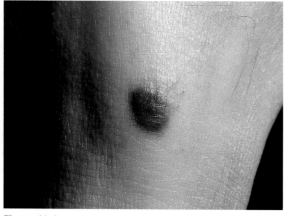

Figure 41-2. Blue nevus on the lower leg. (Courtesy of Fitzsimons Army Medical Center teaching files.)

involvement should be followed closely, because a majority of associated melanomas occur in the ocular region.

14. What is a Mongolian spot?

A Mongolian spot is congenital dermal melanocytoses characterized as a congenital hyperpigmented spot found in the sacrococcygeal region. Most frequently found in black or Asian infants, it also occurs in infants of other races. The pigmentation often improves spontaneously in the first 3 to 5 years of life but may persist to some degree into adulthood. These lesions are believed to represent the delayed disappearance of dermal melanocytes. The deep blue pigmentation is another example of the Tyndall effect.

Snow TM: Mongolian spots in the newborn: do they mean anything? *Neonatal Netw* 24:31–33, 2005.

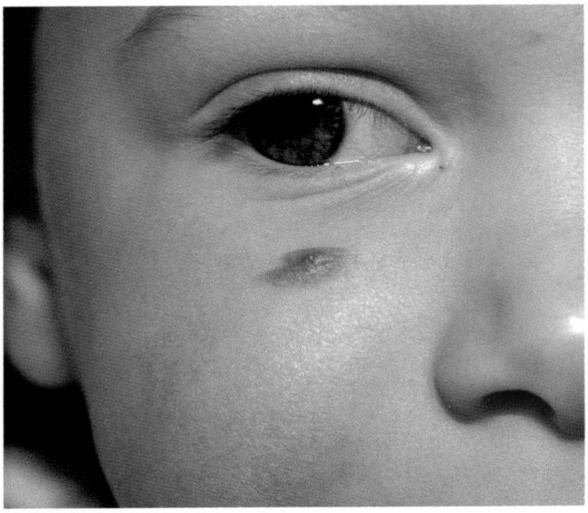

15. What is a Spitz nevus?

A Spitz nevus is a benign melanocytic nevus named in honor of Dr. Sophie Spitz, who initially described this lesion as a *benign juvenile melanoma*. These most commonly occur in children but may occur at any age. Spitz nevi are most commonly acquired but

Figure 41-3. Spitz nevus. Typical red papule on the cheek of a young child. Because of their red color, they are clinically often mistaken for vascular neoplasms. (Courtesy of the William L. Weston, M.D. Collection.)

as many as 7% may be congenital. The lesion usually presents as a small, pink papule or nodule on the face or lower extremities (Fig. 41-3). Histologically, it is composed of nevus cells that are pleomorphic and cytologically atypical; these cells typically demonstrate a spindle or epithelioid appearance that shares many of the histologic characteristics found in melanoma. The histologic differentiation of Spitz nevus from malignant melanoma is one of the most difficult challenges in dermatopathology and, in some cases, the biologic behavior cannot be predicted using current criteria. It is noteworthy that, to date, no *B-Raf* mutations have been detected in Spitz nevi, in contrast to common acquired melanocytic nevi. A small subset of Spitz nevi demonstrate *H-Ras* mutations.

Sulit DJ, Guariano RA, Krivda S: Classic and atypical Spitz nevi: review of the literature, *Cutis* 79:141–146, 2007.
Takata M., Saida, T: Genetic alterations in melanocytic tumors, *J Dermatol Sci* 43:1–10, 2006.

16. Where do Becker's nevi occur?

A Becker's nevus is characterized by an area of hyperpigmentation and often hypertrichosis, most commonly on the upper back, shoulder, or chest of males (Fig. 41-4). The lesions usually become noticeable at puberty. Histologically, there are increased numbers of melanocytes, dermal melanophages, terminal hairs, and hyperpigmentation of the epidermal basal layer. Some lesions can also show increased smooth muscle and have been called smooth muscle hamartomas.

Danarti R, Konig A, Salhi A, et al: Becker's nevus syndrome revisited, *J Am Acad Dermatol* 51:965–969, 2004.

17. What is a dysplastic (atypical) melanocytic nevus?

Dysplastic or atypical nevus is a controversial term that has eluded a precise definition. It has been commonly used to describe an atypical-appearing melanocytic nevus believed to have increased potential for malignant transformation. Since this lesion was first described, the atypical nevus has been the subject of controversy. Argument has centered on the criteria for its histopathologic diagnosis, the incidence of melanomas developing in the lesion, and the histopathologic association of melanoma arising in an atypical nevus.

Naeyaert JM, Brochez L: Clinical practice. Dysplastic nevi. *N Engl J Med* 349:2233–2240, 2003.

18. What is the preferred terminology for dysplastic (atypical) nevi?

The terminology used for this lesion is the subject of controversy. The lesion was first described by Clark et al in 1978, and they used the term "B-K mole syndrome" to refer to the presence of multiple melanocytic lesions that had clinically and

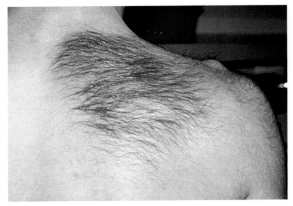

Figure 41-4. A Becker's nevus on the upper back of a young man. This lesion has no potential for malignant degeneration.

histologically distinct features in two families at increased risk of developing melanoma. Since then, various terms have been applied to describe this syndrome and its corresponding lesion, including the B-K mole, precancerous melanosis, atypical melanocytic hyperplasia, Clark's nevus, active junctional nevus, and melanocytic nevus with architectural disorder and cytologic atypia. "Dysplastic nevus" was first coined by Green et al in 1980; however, some authorities have objected to this term and prefer "atypical nevus." The recognition of atypical nevi in the nonfamilial setting has also been reported and termed sporadic dysplastic (atypical) nevi. More recently, an alternative term for dysplastic (atypical) nevi was proposed by a National Institutes of Health consensus group as "nevi with architectural disorder and cytological atypia." The conference also recommended replacing atypical nevus syndrome with familial atypical melanocytic nevus syndrome. Despite their recommendations, this terminology has not been universally accepted among clinicians and pathologists.

Elder DE: Dysplastic naevi: an update, *Histopathology* 56:112–120, 2010.

19. What is the clinical relevance of atypical melanocytic nevi?

The clinical relevance of atypical nevi relates to their association with increased melanoma risk. Several retrospective and prospective case-control studies have established that increasing numbers of atypical nevi confer an independent increasing risk of melanoma ranging from 2- to 71-fold. Patients with atypical nevi and two or more family members with melanoma seem to be at the highest risk for melanoma. Evidence that atypical nevi may be potential precursors of melanoma includes photographically documented examples of change in a preexisting nevus and the observation of histological atypia in proximity to melanomas. About 25% to 50% of melanomas have a histologically associated nevus, and the incidence rate of melanomas arising in association with atypical nevi has been estimated to be ~0.5% to 46%. The most convincing evidence for this association is the demonstration of similar or identical genetic changes in a melanoma and its associated nevus.

Despite the above findings, as well as the documented increased risk of melanoma in patients with atypical nevi, it is important to recognize that most atypical nevi are benign and do not progress to melanoma. In this regard, previous studies have shown that anywhere from 20% to 40% of melanomas arise from a preexisting nevus, 30% to 70% arise de novo and, in almost a quarter, the historical origin cannot be assessed. Therefore, although there is a clear association between nevi and melanoma risk, at present it is not clear whether an atypical nevus is more likely to develop into a melanoma than any other type of nevus. Moreover, it is quite clear that a nevus precursor is not required for the majority of melanomas. It is thought that the discrepancy between melanomas arising in preexisting nevi and de novo melanomas can best be explained by the cancer stem cell theory. In this regard, the risk of melanoma associated with nevi may be due to the potential for secondary mutations within nevi, as well as due to the inherent properties of the stem cell population in individuals with numerous moles.

20. Describe the genetic mutations found in atypical melanocytic nevi.

Mutations in susceptibility genes have been detected in atypical nevi including cyclin-dependent kinase inhibitor 2A (*CDKN2A*) and cyclin-dependent kinase 4 (*CDK4*). Furthermore, a high incidence of *B-Raf* mutations has also been detected in atypical nevi. It is thought that these mutations may be due to ultraviolet radiation because patients with atypical nevi may have a decreased ability to repair ultraviolet light–induced DNA damage.

Weatherhead SC, Haniffa M, Lawrence CM: Melanomas arising from naevi and de novo melanomas: does origin matter? *Br J Dermatol* 156:72–76, 2007.

21. How common are atypical melanocytic nevi?

The exact incidence is unknown, but it is estimated that 2% to 8% of the population have one or more atypical nevus.

22. Is there a difference between an atypical nevus and melanoma in situ?

Yes. The difference is determined by the histopathology. Unfortunately, consensus regarding the histologic definition of atypical nevi is lacking. When an atypical nevus has atypical melanocytic nevus cells at the dermal–epidermal interface, some of these cells may exhibit cytologic atypia, but this is variable and not continuous throughout the lesion. There are also often architectural abnormalities noted between melanocytic nests. In contrast, melanoma in situ has atypical melanocytes, both singly and in small nests scattered through all levels of the epidermis (pagetoid pattern). Further, a typical melanoma is often more asymmetrical; melanocytes present as solitary units in the epidermis rather than in nests, and the melanocytes demonstrate a greater degree of cytologic atypia.

23. What is the recommended treatment for an atypical nevus and melanoma in situ?

Recommended treatment for melanoma in situ is complete full-thickness excision with a minimum of a 0.5-cm margin of normal skin. However some studies suggest that 0.5 cm may be not be the optimal margin for melanoma in situ. Controversy exists regarding the treatment of atypical nevi. Depending on the degree of cytologic atypia, full-thickness excision with margins ranging from 0.2 to 0.5 cm have been recommended. However, for atypical nevi with mild to moderate degrees of cytologic atypia, the question of complete excision is controversial. The latter reflects the lack of consensus about the grading of atypia in nevi, as well as the insufficient data regarding the significance of melanocytic atypia in nevi. It should be stressed that the removal of large numbers of atypical nevi results in significant scarring. Only after thorough evaluation, and when a melanoma cannot be ruled out, should surgical removal be performed. As mentioned above, the vast majority of atypical nevi never become melanomas.

24. Describe the clinical appearance of atypical nevi.

No single feature is diagnostic of atypical nevi; instead, a collection of clinical findings is required for their diagnosis. Atypical nevi are usually larger than ordinary nevi (>6 mm) and have slightly irregular borders that fade into the surrounding normal skin (Fig. 41-5). Variation of color with an asymmetrical pattern is common. The colors vary from shades of brown to black, tan, and light red. The lesions typically have a dark center surrounded by pigment that has poor margination. Atypical nevi most frequently are located on the trunk, scalp, breast (in women) and bathing-trunk areas (in men).

25. Is there a difference between a liver spot and a freckle?

Yes. Liver spot is the term commonly used to refer to a solar or senile lentigo. A lentigo is a hyperpigmented (usually brown or black) macule that is characterized histopathologically by increased numbers of melanocytes at the dermal–epidermal junction and increased amounts of melanin in both the melanocytes and basal keratinocytes. These lesions commonly arise on the dorsal aspects of the hands and face. Although solar lentigines are induced by ultraviolet radiation, they do not increase in pigmentation with exposure to the sun. Polymorphisms in the melanocortin receptor 1 gene (*MCR1*) have been associated with the development of freckles. Freckles (ephelides) are hyperpigmented macules limited to sun-exposed skin. Microscopically, they show increased amounts of melanin in basal keratinocytes, but not increased numbers of melanocytes. Freckles characteristically darken with sun exposure and lighten when the affected areas are protected from ultraviolet radiation.

Key Points: Benign Melanocytic Tumors

1. Benign melanocytic nevi may arise, grow, and regress normally. Rapid change is not normal.
2. There appears to be a small increased risk (1% to 4%) of melanoma in patients with giant CMN.
3. Patients with a large number (>100) of atypical melanocytic nevi should be followed closely for the possible development of melanoma.
4. Between 30% and 70% of malignant melanoma arise de novo independent of a preexisting nevus.
5. Mutations in *CDKN2A, CDK4*, and *B-Raf* have been detected in atypical nevi.
6. Multiple CALMs are most commonly associated with neurofibromatosis.
7. Ephelides and lentigines are not melanocytic nevi.

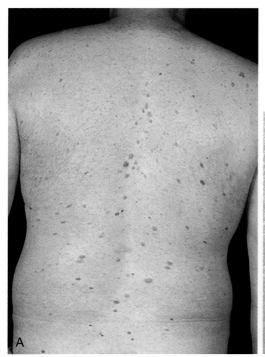
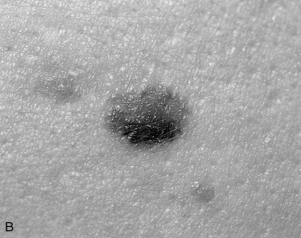

Figure 41-5. Atypical nevi. **A,** Patient with familial atypical melanocytic nevus syndrome demonstrating numerous atypical nevi. **B,** An atypical nevus demonstrating marked variegation in color and loss of normal symmetry.

26. What is a café-au-lait macule?

Café-au-lait macules (CALMs) are uniformly light-brown (the color of coffee with cream) macules that vary in size from 2 to 20 cm and often have irregular borders. They are characterized by increased melanin in both melanocytes and keratinocytes and by giant melanosomes. CALMs grow proportionately to body growth and remain stable in size after body growth has completed. CALMs are found in 10% to 20% of the general population; however, multiple CALMs are relatively rare (0.25% to 0.5%) in the general population and should alert you to the possibility of an associated disease. Multiple CALMs are most commonly associated with neurofibromatosis (see Chapter 5), and large CALMs with the McCune-Albright syndrome (see Chapter 18).

Landau M, Krafchik BR: The diagnostic value of café-au-lait macules, *J Am Acad Dermatol* 40:877–890, 1999.

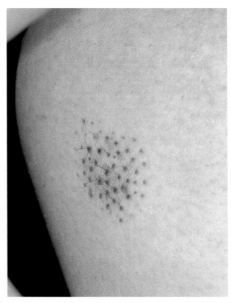

Figure 41-6. Nevus spilus showing a large café-au-lait macule with multiple small pigmented lesions.

27. What is a nevus spilus?

A nevus spilus is an irregularly shaped, light-brown macule with darkly pigmented macules or papules scattered randomly within the macule (Fig. 41-6). The light areas demonstrate the microscopic changes of a café-au-lait macule, and areas of increased melanin with darker pigmentation show the histology of lentigines or junctional nevi. Rare cases have developed malignant melanomas.

Vaidya DC, Schwartz RA, Janniger CK: Nevus spilus, *Cutis* 80:465–468, 2007.

28. Can melanocytic nevi arise in locations other than the skin?

Yes. Melanocytic nevi can occur on the retina, conjunctiva, and oral (and other) mucosal surfaces.

29. What is a labial lentigo?

Labial lentigo (labial melanotic macule) is a hyperpigmented macule that develops on the lip. Seen most commonly in young women, there is thickening of the epidermis and increased melanin in the basal keratinocytes. These typically behave in a benign fashion.

VASCULAR AND LYMPHATIC NEOPLASMS

Joseph G. Morelli, MD

CHAPTER 42

1. Which is the most common benign vascular neoplasm of childhood?

Hemangioma of infancy (HOI), which is a benign tumor of capillary endothelium. This tumor typically presents at ages 2 to 8 weeks and then goes through a rapid growth phase for the first 6 to 9 months of life. It then begins to regress, with complete regression in 50% of patients by age 5 years. Regression does not necessarily imply return of the skin to normal.

Kilcline C, Frieden IJ: Infantile hemangiomas: how common are they? A systematic review of the medical literature, *Pediatr Dermatol* 25:168–173, 2009.

2. What are the clinical subtypes of HOI?

- Superficial: Bright red papules
- Deep: Soft blue nodule (Fig. 42-1)
- Mixed: Combination of the above

Most HOI are clinically the mixed type.

3. Name the complications of hemangiomas.

Obstruction of a vital function (such as vision, breathing, eating, defecation, or urination), ulceration followed by bleeding and infection, and high-output cardiac failure. High-output cardiac failure rarely results from a solitary cutaneous HOI.

4. What is the most common complication of hemangiomas?

Ulceration is the most frequent complication and occurs predominantly in the diaper areas (Fig. 42-2).

5. Are there any residua of hemangiomas after regression?

Hypopigmentation, telangiectasia, excess skin, fibrofatty deposits, and, if ulceration occurred, scarring (Fig. 42-3).

6. What is Kasabach-Merritt syndrome?

Platelet trapping and consumption coagulopathy associated with a vascular tumor.

Rodriguez V, Lee A, Wiltman PM, Anderson PA: Kasabach-Merritt phenomenon: case series and retrospective review of the Mayo Clinic experience, *J Pediatr Hematol Oncol* 31:522–526, 2009.

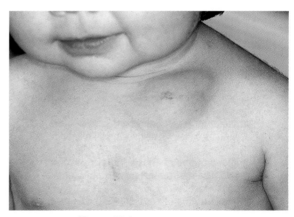

Figure 42-1. Deep hemangioma.

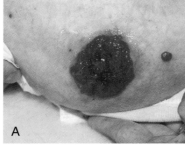 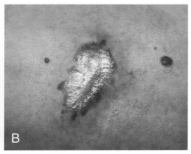

Figure 42-2. A, Ulcerated hemangioma. **B,** The same hemangioma three months after one pulsed dye laser treatment.

7. **Name the two vascular tumors most commonly associated with the Kasabach-Merritt syndrome.**
Kaposiform hemangioendothelioma and tufted angioma.

8. **Port wine stains and lymphangiomas are not neoplasms. What are they?**
They are vascular malformations.

9. **What is the difference between a vascular malformation and a vascular neoplasm?**
A vascular malformation is a developmental error. A vascular neoplasm is a tumor. Vascular malformations stay rather static and grow proportionately with the patient. Vascular tumors grow at a rate greater than the patient does.

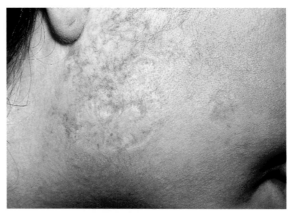

Figure 42-3. Scarring, hypopigmentation, and telangiectasia after regression of a hemangioma.

10. **What is Klippel-Trénaunay syndrome?**
This is overgrowth of an extremity secondary to a vascular malformation. The overgrowth invariably involves soft tissue but can also affect the bone (Fig. 42-4). The vascular malformation may be a capillary malformation (port wine stain), a venous malformation, or a combination of the two.

11. **How does Klippel-Trénaunay-Weber syndrome differ from Klippel-Trénaunay syndrome?**
In Klippel-Trénaunay-Weber syndrome, the vascular malformation must include an arteriovenous malformation.

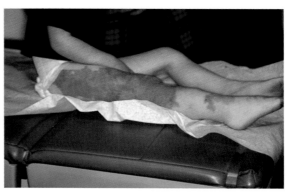

Figure 42-4. Klippel-Trénaunay syndrome. Mixed capillary-venous malformation associated with increased limb size.

12. **What are blue-black hyperkeratotic vascular papules?**
Angiokeratomas. There are five types of angiokeratomas:
- **Localized angiokeratomas:** Usually solitary and found on an extremity
- **Angiokeratoma circumscriptum:** Presents at birth as unilateral plaques on an extremity (Fig. 42-5)
- **Angiokeratoma of Mibelli:** Develops in childhood or adolescence over the dorsal surface of the hands or feet
- **Angiokeratoma of Fordyce:** Most commonly seen on the scrotum
- **Angiokeratoma corporis diffusum (Fabry's disease):** An X-linked recessively inherited disease that results from a deficiency of the lysosomal enzyme α-galactosidase A, leading to the accumulation of glycolipids (mainly globotriaosylceramide) in the cells from various tissues. Multiple skin lesions between the umbilicus and knees. Frequent development of hypohidrosis, paresthesias, cardiac, and renal disease

Rozenfeld PA: Fabry disease: treatment and diagnosis, *IUBMB Life* 26:1043–1050, 2009.

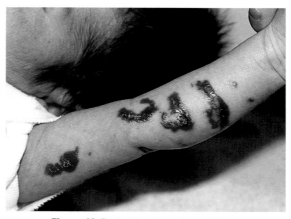

Figure 42-5. Angiokeratoma circumscriptum.

13. **Where and in whom are cherry angiomas most commonly seen?**
Cherry angiomas are extremely common, acquired, 1- to 5-mm, red to purple papules located primarily on the trunk and upper extremities (Fig. 42-6). They are most commonly seen in the middle-aged and elderly. In one study, 75% of the patients over age 64 had cherry angiomas.

14. Where do you find venous lakes?

These are dark blue, slightly raised papules occurring on sun-exposed skin surfaces of elderly patients, most commonly located on the ears, lips, and face. They may be mistaken for melanoma. Twelve percent of patients over age 64 have one or more venous lakes.

15. What is the most common presenting feature of a pyogenic granuloma?

Pyogenic granulomas are 5- to 10-mm soft red papules that bleed easily with minor trauma (Fig. 42-7). They are most common on the skin but may also occur on mucosal surfaces or, rarely, within blood vessels. Granuloma gravidarum is a variant that occurs on the gingiva during pregnancy. The pathogenesis is unknown, but approximately one third will occur after local trauma.

Lin RL, Janniger CK: Pyogenic granulomas, *Cutis* 74:229–233, 2004.

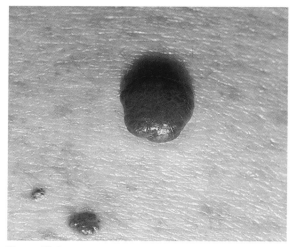

Figure 42-6. Multiple cherry angiomas of variable size. (Courtesy of James E. Fitzpatrick, MD.)

16. Where are you likely to find a lesion of angiolymphoid hyperplasia?

These lesions usually are found on the head and neck. They appear clinically as red-brown papules. Histologically, they demonstrate clusters of vessels with prominent endothelial cells, often accompanied by a nodular lymphocytic infiltrate that may appear as lymphoid follicles. The lesions are at times associated with a peripheral eosinophilia. The etiology is unknown.

17. What vascular tumor is associated with the Sucquet-Hoyer canal?

The Sucquet-Hoyer canal is the arterial segment of the glomus body and may give rise to glomus tumors. A solitary glomus tumor is a painful, purple nodule measuring a few millimeters in diameter. Multiple glomus tumors are inherited in an autosomal dominant fashion, may be much larger than the solitary form, and have been confused with the blue rubber bleb nevus syndrome. The cause of multiple glomus tumors are mutations in the glomulin gene located on chromosome 1p22-p21.

Anakwenze OA, Parker WL, Schiefer TK, et al: Clinical features of multiple glomus tumors, *Dermatol Surg* 34:884–890, 2008.

Key Points: Vascular Neoplasms

1. Hemangiomas of infancy are the most common vascular tumor of childhood.
2. Kasabach-Merritt syndrome is seen with kaposiform hemangioendothelioma and tufted angioma.
3. Multiple angiokeratomas are seen in Fabry's disease.
4. Pyogenic granulomas are acute-onset friable vascular papules that bleed frequently.
5. Multiple matlike telangiectasias are seen in hereditary hemorrhagic telangiectasia.

---

18. Matlike telangiectasias on the face, lips, tongue, ears, hands, and feet associated with internal bleeding is known as what syndrome?

Osler-Weber-Rendu syndrome, or hereditary hemorrhagic telangiectasia. Most patients present with epistaxis. Gastrointestinal telangiectasias are common, and genitourinary, pulmonary, central nervous system (CNS), and hepatic lesions may also occur. It is inherited as an autosomal dominant disease and is caused by mutations in the endoglin or activin receptor, such as kinase genes, which encode for proteins that modulate transforming growth factor–beta superfamily signaling in vascular endothelial cells.

Govani FS, Shovlin CL: Hereditary haemorrhagic telangiectasia: a clinical and scientific review, *Eur J Hum Genet* 17:860–871, 2009.

19. What is the most common cause of acquired facial telangiectasia?

Chronic ultraviolet light exposure is the leading cause of acquired facial telangiectasia. Other common causes include rosacea, connective tissue disease, and abuse of potent topical steroids.

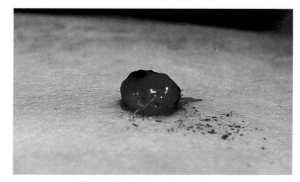

Figure 42-7. Pyogenic granuloma.

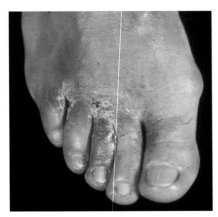

Figure 42-8. Acroangiodermatitis (pseudo-Kaposi's sarcoma) due to underlying arteriovenous malformation. (Courtesy of the Fitzsimons Army Medical Center teaching files.)

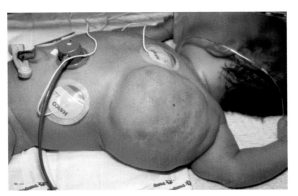

Figure 42-9. Deep lymphatic malformation (cystic hygroma) in a neonate. (Courtesy of the Fitzsimons Army Medical Center teaching files.)

20. Which benign acquired vascular disease is often initially confused with Kaposi's sarcoma?

Acroangiodermatitis: an eruption of purple macules, papules, and plaques usually associated with chronic venous insufficiency. Similar skin lesions can be found overlying arteriovenous malformations (Fig. 42-8).

21. What is a cystic hygroma?

A cystic hygroma is an outdated term for a deep lymphatic malformation (Fig. 42-9).

22. Name the types of lymphatic malformations.

A lymphatic malformation may be either superficial or deep. A superficial lymphatic malformation consists of superficial vesicles containing lymphatic fluid and at times blood. They have been described as looking like frog spawn. Deep lymphatic malformations are flesh-colored, soft, cystic nodules. The cysts may be either small (microcysts) or large (macrocysts).

23. Can you treat deep macrocystic lymphatic malformations?

The best treatment for this type of lesion is percutaneous injection of OK-432 (picibanil). This causes inflammation and subsequent sclerosis and shrinking of the lesion.

Poldervaart MT, Breugem CC, Speleman L, Pasmans S: Treatment of lymphatic malformations with OK-432 (Picibanil): review of the literature, *J Craniofac Surg* 20:1159–1162, 2009.

FIBROUS TUMORS OF THE SKIN

James E. Fitzpatrick, MD

CHAPTER 43

1. What are tumors of fibrous tissue?

Tumors of fibrous tissue are mesenchymal tumors composed of fibroblasts or their variants. Fibroblasts produce normal structural components of the dermis, including collagen, elastin, and ground substance (dermal mucin). Most tumors of fibroblast origin produce collagen, but they may also produce dermal mucin or elastin as the primary product. Some tumors are composed primarily of myofibroblasts, specialized fibroblasts that demonstrate contractile properties because of cytoplasmic actin filaments. Other specialized fibroblasts may demonstrate phagocytosis, and tumors demonstrating this characteristic are referred to as fibrohistiocytic tumors. Tumors of fibrous tissue are conventionally divided into those that are fibrous and those that are fibrohistiocytic (Table 43-1).

2. What is an acrochordon?

An acrochordon (skin tag, fibroma durum) is a soft, flesh-colored to dark brown, often pedunculated, cutaneous papule usually located on the neck, axilla, or groin (Fig. 43-1A). It is probably the most common mesenchymal neoplasm. Acrochordons are often multiple, usually 1 to 4 mm in size, but occasionally 3 cm or larger in diameter. The larger baglike lesions often also contain some fat and are called soft fibromas or fibroepithelial polyps (Fig. 43-1B).

3. Is there a known cause for acrochordons?

An exact cause is not known. The frequent association of acrochordons with diabetes mellitus, obesity, pregnancy, menopause, acanthosis nigricans (see Fig. 43-1A), and certain endocrinopathies suggests that they are hormonally induced. However, the ubiquitous nature of these lesions in healthy older adults has been interpreted by some authorities as simply a manifestation of skin aging.

Demir S, Demir Y: Acrochordon and impaired carbohydrate metabolism, *Acta Diabetol* 39:57–59, 2002.

4. Are any complications associated with acrochordons?

Yes. The most common complications are recurrent trauma to individual lesions (e.g., laceration with a shaving razor) or spontaneous torsion and infarction of a pedunculated lesion. When a pedunculated lesion twists on its stalk, the blood supply is compromised and tissue ischemia occurs. Usually, sudden pain, swelling, necrosis, and even secondary infection result. Often, this sequence of events results in disappearance of the lesion.

5. Are acrochordons associated with intestinal polyposis?

Several widely reported studies asserted a statistically significant association between the presence of acrochordons and colonic polyps. However, other investigators, using methodology that better accounted for the fact that 60% to 70% of the elderly have acrochordons, demonstrated no statistical association. Most dermatologists believe that acrochordons are not a marker for colonic polyps but are simply more common in the elderly population, which is predisposed to colonic polyposis.

6. How can acrochordons be treated?

The simplest way to treat acrochordons is scissors-snip excision (usually without anesthesia). Smaller lesions can be rapidly treated by electrodesiccation or even cryotherapy (beware of postinflammatory dyspigmentation with cryotherapy). Larger lesions (>2 cm) can be shaved off after local anesthesia or excised.

7. What is a hypertrophic scar?

A hypertrophic scar represents excessive collagen deposition at a site of wound healing. Typically, the scars are initially red, raised, firm, and often pruritic. With time, they flatten and become white. Hypertrophic scars do not extend beyond the limits of the original trauma. Scars, including hypertrophic scars, are not usually considered to be neoplasms because they are reactive and eventually regress with time.

8. What is a keloid?

A keloid also represents excessive collagen deposition at a site of wound healing. Clinically, a keloid can be indistinguishable from a hypertrophic scar, though the excess collagen deposition of a keloid is usually more exaggerated. Microscopically, developed keloids can be differentiated from hypertrophic scars by the presence of large eosinophilic collagen fibers and more abundant mucin. Also, unlike hypertrophic scars, keloids uncommonly undergo involution, and they frequently proliferate well beyond the bounds of the original trauma. Some keloids, particularly on the sternum or upper back, even seem to develop without preceding trauma.

Table 43-1. Fibrous Tumors of the Skin

BENIGN FIBROUS TUMORS	MALIGNANT FIBROUS TUMORS	BENIGN FIBROHISTIOCYTIC TUMORS*	MALIGNANT FIBROHISTIOCYTIC TUMORS

Acquired digital fibrokeratoma
Acrochordons
Connective tissue nevus
  (collagenoma, elastoma)
Dermatomyofibroma
Desmoids (extra-abdominal and
  abdominal fibromatosis)
Fibrous hamartoma of infancy
Infantile digital fibromatosis
Knuckle pads
Nodular fasciitis
Keloid
	Fibrosarcoma	Fibrous papule
		Dermatofibroma
		Reticulohistiocytoma
		  (solitary or multiple)
		Xanthogranuloma
		  (including juvenile
		  xanthogranuloma)
		Giant cell tumor of
		  tendon sheath
			Atypical fibroxanthoma
			Dermatofibrosarcoma
			  protuberans
			Malignant fibrous
			  histiocytoma

*Some dermatologists consider atypical fibroxanthoma to be a benign fibrohistiocytic tumor, but this is controversial.

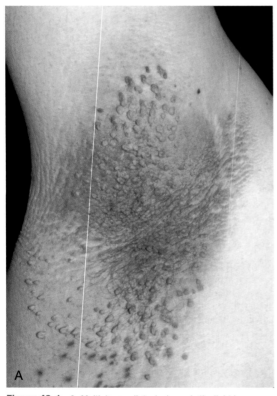

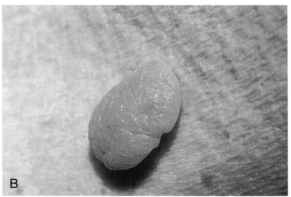

Figure 43-1. A, Multiple, small, typical exophytic, light brown acrochordons of the axilla associated with acanthotisis nigricans. **B,** Typical acrochordon demonstrating skin-colored, soft, pedunculated papule. Exophytic seborrheic keratoses and nevi may resemble acrochordons. (Panel A courtesy of the William L. Weston, M.D. collection.)

9. List the clinical features useful in distinguishing hypertrophic scars from keloids.
In early lesions, it may be impossible to make this distinction, but in developed lesions, the features listed in Table 43-2 are useful.

10. Do any factors predispose to hypertrophic scars and keloids?
Many factors can predispose individuals to develop hypertrophic scars and keloids:
- Certain drugs (e.g., isotretinoin) predispose to hypertrophic scarring, and most dermatologic surgeons defer any elective surgery for at least 1 year following discontinuation of isotretinoin.
- The type of injury and degree of tissue injury also play a role. Thermal burns, with their associated severe tissue damage, commonly produce hypertrophic scars or keloids.

Table 43-2. Clinical Features That Distinguish Hypertrophic Scars from Keloids

HYPERTROPHIC SCAR	KELOID
Any age group, especially children	Adolescents and young adults
All racial and ethnic groups	Blacks and Asians > Caucasians
No familial tendency	Familial tendency
Limited to sites of trauma	Sites of trauma or spontaneous
Onset within 2 months	Onset within 1 year
Any anatomic site	High-risk anatomic site
Dome-shaped lesions	Dome-shaped, exophytic, or crablike extensions
Confined to site of trauma	Extends into normal skin
Improved by corrective surgery	Often worsened by surgery
Spontaneous regression	No spontaneous regression

- Regional variations exist. Skin that is continuously under tension or tightly stretched over bony protuberances and other anatomic peculiarities predispose to the development of hypertrophic scarring and keloids.
- Dark-skinned races are more prone to both hypertrophic scarring and keloid formation. Blacks are 2 to 19 times and Asians 3 to 5 times more likely than Caucasians to develop keloids. The tendency for multiple keloids to occur in families also suggests a genetic predisposition.
- Certain genodermatoses such as Ehlers-Danlos syndrome, Rubinstein-Taybi syndrome, osteogenesis imperfecta, and progeria have all been reported to have increased risk for the development of keloids.

Bayat A, Arscott G, Ollier WE, et al: Keloid disease: clinical relevance of single versus multiple site scars, *Br J Plast Surg* 58:28–37, 2005.

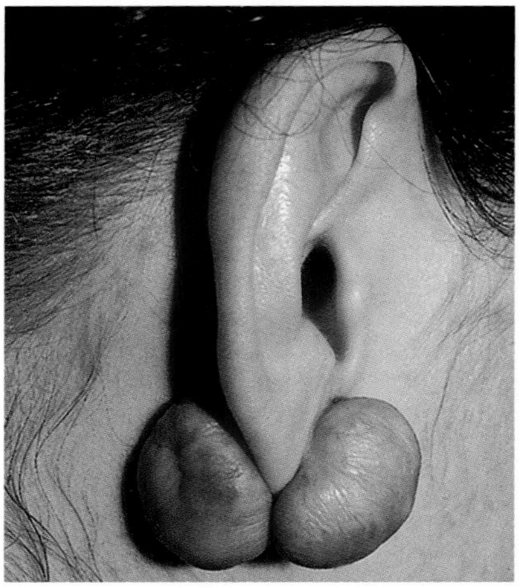

11. List the anatomic regions of the body that are most at risk to develop keloids.
Presternal area, upper back, upper arms, especially over deltoids, beard area, especially over mandibular angle, and earlobes (Fig. 43-2).

Figure 43-2. "Dumbbell" keloids of the earlobe following ear piercing.

12. Are there effective treatments for hypertrophic scars and keloids?
Various traditional and novel modalities for therapy exist. In general, **hypertrophic scars** respond well to less aggressive therapy, such as potent topical steroids, intralesional steroids, chronic pressure dressings, and even chronic occlusive dressings with medical Silastic gel sheeting. Some cases may require surgical revision or dermabrasion.

Keloids demand more aggressive therapy with long-term precautions to prevent recurrence. Surgical excision, corticosteroid injection, and cryotherapy alone can be used but are often not effective. A recent study has suggested that incomplete excision of keloids is associated with an increase chance of recurrence. Radiation has been employed with good results but should be used with caution and only by an experienced physician. Laser excision has theoretical advantages, but long-term studies have not demonstrated an advantage over conventional surgery. Combination approaches appear to work best. Cryosurgery followed by corticosteroid injection is effective in some patients. Surgical excision with subsequent steroid injection is probably the most effective approach. One regimen calls for steroid injection to the surgical site 1 to 4 weeks postoperatively and then monthly for 6 months.

Tan K, Shah N, Pritchard SA, et al: The influence of surgical excision margins on keloid prognosis, *Ann Plast Surg* 64:55–58, 2010.

13. What is an acquired digital fibrokeratoma?
These solitary, firm, hyperkeratotic papules most commonly occur around interphalangeal joints but may occur on any site of the hands or feet. They are typically pedunculated and often demonstrate a collarette of hyperkeratosis at the base (Fig. 43-3). Often, they are mistaken clinically for warts or supernumerary digits. Histologically, they demonstrate overlying hyperkeratosis and thickened collagen bundles.

Baykal C, Buyukbabani N, Yazganoglu KD, Saglik E: Acquired digital fibrokeratoma, *Cutis* 79:129–132, 2007.

14. Has a cause been identified for acquired digital fibrokeratoma?
Some authorities believe that these lesions arise as a reaction to recurring trauma. Often, a history of an activity with recurring trauma to the affected area (e.g., guiding a knitting needle) can be elicited; however, many patients do not recall trauma to the site.

15. How can an acquired digital fibrokeratoma be treated?

Saucerization with secondary healing and simple excision are both effective. Hard cryotherapy is sometimes effective but may require multiple treatments.

16. What is nodular fasciitis?

Nodular fasciitis (pseudocarcinomatous nodular fasciitis) is a rare, benign, fibroblastic tumor that many consider to be a pseudoneoplastic or reactive growth. It may occur at any age but most commonly presents in young adults as a solitary, rapidly growing, subcutaneous nodule on the extremities. The nodule may be painful, is typically 1 to 3 cm in size, and may adhere to the underlying fascia.

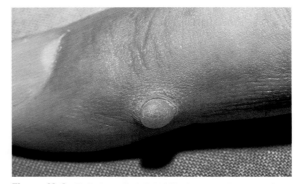

Figure 43-3. Typical acquired digital fibrokeratoma demonstrating an exophytic firm papule with a hyperkeratotic collarette.

Simple excision is curative, but untreated lesions have been documented to regress spontaneously. The importance of this lesion is that, histologically, it may be confused with malignant fibrous neoplasms, because the fibroblasts are large and pleomorphic and mitotic figures are relatively common.

17. What is a connective tissue nevus?

Connective tissue nevus is a term used for cutaneous hamartomas composed primarily of collagen (collagenomas), elastin (elastomas), or a combination of these two. While these are produced by fibroblasts, connective tissue nevi are typically no more cellular than normal dermis. Clinically, they present as one or more dermal papules or plaques. Connective tissue nevi composed primarily of collagen are skin-colored, while those composed primarily of elastin may be skin-colored or yellowish.

18. Why are connective tissue nevi important?

Connective tissue nevi usually do not produce problems, although large lesions may be distressing to the patient for cosmetic reasons. Other patients may become concerned because numerous collagenomas (eruptive collagenomas) develop over a short period of time (Fig. 43-4). However, some of these nevi serve as cutaneous markers for other systemic syndromes. Collagenomas called shagreen patches are frequently seen in patients with tuberous sclerosis. Multiple connective tissue nevi called dermatofibrosis lenticularis disseminata are composed primarily of elastic fibers and are the cutaneous marker for Buschke-Ollendorff syndrome. Buschke-Ollendorff syndrome is an autosomal dominant disorder that presents with osteopoikilosis of the bones and connective tissue nevi.

19. What is the gene defect in Buschke-Ollendorf syndrome?

Recent studies suggest that many but not all patients have a heterozygous, loss-of-function, germline mutation in the *LEMD3* gene on chromosome 12q that encodes for a an inner nuclear membrane called LEMD3 or MAN1. The absence of this mutation in some families suggests that there is genetic heterogeneity and further work needs to be done to clarify the genetics of this disorder.

Yadegari M, Whyte MP, Mumm S, et al: Buschke-Ollendorff syndrome: absence of LEMD3 mutation in an affected family, *Arch Dermatol* 146:63–68, 2010.

20. What is infantile digital fibromatosis?

Infantile digital fibromatosis is a rare tumor composed of myofibroblasts that develops in infancy and early childhood on the fingers and toes. The primary lesion is a skin-colored or red tumor usually located on the lateral or dorsal surface of the digit. Histologically, they consist of myofibroblasts with characteristic eosinophilic cytoplasmic inclusions composed of actin filaments.

Heymann WR: Infantile digital fibromatosis, *J Am Acad Dermatol* 59:122–123, 2008.

21. Describe the natural history of infantile digital fibromatosis.

The tumors of infantile digital fibromatosis may grow up to 2 cm but will eventually regress over a period of years (Fig. 43-5). Occasionally, large lesions may produce functional impairment or joint deformities.

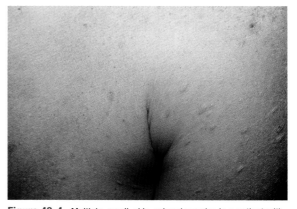

Figure 43-4. Multiple, small, skin-colored papules in a patient with eruptive collagenomas.

The recurrence rate is very high, with up to two thirds of all cases recurring following surgical removal. The importance of this tumor is that physicians not familiar with the natural history of this tumor may become overly aggressive and amputate a digit.

22. What is a dermatofibroma?

A dermatofibroma, or fibrous histiocytoma, is the most common fibrohistiocytic tumor of the skin. Usually, these are small, firm, flat, or exophytic papules on the lower extremities of adults. Although most commonly 2 to 4 mm in diameter, they can occasionally grow to 2 to 3 cm. They may be skin-colored but more commonly demonstrate tan or brown hyperpigmentation and hypertrophy of overlying epidermis. Nondermatologists frequently mistake them for nevi. Other common locations include the sides of the trunk and upper arms.

Microscopically, most dermatofibromas are composed primarily of fibroblasts that produce abundant collagen. Within some, but not all, dermatofibromas, there are often cellular areas composed of cells with round nuclei that phagocytize lipid or hemosiderin. Multinucleated giant cells may also be present. Dermatofibromas that phagocytize abundant hemosiderin molecules are sometimes referred to as hemosiderotic dermatofibromas or sclerosing hemangiomas (Fig. 43-6).

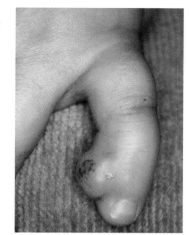

Figure 43-5. Infantile digital fibroma. Firm skin-colored nodule with focal hemorrhage on the finger of an infant. (Courtesy of the Fitzsimons Army Medical Center teaching files.)

23. What is a positive "dimple" sign?

Dermatofibromas characteristically demonstrate a positive "dimple" sign, which is a dimpling of the skin produced when lateral pressure is applied to the dermatofibroma between the thumb and forefinger. This is also called the Fitzpatrick sign, in honor of Dr. Thomas Fitzpatrick (Fig. 43-7).

24. Do dermatofibromas transform into skin cancer?

Dermatofibromas are considered to be benign fibrohistiocytic tumors that do not demonstrate a malignant potential. Though dermatofibromas share clinical and some general histologic similarities with a malignant neoplasm called dermatofibrosarcoma protuberans, histochemical markers show the two are distinct. Although the dermatofibroma itself does not progress into malignancy, the overlying epidermis demonstrates a slight risk to develop into basal cell carcinoma.

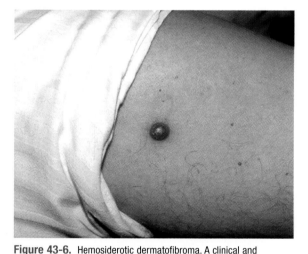

Figure 43-6. Hemosiderotic dermatofibroma. A clinical and histologic variant of dermatofibroma with fibrohistiocytic cells demonstrating phagocytosis of hemosiderin. Because of the color, they are clinically often confused with vascular tumors, but on palpation they are typically firm. (Courtesy of the Fitzsimons Army Medical Center teaching files.)

25. What is the best way to treat a dermatofibroma?

In general, it is best to avoid treating a dermatofibroma. When a lesion is distressing in appearance, painful, or frequently traumatized, simple excision may be indicated. Several authors have reported successful treatment with cryotherapy. The anticipated benefit of treatment should be weighed against the predictable cosmetic outcome of the therapeutic modality.

Key Points: Fibrohistiocytic Tumors

1. Multiple dermatofibromas are associated with an altered immune status, with the most common cause being systemic lupus erythematosus.
2. Dermatofibromas often demonstrate dimpling with lateral pressure. This has been called a "dimple" or "Fitzpatrick" sign.
3. Solitary angiofibromas are commonly found on the nose and are referred to as fibrous papules.
4. Multiple angiofibromas are associated with tuberous sclerosis and are also referred to as adenoma sebaceum.
5. Buschke-Ollendorff syndrome is an autosomal dominant disorder that presents with osteopoikilosis of the bones and connective tissue nevi.

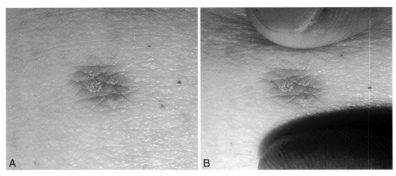

Figure 43-7. A, Characteristic light brown dermatofibroma that is not sharply demarcated. **B,** Dimple or Fitzpatrick sign, demonstrating tendency of dermatofibromas to dimple when compressed laterally.

26. Are multiple dermatofibromas associated with any internal diseases?

Multiple dermatofibromas have been associated with an altered immune status, with the most common cause being systemic lupus erythematosus and, less commonly, myasthenia gravis and malignancies. These associations are rare and only seen in patients with more than six dermatofibromas; patients presenting with isolated dermatofibromas should not be routinely evaluated for these conditions.

Zaccaria E, Rebora A, Rongioletti F: Multiple eruptive dermatofibromas and immunosuppression: report of two cases and review of the literature, *Int J Dermatol* 47:723–727, 2008.

27. What is a "fibrous papule of the nose"?

A fibrous papule of the nose is a relatively common, small (usually 2 to 3 mm), dome-shaped, asymptomatic papule usually located on the lower portion of the nose. The color is variable and may be skin-colored, white, or red. Less commonly, it may occur on other parts of the face. Microscopically, fibrous papules are composed of fibroblasts that may be fusiform, stellate, or multinucleated, and are associated with abundant thick collagen bundles that are oriented around hair follicles or dilated blood vessels. Their greatest significance lies in their clinical similarity to an early basal cell carcinoma. Fibrous papules of the nose are histologically identical to the angiofibromas found in patients with tuberous sclerosis, and most authorities regard fibrous papules to be a solitary form of angiofibroma.

28. How is a fibrous papule of the nose best treated?

Superficial shave excision, cryotherapy, or simple excision is an effective modality.

29. What are "giant cell tumors of the tendon sheath"?

Giant cell tumors of the tendon sheath are benign tumors that arise from the fibrous sheath that surrounds the tendons. They typically occur between the ages of 30 and 50 years. They usually develop on the hand, although they may occur on the feet, ankles, and knees. Although they arise from a structure that is deep to the skin, they not infrequently present initially to the dermatologist. The primary lesion is a subcutaneous nodule that appears to be attached to deeper structures (Fig. 43-8). The overlying skin is usually movable but may be fixed in some cases. X-ray examination, besides revealing a soft tissue tumor, may demonstrate cortical erosion in approximately 10% of cases. The treatment of choice is surgical excision.

Collen J, Mount G, Pollock P, et al: Giant cell tumor of the tendon sheath, *J Clin Rheumatol* 15:85–87, 2009.

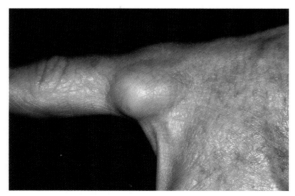

Figure 43-8. Giant cell tumor of the tendon sheath. (Courtesy of the Fitzsimons Army Medical Center teaching files.)

MALIGNANT TUMORS OF THE SKIN

CHAPTER 44

COMMON CUTANEOUS MALIGNANCIES

Mariah Ruth Brown, MD, and Milton J. Schleve, MD

1. How are skin cancers classified?

Primary cutaneous cancers are classified on the basis of their cell of origin within the skin (Table 44-1). Skin cancers are most commonly derived from keratinocytes (e.g., squamous cell carcinoma) or melanocytes (e.g., malignant melanoma), which are normal components of the epidermis. Less commonly, they arise from other cells within the epidermis, dermis, or subcutis.

2. What are the most common nonmelanoma skin cancers (NMSCs)?

Basal cell carcinoma and squamous cell carcinoma. In the United States, over 1 million cases of NMSCs occur yearly, which makes these the most prevalent of all malignancies. Common nonmelanoma skin premalignancies include actinic keratosis, actinic cheilitis, and squamous cell carcinoma in situ (Bowen's disease).

Diepgen TL, Mahler V: The epidemiology of skin cancer, *Br J Dermatol* 146:1–6, 2002.
Nguyen TH, Ho DQ: Nonmelanoma skin cancer, *Curr Treat Options Oncol* 3:193–203, 2002.

3. What is the most important cause of NMSC?

The overwhelming majority of precancerous and cancerous skin lesions are caused by sun exposure. Several observations and epidemiologic studies support the role of ultraviolet light in the production of skin cancers:
1. Most NMSCs develop on skin chronically exposed to the sun, with 85% or more occurring on the head and neck.
2. The incidence of NMSC is lower in more polar latitudes (e.g., Minneapolis) than equatorial latitudes (e.g., Hawaii).
3. Epidemiologic studies clearly demonstrate that NMSCs are much more common in individuals with lighter skin than in individuals with darker skin.
4. NMSC can be induced in animal models by solar irradiation and prevented by the use of sunscreens.

Rigel D: Cutaneous ultraviolet exposure and its relationship to the development of skin cancer, *J Am Acad Dermatol* 58:S129–S132, 2008.
Taylor CR, Sober AJ: Sun exposure and skin disease, *Annu Rev Med* 47:181–191, 1996.

4. Are there any other causes of NMSC?

- Arsenic ingestion
- Chronic ulcers and scars (e.g., burn wounds)
- Environmental pollutants
- Genetic factors (e.g., xeroderma pigmentosum, albinism)
- Local prolonged heat exposure
- Topical exposure to tars and oils
- Viral infection (e.g., some strains of human papillomavirus)
- Radiation treatment (e.g., acne treatment)

5. What special populations are at increased risk of NMSC?

- **Organ transplant patients:** NMSC is the most common malignancy in solid organ transplant recipients. Increased rates of NMSC are seen on average 8 to 10 years after transplantation, and the development of skin cancer in these patients appears to be linked to the duration and degree of immunosuppression required to prevent transplant rejection. The ratio of squamous cell carcinomas (SCCs) to basal cell carcinomas (BCCs) is higher in transplant patients, a reversal of the normal ratio seen in the general population.
- **Human immunodeficiency virus (HIV) patients:** NMSC is the most common nonacquired immune deficiency syndrome (AIDS)–defining cancer seen in HIV-positive patients. HIV-positive patients appear to maintain a normal ratio of BCCs to SCCs, but are two- to sevenfold more likely to develop NMSC than the general population.

Ulrich C, Kanitakis J, Stockfleth E, Euvard S: Skin cancer in organ transplant recipients—where do we stand today? *Am J Transplant* 8:2192–2198, 2008.
Honda K: HIV and skin cancer, *Dermatol Clin* 24:521–530, 2006.

6. How are NMSCs diagnosed?

A cutaneous malignancy should always be considered in any patient who reports a new lesion on the skin, particularly in sun-exposed skin. Currently, the diagnosis is established by shave, punch, incisional, or excisional biopsy, with the choice of biopsy technique depending on the size and location of the suspected malignancy. Current research is focused on developing non-invasive methods of diagnosing NMSC by using techniques such as specialized types of

Table 44-1. Classification of Cutaneous Malignancies

MALIGNANCY	CELL OF ORIGIN
Premalignancies (in situ)	
Actinic keratosis	Keratinocyte
Squamous cell carcinoma in situ (Bowen's disease)	Keratinocyte
Malignant melanoma in situ	Melanocyte
Lentigo maligna (Hutchinson's freckle)	Melanocyte
Common Cutaneous Malignancies	
Basal cell carcinoma	Follicular keratinocyte origin (probable)
Squamous cell carcinoma	Epidermal keratinocyte
Keratoacanthoma	Follicular keratinocyte
Melanomas	
Malignant melanoma	Melanocyte
Lentigo maligna melanoma	Melanocyte
Uncommon Cutaneous Epithelial Malignancies	
Sweat gland carcinoma (numerous variants)	Apocrine or eccrine sweat gland/duct
Follicular carcinomas (several variants)	Follicular epithelial cells
Extramammary Paget's disease	Modified keratinocytes (Toker cell)
Merkel cell carcinoma	Neuroendocrine cell
Cutaneous Mesenchymal Malignancies	
Atypical fibroxanthoma	Fibroblast
Dermatofibrosarcoma protuberans	CD34+ dermal dendrocyte
Fibrosarcoma	Fibroblast
Angiosarcoma	Endothelial cell
Kaposi's sarcoma	Endothelial cell
Hemangiopericytoma	Pericyte
Malignant peripheral nerve sheath tumors	Schwann cells
Liposarcoma	Lipocyte

ultrasonography and microscopy. However, these methods are currently in development and have not replaced skin biopsy with histologic examination as the gold standard for diagnosis.

Mogensen M, Jemec G: Diagnosis of nonmelanoma skin cancer/keratinocyte carcinoma: a review of the diagnostic accuracy of nonmelanoma skin cancer diagnostic tests and technologies, *Dermatol Surg* 33:1158–1174, 2007.

7. How frequently do NMSCs occur?

The exact incidence of NMSCs is unknown, because they are not routinely entered into tumor registries. It is estimated that 1.3 million new cases of NMSC occur each year in the United States, making them by far the most common cancers in this country. The annual cost to Medicare for the management and treatment of NMSCs is 426 million dollars. The lifetime risk of developing NMSC is 1 in 5. Statistically, if a patient develops one NMSC, the risk of another new lesion in 5 years is 30% to 50%.

Chen J, Fleischer A, Smith E, Kancler C, et al: Cost of nonmelanoma skin cancer treatment in the United States, *Dermatol Surg* 27:1035–1038, 2007.

8. How can NMSCs be prevented?

The easy answer is to avoid sun exposure, particularly during childhood. It has been estimated that 25% of the total lifetime dose of solar radiation is received before the age of 18. Sun protection techniques for children and adults alike include avoidance of the midday sun, liberal use of sunscreens, and wearing of protective clothing. Tans, whether received from natural sunlight or tanning booths, represent damaged skin that is more likely to develop NMSC. It is important for health care providers to nurture the idea that pale skin is more attractive than tanned skin.

9. What factors should you consider in treating NMSC?

The method of destruction depends upon the type and subtype of malignancy, degree of invasion, location, health of the patient, potential for recurrence or metastasis, and availability of various methods (Table 44-2).

Neville J, Welch E, Leffell D: Management of nonmelanoma skin cancer in 2007, *Nat Clin Pract Oncol* 4:462–469, 2007.

Table 44-2. Management of Cutaneous Premalignancies and Malignancies

LESION	TREATMENT
Actinic keratosis	Cryosurgery Curettage Fluorouracil, topical Chemical peel Dermabrasion Imiquimod Photodynamic therapy
Actinic cheilitis	Cryosurgery Electrosurgery Chemical peel Laser ablation Lip shave and advancement Imiquimod
Basal cell carcinoma (BCC)	
Superficial spreading	Cryosurgery Curettage ± electrosurgery Laser ablation Imiquimod Photodynamic therapy
Nodular BCC	Cryosurgery Curettage and electrosurgery Excision Radiation therapy Photodynamic therapy Mohs surgery
Morpheaform, aggressive BCC, or recurrent BCC	Excision Mohs surgery
Nonresectable BCC	Cryosurgery Radiation therapy Chemotherapy
Keratoacanthoma	Deep shave plus curettage Curettage plus electrosurgery Intralesional 5-fluorouracil Cryosurgery Excision Mohs surgery
SCC in situ (Bowen's disease)	Curettage ± electrosurgery Fluorouracil, topical Imiquimod Cryosurgery Laser Excision Photodynamic therapy
Squamous cell carcinoma (SCC)	
Small, nonaggressive	Curettage plus electrosurgery Cryosurgery Excision
Large or aggressive	Excision Mohs surgery Radiation therapy Lymph node dissection
Nonresectable SCC	Radiation Chemotherapy

Key Points: Nonmelanoma Skin Cancer

1. Nonmelanoma skin cancers are more common in older, fair-skinned individuals on sun-exposed skin.
2. All new or changing lesions are suspect.
3. Biopsies are the diagnostic test of choice.
4. Treatment of NMSC depends on the tumor type, location, and patient health.

10. What are basal cell carcinomas?

Basal cell carcinomas (BCCs) are the most common cutaneous malignancy and outnumber squamous cell carcinomas by a 4:1 ratio. They are low-grade malignancies of the skin and are microscopically composed of basaloid cells with characteristic peripheral palisading of the nuclei. These basaloid tumor islands usually demonstrate connections to the overlying epidermis or follicular epithelium. BCCs are locally invasive tumors that rarely metastasize. The origin of these common tumors has been debated. The theory with the greatest supporting evidence is that BCCs originate from the follicular epithelium, specifically from the stem cells of the outer root sheath.

Donovan J: Review of the hair follicle origin hypothesis for basal cell carcinoma, *Dermatol Surg* 35(9):1311–1323, 2009.

11. What is the molecular basis for the development of sporadic basal cell carcinoma?

The best evidence suggests that the majority of sporadic BCCs are the result of ultraviolet (UV)-induced alterations in the hedgehog signaling pathway. The most common mutation in sporadic BCCs (90%) occurs in the tumor suppressor gene *PTCH*, found at locus 9q22, that encodes the Ptch1 protein. This protein is a receptor for a secreted protein ligand called sonic hedgehog (Shh), which is important in signaling processes that control cell growth and fate. Another 10% of sporadic BCCs have activating mutations in the smoothened protein (SMO), another participant in the hedgehog signaling pathway. Investigation into this pathway has led to the development of a small molecule inhibitor of the hedgehog pathway called GDC-0449 that shows promise in the treatment of locally advanced and metastatic BCC.

Epstein EH: Basal cell carcinomas: attack of the hedgehog, *Nat Rev Cancer* 8(10):743–754, 2008.
Von Hoff DD, LoRusso PM, Rudin CM, et al: Inhibition of the hedgehog pathway in advanced basal-cell carcinoma, *N Engl J Med* 361(12):1164–1172, 2009.

12. Describe the clinical and histologic appearance of basal cell carcinomas.

BCCs may have more than one clinical or histologic appearance. The most common presentation is as nodular BCCs, which are typically slow-growing lesions with a smooth or pebbly surface. They characteristically appear translucent or pearly and often demonstrate dilated vessels (Fig. 44-1A). They can gradually break down, bleed, and form ulcers (noduloulcerative BCC, Fig. 44-1B). Superficial spreading BCC are thin lesions that demonstrate a horizontal growth pattern. They present as erythematous, minimally indurated, slow-growing plaques with variable scale that are most commonly located on the trunk (Fig. 44-1C). They can be confused with tinea corporis, nummular dermatitis, or other NMSCs such as Bowen's disease.

Morpheaform (also desmoplastic or sclerosing) BCCs are a type of infiltrative lesion that may resemble scars or even normal skin. Microscopically, they are composed of narrow cords and strands of basaloid cells that infiltrate between the collagen bundles. This variant can easily be missed, even by experienced dermatologists, and has a higher rate of recurrence after treatment than other BCC subtypes. Their true extent is often much greater than the appearance suggests.

Basal cell carcinomas can also be completely or focally pigmented and mistaken for malignant melanoma. A rare variant of BCC looks like a large skin tag or fibroma. This variant is usually found on the trunk of older men and is called a *Pinkus tumor* or *fibroepithelioma of Pinkus*.

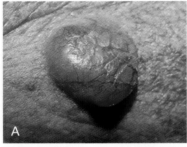

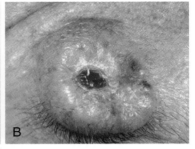

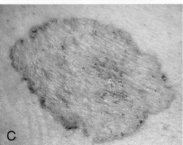

Figure 44-1. Variants of basal cell carcinoma (BCC). **A,** Nodular BCC demonstrating characteristic dilated blood vessels. **B,** Noduloulcerative BCC above the eyebrow, demonstrating pearly appearance and central ulceration. **C,** Large superficial spreading BCC demonstrating multiple small plaques with focal scale and crust. (Panels A and B courtesy of James E. Fitzpatrick, MD.)

13. What is nevoid basal cell carcinoma syndrome?

Nevoid basal cell carcinoma syndrome, also called *Gorlin's syndrome*, is an autosomal dominant inherited disorder characterized by a number of different germline mutations of *PTCH*, the same gene that is found to be mutated in most sporadic basal cell carcinomas. It is characterized by the early onset and continued development of numerous basal cell carcinomas (Fig. 44-2), in addition to other tumors and developmental abnormalities including keratocysts of the jaw, palmar and plantar pits, skeletal abnormalities, medulloblastoma, and calcification of the falx cerebri.

High A, Zedan W: Basal cell nevus syndrome, *Curr Opin Oncol* 17:160–166, 2005.

14. What do typical squamous cell carcinomas look like clinically?

Squamous cell carcinomas (SCCs) may resemble basal cell carcinomas, actinic keratoses, or warts, but often the initial appearance is that of an ill-defined, red lesion with a rough surface (Fig. 44-3A). SCCs are more likely to demonstrate overlying scale than are BCCs. At times, the scale may project above the skin surface, producing a cutaneous horn. Larger lesions may break down and ulcerate. Verrucous carcinomas are a variant of SCC that look like warts and are often misdiagnosed (Fig. 44-3B). Like warts, they often occur on hands and feet but can also appear on the anogenital epithelium and oral mucosa. These tumors are slow growing and rarely metastasize, but they can be extremely locally aggressive.

Rose LC: Recognizing neoplastic skin lesions: a photo guide, *Am Fam Physician* 58:873–884, 887–888, 1998.

15. What is the biologic behavior of cutaneous squamous cell carcinoma?

SCCs are more aggressive than BCCs and are more likely to metastasize. SCCs are currently estimated to metastasize at an overall rate of 2% to 6%. Certain sites have higher rates of metastasis—SCC arising from the lower lip

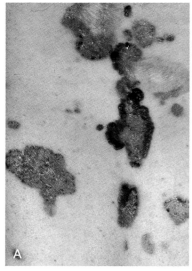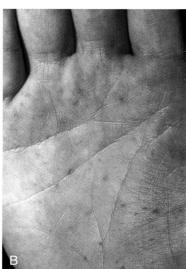

Figure 44-2. Nevoid basal cell carcinoma syndrome. **A,** More than 20 basal carcinomas varying from minute to large are present on the back of this patient with several hundred basal cell carcinomas. **B,** Numerous keratotic palmar pits in a patient with nevoid basal cell carcinoma. (Panel A courtesy of the Fitzsimons Army Medical Center teaching files; panel B courtesy of the John L. Aeling, M.D. collection.)

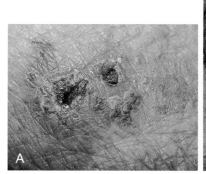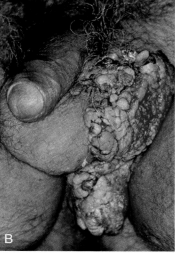

Figure 44-3. Variants of squamous cell carcinoma (SCC). **A,** Early SCC arising in an actinic keratosis. **B,** Large verrucous carcinoma of the genitalia. Verrucous carcinomas often reach large sizes before diagnosis because they are often treated as warts.

metastasize in 10% to 14% of cases, and those arising from the ear metastasize in 11% of cases. Tumors arising in burn scars, draining sinuses, and modified epithelium (e.g., glans penis, vulva) and in immunocompromised patients are also more likely to metastasize. Other factors associated with a higher metastatic rate are increased depth of invasion, perineural invasion and recurrence, with recurrent tumors estimated to metastasize in about 33% of cases. Multiple genetic mutations are associated with the development of cutaneous SCCs, in particular 90% of these tumors have UV-induced mutations in the *p53* tumor suppressor gene.

Rudolph R, Zelac DE: Squamous cell carcinoma of the skin, *Plast Reconstr Surg* 114:82e–94e, 2004.
Black A: The role of p53 in the immunobiology of cutaneous squamous cell carcinoma, *Clin Exp Immunol* 132:379–384, 2003.

16. What are keratoacanthomas?

Keratoacanthomas are relatively common epidermal tumors that almost invariably appear on sun-exposed skin. There is controversy as to whether these lesions should be considered as benign or malignant. Microscopically, the tumor is composed of well-differentiated but cytologically atypical keratinocytes that are difficult for pathologists to separate from squamous cell carcinoma. Clinically, however, keratoacanthomas can behave in a benign fashion and spontaneously regress over a period of weeks or months if left untreated. Clouding the issue is the fact that approximately 10% of lesions that clinically resemble keratoacanthomas develop into invasive SCC. There are also reports of keratoacanthomas that have metastasized. It is not clear whether such lesions are SCC from their inception, keratoacanthomas that have developed into SCC, or more aggressive keratoacanthomas. Currently, the standard of care is to treat keratoacanthomas as well-differentiated squamous cell carcinomas, and many pathologists will describe their distinctive histology as "squamous cell carcinoma, keratoacanthoma type." Solitary keratoacanthomas are the most common variant, but the tumor is also associated with specific genetic syndromes. The site of origin of keratoacanthomas is uncertain, but experimental and epidemiologic studies implicate follicular epithelium.

Karaa A: Keratoacanthoma: a tumor in search of a classification, *Int J Dermatol* 46:671–678, 2007.
Mandrell JC, Santa Cruz D: Keratoacanthoma: hyperplasia, benign neoplasm, or a type of squamous cell carcinoma? *Semin Diagn Pathol* 26:150–163, 2009.

17. How do keratoacanthomas present clinically?

Keratoacanthomas are usually easy to recognize. They appear suddenly, typically on sun-exposed skin, as skin-colored domes that develop a central keratin-filled plug (Fig. 44-4). They grow quickly, often over the course of weeks, and usually reach a size of 1 to 2 cm before regressing. Rarely, they may attain a size of 5 cm or more (giant keratoacanthomas).

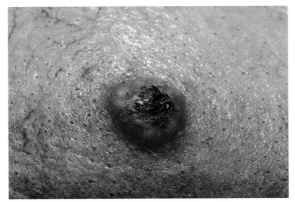

Figure 44-4. Keratoacanthoma demonstrating a crateriform nodule with central keratin plug. (Courtesy of James E. Fitzpatrick, MD.)

18. What is Bowen's disease?

Bowen's disease is an older term for squamous cell carcinoma in situ (Fig. 44-5A). Clinically, SCC in situ presents as persistent, erythematous, slightly indurated plaques with variable scale. It may resemble superficial spreading BCC, Paget's disease, or various inflammatory skin conditions. SCC in situ occurring on the male genitalia has also been described under the name *erythroplasia of Queyrat* and may be associated with human papillomavirus infection (Fig. 44-5B). Microscopically, squamous cell carcinoma in situ demonstrates full-thickness cytologic atypia of the keratinocytes without invasion through the basement membrane.

19. What is an actinic keratosis?

Actinic keratoses (solar keratoses) are sun-induced precancerous lesions of the skin. They are very common in patients with light skin color and significant sun exposure. Microscopically, actinic keratoses are characterized by a proliferation

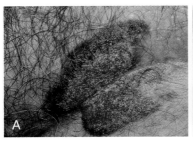

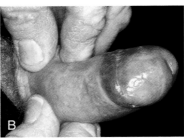

Figure 44-5. A, Squamous cell carcinoma in situ presenting a scaly plaque on the groin. **B,** Squamous cell carcinoma of the penis (erythroplasia of Queyrat) presenting as an erythematous, minimally indurated plaque.

of cytologically atypical keratinocytes that bud off or replace the bottom of the epidermis. The atypical cells do not involve the full thickness of the epidermis. A definitive prospective study has never been done, but epidemiologic and retrospective studies suggest that 6% to 20% of actinic keratoses progress into squamous cell carcinomas if left untreated.

Anwar J, Wrong D, Kimyai-Asadi A, Alam M: The development of actinic keratosis into invasive squamous cell carcinoma: evidence and evolving classifications schemes, *Clin Dermatol* 22:189–196, 2004.

20. What do actinic keratoses look like?

Actinic keratoses initially appear as tiny, palpable bumps on normal sun-exposed skin that gradually enlarge and become red and scaly (Fig. 44-6). The overlying scale may be extensive to the point that markedly exophytic cutaneous horns are produced. Less common variants include atrophic and pigmented actinic keratoses. **Actinic cheilitis** is a term used for actinic keratoses that present on the sun-exposed vermilion lip. Many patients who complain of chronic dry lower lips actually have extensive actinic cheilitis.

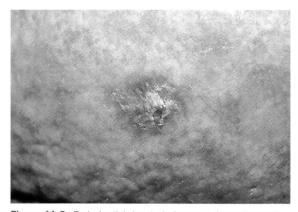

Figure 44-6. Typical actinic keratosis demonstrating scaly papule on an erythematous base.

21. How should premalignant lesions, such as actinic keratoses and actinic cheilitis, be treated?

We should probably first ask, "Why should premalignant lesions be treated?" While a small percentage of actinic keratoses regress spontaneously, up to 20% develop into squamous cell carcinoma. Treating actinic keratosis can therefore prevent the development of SCC. Additionally, small SCCs are difficult to separate from actinic keratoses on clinical exam. The smallest SCCs are often picked up when a suspected actinic lesion does not respond to treatment or a lesion appears in a treated area.

Since actinic lesions can vary from tiny, barely palpable lesions to an entire lip or scalp, treatment modalities depend on the size and location of lesions. Small, individual papules can be treated by cryosurgery or by curettage (usually after local anesthesia). Larger areas can be treated by cryosurgery, curettage, dermabrasion, chemical peels, imiquimod, and topical 5-fluorouracil. Laser ablation (CO_2 laser) and excision with mucosal advancement are reserved for extensive involvement of the lip.

CHAPTER 45

MALIGNANT MELANOMA

Michael R. Campoli, MD, PhD, and Patrick Walsh, MD

1. What is melanoma?

Cutaneous melanoma is a malignant tumor of skin melanocytes. It is differentiated from ocular melanoma, a malignancy of ocular pigment cells. Less common sites of primary melanoma occur in the brain, oral mucosa, nasopharyngeal area, and anal area.

2. How common is malignant melanoma in the United States?

In terms of incidence, melanoma is the most rapidly increasing form of cancer in the United States. Its incidence has increased more than 15-fold over the past 40 years. In 2005, the age-adjusted incidence was 24.6 per 100,000 for men and 15.6 per 100,000 for women. More than 59,000 cases of invasive melanoma and approximately 46,000 new cases of melanoma in situ were diagnosed in the United States in 2005. Malignant melanoma is the fifth and sixth most common form of cancer in men and women, respectively. It is now the most common cancer in young women aged 25 to 29 years. The lifetime risk of developing melanoma has increased from 1 in 1500 for someone born in the early 1900s to 1 in 100 for people born in 1990 to an estimated 1 in 41 to 61 for persons born in the year 2007. Incidence rates differ between genders, ages, ethnic groups, and regions. In this regard, before the age of 40, the incidence of melanoma is higher in young women; subsequently the incidence of melanoma increases rapidly in men, but the rate of increase slows in women.

The mortality rates for melanoma have also continued to increase, although not as greatly as incidence rates. From 1975 to 1990, the mortality rates for women and men increased by 1.6% and 2.2%, respectively. In contrast to women, mortality rates continue to increase in men. In this regard, men older than 65 years have the greatest risk of dying from their disease.

The discrepancy between the rates of increase of incidence and mortality in melanoma has been attributed to improved early detection and the diagnosis of thinner lesions. However, there has been a concurrent increase in thicker, more advanced melanoma lesions, suggesting a true increase in biologically aggressive disease. This issue is likely not going to be resolved until there are better prognostic markers for malignant melanoma.

DevCan: Probability of developing or dying of cancer software, version 6.2.1, Statistical Research and Applications Branch, NCI, 2007. Available at: http://srab.cancer.gov/devcan. Accessed July 28, 2010.

Rager EL, Bridgeford EP, Ollila DW: Cutaneous melanoma: update on prevention, screening, diagnosis, and treatment, *Am Fam Physician* 15:269–276, 2005.

Tucker MA: Melanoma epidemiology, *Hematol Oncol Clin North Am* 23:383–395, 2009.

3. What causes melanoma?

At present the causes of melanoma are not known with certainty, but epidemiologic studies suggest that brief, intense exposure to ultraviolet A (long-wave UVA radiation) contributes to the development of melanoma. Current evidence suggests that long-wave UV radiation (UVA) is more important than short-wave radiation (UVB). Other potential causes include mutations in, or loss of, tumor suppressor genes.

von Thaler AK, Kamenisch Y, Berneburg M: The role of ultraviolet radiation in melanomagenesis, *Exp Dermatol* 19(2):81-88, 2010. [Epub ahead of print, January 7, 2010.]

4. What groups have a genetic predisposition to familial melanoma?

Germline genetic mutations and polymorphisms can predispose to melanoma. The major high-penetrance melanoma susceptibility gene locus associated with familial melanoma is *CDKN2A*, which encodes p16 and p14^{ARF}; p16 and p14^{ARF} regulate retinoblastoma (Rb) nd p53 pathways, respectively. Germline *CDKN2A* mutations are observed in 25% of familial melanoma.

Meyle KD, Guldberg P: Genetic risk factors for melanoma, *Hum Genet* 126:499–510, 2009.

5. List the risk factors for melanoma.

Risk factors for malignant melanoma may be divided into genetic factors, environmental factors, and the interaction between the two.

Genetic factors include past medical history of melanoma, familial medical history of melanoma in a first-degree relative, Fitzpatrick type I or II skin, large congential nevi, the presence of dysplastic (atypical) nevi, >50 benign nevi (>2 mm in size), xeroderma pigmentosum, and familial dysplastic mole syndrome (FDMS). In FDMS, which is defined as occurring in families with atypical nevi and two or more blood relatives with melanoma, the estimated prevalence of melanoma approaches 85% by age 48. It is noteworthy that variations in the melanocortin receptor 1 (*MCR1*) gene, which is a component of pigment diversity, also confer an increased risk of melanoma. Variants differ in their associations with melanoma and nonmelanoma skin cancer, but both red hair and non–red hair variants confer increased risk.

Environmental factors include intermittently high-intensity exposure of fair skin to UVA and UVB radiation (especially at a young age), sunburns, immune suppression, and residence in equatorial latitudes. Ephelides (freckles), which are a reflection of sun exposure, are associated with a two- to threefold increased risk of melanoma.

MacKie RM, Hauschild A, Eggermont AM: Epidemiology of invasive cutaneous melanoma, *Ann Oncol* 20(Suppl 6):vi1–vi7, 2009.

6. List the high-risk groups for developing melanoma.
- Persons with a persistently changing nevus
- Persons with FDMS
- Persons with *CDKN2A* mutations
- Persons with large numbers of atypical nevi
- Persons with >50 benign nevi or a large congential nevus
- Persons with a past medical history of melanoma or a family history of melanoma in a first-degree relative
- Persons with xeroderma pigmentosum

MacKie RM, Hauschild A, Eggermont AM: Epidemiology of invasive cutaneous melanoma, *Ann Oncol* 20(Suppl 6):vi1–vi7, 2009.
Meyle KD, Guldberg P: Genetic risk factors for melanoma, *Hum Genet* 126:499–510, 2009.

7. Do all melanomas develop from atypical nevi?
In the past, the development of melanoma has been modeled as a stepwise process from a cutaneous melanocyte through nevus through atypical nevus stages to melanoma in situ and eventually invasive melanoma. However, around 40% to 75% of melanomas develop in normal skin de novo and, of those melanomas that develop in association with a preexisting nevus, <50% of the nevi are atypical. At present it is difficult to determine whether an atypical nevus is any more likely to become a melanoma than any other nevus or isolated melanocyte. Moreover, it is now clear that a preexisting nevus is not required for a melanoma to develop. It is thought that the discrepancy between melanomas arising in preexisting nevi and de novo melanomas can best be explained by the cancer stem cell theory. In this regard, the risk of melanoma associated with nevi may be due to the potential for secondary mutations within nevi, as well as due to the inherent properties of the stem cell population in individuals with numerous moles. Therefore, although there is a clear association between nevi and melanoma risk, only a portion of this risk may be related to the acquisition of genetic mutations within the nevi. The majority of the risk may be associated with the inherent properties of melanocyte stem cell populations in individuals with numerous nevi.

Friedman RJ, Farber MJ, Warycha MA, et al: The "dysplastic" nevus. *Clin Dermatol* 27:103–115, 2009.
Elder, DE: Dysplastic nevi: an update, *Histopathology* 56:112–120, 2010.

8. What are cancer stem cells?
In recent years, there has been increasing evidence demonstrating that melanoma, as well as other solid tumors, contain a subpopulation of cancer stem cells (CSCs). CSCs are rare cells within tumors with the ability to self-renew, drive tumorigenesis, and give rise to a phenotypically diverse tumor cell population. They are considered the source of the primary tumor mass and are thought to be responsible for drug resistance and cancer recurrence. Experimental evidence supports the existence of CSCs in leukemia and melanoma, as well as in breast, brain, colon, pancreatic, and ovarian cancer. Although controversy exists regarding the location of melanoma stem cells in the skin, it has been hypothesized that most melanomas arise from mutations that accumulate in a common precursor CSC, which subsequently drives the establishment of primary and metastatic lesions. This CSC-like precursor is thought to be responsible for the metastatic process, while the less stable progeny are unable to spread locally or distantly. Although definitive markers are still lacking for melanoma CSC, CD133, ABCB5, and ABCG2 have been identified as potential markers.

Sabatino M, Stroncek DF, Klein H, et al: Stem cells in melanoma development, *Cancer Lett* 279:119–125, 2009.
La Porta C: Cancer stem cells: lessons from melanoma, *Stem Cell Rev* 5(1):61–65, 2009.
Frank NY, Schatton T, Frank MH: The therapeutic promise of the cancer stem cell concept, *J Clin Invest* 120:41–45, 2010.

9. Is melanoma a single disease?
No. Melanoma has historically been divided into major subsets based on the clinical and histologic appearance and varied associations with skin color, sun exposure, and anatomic site. However, recent molecular investigations have demonstrated biologically distinct subsets of the disease that vary in their relationship to anatomic site, sun exposure, nevus phenotype, and mutational analysis.

Key Points: Diagnosis of Malignant Melanoma

1. Melanoma, the most aggressive malignant neoplasm arising in the skin, has one of the most rapidly increasing incidence rates of all human malignancies.
2. When diagnosed early and treated appropriately, melanoma has high cure rates.
3. High-risk patients include those with FDMS, *CDKN2A* mutations, atypical nevi, >50 benign nevi, large congential nevi, a past medical history of melanoma or a family history of melanoma in a first-degree relative, and xeroderma pigmentosum.
4. Patients with dark complexions (skin types IV and V) can develop melanoma.
5. Melanomas do not always arise within a preexisting nevus.
6. CSCs are rare cells within tumors having the ability to self-renew and drive tumorigenesis.
7. Melanoma is not a single disease:
   - *B-Raf* mutations are often found in younger patients on intermittently sun-exposed skin.
   - *N-Ras* mutations are often found in older patients on chronically sun-exposed skin.
   - *c-Kit* mutations are often found in mucosal and acral melanomas.

10. What are the molecular pathways in melanoma?

Major molecular pathways that have been implicated in melanoma include p16 (25% to 50%) and p14[ARF] (25% to 50%), microphthalmia-associated transcription factor (MITF) (50% to 75%), B-Raf (50% to 60%), and PTEN (15% to 25%). Furthermore, the antiapoptotic factor Bcl-2 is often overexpressed in melanoma. It should be stressed, that as noted above, not all melanomas are the same. In this regard, those melanomas that develop in younger patients on intermittently sun-exposed skin demonstrate a greater percentage of *B-Raf* mutations (>60%) than those melanomas that develop on chronically sun-exposed skin in older patients (<15%). In contrast, those melanomas that develop on chronically sun-exposed skin in older patients demonstrate a greater percentage of *N-Ras* mutations (20% to 40%). Along the same lines, melanomas that develop on acral and mucosal sites more demonstrate a greater percentage of *c-Kit* mutations (~40%) compared to non–sun-exposed (0%) and sun-exposed (30%) melanomas. Further, acral and mucosal melanomas demonstrate a lower percentage of *B-Raf* mutations (~20% and ~10%, respectively).

Bauer J, Bastian B: Genomic analysis of melanocytic neoplasia, *Adv Dermatol* 21:81–99, 2005.

Fecher LA, Cummings SD, Keefe MJ, Alani RM: Toward a molecular classification of melanoma, *J Clin Oncol* 25:1606–1620, 2007.

Mocellin S, Verdi D, Nitti D: DNA repair gene polymorphisms and risk of cutaneous melanoma: a systematic review and meta-analysis, *Carcinogenesis* 30:1735–1743, 2009.

Curtlin JA, Busam K, Pinkel D, Bastian BC: Somatic activation of KIT in distinct subtypes of melanoma, *J Clin Oncol* 24:4340–4346, 2006.

Miller AJ, Mihm MC: Melanoma, *N Engl J Med* 355:51–65, 2006.

Dhomen N, Marais R: BRAF signaling and targeted therapies in melanoma, *Hematol Oncol Clin North Am* 23:529–545, 2009.

11. Is there a host immune response to melanoma?

Yes. Observations such as incomplete or complete regression of melanoma, occurrence of vitiligo and halo nevi in patients, as well as increased rates of melanoma in immune suppressed patients indicate that immunologic events appear to play a role in the clinical course of the melanoma and may occasionally cause clinical regressions. Tumor antigen (TA)–specific T cells have been shown to play an active role in eliminating tumors and metastases, as well as in inducing TA-specific T-cell memory responses in a wide range of animal tumor models. Similarly, in vitro studies employing human peripheral blood lymphocytes (PBL) isolated from patients with melanoma have been reported to contain TA-specific CD8+ and CD4+ T-cell precursors, as well as natural killer (NK) cells and macrophages that are capable of killing tumor cell targets after appropriate in vitro activation. CD8+ T cells are believed to play a major role in control of melanoma growth. It is thought that this immunosurveillance of melanoma often fails in patients. This has been the rationale for the development of immunotherapy of melanoma.

Parmiani G, Castelli C, Santinami M, Rivoltini L: Melanoma immunology: past, present and future, *Curr Opin Oncol* 19:121–127, 2007.

12. Describe the clinical appearance of melanoma.

Cutaneous melanoma can have a number of different appearances. Malignant melanomas can begin in a preexisting melanocytic nevus; however, as noted above, the exact percentage of malignant melanomas arising in preexisting nevi versus those arising de novo is controversial. When malignant melanoma arises in a preexisting nevus, the nevus usually demonstrates a change in appearance, such as an increase in size or change in shape, or it may bleed easily when traumatized. **A changing nevus is the most important risk factor for melanoma**. The development of a new pigmented nevus in any patient over 35 years of age should be evaluated. Classically, early melanoma lesions are characterized by containing different colors, such as different hues of brown, black, red, and blue. Melanoma may also appear as a brown or black discoloration of the nail or as a skin ulcer that does not heal.

13. What are the ABCDEs of melanoma?

The development of a new or changing pigmented lesion is the classic initial presentation of melanoma. A lesion that demonstrates a noticeable increase in size over a period of weeks to months or development of pigment irregularity (black, hues of brown, red, blue, or white) should be evaluated by a physician and biopsied. The ABCDEs of melanoma (Fig. 45-1) are a helpful guideline for determining which moles could be suspicious for melanoma:

- **A**symmetry. Any mole that appears unusual or shows asymmetry in shape should be evaluated.
- **B**order and bleeding. The border of any melanocytic nevus should be relatively smooth, with a clear demarcation between the nevus and surrounding normal skin. Nevi that develop irregular or ill-defined borders should be evaluated. B is also for bleeding, and any mole that bleeds needs careful evaluation.
- **C**olor. Most moles have a homogeneous tan or brown color. Moles that develop pigment variegation within an otherwise homogeneous background should be evaluated.
- **D**iameter. Most melanomas are 0.6 mm in diameter, but an otherwise suspicious lesion that is small might also be malignant.
- **E**volving. This emphasizes the need to evaluate any melanocytic nevus is whether the nevus has changed in terms of the ABCDs over a relatively short time (weeks to months).

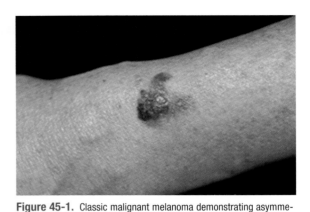

Figure 45-1. Classic malignant melanoma demonstrating asymmetry, irregular notched border, multiple colors, wide diameter, and a history of change and growth (evolution).

It should be stressed that the ABCDEs are meant strictly as guidelines and cannot take the place of a thorough evaluation. Some physicians stress utilizing the "ugly duckling" sign. The latter refers to the fact that nevi in an individual generally tend to share a similar appearance, so one that does not share the same characteristics should be considered for biopsy.

Abbasi NR, Shaw HM, Rigel DS, et al: Early diagnosis of cutaneous melanoma: revisiting the ABCD criteria, *JAMA* 292:2771–2776, 2004.

14. What is dermoscopy?

Dermoscopy, also known as skin surface microscopy, or epiluminescence microscopy, is a noninvasive tool to assist in the diagnosis of melanocytic and nonmelanocytic tumors. A number of dermoscopy algorithms have been developed to aid in the diagnosis of melanocytic tumors. However, these algorithms cannot be applied to lesions located on the face, acral and mucosal surfaces, and the nails. The sensitivity of dermoscopy in the diagnosis of melanoma ranges from 70% to 95%, compared to clinical investigation with the unaided eye, which ranges from 60% to 90%. It is noteworthy that the success of dermoscopy depends critically on appropriate training.

Campos-do-Carmo G, Ramos-e-Silva M: Dermoscopy: basic concepts, *Int J Dermatol* 47:712–719, 2008.

15. Where on the body does melanoma most commonly arise?

Melanoma can arise on any part of the body. Primary tumors are most common on the trunk in men and on the lower extremity in women.

16. Are there different types of melanoma?

There are several different types of melanoma, and each may appear somewhat differently:

- **Superficial spreading malignant melanoma** (SSMM) is the most common form of melanoma in Caucasians (~70% of cases). It is most commonly diagnosed in the fourth or fifth decade. It usually presents as a slowly enlarging, brown (usually) or black spot that may have both a macular and papular component. The lesion may show color variegation and irregular borders (Fig. 45-2A). About 30% arise in a preexisting nevus, and 75% of these lesions demonstrate regression on clinical exam.
- **Nodular melanoma** is the second most common type of melanoma and represents about 15% to 20% of all cases. It is most commonly diagnosed in men between the fifth and sixth decade. Nodular melanoma usually presents as a pigmented (usually brown or black) papule that slowly enlarges and frequently ulcerates. These lesions most commonly present on the head, neck or trunk. Nodular melanomas may ulcerate, presenting as a nonhealing skin ulcer (Fig. 45-2B).
- **Lentigo maligna melanoma,** also known as the Hutchinson freckle, represents ~15% of all cases of melanoma. It usually presents as an irregularly shaped, flat, pigmented lesion on actinically damaged skin. It is seen most frequently on the face or other sun-exposed sites. Most patients are in their seventh decade. More advanced lesions can develop papules or nodules, indicating the lesions have developed a vertical or downward growth component.
- **Acral lentiginous melanoma** represents 5% to 10% of all cases of melanoma. It is the most common form of melanoma in African-Americans, Asians, and Hispanics (Fig. 45-2C). The latter does not reflect an increase incidence of acral lentiginous melanoma in these races. It usually appears as brown or black macules arising on the glabrous (non–hair-bearing) skin of an extremity (palms, soles, or nail beds). It can also occur on mucosal surfaces. The latter have an extremely poor prognosis.

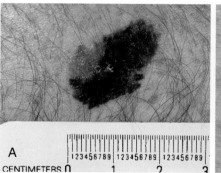
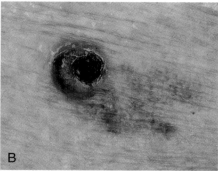
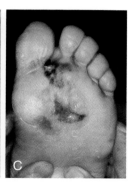

Figure 45-2. A, Superficial spreading malignant melanoma. The lesion shows asymmetry, notched borders, and shades of light brown. **B,** Superficial spreading malignant melanoma that has developed a nodular melanoma. **C,** Acral lentiginous melanoma on the sole of the foot demonstrating a macular and focally nodular pigmented lesion with multiple shades of black and gray with a very irregular border. (Panel A courtesy of James E. Fitzpatrick, MD; panel C courtesy of Fitzsimons Army Medical Center teaching files.)

- **Amelanotic melanoma** is usually considered a non–pigment-producing variant of nodular melanoma. Amelanotic melanoma can be confused with other benign skin lesions, such as pyogenic granuloma. Amelanotic melanoma often evades early diagnosis and results in a poorer prognosis.

17. What are Clark's levels?

A system used to describe the depth of invasion of a melanoma that was originally described by Dr. Wallace H. Clark, Jr. The system provides a helpful means to determine the probability of developing progressive disease. Primary tumors are classified according to the degree of invasion into the various anatomic levels of the skin. This classification scheme has been shown to correlate well with 5-year survival rates; however, the new 2009 AJCC Melanoma Staging and Classification System, for the first time, has removed the Clark's level as a recommended parameter.

- **Level I:** Tumor cells in epidermis only (melanoma in situ)
- **Level II:** Tumor cells extend from epidermis into (but do not fill) papillary dermis
- **Level III:** Tumor cells extend from epidermis into and fill papillary dermis
- **Level IV:** Tumor cells extend into reticular dermis
- **Level V:** Tumor cells extend through the dermis into underlying subcutaneous fat

18. What is Breslow's depth?

This is a more precise way of measuring the level of invasion of primary malignant melanoma. An ocular micrometer is used to directly measure the distance that tumor cells have invaded. The distance of invasion is measured from the top of the granular layer of the epidermis, or in ulcerated lesions, the base of the ulcer to the point of deepest invasion by the tumor cells. This measurement appears to be more easily reproducible among institutions and more objective than Clark's levels. The Breslow tumor thickness is the strongest predictor of survival.

Payette MJ, Katz M 3rd, Grant-Kels JM: Melanoma prognostic factors found in the dermatopathology report, *Clin Dermatol* 27:53–74, 2009.

19. What other findings should be reported in the histopathologic diagnosis of melanoma?

The World Health Organization, as well as the American Joint Committee on Cancer (AJCC), recommends reporting the following when reporting on the histologic diagnosis of melanoma: thickness (Breslow depth), mitoses/mm^2, level of invasion (Clark's level), regression, tumor-infiltrating lymphocytes, ulceration, vascular invasion, microscopic satellites, associated nevus, and margins. Because the most recent AJCC staging system for melanoma has deleted the Clark's level, many pathologists and dermatopathologists no longer include this finding in their reports.

Payette MJ, Katz M 3rd, Grant-Kels JM: Melanoma prognostic factors found in the dermatopathology report, *Clin Dermatol* 27:53–74, 2009.

20. What are the common immunohistochemical (IHC) markers utilized in the diagnosis of melanoma?

Most melanomas can be diagnosed on routine histology, but IHC staining can be useful in the difficult cases. A wide range of melanoma- and melanocyte-associated antigens have been identified for use in IHC staining. The most commonly utilized ones are as follows:

- **S100:** A calcium-binding protein that is expressed in melanocytes, Schwann cells, glial cells, chondrocytes, adipocytes, myoepithelial cells, macrophage, Langerhans cells, and dendritic cells. Despite its low specificity, S100 has a high sensitivity for melanocytes and melanoma.

- **gp100:** A glycoprotein considered to part of the premelanosome complex. HMB45 is the most commonly utilized antibody to detect gp100. HMB45 has a higher specificity for melanocytes and nevus cells, but its use is limited by its sensitivity, with false negative rates up to 35%.
- **MART1:** A melanocyte differentiation antigen known as **m**elanoma **a**ntigen **r**ecognized by **T** cells–1. It represents a protein associated with melanosomes. MART1 is more specific than S100 and HMB45, as well as more sensitive than HMB45.

  Other less commonly used markers include microphthalmia-associated transcription factor (MITF) and tyrosinase, but their utility is limited to determining the melanocytic origin of a lesion.

  Piris A, Mihm MC Jr: Progress in melanoma histopathology and diagnosis, *Hematol Oncol Clin North Am* 23:467–480, 2009.

21. Are there other factors with prognostic impact in patients with melanoma?

The strongest predictors of prognosis are Breslow's depth, presence of ulceration in the primary tumor, and presence of nodal disease. Secondary predictors of prognosis include the number of positive lymph nodes, extension of the tumor into extranodal soft tissue, age at time of diagnosis, sex (women > men), and anatomic site of primary tumor. In this regard, extremities, excluding the hands and feet, have the most favorable prognosis, while lesions on the scalp, hands, feet, and mucosal surfaces have the worst.

Balch CM, Seng-Jaw S, Gershenwald JE, et al: Prognostic factors analysis of 17,600 melanoma patients: validation of the American Joint Committee on Cancer Staging System, *J Clin Oncol* 19:3622–3634, 2001.

Mohr P, Eggermont AM, Hauschild A, Buzaid A: Staging of cutaneous melanoma, *Ann Oncol* 20(Suppl 6):vi14–vi21, 2009.

22. How are patients with melanoma evaluated after the initial diagnosis?

Baseline evaluations then should be performed to determine if there are any detectable secondary primary tumors, local extension of the first primary, or if metastatic disease is present. These evaluations should include a complete physical examination—a complete skin evaluation and lymph node exam; a chest x-ray; and may include baseline laboratory tests such as a complete blood count, blood chemistry studies, liver function tests, and possibly serum lactate dehydrogenase. It should be stressed that there is significant evidence to suggest that routine imaging studies and blood work have limited, if any, value in the initial evaluation of asymptomatic patients with a primary cutaneous melanoma 4 mm or less in thickness. The American Academy of Dermatology recommends that these tests should be optional and directed based on a thorough medical history and physical examination. Exceptions for asymptomatic patients include those with a primary tumor > 4 mm and in the setting of clinical trials. Any abnormality detected with these exams should be more fully investigated with the proper diagnostic procedure (e.g., a fine-needle aspirate to assess an enlarged lymph node or computerized tomography of the abdomen for abnormal liver chemistry).

23. What is the most current system for staging melanoma?

The current and preferred staging system for melanoma is that of the American Joint Commission on Cancer (AJCC) from 2009. It is based on the TNM (tumor, lymph node, metastasis) system, which allows the assessment of patients based on the thickness of the primary tumor and whether lymph node or other metastases are present. Staging and survival rates for cutaneous melanoma are summarized in Table 45-1.

Balch CM, Gershenwald JE, Soong SJ, et al: Final version of the 2009 AJCC Melanoma Staging and Classification, *J Clin Oncol* 27:6199–6206, 2009.

Table 45-1. 2009 AJCC Stage Groupings and 5-Year Survival for Primary Cutaneous Melanoma*

STAGE	TUMOR	NODE	METASTASES	5-YEAR SURVIVAL
0	Tis	N0	M0	99.5%–100%
IA	T1a	N0	M0	97%–99%
IB	T1b, 2a	N0	M0	90%-92%
IIA	T2b, 3a	N0	M0	78%–82%
IIB	T3b, 4a	N0	M0	68%–71%
IIC	T4b	N0	M0	53%–56%
IIIA	T1–4a	N1a–2a	M0	78%
IIIB	T1–4b	N1a–2b	M0	50%–68%
IIIC	T1–4b	N1b–3	M0	27%–52%
IV	Any T	Any N	M1a–c	9%–18%†

*Range reflects the prognostic impact of tumor burden (micrometastasis versus macrometastasis), number of nodes involved, and whether there was extracapsular extension. Patients with in-transit metastases/satellite lesions without metastatic lymph nodes are classified as N2c.
†Range reflects the prognostic impact of lung metastasis and/or elevated lactate dehydrogenase (LDH).
AJCC, American Joint Committee on Cancer.
Data from Greene FL, Page DL, Fleming ID, et al, editors: *AJCC cancer staging manual,* ed 7, New York, 2009, Springer Verlag.

24. How is melanoma treated?

The standard of care for treating melanoma is to:
1. Establish a histologic diagnosis of the suspect lesion.
2. Completely excise the tumor with adequate margins.
3. Assess for the presence of detectable metastatic disease.
4. Conduct follow-up evaluations for the rest of the patient's life.

Pathology remains the gold standard for the diagnosis of melanoma. To establish a histologic diagnosis, the suspect lesion should be completely excised with a 1- to 3-mm margin of skin to the depth of the subcuticular fat. If this is not possible, due to anatomic location or size of the lesion, an incisional or punch biopsy to the depth of the subcuticular fat should be performed on the thickest or most atypical portion of the lesion. It is noteworthy that biopsy of lentigo maligna can be problematic, because there are often skip areas, as well as areas of regression, in these lesions that may lead to misdiagnosis. The best biopsy technique to establish the diagnosis of lentigo maligna is usually multiple punch biopsies from different sites or broad shave biopsy from multiple areas.

Once a diagnosis of melanoma is established, wide local excision of the primary tumor to the muscle fascia is recommended. It should be noted that no randomized trials have compared this approach with excision to the deep subcutaneous fat.

Aloia TA, Gershenwald JE: Management of early-stage cutaneous melanoma, *Curr Probl Surg* 42:455–534, 2005.
McKenna JK, Florell SR, Goldman GD, Bowen GM: Lentigo maligna/lentigo maligna melanoma: current state of diagnosis and treatment, *Dermatol Surg* 32:493–504, 2006.

25. How wide should surgical margins be?

There is ongoing controversy regarding the width of normal-appearing skin that should be excised. At one time, 5.0-cm margins were recommended. With the exception of only four prospective multicenter trials, surgical margins were originally based, at least in part, on consensus decision and tradition. A National Institutes of Health Consensus Conference on Melanoma has recommended surgical margins based on the depth of invasion of the primary tumor. Malignant melanoma in situ should be excised with a 0.5-cm border of normal skin. Lesions that have a Breslow's depth of 1.0 mm should have wide local reexcision with 1.0-cm margins. Lesions that are 1 to 2 mm thick should be excised with 1- to 2-cm margins (2 cm, if primary closure can be achieved, or no significant difference exists in reconstruction between a 1- and 2-cm margin of excision). Lesions that are intermediate, 2 to 4 mm thick, are excised with 2-cm margins. Lesions 4.0 mm thick should be excised with 2- to 3-cm margins; there are no randomized trials that have determined the optimal margins for excision of melanoma > 4 mm in thickness. These recommendations are meant only as general guidelines, and individual patient considerations must be taken into account. It should be stressed that there are several studies demonstrating that 0.5-cm margins are inadequate for most malignant melanoma in situ on the head, neck, hands, and feet. Moreover, there is evidence to suggest that tumor thickness should not influence surgical margins.

Studies suggest that definitive surgical treatment may be delayed up to 3 weeks after biopsy of the primary lesion without adversely affecting the 5-year survival rate.

Landthaler M, Braun-Falco O, Leitl A, et al: Excisional biopsy as the first therapeutic procedure versus primary wide excision of malignant melanoma, *Cancer* 64:1612–1616, 1989.
Zitelli JA: Surgical margins for lentigo maligna, *Arch Dermatol* 2004 140:607–608, 2004.
Bricca GM, Brodland DG, Ren D, Zitelli JA: Cutaneous head and neck melanoma treated with Mohs micrographic surgery, *J Am Acad Dermatol* 52:92–100, 2005.
Thompson JF, Scolyer RA, Uren RF: Surgical management of primary cutaneous melanoma: excision margins and the role of sentinel lymph node examination, *Surg Oncol Clin N Am* 15:301–318, 2006.

26. What is the most important risk factor for local recurrence of primary melanoma?

Ulceration of the primary tumor is the most significant prognostic factor for increased risk of local recurrence.

Balch CM, Seng-Jaw S, Gershenwald JE, et al: Prognostic factors analysis of 17,600 melanoma patients: validation of the American Joint Committee on Cancer Staging System, *J Clin Oncol* 19:3622–3634, 2001.
Mohr P, Eggermont AM, Hauschild A, Buzaid A: Staging of cutaneous melanoma, *Ann Oncol* 20(Suppl 6):vi14–vi21, 2009.

27. Does a biopsy of melanoma increase the risk of spreading tumor cells or causing metastases?

Two independently conducted studies of this question have concluded that incisional biopsies of melanoma do not cause the tumor to spread locally or metastasize.

Lederman JS, Sober AJ: Does biopsy type influence survival in clinical stage I cutaneous melanoma? *J Am Acad Dermatol* 86:983–987, 1985.

28. Describe the recommended follow-up for a patient with melanoma.

Routine follow-up evaluations vary, depending on the depth of the primary tumor (Table 45-2). It is important to stress that unlike many malignancies, melanoma has a tendency to recur many years after the primary tumor is removed. Therefore, patients at high risk for recurrence need to be followed very closely for long periods of time.

Table 45-2. Recommended Follow-up Schedules for Patients with Cutaneous Melanoma

STAGE	FOLLOW-UP	DURATION	THEREAFTER
0	Every 12 months	2 years	Variable
Ia	Every 6–12 months	2 years	Variable
Ib	Every 6–12 months	5 years	Variable
II	Every 3–6 months	2–3 years	Every 6–12 months for life
IIb–IV	Every 3-6 months	3 years	Every 6–12 months for life, consider CXR, LDH

CXR, Chest x-ray; *LDH*, lactate dehydrogenase.

29. Which tests or examinations are conducted during the routine follow-up of patients who have had melanoma?

There is no general consensus regarding the routine follow-up of patients with malignant melanoma. Close follow-up is recommended because the risk of developing a second primary melanoma is around 3% to 4.5%. Follow-up recommendations vary from 1 to 4 times per year during the first 2 years after diagnosis. During the follow-up evaluations, patients should receive a physical exam directed toward the detection of a local recurrence of the primary tumor, the development of metastatic disease in the surrounding skin or the draining lymphatic system, or development of a second primary melanoma. As in the initial staging evaluation, any abnormality detected by physical exam, review of systems, or laboratory tests is more fully investigated. If no abnormalities are detected by routine physical exam and review of systems, repeat laboratory tests, and chest x-ray are often dictated by stage of the patient's disease.

Brobeil A, Rapaport D, Wells K, et al: Multiple primary melanomas: implications for screening and follow-up programs for melanoma, *Ann Surg Oncol* 4:19–23, 1997.

Aloia TA, Gershenwald JE: Management of early-stage cutaneous melanoma, *Curr Probl Surg* 42:455–534, 2005.

McKenna JK, Florell SR, Goldman GD, Bowen GM: Lentigo maligna/lentigo maligna melanoma: current state of diagnosis and treatment, *Dermatol Surg* 32:493–504, 2006.

30. Does local tumor recurrence influence overall survival?

No. Local recurrence is defined as any recurrence of a primary tumor within 2 cm of the excisional scar of a primary melanoma. Most (~95%) recurrences occur within the first 5 years after excision, and the overall risk for local recurrence is usually depends on ulceration and anatomical sites. In this regard, the risk of local recurrence is increased in ulcerated primary tumors, as well as tumors on the head, neck, hands, and feet. Local recurrence is associated with the development of in-transit, regional, and distant metastatic disease but is not an independent prognostic indicator of survival.

Karakousis CP, Bartolucci AA, Balch C: Local recurrence and its management. In Balch CM, Houghton AN, Sober AJ, Soon S-J, editors: *Cutaneous melanoma*, ed 3, St Louis, Quality Medical Publishing, 1998, pp 155–162.

Bricca GM, Brodland DG, Ren D, Zitelli JA: Cutaneous head and neck melanoma treated with Mohs micrographic surgery, *J Am Acad Dermatol* 52:92–100, 2005.

Thompson JF, Scolyer RA, Uren RF: Surgical management of primary cutaneous melanoma: excision margins and the role of sentinel lymph node examination, *Surg Oncol Clin N Am* 15:301–318, 2006.

31. What is elective lymph node dissection (ELND)? When is it indicated?

ELND is the dissection of the draining lymph node basin in patients with deep primary melanomas who are felt to be at high risk for development of metastasis to the lymph nodes. ELND is based on the notion that melanoma cells migrate in an orderly fashion toward the draining lymph node. Therefore, surgical excision of all involved nodes in patients with stage III disease was postulated to prevent the spread of tumor to other organs. However, five multicenter randomized prospective trials in patients with primary melanoma have not shown a survival benefit for patients treated with ELND plus wide excision as compared to wide excision alone. Most large melanoma centers do not routinely perform ELND.

Balch CM, Cascinelli N, Sim FH, et al: Elective lymph node dissection: results of a prospective randomized surgical trial. In Balch CM, Houghton AN, Sober AJ, Soong S-J, editors: *Cutaneous melanoma*, ed 3, St Louis, Quality Medical Publishing, 1998, pp 209–215.

Medalie NS, Ackerman AB: Sentinel lymph node biopsy has no benefit for patients with primary cutaneous melanoma metastatic to a lymph node: an assertion based on comprehensive, critical analysis: part I, *Am J Dermatopathol* 25:399–417, 2003.

Medalie NS, Ackerman AB: Sentinel lymph node biopsy has no benefit for patients with primary cutaneous melanoma metastatic to a lymph node: an assertion based on comprehensive, critical analysis: part II, *Am J Dermatopathol* 25:473–484, 2003.

32. What is sentinel lymph node biopsy? When is it indicated?

In 1990, Morton introduced intraoperative lymphatic mapping and selective lymph node dissection or sentinel lymph node biopsy (SLNB) as an alternative to ELND for melanoma patients. He showed that the histology of the SLN reflects the histology of the entire lymph node basin, because when it is negative, the other lymph nodes within that basin are almost always also negative. The initial data from large series show substantial differences in the survival curves of patients, depending on their SLN status, and, in multivariate analysis, the status of the SLN has been confirmed as the most important prognostic factor for patients with primary melanoma.

SLNB are now being performed in clinical practice in many centers in the United States and abroad. The status of the SLN often guides further therapeutic interventions including complete lymphadenectomy and adjuvant chemotherapy or radiation therapy. Nevertheless, like ELND the theoretical value of SLNB dissection is based on the notion that melanoma cells migrate in an orderly fashion toward the draining lymph node.

To date there is little evidence that early dissection in SLN positive patients improves their survival compared to patients who receive nodal dissection when clinically detectable nodes develop. SLN remains a very controversial topic, and several points need to be emphasized. First, there is little evidence to suggest that melanoma cells migrate in an orderly fashion toward the draining lymph node, and the presence of melanoma cells within a lymph node may merely be an indicator of systemic metastatic disease. Second, surgical alteration of a patient's regional lymphatic structure may impair the body's immune response to melanoma. Third, at present we are unable to determine what constitutes relevant nodal disease. In this regard, 60% of patients with primary melanoma <1.0 mm in depth demonstrate positive SLN through polymerase chain reaction (PCR) analysis. These patients have a very favorable survival rate and rarely go on to develop nodal disease. Therefore, the presence of microscopic metastases does not correlate with the clinical course. Fourth, SLN biopsies require close collaboration between the nuclear radiologist, surgeon, and pathologist. Patient selection is also paramount. This procedure is less reliable if a wide excision has been performed; therefore, patients considered candidates should be referred for this procedure prior to the wide excision, which can be carried out simultaneously with the SLNB. Fifth, lymphatic flow is markedly varied in different persons, and it is difficult to predict with any degree of certainty which nodal basin serves a particular area of skin. Lastly, proponents of SLNB argue that SLN may identify patients who may be candidates for adjuvant therapy (see below). Nevertheless, to date no effective adjuvant therapy exists for metastatic melanoma.

Despite the controversies surrounding SNL, the AJCC recommends that all patients with primary melanoma >1 mm in tumor thickness have SNL biopsy performed prior to entry into melanoma clinical trials.

Amersi F, Morton DL: The role of sentinel lymph node biopsy in the management of melanoma, *Adv Surg* 41:241–256, 2007.
Medalie NS, Ackerman AB: Sentinel lymph node biopsy has no benefit for patients with primary cutaneous melanoma metastatic to a lymph node: an assertion based on comprehensive, critical analysis: part I, *Am J Dermatopathol* 25:399–417, 2003.
Medalie NS, Ackerman AB: Sentinel lymph node biopsy has no benefit for patients with primary cutaneous melanoma metastatic to a lymph node: an assertion based on comprehensive, critical analysis: part II, *Am J Dermatopathol* 25:473–484, 2003.
Zitelli JA: Sentinel lymph node biopsy: an alternate view, *Dermatol Surg* 34:544–549, 2008.

33. What is linear melanonychia?

A linear, pigmented streak of the nail (Fig. 45-3). Among the many potential causes, subungual melanoma is the most serious. A biopsy of the nail matrix is required if melanonychia develops rapidly, if it involves only a single digit, or if other causes of the abnormal pigmentation cannot be determined. This is a more common presentation of melanoma in blacks than in whites.

Note that longitudinal pigmented nail bands are commonly seen in darkly pigmented patients but are less common in light-skinned patients. If a pigmented nail band involves only one nail, occurs in a middle-aged or elderly white patient, shows progressive widening or darkening, or has an extension of pigment onto the surrounding nail fold, a biopsy is indicated to rule out melanoma.

34. What is Hutchinson's sign?

The development of pigmentation at the base of linear melanonychia involving the proximal nail fold and periungual skin (Fig. 45-4). This sign is felt to be a very specific indication that the linear melanonychia is due to melanoma.

Baran R, Kechijian P: Hutchinson's sign: a reappraisal, *J Am Acad Dermatol* 44:87–90, 2001.

35. What is Hutchinson's freckle?

Lentigo maligna, the precursor lesion of lentigo maligna melanoma. The lesion appears as a relatively large (usually greater than 1.0 cm), irregularly shaped, hyperpigmented macule that arises on sun-damaged skin (Fig. 45-5).

36. Are there any new ways to assess prognosis in patients with melanoma?

Some recently reported experimental tests may prove helpful in the early detection of metastatic disease. One such test is a reverse transcriptase

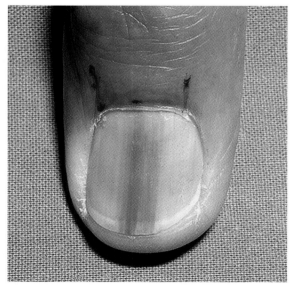

Figure 45-3. Linear melanonychia demonstrating linear brown streak of pigment. (Courtesy of James E. Fitzpatrick, MD.)

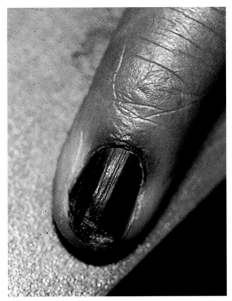

Figure 45-4. Acral lentiginous melanoma in situ arising from the nail bed of a black woman. Note the presence of pigment in the periungual tissue (positive Hutchinson's sign). (Courtesy of James E. Fitzpatrick, MD.)

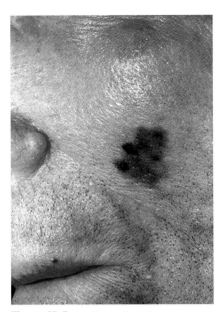

Figure 45-5. Lentigo maligna. These lesions remain superficial at the dermal–epidermal interface, often for many years, before they develop a vertical growth phase and become lentigo maligna melanoma. They are most commonly seen in elderly patients on sun-exposed skin.

polymerase chain reaction test used to detect circulating melanoma cells in the peripheral blood. Two groups have found that this test correlates positively with stage of disease and may be helpful in identifying patients who will eventually develop metastasis. Another test being developed is a positron emission tomography using a glucose analog coupled to a positron emitter. This test also is capable of identifying clinically undetectable lymph node and visceral metastases. Both of these tests may allow earlier detection and thereby more successful treatment of metastatic disease.

Palmieri G, Casula M, Sini MC, et al: Issues affecting molecular staging in the management of patients with melanoma, *J Cell Mol Med* 11:1052–1068, 2007.

Fusi A, Collette S, Busse A, et al: Circulating melanoma cells and distant metastasis-free survival in stage III melanoma patients with or without adjuvant interferon treatment (EORTC 18991 side study), *Eur J Cancer* 45:3189–3197, 2009.

37. What forms of chemotherapy are used in the treatment of metastatic melanoma?

Chemotherapy in metastatic melanomas yielded disappointing results with 5-year survival rates for treated patients ranging from 3% to 14%. There are currently no curative forms of therapy for patients with metastatic disease. Dacarbazine has shown some efficacy as single-agent therapy. Response rates average around 10% to 20%, with durations averaging 6 months, and a complete response rate of about 5%. Newer agents such as temozolomide (TMZ) are similar to dacarbazine but offer the advantages of oral administration, as well as penetration through the blood–brain barrier. Nevertheless, response rates average ~15%. Temozolomide has also been tried in combination with IFN-α and thalidomide; however, no increase in survival rates has been observed. Cisplatin has been shown to be somewhat effective as single-agent therapy, but it has significant toxicities. Other studies have shown that the nitrosoureas (carmustine, lomustine, and semustine) have an overall response rate ranging from 13% to 18%. Similarly, tubular toxins such as vinblastine, vincristine, and Taxol (paclitaxel) have led to response rates of between 12% and 15%. The combination of carboplatin and paclitaxel is currently under investigation.

Wolchok JD, Saenger YM: Current topics in melanoma, *Curr Opin Oncol* 19:116–120, 2007.

38. Is radiation therapy effective for melanoma?

No. High-dose radiation is utilized for palliative care of cerebral metastases and for local control of unresectable disease.

Testori A, Rutkowski P, Marsden J, et al: Surgery and radiotherapy in the treatment of cutaneous melanoma, *Ann Oncol* 20(Suppl 6): vi22–vi29, 2009.

Key Points: Treatment of Malignant Melanoma

1. Immunologic events appear to play a role in the clinical course of the melanoma.
2. Thickness and ulceration are key prognostic factors of the primary tumor.
3. At present there is no effective treatment for advanced-stage melanoma.
4. Early dissection in SLN-positive patients does not improve survival.
5. The presence of pigmentation extending onto the nail fold from a band of linear melanonychia (Hutchinson's sign) is a strong indication for biopsy and histopathologic evaluation of the nail matrix.

39. How effective is immunotherapy in malignant melanoma?

The lack of effective treatment for advanced-stage melanoma by conventional therapies, such as radiation and chemotherapy, has highlighted the need to develop alternative therapeutic strategies. Among them, immunotherapy has attracted much attention because immunologic events appear to play a role in the clinical course of the disease and may occasionally cause clinical regressions.

Monoclonal antibody (mAb) therapy has been investigated using a variety of nonconjugated and conjugated (linked to toxins or radioisotopes) mAb directed against glycolipids, glycoproteins, and proteoglycans expressed by melanoma cells. Occasional dramatic responses have been reported, but the overall efficacy is quite limited, and responses have been noted only in about 10% to 12% of treated patients. More recent studies have investigated the use of mAb that targets immunomodulatory pathways that regulate immune effector cells. In this regard, considerable attention has been given toward targeting either CD28 or CTLA-4 on immune effector cells. It should be stressed that targeting the CD28/CTLA-4 pathway is fraught with hazard, because affinity and concentration of the administrated mAb must be balanced to prevent superinflammatory responses. The CTLA-4–specific ipilimumab (MDX-010) and tremelimumab (CP-675,206), which are fully human IgG1 and IgG2 mAbs, respectively, are being tested in patients with metastatic melanoma. The use of tremelimumab is also currently being investigated in a phase I trial in stage IV melanoma patients in combination with the Toll-like receptor (TLR)9 agonist PF-3512676.

A number of new mAbs are directed against various targets, including vascular endothelial growth factor (VEGF), tumor necrosis family costimulatory receptors (e.g., DR4, DR5, glucocorticoid-induced tumor necrosis factor receptor [GITR], CD134 [OX40], CD137 [4-1BB], and CD40), and integrins also are currently being investigated in clinical trials.

Recently, T-cell–based immunotherapy has been emphasized, because there have been disappointing results in the clinical trials implemented with mAbs, and because T cells are believed to play the major role in the control of tumor growth. In general, these vaccines have been relatively successful in animals; however, these results have not translated into human trials. These studies have demonstrated that cell-based, heat shock protein–based, T-cell–defined peptide epitopes and dendritic cell–based vaccinations can effectively induce tumor-specific immune responses. Nonetheless, a lack of clinical response and/or recurrence of disease occurs frequently, in spite of induction and/or persistence of TA-specific immune responses. This lack of correlation is caused, at least in part, by the multiple immune escape mechanisms utilized by melanoma cells.

An additional means of cellular immunotherapy is the adoptive transfer of immune effector cells into patients. The ex vivo expansion of lymphokine-activated killer (LAK) cells or tumor-infiltrating lymphocytes (TIL), with or without interleukin-2 (IL-2), has achieved some remarkable response rates in cancer patients.

The use of biologic response modifiers, such as interferon (IFN) and other cytokines, has had modest success. The use of IFN-α as a single-agent treatment has yielded response rates of 15% to 20% and complete response rates in up to 5% of patients. However, it should be stressed that the use of IFN-α remains controversial because its use has only been associated with an increase in disease-free interval but not an increase in overall survival in treated patients.

Combination therapy with the chemotherapeutic drugs dacarbazine and cisplatin, along with immunotherapeutic agents such as IFN-α and IL-2, has yielded significantly higher response rates, variously reported in the 40% to 50% range. Most of these cases, however, were limited to metastases involving soft tissues, including lymph nodes and subcutaneous tissue or the lung. Very few responses have been recorded in patients with liver or other visceral metastases. Furthermore, there has been little prolongation of survival with the use of combination therapy.

Campoli M, Ferrone S: T-cell-based immunotherapy of melanoma: what have we learned and how can we improve? *Expert Rev Vaccines* 3:171–187, 2004.

Terando AM, Faries MB, Morton DL: Vaccine therapy for melanoma: current status and future directions, *Vaccine* 25(Suppl 2):B4–B16, 2007.

Campoli M, Ferrone S: Immunotherapy of malignant disease: the coming age of therapeutic monoclonal antibodies. In De Vita V, Hellman S, Rosenberg S, editors: *Cancer: principles and practice of oncology*, New York, 2009, Lippincott Williams & Wilkins, 23:1–18.

Schadendorf D, Algarra SM, Bastholt L, et al: Immunotherapy of distant metastatic disease, *Ann Oncol* 20(Suppl 6):vi41–vi50, 2009.

Rosenberg SA, Dudley ME: Adoptive cell therapy for the treatment of patients with metastatic melanoma, *Curr Opin Immunol* 21: 233–240, 2009.

40. Does gene therapy offer any better results?

Several different strategies are being explored that are generically termed "gene therapy." One strategy involves the genetic modification of tumor-infiltrating lymphocytes to make them more effective at killing tumor cells. Another strategy involves the genetic modification of the tumor cells so that they produce immunostimulatory cytokines, which attract and stimulate cells involved in the immune response. Yet another approach involves the in situ genetic modification of tumor nodules so that they produce nonself human leukocyte antigens; the immune system recognizes and rejects these modified tumor nodules in a manner similar to that in which transplanted organs are rejected.

All three approaches have generated promising results in laboratory and/or clinical trials, but all are still in the early investigational phases.

Pavlick AC, Adams S, Fink MA, Bailes A: Novel therapeutic agents under investigation for malignant melanoma, *Expert Opin Investig Drugs* 12:1545–1558, 2003.

41. How about local perfusion?

The treatment of localized cutaneous and lymphatic metastases by isolated hyperthermic limb perfusion using a combination of chemotherapeutic and immunotherapeutic agents has generated renewed interest following a successful European trial. In this treatment, the circulation of the affected limb is isolated, the blood slowly heated, and then it is returned to the limb along with high doses of melphalan with or without tumor necrosis factor or gamma-interferon. Because the circulation of the limb is isolated from the remaining systemic circulation, much higher doses of the therapeutic agents can be administered than what could be tolerated systemically.

Kroon BB, Noorda EM, Vrouenraets BC, et al: Isolated limb perfusion for melanoma, Surg *Oncol Clin N Am* 17:785–794, 2008.

42. What are some newer targeted therapies for melanoma?

The available information regarding the molecular mechanisms underlying melanoma has increased greatly over the past several years. As noted above, the major molecular pathways that have been implicated in melanoma include p16 and p14[ARF], B-Raf, N-Ras, microphthalmia-associated transcription factor (MITF), PTEN, and Bcl2. Of particular clinical relevance is the RAS-RAF-MEK-ERK (MAP kinase) signaling pathway. Sorafenib and imatinib are oral multikinase inhibitors that inhibit MAP kinase pathway signaling. Trials of sorafenib or imatinib in combination with dacarbazine and carboplatin/paclitaxel are currently underway. Trials are also underway investigating the Bcl-2 antisense molecule, oblimersen, in combination with dacarbazine. Newer small molecular inhibitors are currently under investigation.

Tawbi H, Nimmagadda N: Targeted therapy in melanoma, *Biologics* 3:475–484, 2009.
Dhomen N, Marais R: BRAF signaling and targeted therapies in melanoma, *Hematol Oncol Clin North Am* 23:529–545, 2009.

LEUKEMIC AND LYMPHOMATOUS INFILTRATES OF THE SKIN

Theresa R. Pacheco, MD

CHAPTER 46

1. Define lymphoma.

A lymphoma is a malignancy of the immune system that is characterized by an abnormal proliferation of lymphocytes and related cell types. Most lymphomas begin in lymph nodes and are divided into Hodgkin's and non–Hodgkin's lymphomas. The non–Hodgkin's lymphomas are further subdivided into T-cell and B-cell subtypes.

Willemze R: New concepts in the classification of cutaneous lymphomas, *Arch Dermatol* 131:1077–1080, 1995.

MYCOSIS FUNGOIDES

2. Is there a lymphoma that begins in the skin?

Yes. Mycosis fungoides begins in the skin and often remains localized there for many years. Rarely, other T- and B-cell lymphomas also can present with skin lesions.

3. What type of lymphoma is mycosis fungoides?

Mycosis fungoides is a low-grade T-cell lymphoma. Histologically, it has a polymorphous cellular infiltrate with polymorphonuclear leukocytes, eosinophils, lymphocytes, and atypical mononuclear cells. The atypical mononuclear cells are moderately large and have a folded (cerebriform) nucleus. These cells are typically seen within the epidermis either singly or in small clusters (Pautrier's microabscesses). The mycosis cells are primarily CD4-positive helper T cells.

4. How common is mycosis fungoides?

The incidence of cutaneous T-cell lymphoma (CTCL) in the United States is approximately 1,500 new cases per year. The prevalence of CTCL in the United States ranges from 16,000 to 20,000 cases.

Cutaneous Lymphoma Foundation. CTCL-MF fast facts. Available at: http://www.clfoundation.org/publications/publications.htm. Accessed December 6, 2006.

5. How does mycosis fungoides begin?

Typically, mycosis fungoides begins with persistent scaly patches (Fig. 46-1A) that respond poorly to topical therapy with emollients and topical steroids. In the early stages, skin biopsy is frequently not diagnostic. The average time from onset of skin lesions to diagnosis is 7 years. In this early phase of the disease, a diagnosis of parapsoriasis en plaque is often made. In time, the patches thicken and become plaques. Eventually, skin tumors develop (Fig. 46-1B,C) and the lymph nodes can become involved. Visceral disease is a late occurrence in this low-grade lymphoma. Median survival for persons with patch- and plaque-stage disease is 12 years; for tumor-stage disease, it is 5 years; and for nodal or visceral disease, it is 3 years.

Epstein E, Levin D, Croft J, et al: Mycosis fungoides: survival, prognostic features, response to therapy, and autopsy findings, *Medicine* 51:61–72, 1972.

6. What is parapsoriasis?

The skin diseases included under this diagnosis are poorly understood and encompass a morass of confusing terms. The "splitters" have described over a dozen varieties of parapsoriasis, while the "lumpers" limit this designation to only a few types. This discussion supports the "lumpers" viewpoint.

Small-plaque parapsoriasis is characterized by chronic, well-marginated, mildly scaly, slightly erythematous, and round to oval skin lesions measuring <4 to 5 cm in diameter. The long axes of the lesions are arranged in a parallel configuration, and the lesions occur on the trunk and proximal extremities in a pityriasis rosea–like pattern. The lesions have been likened to fingerprints and reported under the descriptive term of *digitate dermatoses*. This form of parapsoriasis does not progress to lymphoma.

Large-plaque parapsoriasis presents as palm-sized or larger lesions located most frequently on the thighs, buttocks, hips, lower abdomen, and shoulder girdle areas (Fig. 46-2). The lesions may be pink, red-brown, or salmon-colored. They often have fine scale and show epidermal atrophy with cigarette-paper wrinkling. Some patients may have lesions with a netlike or reticular pattern with telangiectasia and fine scale. This clinical type of lesion is referred to as *retiform parapsoriasis* or *poikiloderma atrophicans vasculare*. Between 15% and 20% of patients with large-plaque parapsoriasis eventually develop mycosis fungoides.

Sehgal VN, Srivastava G, Aggarwal AK: Parapsoriasis: a complex issue, *Skinmed* 6:280–286, 2007.

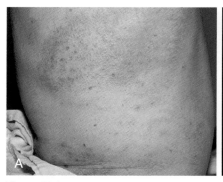
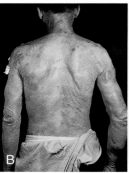
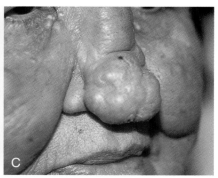

Figure 46-1. Mycosis fungoides. **A,** A 12-year-old boy with extensive patch-stage mycosis fungoides. **B,** A patient with extensive patch-, plaque-, and tumor-stage mycosis fungoides. **C,** Tumor-stage mycosis fungoides. This patient had skin lesions for 18 years before tumors developed and a diagnosis was made.

7. What type of skin lesions are seen in patients with mycosis fungoides?

Although the classic skin lesions are scaly patches, plaques, and tumors, a wide variety of skin lesions have been reported, such as follicular papules and pustules with or without alopecia (alopecia mucinosa). Bullous, erythrodermic, hypopigmented, vasculitic, and hyperkeratotic lesions also have been described.

A rare variant of mycosis fungoides is granulomatous slack skin disease (Fig. 46-3). This disorder is characterized by the slow development of lax erythematous skin that eventually develops large pendulous folds of redundant integument. Histologic examination shows a dense atypical granulomatous infiltrate with destruction and phagocytosis of elastic tissue.

8. Describe the three subtypes of mycosis fungoides.

- **Sézary syndrome** (Fig. 46-4) presents with the classic triad of erythroderma, lymphadenopathy, and atypical circulating mononuclear cells (Sézary cells). These cells are moderately large mononuclear cells with hyperconvoluted nuclei. They resemble activated T cells, and when >15% of circulating lymphocytes are atypical, it is considered significant, with 10% to 15% being considered borderline. However, the finding of circulating Sézary cells must be evaluated in context with the clinical picture and skin biopsy. Severe pruritus, ectropion, nail dystrophy, peripheral edema, alopecia, and keratoderma of the palms and soles are common associated features. The disease tends to wax and wane and generally progresses faster and is more resistant to treatment than typical mycosis fungoides.
- **Pagetoid reticulosis (Woringer-Kolopp disease)** is characterized by single or grouped hyperkeratotic skin lesion(s). Skin biopsy shows striking epidermotropism, with numerous atypical mononuclear cells, both singly and in clusters, scattered through all levels of the epidermis. The disease tends to be slowly progressive and responds well to local radiation.
- The **tumor d'emblee** form was initially thought to be a type of mycosis fungoides that began with skin tumors without the usual progression through a patch-and-plaque stage. Recent reports suggest that some of these cases are B-cell primary cutaneous lymphomas and some represent Ki-1–positive primary cutaneous T-cell lymphomas.

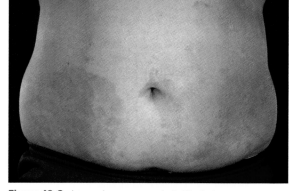

Figure 46-2. Large-plaque parapsoriasis. The lesion was unresponsive to topical treatment. (Courtesy of the Fitzsimons Army Medical teaching files.)

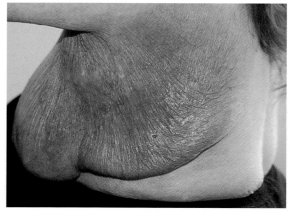

Figure 46-3. A young woman with granulomatous slack skin, a rare variant of mycosis fungoides.

9. What is the TNM classification of mycosis fungoides?

See Table 46-1.

Hoppe R, Wood G, Able E: Mycosis fungoides and the Sézary syndrome: pathology, staging, and treatment, *Curr Probl Cancer* 14:295–371, 1990.
Lamberg SI: Clinical staging for cutaneous T-cell lymphoma, *Ann Intern Med* 100:187–192, 1984.

10. How is mycosis fungoides treated?

There are many treatments for mycosis fungoides. Treatments can be classified as skin-directed therapy or systemic therapy.

SKIN-DIRECTED

- Topical corticosteroids
- Topical chemotherapy
  - Nitrogzen mustard (Mustargen)
  - Carmustine (BCNU)
- Topical retinoids: Bexarotene gel (Targretin gel)
- Phototherapy
  - Narrow-band ultraviolet B (NBUVB)
  - Psoralen with ultraviolet A (PUVA)
- Radiation therapy
  - Total-skin electron beam therapy (TSEBT)
  - Site-directed radiation

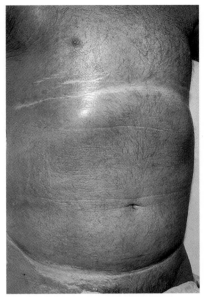

Figure 46-4. A patient with Sézary syndrome.

SYSTEMIC

- Vorinostat (ZOLINZA)
- Bexarotene capsules (Targretin)
- Denileukin diftitox (Ontak)
- Alemtuzumab (Campath)
- Interferon-α
- Extracorporeal photochemotherapy
- Chemotherapy? (single agent)
  - Chlorambucil (Leukeran)
  - Cladribine (Leustatin)
  - Fludarabine (Fludara)
  - Methotrexate (Trexall, Rheumatrex)
  - Gemcitabine (Gemzar)
  - Pegylated doxorubicin (Doxil)
  - Pentostatin (Nipent)
- Combination chemotherapies
  - CHOP
  - ESHAP
  - EPOCH

National Cancer Institute. Mycosis fungoides and the Sézary syndrome treatment. Available at: http://www.cancer.gov/cancertopics/pdq/treatment/mycosisfungoides/healthprofessional/allpages. Accessed December 6, 2006.

Table 46-1. TNM Classification of Mycosis Fungoides			
STAGE	**TNM CLASSIFICATION**		
IA	T1	N0	M0
IB	T2	N0	M0
IIA	T1-T2	N1	M0
IIB	T3	N0-N1	M0
III	T4	N0-N1	M0
IVA	T1-T4	N2-N3	M0
IVB	T1-T4	N0-N3	M1

11. Describe topical nitrogen mustard (HN₂) therapy.

This treatment is one of the most common for mycosis fungoides in the United States, and it has been used extensively in this disease since the early 1960s. It is easy to learn, can be applied by the patient at home, and has few side effects. The treatment consists of the topical application of 10 mg of nitrogen mustard in 60 mL of water every day to the entire skin surface except the eyelids and genitalia. Complete response rates for stage 1 disease are >50%. The treatment is well tolerated with few side effects and no severe systemic side effects. Over 50% of patients will develop allergic contact dermatitis to the topical medication, and there is a long-term risk for basal and squamous cell carcinoma. Some physicians prefer to use the medication in an ointment base.

Vonderheid E, Tan E, Kantor A, et al: Long-term efficacy, curative potential, and carcinogenicity of topical mechlorethamine chemotherapy in cutaneous T-cell lymphoma, *J Am Acad Dermatol* 20:416–428, 1989.

12. If a patient develops allergic contact dermatitis to topical nitrogen mustard, does the treatment have to be permanently discontinued?

No. The medication should be temporarily discontinued, and the dermatitis treated with either topical or systemic steroids. When the dermatitis has cleared, the patient can then be restarted on dilute HN₂. Usually, the patient will tolerate 10 mg of HN₂ in 1 gallon of water. The concentration of the HN₂ can be slowly increased over several months without a flare of the dermatitis. On a rare occasion, a patient may develop immediate contact urticaria to topical HN₂, requiring discontinuation of treatment.

13. Is photochemotherapy an effective treatment of mycosis fungoides?

Yes. The response rates to psoralen plus ultraviolet A (PUVA) are at least equal to those with topical nitrogen mustard. Ultraviolet light irradiation required special instruments for whole skin irradiation of UVA light. Adding psoralens potentiates the effects of UVA light (PUVA). A study from Sweden, where PUVA is the treatment of choice, showed a 50% decrease in mortality from mycosis fungoides after the introduction of PUVA. UVB therapy may work in some patients with early patches and plaques. Newer NBUVB (311- to 313-nm range) phototherapy has certain advantages over PUVA: no oral premedication required, eliminating systemic side effects, and long-term skin carcinogenic effects may be decreased. Small studies of PUVA and oral and topical bexarotene (Targretin) indicate a combination treatment of light and retinoids may have synergistic benefit.

Swanbeck G, Roupe G, Sandstrom MH: Indications of a considerable decrease in the death rate in mycosis fungoides by PUVA treatment, *Acta Derm Venereol* (Stockh) 74:465–466, 1994.

14. What are the major side effects of bexarotene in the treatment of patients with cutaneous T-cell lymphoma?

Bexarotene (Targretin) is a synthetic retinoid that selectively activates retinoid X receptors. The drug is given orally at a recommended dose of 300 mg/m². Partial response rate (50% improvement) was 67% and complete response occurred in 7% of patients. Like other retinoid drugs, Targretin is teratogenic and should not be given to pregnant women. In a study of 58 patients with patch and plaque stage disease, side effects included hyperlipidemia in 83%, neutropenia in 47%, central hypothyroidism in 74%, and hypercholesteremia in 47% of patients.

Duvic M, Martin AG, Kim Y, et al: Oral Targretin (bexarotene) capsules are safe and effective in refractory or persistent early-stage cutaneous T-cell lymphoma: results of the phase 2–3 clinical trial, Presented at the American Society of Hematology Annual Meeting, New Orleans, 1999.

15. How does one manage the side effects of bexarotene?

Hypothyroidism caused by bexarotene (Targretin) results in a low thyroid-stimulating hormone level because the drug stops RNA transcription. Central hypothyroidism is managed with levothyroxine replacement. It is recommended that one start and stop levothyroxine and bexarotene together. Measure free T4 at baseline, at 2 weeks, then monthly. Normalizing free T4 helps clear plasma lipids.

Hyperlipidemia caused by bexarotene (Targretin) can be managed with lipid-lowering agents. The preferred lipid-lowering agents include atorvastatin (Lipitor), an HMG CoA reductase inhibitor (statin), and fenofibrate (Tricor), which acts by increasing lipolysis through activation of lipoprotein lipase. Other statins include simvastatin (Zocor), pravastatin (Pravachol), fluvastatin (Lescol), lovastatin (Mevacor), and rosuvastatin (Crestor). It is recommended that one start the preferred statin 1 week before starting bexarotene.

16. Are interferons effective in treating mycosis fungoides?

Yes. Of the interferon group of drugs, recombinant interferon-α has been the most promising. Both complete remissions and partial remissions have been reported. Low-dose treatment protocols are as effective as high-dose protocols and have fewer side effects. The recommended dose is 3 million units, given subcutaneously, three times weekly.

17. Is chemotherapy an effective treatment of mycosis fungoides?

Yes. Both partial and complete remissions can be achieved with both single-drug and multidrug chemotherapy protocols. However, the remissions are short-lived, and no one drug or combination of drugs appears to be superior. In a large blinded study, 103 patients randomized to 3000 cGy of electron-beam therapy followed by chemotherapy with cyclophosphamide, daunorubicin, etoposide, and vincristine were compared to a group of patients treated with topical

HN$_2$ progressing to PUVA if necessary. After a median follow-up of 75 months, there was no difference in response rates or survival in the two groups.

Kaye F, Bunn P, Steinberg S, et al: A randomized trial comparing combination electron-beam radiation and chemotherapy with topical therapy in the initial treatment of mycosis fungoides, *N Engl J Med* 321:1784–1790, 1989.

18. What is extracorporeal photophoresis?

Extracorporeal photopheresis (ECP) is a treatment in which peripheral blood is exposed in an extracorporeal circuit to UVA following administration of 8-methoxypsoralen. Response rates of 50% to 80% have been observed in CTCL. ECP is also used as a treatment for chronic graft-versus-host disease (GVHD) in allogeneic stem cell transplant recipients. The mechanism of action is thought to be activation of cellular apoptosis and possible immunomodulatory effects. The treatment is expensive, requires the availability of specialized equipment, and is administered on an outpatient basis in a hospital setting. It is the only Food and Drug Administration (FDA)–approved treatment for mycosis fungoides.

Bisaccia E, Gonzalez J, Palangio M, et al: Extracorporeal photochemotherapy alone or with adjuvant therapy in the treatment of cutaneous T-cell lymphoma: a 9-year retrospective study at a single institution, *J Am Acad Dermatol* 43:263–271, 2000.

Key Points: Mycosis Fungoides

1. Mycosis fungoides is a low-grade T-cell lymphoma with a median survival of 12 years for patients with patch- or plaque-stage disease.
2. Sézary syndrome is the term applied to the leukemic variant of cutaneous T-cell lymphoma.
3. Management of mycosis fungoides is best accomplished by the involvement of several specialists, such as those in dermatology, dermatopathology/pathology, hematology/oncology, and radiation oncology.

---

19. Are there any other FDA-approved treatments for cutaneous T-cell lymphoma?

Yes. Denileukin diftitox (Ontak) is interleukin-2 (IL-2) conjugated to diphtheria toxin. The drug is given intravenously only to patients whose malignant cells express CD25, the IL-2 receptor. The drug can be associated with significant toxicity, including capillary leak syndrome, acute hypersensitivity–type reactions, hypoalbuminemia, and hypotension. Flulike symptoms for several weeks following infusion are frequently noted. Partial responses are reported in 30% and complete responses in 10% of patients.

Histone deacetylase inhibitors (HDACi) inhibit the deacetylation of histone proteins associated with DNA and nonhistone proteins. The exact mechanism involving the treatment of CTCL is unknown, but DNA microarray studies show that HDACi affects the expression of numerous genes and proteins involved in cell proliferation, migration, and apoptosis. Oral Vorinostat (suberoylanilide hydroxamic acid) targets HDAC class 1 and class 2 HDAC enzymes and is FDA-approved for the treatment of refractory CTCL, with response rates of 24% to 30%. Ongoing studies are looking at HDACi used in combination with other therapies (phototherapy, ECP, and oral bexarotene).

Gardner JM, Evans KG, Musiek A, et al: Update on treatment of cutaneous T-cell lymphoma, *Curr Opin Oncol* 21(2):131–137, 2009.

OTHER LYMPHOMAS AND LEUKEMIAS

20. Outline the Ann Arbor clinical staging system for Hodgkin's disease.

- **Stage I:** Single lymph node or extralymphatic site
- **Stage II:** Two or more lymph node regions on the same side of the diaphragm or nodal involvement with a contiguous extralymphatic site
- **Stage III:** Nodal involvement on both sides of the diaphragm, with or without a contiguous extralymphatic site
- **Stage IV:** Multiple extralymphatic tissue sites, with or without nodal involvement
  - **A:** Absence of B symptoms
  - **B:** Presence of B symptoms (fevers, drenching night sweats, or >10% weight loss over past 6 months)

21. What is a Reed-Sternberg cell?

It is a large cell with two mirror-image nuclei with large distinct nucleoli, often with surrounding halos (owl's eye cells). It is considered to be the malignant cell of Hodgkin's disease, and its presence confirms the histologic diagnosis. The origin of the cell is debated, with marker studies having shown both T- and B-cell immunoenzymatic staining.

22. What are the histologic classes of Hodgkin's disease?

- **Nodular sclerosis** is the most common type, accounting for 35% of all patients with Hodgkin's disease. It is more common in women and has a relatively good prognosis. It is characterized by a particular type of Reed-Sternberg cell, called the lacunar cell, which is a large cell with a hyperlobulated nucleus and multiple nucleoli surrounded by a clear space (lacunae).
- **Mixed cellularity** represents a histologic type that is intermediate between lymphocyte-predominance and lymphocyte-depletion types. It is the second most common type. Reed-Sternberg cells are prominent.
- **Lymphocyte-predominance** type has a diffuse or slightly nodular histologic pattern (popcorn pattern). Reed-Sternberg cells are rare. It is the most common pattern found in young men, and the prognosis is excellent. The anti–CD20

monoclonal antibody, rituximab, which is usually used in non–Hodgkin's lymphoma, has been shown to produce over a 50% complete response rate for this subtype of Hodgkin's disease.
- **Lymphocyte-depletion** pattern is characterized by a paucity of lymphocytes and numerous Reed-Sternberg cells or their variants. There is a diffuse fibrotic and a reticular variant of the lymphocyte-depleted subtype. This type tends to occur in older patients, with disseminated involvement and a poor prognosis.

23. Does Hodgkin's disease occur in the skin?

Yes, but very rarely. One series of 1800 cases reported a <5% incidence of specific skin lesions in patients with Hodgkin's disease. Many of the early reports of Hodgkin's disease presenting with skin lesions with no nodal involvement probably represent Ki-1–positive, T-cell lymphomas. Nonspecific skin lesions are common and include pruritus, pigmentation, prurigo, ichthyosis, alopecia, and herpes zoster.

Fernandez-Flores A: The early reports on cutaneous involvement of Hodgkin lymphoma, *Am J Dermatopathol* 31:853–854, 2009.

24. How are cells immunophenotyped? What does the CD nomenclature mean?

"CD" stands for *cluster designation* and is a nomenclature for identification of specific cell surface antigens defined by monoclonal antibodies. The procedure can be applied to both formalin-fixed and frozen tissue. It is very helpful in identifying subpopulations of T- and B-cell lymphocytes (Table 46-2).

25. What is lymphomatoid papulosis?

This chronic recurrent skin eruption is characterized by papules and/or nodules that frequently crust or ulcerate and self-heal, often with atrophic scars (Fig. 46-5). There are three histopathologic types. Type A has large Reed-Sternberg–like cells, which are often CD30 (Ki-1) positive. Type B has moderately large atypical cells with cerebriform nuclei similar to the cell type found in mycosis fungoides. These cells are usually CD30 negative. Type C is composed of sheets of cells that resemble the cells of anaplastic T-cell lymphoma. About 15% to 20% of patients with lymphomatoid papulosis will develop a lymphoma.

El Shabrawi-Caelen L, Kerl H, Cerroni L: Lymphomatoid papulosis: reappraisal of clinicopathologic presentation and classification into subtypes A, B, and C, *Arch Dermatol* 140:441–447, 2004.

26. Are CD30-positive cells specific for lymphomatoid papulosis?

No. The monoclonal antibody CD30 (Ki-1) was first described in 1982 with positive staining of Reed-Sternberg cells of Hodgkin's disease. Positive staining was also found in the paracortical cells of reactive lymph nodes. Ki-1 positivity can

Table 46-2. Cells Marked by CD Antigens	
CD2	T cells (E rosette receptor)
CD3	T-cell receptor
CD4	Helper T cells
CD5	Mature thymocytes, some B-cell subsets
CD7	T cells, natural killer (NK) cells
CD8	T cells, NK cells
CD10	Pre-B cells, lymphoblastic leukemia cells
CD14	Monocytes
CD15	Reed-Sternberg cells, myeloid cells
CD19	Pan-B cells
CD20	Pan-B cells, dendritic cells
CD21	Receptor for complement 2 and Epstein-Barr virus
CD23	Activated B cells, monocytes, eosinophils, and platelets
CD25	Activated T and B cells, monocytes (interleukin-2 receptor)
CD30	Ki-1–related cells, Reed-Sternberg cells, T-cell NHL
CD34	Lymphoid and myeloid precursor cells
CD43	T cells, myeloid cells
CD45	Leukocytes
CD45R	T cells, myeloid cells
CD56	NK cells
CD74	HLA-invariant chain
CD75	Follicular center cells

CD, Cluster of differentiation; *HLA*, histocompatibility locus antigen; *NHL*, non-Hodgkin's lymphoma.

be seen in primary T-cell lymphomas, anaplastic large-cell lymphomas, regressing atypical histiocytosis, and occasionally pityriasis lichenoides et varioliformis acuta (Mucha-Habermann disease). Ki-1–positive primary cutaneous lymphomas have a better prognosis than Ki-1–negative primary cutaneous lymphomas.

Borchmann P: CD30+ diseases: anaplastic large-cell lymphoma and lymphomatoid papulosis, *Cancer Treat Res* 142:345–365, 2008.

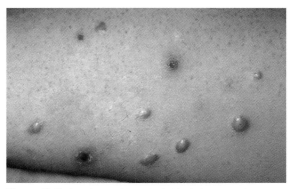

Figure 46-5. Lymphomatoid papulosis. The lesions occur in crops and self-heal. (Courtesy of the Fitzsimons Army Medical teaching files.)

27. What is HTLV-1 virus? What is its significance?

HTLV-1 is a type C retrovirus associated with T-cell lymphoma and leukemia. It was initially isolated from a patient diagnosed with mycosis fungoides. The virus is endemic in Japan, the Caribbean, and northeastern South America; a few cases have been reported in the United States. It can be transmitted by blood transfusions, intravenous drug abuse, breast feeding, and, less commonly, sexual contact. A small subset of patients who are HTLV-1–antibody positive (<5%) will develop lymphoma or lymphocytic leukemia. The disease is characterized by immunosuppression, lymphadenopathy, cutaneous lesions, and hypercalcemia.

28. Can multiple myeloma present with skin lesions only?

Yes. However, it is extremely rare for myeloma to begin with only skin lesions. Extraosseous lesions in association with osseous myeloma are common, and the skin is one of the extraosseous sites. There are many skin diseases associated with monoclonal gammopathy, including pyoderma gangrenosum, scleromyxedema, scleroderma adultorum, leukocytoclastic vasculitis, collagen-vascular disease, xanthomas, Waldenström's macroglobulinemia, subcorneal pustular dermatosis, pustular psoriasis, and even urticaria. The diagnosis of multiple myeloma is confirmed when there are lytic bone lesions, anemia, hypercalcemia, elevated serum and/or urine monoclonal protein spike, and bone marrow plasma cells exceeding 10%. Subcutaneous myeloma is much more common during late-stage, relapsed disease.

Requena L, Lutzner H, Palmedo G, et al: Cutaneous involvement in multiple myeloma: a clinicopathologic, immunohistochemical, and cytogenetic study of 8 cases, *Arch Dermatol* 139:475–486, 2003.

29. What is pseudolymphoma of the skin?

This term represents several clinical entities that probably have multiple etiologies. Included are lymphocytoma, Spiegler-Fendt sarcoid, lymphadenosis benigna cutis, and Jessner's benign lymphocytic infiltrate. In most cases, the etiology is unknown, although chronic arthropod bite reactions are an etiologic stimulus in some cases. The lesions present as indolent single or grouped, red or purple nodules or plaques on the head, neck, and upper trunk, and other anatomic sites can be involved (Fig. 46-6). The infiltrate may show either B- or T-cell predominance. Some cases can be difficult to differentiate from lymphoma, and the patient must be followed before a definite diagnosis can be made.

Ploysangam T, Breneman DL, Mutasim DF: Cutaneous pseudolymphomas, *J Am Acad Dermatol* 38:877–895, 1998.

30. Can B-cell lymphomas present with skin lesions?

Yes. Most benign and malignant cutaneous lymphocytic infiltrates are predominantly T cell in origin. Cutaneous involvement occurs in >5% of patients with B-cell nodal lymphoma. Also, an entity termed SALT (skin-associated lymphoid tissue) lymphoma, or primary cutaneous B-cell lymphoma (PCBCL) may present as solitary or multiple, red to violaceous nodules or plaques (Fig. 46-7). The treatment of choice is local radiation therapy.

Some primary cutaneous B-cell lymphomas (approximately 8%) are associated with Lyme disease (*Borrelia* spp.), and some reports suggest an improvement with Lyme disease therapy, analogous to results with *Helicobacter pylori* treatment and

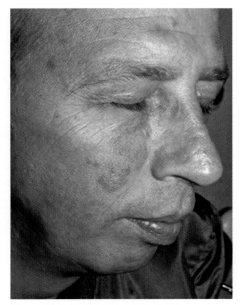

Figure 46-6. Pseudolymphoma. Patient with plaques on nodules of the right cheek and forehead. (Courtesy of the Fitzsimons Army Medical teaching files.)

regression of mucosa-associated lymphoid tissue (MALT) lymphoma. Patients with PCBCL should be screened for positive Lyme serologies.

Jelic S, Filipovic-Ljeskovic I: Positive serology for Lyme disease borrelias in primary cutaneous B-cell lymphoma: a study in 22 patients; is it a fortuitous finding? *Hematol Oncol* 17:107–116, 1999.

Santucci M, Pimpinelli N, Arganini L: Primary cutaneous B-cell lymphoma: a unique type of low-grade lymphoma, *Cancer* 67:2311–2326, 1991.

31. What is the most common type of leukemia in adults?

Chronic lymphocytic leukemia. It is the most common cause of specific leukemic skin lesions, which are usually multiple and may present with papules, nodules, plaques, erythema, and, rarely, bullae (Fig. 46-8A). This neoplastic proliferation of lymphocytes is usually B cell in origin.

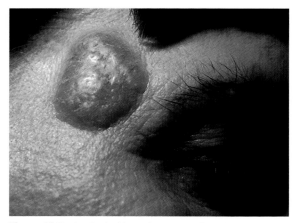

Figure 46-7. A patient with purely cutaneous B-cell lymphoma presenting with a single purple nodule on the temple.

32. Can leukemia present with specific skin lesions?

Yes. Although uncommon, skin infiltration with neoplastic leukemia cells can be a presenting finding and precede the leukemic phase of the disease by several months. This is most common with acute myeloid leukemia (AML). Often, this phenomenon is preceded by a myelodysplastic or myeloproliferative syndrome. The skin lesions may present as red or purple papules, nodules, or plaques.

Aractingi S, Bachmeyer C, Miclea J, et al: Unusual specific cutaneous lesions in myelodysplastic syndromes, *J Am Acad Dermatol* 33:187–191, 1995.

33. What are some nonspecific skin lesions seen in patients with leukemia?

Nonspecific skin lesions are quite common in patients with all types of leukemia and preleukemia. The most common skin findings are petechiae, purpura, pruritus, papular eruptions, vasculitis, urticaria, herpes zoster, and erythroderma. Approximately 5% to 10% of patients with pyoderma gangrenosum have or will develop leukemia, usually of the myelocytic type. Gingival hyperplasia is a common association with acute myelomonocytic leukemia (FAB subtypes M4 and M5) (Fig. 46-8B).

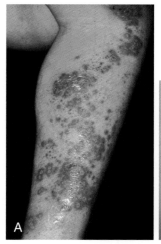
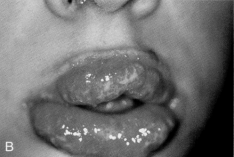

Figure 46-8. Cutaneous manifestations of leukemia. **A,** A patient with lymphocytic leukemia and multiple nodules on the lower extremity. **B,** A young child with myelomonocytic leukemia and severe gingivostomatitis.

UNCOMMON MALIGNANT TUMORS OF THE SKIN

Renata Prado, MD, and J. Ramsey Mellette, MD

EPITHELIOID SARCOMA

1. What is an epithelioid sarcoma?

Epithelioid sarcoma is an exceedingly rare high-grade malignancy of unknown lineage with no normal cellular counterpart. The tumor has an indolent course but a high potential to metastasize. It is remarkable for being a difficult diagnosis, both clinically and histologically, resulting in a high frequency of initial misdiagnosis. Diagnosis is reached on average 8 years after initial clinical presentation.

2. Why is it called "epithelioid" sarcoma?

"Epithelioid" describes the histologic appearance of the large, plump, epithelium-like tumor cells that are focally present in the tumor.

3. How does epithelioid sarcoma present?

It presents as a painless, firm, slow-growing, intradermal or subcutaneous nodule, often ulcerated, usually on the volar surface of the fingers or palms. It occurs most frequently on the distal upper extremity, but it may also occur on the lower extremities and occasionally in the trunk or head and neck region. Epithelioid sarcoma has a tendency to spread locally through lymphatic channels or along fascial planes, and may give rise to multiple local nodules. The clinical differential diagnosis includes mycobacterial or deep fungal infection, squamous cell carcinoma, and other soft tissue sarcomas. The male-to-female ratio is approximately 2:1, and it affects mainly young adults.

Burgos AM, Chávez JG, Sánchez JL, Sánchez NP: Epithelioid sarcoma: a diagnostic and surgical challenge, *Dermatol Surg* 35:687–691, 2009.

4. How is the diagnosis of epithelioid sarcoma made?

The diagnosis of epithelioid sarcoma is made by typical histologic features. The tumor is composed of malignant, eosinophilic, epithelioid and spindle cells arranged in nodules that often demonstrate central necrosis. Immunohistochemistry, special stains, and tissue culture are used to assist the diagnosis. The tumor cells demonstrate staining with both mesenchymal markers (vimentin), as well as epithelial markers (keratins and epithelial membrane antigen).

5. How are epithelioid sarcomas treated?

Early radical local excisional surgery is required. The local recurrence rate has been reported to range from 35% to 77%. Multifocal recurrences are common because the tumor spreads insidiously along tendons, fascial planes, nerves, and blood vessels. Adjuvant radiotherapy is often used to lower the risk of local recurrence; however, amputation is sometimes required. Chemotherapy with ifosfamide and doxorubicin is recommended for metastatic disease.

Jawad MU, Extein J, Min ES, Scully SP: Prognostic factors for survival in patients with epithelioid sarcoma: 441 cases from the SEER database, *Clin Orthop Relat Res*, 467:2939–2948, 2009.

6. Can epithelioid sarcoma metastasize?

Yes. The recurrent spreading tumor can develop nodules and plaques along the forearm. Forty-five percent of patients develop metastases, mostly to the lymph nodes and lungs.

7. What are the prognostic factors of epithelioid sarcoma?

The recognized adverse prognostic factors include male sex, older age, large size, multifocality, proximal or axial location, depth of invasion, mitotic activity, necrosis, vascular invasion, tumor hemorrhage, nodal involvement, rhabdoid cytomorphology, and inadequate excision.

Chbani L, Guillou L, Terrier P, et al: Epithelioid sarcoma: a clinicopathologic and immunohistochemical analysis of 106 cases from the French sarcoma group, *Am J Clin Pathol* 131:222–227, 2009.

ANGIOSARCOMA

8. What is angiosarcoma?

Angiosarcoma of the skin is a highly malignant tumor of vascular endothelial cells.

9. Is there more than one type of angiosarcoma?

Yes. The three types are as follows:
- Angiosarcoma of the face and scalp in the elderly
- Angiosarcoma associated with chronic lymphedema; most commonly occurs in the upper extremity following radical mastectomy (Stewart-Treves syndrome)
- Postirradiation angiosarcoma

10. How does angiosarcoma of the scalp and face in the elderly present?

It presents as an erythematous or hemorrhagic bruiselike patch on the central face or scalp, which spreads centrifugally and evolves into nodules that bleed easily and ulcerate (Fig. 47-1). There is often extensive infiltration, and the extent of the tumor is often underestimated clinically.

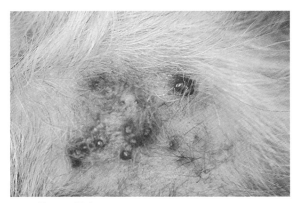

Figure 47-1. Angiosarcoma of the scalp in the elderly.

11. What are the clinical course and prognosis for angiosarcoma?

In the largest reported series of 72 patients, only 12% survived for 5 years. Metastases to the cervical nodes and hematogenous metastases to the lungs, liver, and spleen occur. Because of their rarity, there are no clear definitive or significant prognostic factors identified for angiosarcoma, but histologic grade, tumor diameter, depth of invasion, positive margins, metastases, and tumor recurrence are potential predictors of outcome.

Köhler HF, Neves RI, Brechtbühl ER, et al: Cutaneous angiosarcoma of the head and neck: report of 23 cases from a single institution, *Otolaryngol Head Neck Surg* 139:519–524, 2008.

12. Is there an effective treatment for angiosarcoma?

Early diagnosis and complete surgical excision offer the best chance of survival. However, because the lesions tend to be multicentric, extensive, and rapidly growing over the face and scalp, surgical excision is rarely successful. A combined-modality approach is often used, including excision of disease with negative margins if possible, with adjuvant radiotherapy. Chemotherapy is usually recommended in cases of systemic disease.

13. What is the clinical presentation of angiosarcoma arising in chronic lymphedema?

This rare tumor, also called Stewart-Treves syndrome, arises as cutaneous and subcutaneous firm, coalescing, violaceous nodules on a background of nonpitting edema, often in the inner aspect of the upper arm. It occurs on average 10 years following mastectomy and lymphadenectomy (range 1 to 30 years). It is less commonly associated with filarial, congenital, traumatic, or idiopathic lymphedema.

Hallel-Halevy D, Yerushalmi J, Grunwald MH, et al: Stewart-Treves syndrome in a patient with elephantiasis, *J Am Acad Dermatol* 41:349–350, 1999.

14. What are the clinical course and prognosis of angiosarcoma?

The tumor grows rapidly and often ulcerates. Metastases occur early, especially to the lungs, pleura, and chest wall. Death usually occurs within 1 to 2 years as a result of the disease, with widespread pulmonary, cardiac, and/or brain metastases.

15. What are the histologic features of angiosarcomas?

Angiosarcomas are composed of an anastomosing network of well-formed, irregular vascular channels, often lined by flattened endothelial cells. They exhibit a highly infiltrative pattern, dissecting and splitting collagen bundles. Poorly differentiated angiosarcomas may closely resemble carcinomas or other soft tissue sarcomas, with only subtle vascular lumen formation.

MERKEL CELL CARCINOMA

16. What is Merkel cell carcinoma (MCC)?

Merkel cell carcinoma (MCC), also known as primary neuroendocrine carcinoma of the skin, is an aggressive malignant neoplasm. The tumor was initially thought to arise from Merkel cells, receptors of mechanical stimuli with a high density on hairless skin. However, the tumor is now thought to arise from a less–well-differentiated progenitor cell of probably epithelial origin.

17. Describe the clinical presentation of MCC.

Over 50% of patients present with a solitary, rapidly growing, erythematous to violaceous nodule approximately 0.5 to 5.0 cm in diameter on the head, face, or neck. Other areas may be involved, including the extremities and trunk (Fig. 47-2). Most cases are seen in caucasians.

18. What is the pathogenesis of MCC?

MCC is extremely rare before age 50 years, and the incidence increases steeply after 65 years of age, suggesting an accumulation of oncogenic events. Immunosuppression is likely involved in the pathogenesis, as MCC incidence is increased approximately 11-fold for persons with AIDS and 5-fold for persons who have undergone organ transplantation. The majority of tumors present on sun-exposed areas, and the risk of MCC may be particularly high with prior psoralen and ultraviolet A treatment (PUVA) suggesting that UV radiation contributes to the etiology of this malignancy. More recently, the viral genome of polyomavirus (Merkel cell polyomavirus) was detected in MCC, and there is accumulating evidence to suggest a direct mechanistic role for the virus in the pathogenesis of MCC.

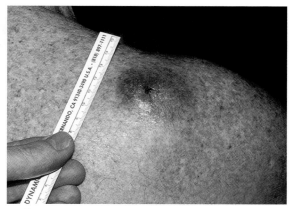

Figure 47-2. Merkel cell carcinoma presenting on the trunk.

Feng H, Shuda M, Chang Y, Moore PS: Clonal integration of a polyomavirus in human Merkel cell carcinoma, *Science* 319:1096–1100, 2008.

19. Can any other tumors be microscopically confused with MCC?

Yes. MCC is composed of undifferentiated basaloid, small, blue cells with hyperchromatic nuclei, scant cytoplasm, and frequent mitotic figures, and it may be confused with metastatic small cell carcinoma (oat-cell carcinoma) of the lung, malignant lymphoma, sweat gland carcinoma, metastatic carcinoid tumors, and Ewing's sarcoma. Electron microscopy may be helpful in order to highlight the dense core neurosecretory granules seen in MCC.

20. What special stains are available to diagnose MCC?

MCC often has a characteristic paranuclear "dot" that stains with cytokeratin, especially cytokeratin 20. MCC also stains positively for various neuroendocrine markers, such as synaptophysin, chromogranin A, neuron-specific enolase, calcitonin, and vasoactive intestinal peptides. Epithelial membrane antigen is also often positive. MCC are usually not decorated with thyroid transcription factor–1 (TTF-1), which is an important finding because most small cell carcinomas of the lung are TTF-1 positive.

21. How do you treat MCC?

Wide local excision with surgical margins up to 3.0 cm has been recommended. In cosmetically sensitive areas, Mohs surgery may be helpful, although research is limited. Other considerations at the time of surgery include assessment of regional lymph nodes (lymph node dissection) and irradiation. Chemotherapy is used for nodal, metastatic, and recurrent MCC, and common agents used are cyclophosphamide, anthracyclines, and cisplatin. Local recurrences occur in 40% of patients.

Eng TY, Naguib M, Fuller CD, et al: Treatment of recurrent Merkel cell carcinoma: an analysis of 46 cases, *Am J Clin Oncol* 27:576–583, 2004.

22. Does MCC metastasize?

Yes. Up to 75% of patients develop regional lymph node metastases at some time during the course of their disease. Distant metastases occur to the lungs and other sites in 30% to 40%.

23. What is the overall prognosis?

The prognosis of MCC is related to the stage of disease, with a 5-year survival rate ranging from 81% in patients with localized small tumors, to 11% in patients with metastatic disease. More than half of patients experience recurrence, usually within 1 year of treatment. All patients need close follow-up after excision.

Allen PJ, Bowne WB, Jacques DP, et al: Merkel cell carcinoma: prognosis and treatment of patients from a single institution, *J Clin Oncol* 23:2300–2309, 2005.

MICROCYSTIC ADNEXAL CARCINOMA

24. What are the clinical features of microcystic adnexal carcinoma (MAC)?

MAC is a locally aggressive tumor that shows histologic evidence of follicular and sweat duct differentiation. It classically presents as a slow-growing, firm, ill-defined plaque or nodule on the head and neck, most often on the upper lip (Fig. 47-3). Numbness, paresthesia, burning, discomfort, or, rarely, pruritus of the affected area may be reported, and are likely related to the fact that the tumor frequently exhibits perineural invasion. Histologically, it must be differentiated from morpheaform basal cell carcinoma, desmoplastic trichoepithelioma, or syringoma.

Wetter R, Goldstein GD: Microcystic adnexal carcinoma: a diagnostic and therapeutic challenge, *Dermatol Ther* 21:452–458, 2008.

25. How is MAC treated?

Surgical excision by the Mohs technique is the treatment of choice. Frequent recurrences, often resulting from perineural invasion, tend to occur in cases treated by standard surgical excision.

26. What is the prognosis?

Excellent with adequate excision. Metastases have been reported but are rare.

DERMATOFIBROSARCOMA PROTUBERANS

27. What is dermatofibrosarcoma protuberans?

Dermatofibrosarcoma protuberans (DFSP) is a firm, locally aggressive tumor that exhibits massive proliferation of spindle cells in the dermis and subcutaneous fat. These cells form intersecting bundles with a characteristic storiform (cartwheel) arrangement. The pigmented variant is called Bednar tumor.

28. Is a special stain available to identify DFSP?

Yes. DFSP stains positively for the human hematopoietic progenitor cell antigen CD34, which helps to differentiate it from other fibrous tumors.

29. Describe the clinical features of DFSP.

DFSP presents as a slow-growing, elevated, and indurated (often multinodular) plaque that is flesh-colored to red-brown or blue (Fig. 47-4). It may occasionally present as an atrophic lesion and be mistaken for a scar. It most commonly occurs on the trunk and extremities on young to middle-aged adults, but it may be seen on the head and neck.

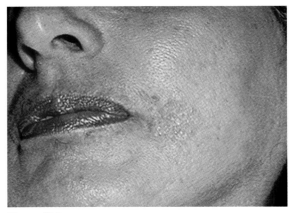

Figure 47-3. Middle-aged woman with a typical microcystic adnexal carcinoma.

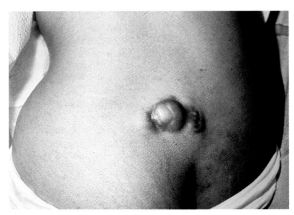

Figure 47-4. Multinodular dermatofibrosarcoma protuberans in a young woman.

30. Do DFSPs have a tendency to recur?

Yes. Local recurrence occurs following incomplete removal. Metastases rarely occur in recurrent lesions.

31. How is DFSP treated?

Adequate local excision is the treatment of choice. Mohs micrographic surgery affords the highest cure rates (>95%). Patients with locally aggressive tumors that are not resectable or with metastatic disease are most commonly treated with imatinib mesylate, which targets a specific translocation between chromosomes 17 and 22 that is found in most cases of DFSP.

Llombart B, Sanmartin O, López-Guerro JA, et al: Dermatofibrosarcoma protuberans: clinical, pathological, and genetic (COL1A1-PDGFB) study with therapeutic implications, *Histopathology* 54:860–872, 2009.

Wacker J, Khan-Durani B, Hartschuh W: Modified Mohs micrographic surgery in the therapy of dermatofibrosarcoma protuberans: analysis of 22 patients, *Ann Surg Oncol* 11:438–444, 2004.

ATYPICAL FIBROXANTHOMA

32. What is an atypical fibroxanthoma (AFX)?

AFX is a superficial mesenchymal dermal tumor that microscopically shows high-grade cytologic atypia. It most commonly presents in the elderly as a nondistinct solitary dome-shaped nodule in sun-damaged skin, usually of the head and neck (Fig. 47-5). Ulceration is variably present. Histologically, it demonstrates a cellular dermal tumor with an epidermal collarette. Skin adnexa are generally surrounded but not destroyed by the tumor, and the deep margin is generally pushing rather than infiltrative. The tumor is composed of spindle and epithelioid cells arranged in disordered fascicles, with striking pleomorphism and atypia of the cells and numerous mitosis.

33. What is the clinical course?

Despite high-grade cytologic atypia and malignant histologic appearance, most tumors demonstrate indolent behavior with local extension and a benign course. Rare cases demonstrate metastatic behavior.

Cooper JZ, Newman SR, Scott GA, Brown MD: Metastasizing atypical fibroxanthoma (cutaneous malignant histiocytoma): report of five cases, *Dermatol Surg* 31:221–225, 2005.

34. What are the treatment and the prognosis?

Complete surgical excision is usually curative. Mohs micrographic surgery has been used to successfully treat these lesions. The prognosis with either method is excellent.

MALIGNANT FIBROUS HISTIOCYTOMA

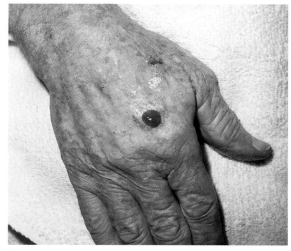

Figure 47-5. Atypical fibroxanthoma arising on a sun-damaged hand.

35. What is a malignant fibrous histiocytoma (MFH)?

MFH is a malignant soft tissue tumor arising in the deep soft tissue. It is thought by several authors not to represent a diagnostic entity, but a common, final pathway of many tumors, as its features are shared by a variety of poorly differentiated malignant neoplasms. The term MFH is now reserved for the small group of truly undifferentiated pleomorphic sarcomas. The histogenesis has been a cause of an ongoing debate, but it is now accepted that the histiocyte is most likely not the cell of origin of the tumor. More recent studies suggest that MFH is a sarcoma of a poorly defined mesenchymal cell, which may differentiate along histiocytic and fibrocytic lines. The term MFH is being substituted by pleomorphic sarcoma. Histologically, the tumor demonstrates a variable appearance with five subtypes: pleomorphic-storiform, myxoid (also called myxofibrosarcoma), giant cell, angiomatoid, and inflammatory. The histologic diagnosis is one of exclusion based on the histologic appearance and special stains, because these histologic patterns may be mimicked by other soft tissue tumors.

Al-Agha OM, Igbokwe AA: Malignant fibrous histiocytoma: between the past and the present, *Arch Pathol Lab Med* 132:1030–1035, 2008.

36. Do they arise in the skin?

Yes. Ten percent arise in the superficial subcutis, but most tumors arise from the deep soft tissue of the extremities or trunk, and some of them from the retroperitoneum.

37. What are the prognosis and treatment?

Small superficial tumors have a much better prognosis than do deep ones. Ten percent of the superficial tumors above the fascia metastasize. Adequate surgical excision is necessary.

EXTRAMAMMARY PAGET'S DISEASE

38. What are the clinical features of extramammary Paget's disease (EMPD)?

EMPD is a malignant epithelial tumor most often found in the genital region or perineum, which also uncommonly occurs on the axillae, eyelid, ear, anterior chest, and accessory nipples. Nearly all cases of EMPD occur in areas that contain apocrine glands, and, although the histogenesis is not proven, current evidence suggests that they arise from Toker cells. The function of Toker cells is not entirely understood, but based on their distribution, they are likely involved in apocrine gland and breast development. Clinically, EMPD presents as a pruritic, erythematous patch or plaque with oozing and crusting (Fig. 47-6A), which can be confused with dermatitis. It occurs in older adults.

Wilman JH, Golitz LE, Fitzpatrick JE: Vulvar clear cells of Toker: precursors of extramammary Paget's disease, *Am J Dermatopathol* 27:185–188, 2005.

39. Is EMPD associated with underlying malignancies?

Yes. Some cases with a similar clinical and histologic presentation arise when an underlying gastrointestinal or genitourinary adenocarcinoma demonstrates a similar pagetoid spread of epithelial cells. Some authorities refer to those cases that arise in the epidermis without an underlying carcinoma as "primary extramammary Paget's disease," and those that arise from an underlying malignancy as "secondary extramammary Paget's disease."

40. What is meant by "pagetoid" growth?

This is a histologic term used to describe large, pale cells that demonstrate a scattered growth pattern through the epidermis (Fig. 47-6B). In addition to extramammary Paget's disease, pagetoid growth is also seen in Paget's disease

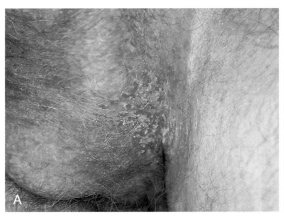
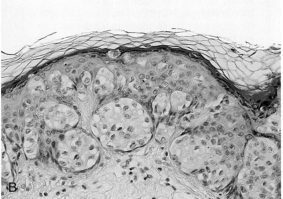

Figure 47-6. Primary extramammary Paget's disease. **A,** Typical extramammary Paget's disease arising in the groin. **B,** Typical large, pale, atypical epithelial cells that demonstrate a scattered growth pattern, both as single cells and as small aggregates throughout the epidermis (hematoxylin and eosin [H&E], ×400).

of the breast, squamous cell carcinoma in situ (Bowen's disease), malignant melanoma, and, rarely, sebaceous gland carcinomas. Paget's disease is named after Sir James Paget (1814–1894), who was among the first to describe this disease in the breast.

41. How is it treated?
Surgical excision with careful margin control. Mohs micrographic surgery can be useful, but the tumor can be multifocal and local recurrences occur.

Hendi A, Brodland DG, Zitelli JA: Extramammary Paget's disease: surgical treatment with Mohs micrographic surgery, *J Am Acad Dermatol* 51:767–773, 2004.

Key Points: Uncommon Malignant Tumors of the Skin

1. Epithelioid sarcoma is an aggressive tumor that presents on the volar distal extremities of young adults as a slow-growing dermal or subcutaneous nodule.
2. Merkel cell carcinoma is a rapidly growing tumor of the head, face, and neck that frequently metastasizes to regional lymph nodes and is treated with wide local excision (with 3-cm margins), lymph node dissection, and irradiation.
3. Dermatofibrosarcoma protuberans is a slow-growing, multinodular, flesh-colored to red-brown or blue plaque of the trunk and extremities that has a high local recurrence rate after incomplete excision.
4. Extramammary Paget's disease is characterized by an erythematous patch or plaque in the anogenital region of older adults.
5. Sebaceous carcinoma most commonly arises from the meibomian glands of the eyelid and presents as a firm nodule that may mimic a chalazion.

SEBACEOUS CARCINOMA

42. Where do sebaceous carcinomas occur?
They occur in both ocular (most commonly) and extraocular sites. Ocular lesions often arise from the meibomian glands of the eyelid and are more aggressive than tumors at extraocular sites.

43. How does sebaceous carcinoma present?
Ocular tumors present as firm nodules (Fig. 47-7). Because they may mimic a chalazion, it is important to biopsy persistent or unusual lesions. Extraocular tumors occur on the head and neck of the elderly. Sebaceous carcinoma is more common in Asians.

44. What are the treatment and prognosis?
Treatment is complete surgical removal, and Mohs surgery has a lower recurrence rate than standard excision. Up to one third of patients with ocular

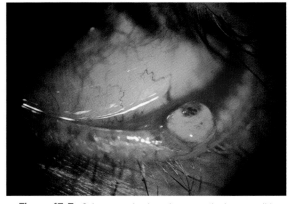

Figure 47-7. Sebaceous gland carcinoma on the lower eyelid.

tumors develop metastases to cervical lymph nodes. Muir-Torre syndrome should be considered in patients presenting with sebaceous carcinoma.

LEIOMYOSARCOMA

45. What is leiomyosarcoma?

It is a malignant tumor of smooth muscle. Dermal tumors occur in erector pili, dartos (scrotum), and vascular smooth muscles.

46. Describe dermal leiomyosarcoma.

This solitary tumor has a nonspecific appearance, presenting as a red-pink nodule of 0.5 cm to >3.0 cm, and may be painful. It exhibits a predilection for proximal extremity extensor surfaces and areas of greatest hair distribution. The tumors may occasionally be ulcerated (Fig. 47-8).

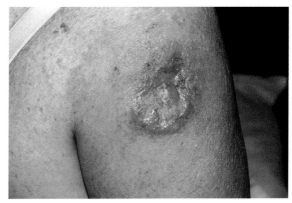

47. What histologic stains help identify leiomyosarcoma?

Smooth muscle stains such as Masson, trichrome, smooth muscle–specific actin, muscle-specific actin, calponin, and desmin.

48. What are the treatment and prognosis?

Early detection and adequate surgical excision is necessary. Dermal tumors metastasize rarely, whereas subcutaneous tumors metastasize in about one third of patients.

Humphreys TR, Finkelstein DH, Lee JB: Superficial leiomyosarcoma treated with Mohs micrographic surgery, *Dermatol Surg* 30:108–112, 2004.

Figure 47-8. Leiomyosarcoma. Ulcerated leiomyosarcoma of the upper arm in a woman. (Courtesy of the Fitzsimons Army Medical Center teaching files.)

CUTANEOUS METASTASES

Martin B. Giandoni, MD, and James E. Fitzpatrick, MD

1. How often do internal malignancies metastasize to the skin?

Cutaneous metastases of internal malignancies are relatively uncommon. An autopsy study including 7500 patients with internal malignancies demonstrated cutaneous metastases in 9% of patients. Most cases occur late in the course of the disease, but cutaneous metastasis may also be the initial presentation of an internal malignancy.

Lookingbill DP, Spangler N, Helm KF: Cutaneous metastases in patients with metastatic carcinoma: a retrospective study of 4020 patients, *J Am Acad Dermatol* 29:228–236, 1993.

2. By what three routes do internal malignancies metastasize to the skin?

They extend by local infiltration, lymphatic spread, or hematogenous spread. Breast carcinoma and oral cancer are the most likely to demonstrate direct extension into the skin. It is assumed that the fundamental mechanisms are similar to those of metastasis to parenchymal organs, but this has not been investigated. Rare cases have been inoculated by local procedures such as needle biopsies.

Jilani G, Mohamed D, Wadia H, et al: Cutaneous metastasis of renal cell carcinoma through percutaneous fine needle aspiration biopsy: case report, *Dermatol Online J* 15:10, 2010.

3. How do malignant cells invade and metastasize?

The genetic and molecular events that allow cells to invade and metastasize are a complex issue that is being studied in numerous laboratories. Malignant cells must be able to detach from adjacent cells (i.e., downregulate adhesion molecules), adhere to the adjacent matrix by the development of receptors to matrix molecules, such as fibronectin; lyse the extracellular matrix by the production of various enzymes; and migrate by the production of motility factors, such as hepatocyte growth factor. Once the tumor cells gain access to lymphatic spaces or blood vessels, they must be able to express adhesion molecules on their surface, which then allows them to attach to endothelial cells (e.g., CD44). There is also evidence that certain normal tissues produce chemoattractants that may attract tumor to a specific site.

Nguyen TH: Mechanisms of metastasis, *Clin Dermatol* 22:209–216, 2004.
Nomura T, Katunuma N: Involvement of cathepsins in the invasion, metastasis, and proliferation of cancer cells, *J Med Invest* 52:1–9, 2005.

4. What are the most common cancers that metastasize to the skin in women?

Different gender and age groups are affected by somewhat different metastatic malignancies. In a large study done at the Armed Forces Institute of Pathology in the early 1970s, the most common etiologies of cutaneous metastases in women were:

- Breast carcinoma: 69%
- Colon: 9%
- Malignant melanoma: 5%
- Ovary: 4%
- Lung: 4%

Because of the rapid increase in the incidence of lung carcinoma and malignant melanoma in women, it is likely that metastatic disease from these two malignancies is now more common than reported in this study.

Brownstein MH, Helwig EB: Spread of tumors to the skin, *Arch Dermatol* 107:80–86, 1973.

5. What are the most common cancers that metastasize to the skin in men?

In the same study, the five most common causes of skin metastases in men were:

- **Lung:** 24%
- **Colon:** 19%
- **Malignant melanoma:** 13%
- **Oral squamous cell carcinoma:** 12%
- **Kidney:** 6%

In a more recent study, malignant melanoma was the most common cause of cutaneous metastases, accounting for 32% of all cases (Fig. 48-1).

6. Do metastases to the skin typically occur in random patterns?

No. Different tumors demonstrate characteristic patterns of metastases (Table 48-1). A well-known example is ocular malignant melanoma, which frequently demonstrates metastasis to the liver. As a rule, cutaneous metastases usually appear in skin that is near the primary tumor (Fig. 48-2). Most regional metastases are probably spread through the lymphatic system, while distant metastases are more likely to occur via the hematogenous route.

7. Describe the most common presentations of malignancies metastatic to the skin.

Cutaneous metastases most commonly present as a cutaneous nodule or group of nodules that may be movable or fixed to underlying structures. Less commonly, they may present as indurated plaques. They may be skin-colored (Fig. 48-3), violaceous, erythematous, or, rarely, pigmented (malignant melanoma). The overlying epidermis is usually intact, but large metastatic lesions may be eroded or ulcerated. Clinically, they may mimic primary cutaneous lesions, including epidermoid cysts, lipomas, primary cutaneous malignancies, neurofibromas, scars, pyogenic granulomas, cellulitis, and even dermatitis. Metastatic breast carcinoma may uncommonly present with distinct patterns, including carcinoma erysipelatoides (inflammatory carcinoma; Fig. 48-4), carcinoma telangiectaticum (a variant of inflammatory carcinoma), and carcinoma en cuirasse (a sclerodermoid pattern).

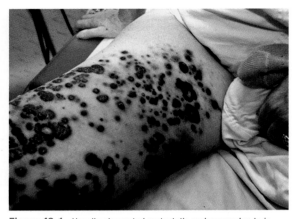

Figure 48-1. Heavily pigmented metastatic melanoma due to in transit metastases from a primary tumor on the lower extremity. (Courtesy of Rene Gonzalez, MD.)

8. What is alopecia neoplastica?

The scalp appears to be a unique site for cutaneous metastasis, and often cutaneous metastases to the scalp are a presenting sign for internal malignancy. One characteristic clinical presentation is that of an isolated, indurated plaque

Table 48-1. Characteristic Sites of Cutaneous Metastases	
PRIMARY TUMOR	SITE OF METASTASES
Oral squamous cell carcinoma	Head and neck
Thyroid carcinoma	Neck
Lung	Chest wall
Breast	Anterior chest wall
Renal cell carcinoma	Head
Gastrointestinal carcinoma	Abdomen
Genitourinary carcinoma	Lower abdomen

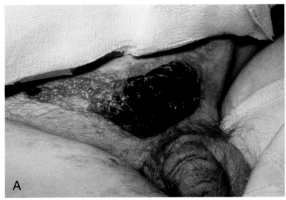
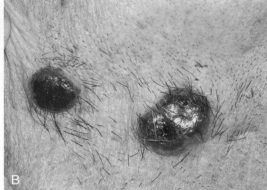

Figure 48-2. A, Large metastatic nodule of prostate carcinoma. The lower abdomen and pubic area are common sites for metastases of genitourinary cancers. **B,** Lung carcinoma metastatic to the chest wall, which is the most common site. (Courtesy of Paul Thompson, MD.)

in the scalp with associated alopecia (Fig. 48-5). Biopsy of this site will demonstrate cutaneous metastasis of a visceral malignancy and loss of hair follicles. The most common tumors to metastasize to the scalp are those of the breast, lung, and kidney.

9. What is a Sister Mary Joseph's nodule?

It is a nodular umbilical metastatic tumor (Fig. 48-6). This sign is named in recognition of Sister Mary Joseph, who was the superintendent of St. Mary's Hospital in Rochester, Minnesota, and served as the first surgical assistant to Dr. W.J. Mayo. She is credited with recognizing that patients with this finding had a poor prognosis.

Albano EA, Kanter JL: Images in clinical medicine. Sister Mary Joseph's nodule, *N Engl J Med* 352:1913, 2005.

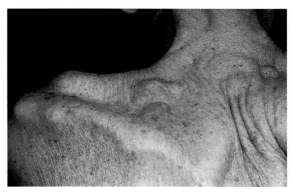

Figure 48-3. Metastatic adenocarcinoma of the gastrointestinal tract presenting as skin-colored dermal and subcutaneous nodules.

10. Which tumors usually present as a Sister Mary Joseph's nodule?

The four most common tumors to present with this sign are stomach (20%), large bowel (14%), ovary (14%), and pancreatic tumors (11%). In about one fifth of patients, the primary site cannot be determined.

11. Does basal cell carcinoma ever metastasize?

Yes. Basal cell carcinoma is the most common cutaneous malignancy in the United States with over 1 million new cases per year. It has been estimated that the overall metastatic rate is 0.03% with the majority of cases occurring in large destructive tumors that have been present for many years. Basal cell carcinomas most commonly metastasize to regional lymph nodes followed by the lungs, bones, and skin. The 5-year survival for metastatic basal cell carcinoma is grave and is estimated to be about 10%.

Spates ST, Mellette JR Jr, Fitzpatrick J: Metastatic basal cell carcinoma, *Dermatol Surg* 29:650–652, 2003.

12. How do you diagnose a cutaneous metastasis?

The diagnosis is best established by doing an excisional, incisional, or punch biopsy, and by submitting the specimen in formalin for routine processing. In addition to hematoxylin and eosin (H&E) stains, the pathologist can perform special histochemical stains (e.g., mucicarmine for mucin, Fontana-Masson for melanin) or immunoperoxidase studies (e.g.,

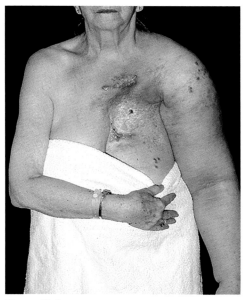

Figure 48-4. Inflammatory breast carcinoma presenting as an erythematous plaque on the anterior chest wall and red dermal papules on the shoulder.

prostate-specific antigen for prostate cancer and calcitonin for medullary thyroid carcinoma). Problematic cases may require submission of part of the tumor for electron microscopy, or frozen for immunoperoxidase studies that cannot be done on formalin-fixed tissue. Less commonly, the tumor specimen is obtained by a fine-needle aspiration.

Key Points: Cutaneous Metastatic Tumors

1. Approximately 9% of all patients who die from internal malignancy will demonstrate metastatic tumors in the skin.
2. Cutaneous metastasis may be the initial presentation of an internal malignancy.
3. Sister Mary Joseph's nodule is a nodular umbilical metastatic tumor.
4. Cutaneous metastasis is usually a poor prognostic sign, and most patients are dead within 1 year.

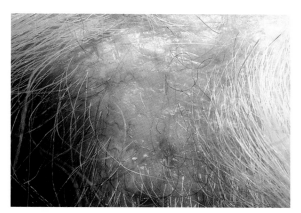

Figure 48-5. Alopecia neoplastica secondary to metastatic breast carcinoma. On palpation, the lesion was firm and indurated.

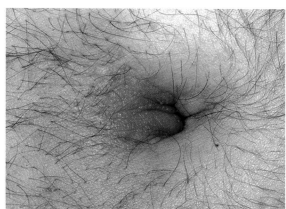

Figure 48-6. Sister Mary Joseph's nodule of the umbilicus. The primary malignancy was never detected.

13. What is the prognosis of a patient with a cutaneous metastasis?

Cutaneous metastasis is usually a poor prognostic sign and often reflects preexisting widespread internal metastasis. In one study, the average life expectancy after development of skin metastases was only 3 months. The prognosis is ultimately dependent on the primary tumor, and some patients do survive for years.

Carroll MC, Fleming M, Chitambar CR, Neuburg M: Diagnosis, workup, and prognosis of cutaneous metastases of unknown primary origin, *Dermatol Surg* 28:533–535, 2002.

SUNSCREENS AND PREVENTION OF SKIN CANCER

Joseph Yohn, MD

1. List some of the important facts about skin cancer.

- Most people receive nearly 50% of their cumulative lifetime sun exposure by age 40.
- Sun exposure causes at least 90% of all skin cancers.
- One in five Americans will develop skin cancer during his or her lifetime.
- In the United States, over 1 million new cases of skin cancer are diagnosed annually, afflicting more people than any other cancer.
- In 2009, according to the American Cancer Society, 68,720 Americans will develop malignant melanoma, and there will be 8,650 melanoma-related deaths.
- Melanoma accounts for about 4% of skin cancer cases, but it causes about 79% of skin cancer deaths.
- The incidence of melanoma is increasing at a rate faster than that of any other cancer, having nearly doubled in the last decade.

American Academy of Dermatology. Available at: http://www.aad.org. Accessed August 3, 2010.
American Cancer Society. Available at: http://www.cancer.org. Accessed August 3, 2010.
Skin Cancer Foundation. Available at: http://www.skincancer.org. Accessed August 3, 2010.

2. How does skin type affect the risk for skin cancer?

Anyone can get skin cancer, although some people are at greater risk than others. The skin phototype (SPT) system was developed to identify people who are prone to develop skin cancer. The SPT system is a six-point scale based on a person's skin color and ability to tan (Table 49-1). Individuals who fall into SPT groups I and II are at highest risk for the development of skin cancer. These two groups of people are especially prone to develop basal cell and squamous cell carcinoma and are at high risk for developing melanoma. Skin types III and IV are less prone to develop basal cell and squamous cell carcinoma but are still at risk for developing melanoma. Basal cell carcinoma, squamous cell carcinoma, and melanoma are rare in skin types V and VI. If patients in groups V and VI develop melanoma, it usually occurs on the palms and soles (acrolentiginous melanoma) or on mucosal surfaces, such as in the mouth or on the genitalia.

3. What are the other risk factors for skin cancer?

Strong skin cancer risk factors include family history, total cumulative sun exposure, the number of blistering sunburns, multiple atypical moles, immunosuppression, and occupational exposure to coal tar, pitch, creosote, arsenic compounds, or radium. Lifetime cumulative sun exposure directly correlates with basal cell and squamous cell carcinoma risk. Individuals who are exposed to the sun on a daily basis, such as farmers, fishermen, and construction workers, are at high risk for developing nonmelanoma skin cancer. Sunburns are directly related to melanoma risk. One study reported a 2.5- to 6.3-fold increased melanoma risk for a person with a history of three or more blistering sunburns. For this reason, indoor workers such as health care professionals and office workers who experience intense, intermittent sun exposure are more prone to developing melanoma.

4. Do hereditary factors affect skin cancer risk?

Skin cancer appears to have a hereditary component. The prototype syndrome of genetically determined increased skin cancer risk is xeroderma pigmentosum (XP). XP patients suffer from an autosomal recessive defect in DNA repair that results in sun sensitivity and early onset of basal cell carcinoma, squamous cell carcinoma, and melanoma. Although much of the molecular genetics of XP is understood, further study is necessary to better understand the genetics of other types of skin cancer-prone families. However, a useful recommendation is to have all first-degree relatives (parents, siblings, and children) of a skin cancer patient examined for skin cancer and taught sun-protection measures.

5. What age or sex factors are important in skin cancer risk?

- Basal cell and squamous cell carcinoma incidences peak in the seventh decade of life. Melanoma incidence peaks around age 50.
- Overall, men develop more skin cancer than do women, but in the third and fourth decades of life, almost as many women develop skin cancer as men.
- Melanoma occurs most frequently on the chest, shoulders, and back in males and in young women (ages 15 to 29). Melanoma is most commonly found on the legs of adult women 30 years and older.
- For both sexes, basal cell and squamous cell carcinoma develop most often on chronically sun-exposed areas, including the head, neck, shoulders, arms, and hands.

Table 49-1. Human Skin Phototypes

SKIN PHOTOTYPE*	UNEXPOSED SKIN COLOR	SUN RESPONSE HISTORY
I	White	Always burns, never tans
II	White	Always burns, tans minimally
III	White	Burns minimally, tans gradually and uniformly
IV	Light brown	Burns minimally, always tans well
V	Brown	Rarely burns, tans darkly
VI	Dark brown	Never burns, tans darkly

*Based on the first 30 to 60 minutes of sun exposure of untanned skin after the winter season.

- One caveat: Patients should have a total skin exam, because skin cancer of all types can occur on infrequently sun-exposed or non–sun-exposed areas, such as scalp, buttocks, and between the toes.

6. What should physicians teach patients about skin cancer prevention?
Basically, two things: sun protection and the self-skin exam.

7. What warning signs of possible skin cancer should be looked for in the self-skin exam?
The self-skin exam is an important part of skin cancer prevention for two reasons: Studies have shown that abnormal skin lesions are frequently discovered first by the patient, and skin cancer, when treated early, is curable. Patients should be encouraged to examine their entire skin surface on a monthly basis, remembering to include the scalp and normally non–sun-exposed sites, including the buttocks, genitalia, and feet. Warning signs of a possible skin cancer include
- An open sore that does not heal in 3 weeks
- A spot or sore that persistently itches, burns, stings, crusts, scabs, or bleeds
- Any mole or brown spot that changes in size, thickness, or texture or develops an irregular border
- A skin lesion that increases in size and appears pearly, translucent, tan, brown, black, or multicolored

8. How is ultraviolet light classified?
Ultraviolet (UV) light is broken down into bands of light according to its physical characteristics and biologic effects:
- **UVC: 100 to 290 nm wavelength.** High-energy radiation that injures cells through direct DNA damage and the generation of free-radical species. Fortunately, UVC radiation is filtered by atmospheric ozone and does not reach the earth's surface.
- **UVB: 290 to 320 nm wavelength.** Midrange radiation that is not completely filtered by atmospheric ozone, called the "burning" rays because it causes sunburn. UVB injures skin cells primarily through formation of DNA thymine dimers and 6 to 4 photoproducts that, if not repaired properly, cause gene mutations and lead to altered cell function and carcinogenesis.
- **UVA: 320 to 400 nm wavelength.** Long-wave radiation that is the lowest energy spectrum of ultraviolet. UVA is not filtered by atmospheric ozone, and a 150-fold greater amount of UVA strikes the surface of the earth compared to UVB. UVA damages skin cells predominantly through the formation of free radicals. UVB penetrates to the basal layer of the epidermis, whereas UVA penetrates to the middermis. Skin wrinkling following chronic sun exposure is due to UVA injury of dermal fibroblasts, resulting in altered collagen and elastin synthesis.

Combined, UVB and UVA are carcinogenic. Thus, it is imperative to warn patients about the damaging effects of ultraviolet radiation and how to properly protect against its adverse effects.

Key Points: Adverse Effects of Acute Sun Exposure
1. Sunburn
2. Transient immune suppression
3. Drug-induced phototoxic reactions
4. Exacerbation of an underlying photosensitivity disorder (e.g., lupus erythematosus)

Key Points: Adverse Effects of Chronic Sun Exposure
1. Skin wrinkles
2. Abnormal pigmentation
3. Precancers (actinic keratoses)
4. Impaired immune surveillance of preskin cancer and skin cancer
5. Cataracts
6. Basal cell carcinoma
7. Squamous cell carcinoma
8. Melanoma

Key Points: Health Benefits of Solar Radiation

1. Health benefits of solar radiation are few.
2. Skin exposure to ultraviolet B is necessary for the conversion of 7-dehydrocholesterol into previtamin D_3, which then isomerizes to vitamin D_3.
3. Periodic exposure to the visible spectrum of solar radiation is believed to enhance psychological well-being.
4. Lastly, the ultraviolet spectrum of solar radiation is used for the treatment of skin disorders, such as psoriasis, vitiligo, eczema, and cutaneous T-cell lymphoma.

9. List the 13 basic facts regarding sun protection.

1. Sun damage is cumulative. Each dose of ultraviolet radiation (UVR), large and small, adds up, leading to skin wrinkling, dyspigmentation, and skin cancer.
2. There is no such thing as a "healthy tan." Skin tanning is a response to UVR skin injury.
3. Avoid sun exposure between the hours of 10 AM and 2 PM (11 AM to 3 PM daylight savings time), when UVB is most intense. Plan outdoor activities for early morning or late afternoon.
4. Protect the skin with clothing first, and apply sunscreen to any remaining unprotected skin.
5. Beware of high-altitude sun exposure, where there is less (thinner) atmosphere to absorb UVR, and therefore the risk of sunburn is greater.
6. UVR is stronger near the equator, where the sun's rays strike the earth most directly.
7. Use protective clothing and apply sunscreens even on overcast days. Although UVR is less intense on overcast days, it is still present and adds to cumulative skin damage.
8. UVR is reflected off of sand, concrete, and snow and adds to the total UVR exposure. Because UVR is reflected and scattered, sitting in the shade is not totally protective and sunburn can occur.
9. Do not use tanning beds. Although tanning beds emit primarily UVA, overexposure can cause sunburn, and their use enhances skin aging and the risk for skin cancer.
10. People at high risk for skin cancer (persons with skin types I and II, outdoor workers, and persons with a history of skin cancer or a photosensitivity disorder) should apply sunscreens daily.
11. Some medications (sulfonamides, tetracyclines, and birth control pills, as well as over-the-counter products) and cosmetic ingredients (lime oil) can be photosensitizing.
12. Keep infants and children out of direct sunlight. Begin using sunscreens on children after they learn to walk, and then allow sun exposure with moderation.
13. Teach children sun protection early.

10. What type of clothing is considered sun-protective?

Optimal sun protection includes wearing a hat, sunglasses, a long-sleeved shirt, and long pants. Be sure to choose the correct type of clothing for sun protection. Weave and construction of the fabric is more important than the fiber. Choose tightly woven materials for greater protection from UVR.

Edlich RF, et al: Recent technologic advances in sun-protective clothing to prevent the development of skin cancer. In Martakis IK, editor: *Cancer research at the leading edge*, New York, 2008, Nova Science Publishers, pp 171–181.

11. What are sunscreens?

In the broadest terms, sunscreens are agents that block ultraviolet radiation absorption by the skin. Sunscreens can be in the form of clothing, hats, sunglasses, or chemical or physical agents, including lotions, creams, pastes, and gels.

12. Compare the advantages and disadvantages of the physical and chemical sunscreens.

Physical sunscreens are agents that scatter and reflect UVR, while chemical sunscreens absorb UVR through a photochemical reaction. Physical sunscreens include zinc oxide and titanium dioxide and have advantages over chemical sunscreens. Physical sunscreens are inert, they do not break down over time, and they do not cause contact dermatitis or photodermatitis. They block both UVB and UVA (Table 49-2). However, physical sunscreens have one drawback: they leave a slight makeup base appearance to the skin that some people find unappealing.

Although chemical sunscreens do carry a risk for contact dermatitis and photodermatitis, the risk is quite low (0.1% to 2.0%). Another disadvantage of chemical sunscreens is that they degrade with sun exposure, requiring reapplication every 2 hours. However, for many people, the advantages of chemical sunscreens outweigh the disadvantages. Chemical sunscreens are available in a plethora of formulations, such as creams, lotions, and gels. There are formulations for use on the face, lips, and small children. Today, there are chemical sunscreen formulations that block both UVB and UVA, and these formulations should be recommended to patients.

13. What chemicals are used in chemical sunscreens?

See Table 49-3.

Table 49-2. Sunscreens That Block UVB and UVA

PRODUCT NAME	SPF	MANUFACTURER
Aveeno Continuous Protection	30, 50, 55, 70	Johnson and Johnson
Aveeno Baby	55	Johnson and Johnson
Banana Boat	15, 30, 50	Sun Pharmaceutical
Bull Frog	36, 50	Chattem
Clinique Sunblock	15, 30, 45, 50	Clinique
Coppertone Water Babies	50, 70	Schering-Plough
Coppertone Nutrashield	30, 70	Schering-Plough
Coppertone Sport	15, 30, 50, 70	Schering-Plough
Estee Lauder	15, 30	Estee Lauder
Hawaiian Tropic Shear Touch	15, 30, 50	Tanning Research
Hawaiian Tropic Ultimate	55, 70, 80	Tanning Research
Hawaiian Tropic Baby Faces	50, 60	Tanning Research
Neutrogena Ultra Sheer	55, 70, 85	Neutrogena
Neutrogena Sensitive Skin	30	Neutrogena
Neutrogena Baby	60	Neutrogena
No-Ad	15, 30, 45	Sun and Skin Care Research
No-Ad Babies	50	Sun and Skin Care Research
Pre Sun	27, 30	Bristol Myers
Mary Kay Sunscreen	15, 30	Mary Kay
Vanicream Sunscreen Sport	35	Pharmaceutical Specialties

Table 49-3. Chemicals Used in Sunscreens

CHEMICAL	MAXIMUM CONCENTRATION USED (%)
Aminobenzoic acid	15
Avobenzone	3
Cinoxate	3
Dioxybenzone	3
Homosalate	15
Menthyl anthranilate	5
Octocrylene	10
Octyl methoxycinnamate	7.5
Octyl salicylate	5
Oxybenzone	6
Octyl dimethyl PABA	8
Phenylbenzimidazole sulfonic acid	4
Sulisobenzone	10
Titanium dioxide	25
Trolamine salicylate	12
Zinc oxide	25

14. What factors should be considered in selecting a sunscreen?
- The sunscreen should block both UVB and UVA and have a sun protection factor (SPF) rating of 15 or greater.
- Avoid sunscreens that contain fragrance, which can be a source of contact dermatitis or photodermatitis and can attract stinging insects. Para-aminobenzoic acid (PABA) also can cause contact dermatitis; all sunscreen products are now PABA-free.

- Although some sunscreens claim to be waterproof and rub-proof or offer "all-day protection," these sunscreens should be reapplied after sweating or swimming.

15. How is an SPF determined?

Sunscreen SPF is defined as the ratio of the minimal dose of sunlight needed to cause redness of sunscreen-protected skin divided by the minimal dose of sunlight needed to cause redness of unprotected skin. SPFs of 15, 30, and 50 effectively reduce UV skin absorption by 94%, 97%, and 98%, respectively.

16. How much sunscreen should be applied? How often should it be reapplied?

Warn your patients that most people apply too little sunscreen. To cover the face, arms, legs, and upper torso of an average-sized adult requires 1 ounce of sunscreen, which is generally a handful. A smaller person or child needs proportionally less. Sunscreen should be applied evenly and rubbed into all exposed skin. It should be applied 30 to 60 minutes before sun exposure. Then a second layer should be applied at the beginning of sun exposure and, under normal conditions, reapplied every 2 hours. Sunscreen should be reapplied more often if swimming, sweating, or rubbing has removed some of the product. Warn patients that reapplication does not double the SPF and to not rely on redness as a signal to reapply sunscreen. Skin damage occurs before sunburn appears.

17. Can sunscreens be safely used in children?

Yes. Most major cosmetic and pharmaceutical companies make sunscreen products for children. All recommendations for sunscreen use in adults should be followed for children. However, sunscreens need not be used in children less than 6 months of age. Any child who has not yet learned to crawl should be protected with long sleeves, long pants, and a hat and should be kept away from direct sunlight.

18. Why are sunglasses included in sun-protection recommendations?

Sunglasses protect the eyelids, sclera, cornea, and lens from UVR injury. Intense, acute UVR eye injury results in sunburn of the eyelids, sclera, and cornea, whereas chronic sun exposure causes cataracts and skin cancer of the periorbital skin. Patients should be instructed to buy sunglasses that absorb UVB and UVA. Also, a large frame area better protects the skin around the eyes.

19. Are tanning pills safe to use?

Not entirely. Canthaxanthin, the active ingredient in most tanning pills, is not approved by the U.S. Food and Drug Administration. While most patients do not have significant side effects, some patients have developed nausea, diarrhea, pruritus, skin eruptions, night blindness, and drug-induced hepatitis. There has been one reported death due to aplastic anemia in a woman who took tanning pills.

20. What about "tan-in-a-bottle" lotions?

Self-tanning lotions are skin dyes and are safe to use; however, skin-coloring agents do not protect the skin from UVR injury. Therefore, sun-protection measures must be followed by people using self-tanning products.

21. What is the relationship between UVR, the skin, and vitamin D?

Two primary sources of vitamin D are the diet and cutaneous UVB exposure. The inactive form of vitamin D (7-dehydrocholesterol) contained within epidermal keratinocytes is converted photochemically by UVB radiation to previtamin D3. Previtamin D3 then spontaneously isomerizes to vitamin D3 (3-cholecalciferol). Vitamin D3 is then hydroxylated by the epidermis and the liver to 25-hydroxy vitamin D3, which is then further hydroxylated to the active form 1,25-hydroxy vitamin D3 or calcitriol.

Anything that interferes with ambient UVB levels (latitude, time of day, season of the year, cloud cover, smog) or cutaneous UVB penetration (clothing, melanin, sunblock) will reduce vitamin D production.

22. If UVB is required for vitamin D metabolism, how would one maintain normal vitamin D levels with restricted sun exposure? How much sun exposure is necessary?

In the southern United States, daily short UVB exposure (5 minutes for lightly pigmented people and 10 minutes for darkly pigmented people) of a small area of skin (face, hands, and arms) will supply ample vitamin D for the body's needs. However, at latitudes greater than 40 degrees, winter sun exposure does not produce active vitamin D. Therefore, residents of the northern United States should take supplemental vitamin D of at least 400 IU daily. Fortunately, proper vitamin D levels can be easily maintained by eating a vitamin D–fortified diet. Eggs, beef liver, and oily fish, such as salmon, catfish, herring, mackerel, and tuna, are excellent sources of vitamin D. Many foods, such as milk, cereals, and bread are fortified with vitamin D, and most multivitamins contain vitamin D.

Cicarma E, Porojnicu AC, Lagunova Z, et al: Sun and sun beds: inducers of vitamin D and skin cancer, *Anticancer Res* 29 (9):3495–3500, 2009.

Weinstock MA, Moses AM: Skin cancer meets vitamin D: the way forward for dermatology and public health, *J Am Acad Dermatol* 61(4):720–724, 2009.

23. What is proper sunburn treatment?

Take aspirin or ibuprofen as soon as sunburn is detected to help reduce inflammation and control pain. Tylenol helps control pain but is not antiinflammatory. Cool, wet compresses, or tub soaks for 20 minutes, four or five times daily will help with pain control. Do not use butter or heavy ointments, because they can cause skin irritation, and do not use benzocaine sprays, because they can cause contact dermatitis. Light creams and lotions containing pramoxine will soothe the skin and reduce pain. Increased fluid loss can occur through sunburned skin. Therefore, fluid replenishment with an isotonic sport drink is recommended. Because sun-damaged skin is more susceptible to subsequent burns, sun exposure should be avoided until the skin completely heals in 1 to 2 weeks.

CHAPTER 50

TOPICAL STEROIDS

T. Minsue Chen, MD

1. When were corticosteroids discovered? When were they first used therapeutically?
- **1935:** Discovery of compound E (cortisone)
- **1948:** First reported use of cortisone and adrenocorticotropic hormone (ACTH) in the treatment of rheumatoid arthritis
- **1951:** First report of cortisone and ACTH used in the treatment of inflammatory dermatoses
- **1952:** First report of using compound F (hydrocortisone) topically

   Corticosteroids are synthetic relatives of the hormones produced by the adrenal glands, such as cortisone. Since the mid-1950s, there have been numerous modifications of the corticosteroid molecule that have dramatically increased the potency of this topical therapy (i.e., halogenation, esterification, hydroxylation, modification of side chains, and improvements in delivery systems). As the potency of the molecule has increased, so has the likelihood of side effects.

2. Describe the basic steroid nucleus.
See Fig. 50-1.

3. How is the potency of topical steroid medications determined?
At present, the most widely used topical steroid ranking system of potency is based on the vasoconstrictor assay, where test medications are applied in serial dilutions to the forearms of the volunteers for a standard length of time. Many believe that this one measure of biologic function correlates with clinical effectiveness. Although it is difficult to compare studies because of a lack of standardization, a recent study demonstrated that therapeutic index did not correlate with the vasoconstrictor assay or clinical outcome.

Hepburn DJ, Aeling JL, Weston WL: A reappraisal of topical steroid potency, *Pediatr Dermatol* 13(3):239–245, 1996.

4. How do topical steroids inhibit cutaneous inflammation?
The steroid molecule binds to specific cytoplasmic steroid receptors that are transported to the cell nucleus, where it interacts with high-affinity binding sites on nuclear DNA. Steroid-induced proteins, called lipocortins, are then synthesized by the target cells. There is good evidence that these proteins inhibit phospholipase A_2, an enzyme necessary for formation of inflammatory mediators (e.g., arachidonic acid, prostaglandins, leukotrienes, and platelet-activating factor) that decrease vascular permeability. Another immediate effect of topical steroids is to produce vasoconstriction, thus decreasing tissue edema, erythema, and heat. The steroid molecule can also bind to cell membranes, altering their function. Inflammatory cells show reduced migration and function at sites of inflammation.

5. How are topical corticosteroids classified as to potency?
Many authors in the United States classify topical corticosteroids into seven categories of potency: 1) superpotency, 2) high potency, 3) high midpotency, 4) midpotency, 5) low midpotency, 6) mildly potent, and 7) low potency. The authors of this book prefer to rank them into four classes of potency (Table 50-1).

6. How many topical steroid medications are available in the United States?
Epocrates Rx lists over 100 brand name and generic topical products that contain corticosteroids; this does not include the various vehicles and concentrations. It is not necessary to learn all of the steroid names and preparations. Familiarity with one preparation in each potency class is often sufficient.

Epocrates Rx (database for Parental Drug Association [PDA]), Version 1.0: Epocrates, Inc, San Mateo, CA. Copyright 2006 [updated Dec 14, 2009; cited Dec 14, 2009]. Available from: http://www.epocrates.com.

7. What are the differences between brand name and generic topical steroid products?
When brand name and generic products are compared, pharmacology, vasoconstriction assay, clinical response, and cost are variable. Ingredients may be different (e.g., perfume, preservative, vehicle).

Puavilai S, Krisadaphong P, Leenutaphong V, et al: Comparative study of the efficacy of topical corticosteroid: five locally made and one brand name cream (abstract), *J Med Assoc Thai* 85(7):789–799, 2002.

8. With so many products available, how do you decide which product to prescribe for your patient?
There are anatomic site differences in relative absorption: forearm = 1, back = 1.7, sole = 0.14, palm = 0.83, scalp = 3.5, cheek = 13, eyelid and scrotum = 42. A multitude of additional factors must be considered, including: chronicity of disease being treated, percentage of body surface involvement, patient age, specific medication, vehicle, frequency of application and

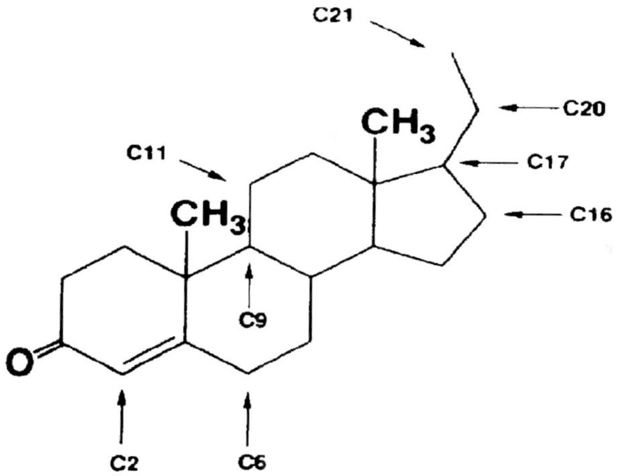

Figure 50-1. Structure of steroid nucleus.

Table 50-1. Topical Steroid Potency[*]

Group I: Super Potency (antiinflammatory activity = 500)
- Clobetasol diproprionate 0.05% (Temovate)
- Betamethasone diproprionate 0.25% (Diprolene)
- Halbetasol proprionate 0.05% (Ultravate)
- Diflorasone diacetate 0.05% (Psorcon)

Group II: High Potency (antiinflammatory activity = 100–500)
- Fluocinonide 0.05% (Lidex)
- Halcinonide 0.05% (Halog)
- Amcinonide 0.05% (Cyclocort)
- Desoximetasone 0.25% (Topicort)

Group III: Midpotency (antiinflammatory activity = 10–100)
- Fluocinolone acetonide 0.01%–0.2% (Synalar, Synemol, Fluonid)
- Hydrocortisone valerate 0.2% (Westcort)
- Hydrocortisone butyrate 0.1% (Locoid)
- Triamcinolone acetonide 0.01%–0.5% (Kenalog, Aristocort)
- Betamethasone valerate 0.1% (Valisone)
- Clocortolone pivalate 0.1% (Cloderm)
- Flurandrenolide 0.05% (Cordran)
- Betamethasone benzoate 0.028% (Benisone, Uticort)
- Mometasone furoate 0.1% (Elocon)
- Diflorasone diacetate 0.05% (Florone, Maxiflor)
- Fluticasone proprionate 0.005% (Cutivate)
- Betamethasone diproprionate 0.005% (Maxivate)

Group IV: Low Potency (antiinflammatory activity = 1–10)
- Hydrocortisone acetate 0.25%–2.5% (1% is OTC; 0.1% is prescription)
- Desonide 0.05% (DesOwen, Tridesilon)
- Aclometasone 0.05% (Aclovate)
- Prednisolone 0.5% (Meti-Derm)
- Dexamethasone 0.1% (Decadron)
- Methylprednisolone 1% (Medrol)

*The individual steroid molecules can be moved up or down in the potency ranking by changing the vehicle of the topical formulation.
OTC, Over-the-counter.

technique, potential side effects, presence of coexisting factors, and cost. Importantly, if the product is unpleasing, patient compliance may be compromised.

9. What specific directions should be provided when prescribing super-, high-, and midpotency topical steroids?

Education is imperative. Side effects should be discussed, as well as correct application methods to avoid misuse. Failure to do so may result in nonadherence and irrational steroid phobia. Timely follow-up should be scheduled to monitor for treatment and side effects.

The directions should specify that the potent topical steroid should *not* be used in areas of thin skin (e.g., face, neck), and in intertriginous locations where skin touches skin (e.g., axilla, inframammary, infrapannus, groin). Areas of thinner epidermis provide less resistance and facilitate absorption. In addition, apposition of two skin surfaces simulates an occlusive dressing, which greatly enhances penetration and absorption of medication.

Because it is common for patients to distribute their medication to other family members or friends, or save it for use on another skin problem in the future, instructions should include exclusive use by the patient only and for this particular rash only.

Charman CR, Morris AD, Williams HC: Topical corticosteroid phobia in patients with atopic eczema, *Br J Dermatol* 142(5):931–936, 2000.

10. Why is the vehicle important when recommending a topical corticosteroid?
The choice of vehicle may affect several factors that relate to potency, including bioavailability, lipid solubility, and the partition coefficient of each product. A vehicle should also be selected based on indication, disease severity and extent, body region to be treated, as well as patient preference. A steroid molecule in an ointment base will result in the most potent preparation, because it is the most occlusive with the greatest penetration. This is followed by creams, lotions, solutions, gels, and sprays. Compounding, dilution, or addition of ingredients to a proprietary product should be discouraged. This practice can affect the uniformity, stability, and/or bioavailability of the active ingredient. Also, the cost is greater because additional labor is required.

11. Are certain vehicles preferred for particular types of lesions or anatomic sites?
Ointments work best on chronic, thickened skin lesions and should be avoided when the dermatosis is acute, vesicular, and weeping. Solutions, gels, sprays, or foams are recommended for dermatoses in hairy areas. Creams or lotions are best for intertriginous locations. Gels and sprays can also be used to treat inflammatory lesions on mucosal surfaces.

12. A patient has 5% total body surface area (TBSA) involvement. How much topical steroid should be prescribed for twice daily application for a 1-week-on and 1-week-off treatment cycle? The patient will return in 4 weeks for follow-up.
Topical medications are frequently under- or overprescribed, and only a thin layer of medication is necessary. Use the fingertip unit (FTU) application technique and percent of TBSA to calculate the amount needed: 1 FTU equals approximately 0.5 gm of medication and will treat 2% TBSA in the average adult. The patient will need approximately 35 grams for the next 4 weeks. Calculation: (5% TBSA/1 application) × (1 FTU/2% TBSA) × (0.5 grams/1 FTU) × 14 day × (2 applications/1 day) = 35 grams.

NOTE: One FTU is the amount of medication expressed from a tube with a 5-mm opening that extends from the distal interphalangeal crease to the tip of the finger (Fig. 50-2). One palm size, including fingers, represents 1% TBSA.

13. How should the FTU application technique be applied to children?
Use the adult FTU to calculate the amount needed. The quantity, however, should be reduced to 25% for a 1-year-old and 33% for a 4-year-old child.

14. When are combination topical steroid and antiinfective products indicated?
The combination products are often marginally effective and expensive. The most commonly prescribed products are Mycolog II (nystatin/triamcinolone) and Lotrisone (clotrimazole/betamethasone). Lotrisone is approved by the U.S. Food and Drug Administration (FDA) for tinea cruris/corporis/pedis in adults and children more than 12 years of age.

Few nondermatology physicians recognize the steroid component to be fluorinated and high-/midpotency. They are also more likely to prescribe this product to children less than 5 years of age for use on genital skin. A baby's diaper is occlusive, enhancing absorption, as well as the likelihood of side effects. Use of these products may lead to persistent and recurrent disease.

Alston SJ, Cohen BA, Braun M: Persistent and recurrent tinea corporis in children treated with combination antifungal/corticosteroid agents, *Pediatrics* 111(1):201–203, 2003.

Railan D, Wilson JK, Feldman SR, Fleischer AB: Pediatricians who prescribe clotrimazole-betamethasone diproprionate (Lotrisone) often utilize it in inappropriate settings regardless of their knowledge of the drug's potency, *Dermatol Online J* 8(2):3, 2002.

Shaffer MP, Feldman SR, Fleischer AB Jr: Use of clotrimazole/betamethasone dipropionate by family physicians, *Fam Med* 32(8):561–565, 2000.

15. What is tachyphylaxis and how can it be prevented?
Resistance to treatment (tachyphylaxis) is a common problem with prolonged use of topical steroids.

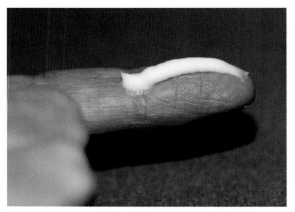

Figure 50-2. Demonstration of a fingertip unit (FTU), which is approximately 0.5 grams of medication. (Courtesy of the John L. Aeling, M.D. Collection.)

Topical steroid holidays (i.e., intermittent pulse dosing of 1 week "on" and 1 week of "rest") or alternate nonsteroid treatments should be considered for difficult chronic skin disease.

16. What are the local cutaneous side effects of topical steroids?

Local cutaneous side effects are the most common problem associated with topical steroids. They may develop quickly with potent topical steroids, especially when applied to thin-skinned or intertriginous areas (Table 50-2). Therefore, prolonged use is not recommended.

17. What are the effects of topical steroids on the epidermis?

Thinning of the epidermis can occur within 7 days of use of superpotent topical steroids. After 3 weeks of potent topical steroid use, all layers of the epidermis are reduced in thickness by about one half. The thinning of the epidermis, particularly the stratum corneum, impairs the barrier function of the epidermis, thus increasing transepidermal water loss and skin irritancy.

18. What are the effects of topical steroids on the dermis?

Within 1 to 3 weeks of using superpotent topical steroids, the dermal volume is measurably reduced. This is due to decreased fibroblast production of dermal ground substance, primarily hyaluronic acid, and decreased dermal water content. Abnormal synthesis of collagen and elastin results in dermal atrophy (Fig. 50-3), skin fragility, striae (Fig. 50-4), telangiectasias, poor vascular support with skin purpura, and decreased wound healing.

19. What are the systemic side effects of topical steroid therapy?

The superpotent topical steroids are over a thousand times more potent than hydrocortisone. Infants and children are more at risk for systemic side effects because they have greater surface-to-body ratio than adults, and they may not be able to metabolize the steroid molecule efficiently.

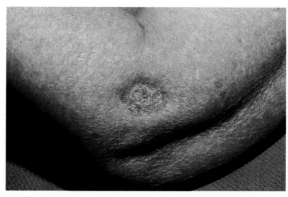

Figure 50-3. Cutaneous atrophy and slight hypopigmentation from intralesional corticosteroids. (Courtesy of the Fitzsimons Army Medical Center teaching files.)

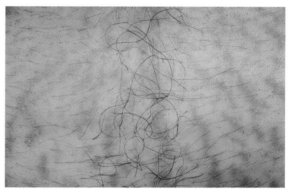

Figure 50-4. Striae associated with midpotency topical steroid use.

Table 50-2. Topical Steroid Side Effects	
LOCAL CUTANEOUS SIDE EFFECTS	**SYSTEMIC SIDE EFFECTS**
Acne vulgaris, acne rosacea, periorificial dermatitis	Cushing's syndrome
Atypical presentation of skin diseases (i.e., tinea incognito)	Fluid retention
Burning, stinging, erythema, peeling	Growth retardation, failure to thrive
Contact dermatitis	Hypothalamic-pituitary-adrenal (HPA) axis suppression
Delayed wound healing	Hypertension
Dermal atrophy with skin "dents/potholes"	Increased blood sugar
Epidermal atrophy with telangiectasia and purpura	Ocular hypertension, glaucoma, cataracts
Exacerbation of psoriasis with rebound phenomenon	
Exacerbation of skin infections and infestations	
Folliculitis	
Granuloma gluteal	
Hirsutism	
Hypopigmentation	
Skin blanching	
Steroid addiction syndrome	
Striae	
Susceptibility to skin infections	

Adults can show hypothalamic-pituitary-adrenal (HPA) axis suppression within 3 to 4 days by use of as little as 7.5 gm of superpotent topical steroid daily. However, it is rare to see clinical Cushing's syndrome in an adult patient. Superpotent topical steroids are not recommended for children under age 12 (see Table 50-2).

20. Are there topical steroid addicts?

Yes. These patients often present with a mild dermatitis that respond well to topical steroids. However, when the topical steroid is discontinued, the symptoms quickly return and are more profound. Thus, the patient is reluctant to discontinue the steroid use despite the perpetuation of the syndrome.

The topical steroid addiction syndrome is a frustrating side effect that occurs most commonly on the face or anogenital skin. Topical moisturizers, soaps, sunscreens, and makeup are poorly tolerated. Patients complain of burning and stinging as a result of thinning of the stratum corneum and epidermis. Treatment is discontinuation of the topical steroid medication; the patient should be warned that the symptoms will flare and may take weeks or even months to completely clear.

21. What is periorificial dermatitis?

Periorificial dermatitis is frequently associated with the inappropriate use of topical steroids (Fig. 50-5). It occurs most commonly in adult, fair-skinned caucasian women who have a family history of rosacea. The rash is characterized by inflammatory follicular papules and pustules with a background of erythema and scaling located on the chin, perioral, and perinasal skin, and less commonly on the eyelids. Most patients respond well to discontinuation of the topical steroid and oral antibiotics of the tetracycline class for 4 to 6 weeks. Some patients flare when the steroid is discontinued, and some have recurrences.

22. What is tinea incognito?

The symptoms produced by dermatophyte infections are due to the body's immune response to the offending fungal organism. Topical steroids decrease the inflammatory response and initially alleviate the symptoms. In decreasing the body's defense mechanisms, however, they allow the organism to proliferate, alter the typical clinical picture, and delay the correct diagnoses.

Key Points: Topical Steroids

1. Approximately 2% total body surface area (TBSA) requires 1 fingertip unit (FTU) or 0.5 gram of topical steroid medication. One percent of the patient's TBSA can be estimated as 1 palmar surface, including the fingers.
2. Provide written instructions *and* demonstration of proper FTU application technique to enhance compliance when using topical steroids. Specifically indicate that *only* low-potency topical steroids may be used in areas of thin skin (i.e., face, neck, axilla, inframammary, infrapannus, groin).
3. Tachyphylaxis may develop with prolonged use of topical steroids. To avoid this, recommend intermittent pulse dosing (i.e., 1 week of "rest" between weekly treatment periods).
4. Monitor the patient for topical corticosteroid side effects, especially potentially irreversible ones (e.g., atrophy, telangiectasia, striae). Discourage long-term use.
5. If the presumed inflammatory skin disease remains unresponsive, deteriorates, or the morphology changes after topical steroids use, reconsider the diagnosis and/or consider the possibility of contact dermatitis, bacterial infection, presence of dermatophytes or yeast, and noncompliance.

---

23. Can topical steroid medications cause contact dermatitis?

Yes. Contact dermatitis can be either irritant or allergic. Irritant reactions are frequent and most commonly are due to propylene glycol in the topical preparation. The patient complains of immediate burning or stinging after application.

True allergic contact dermatitis should be suspected when a patient does not respond predictably with appropriate topical steroid therapy. It can be due to the vehicle, preservative, fragrance, or the steroid molecule itself, and there is often cross-reactivity. Contact allergies are most common with hydrocortisone, budesonide, and tixocortol and are least common with betamethasone, clobetasol, mometasone, and triamcinolone. Patch testing may be needed to identify the allergen.

Figure 50-5. Perioral dermatitis (steroid rosacea). **A,** A prepubertal child with typical perioral dermatitis. **B,** A prepubertal child with perioral dermatitis and steroid vasoconstriction related to a midpotency topical steroid. (Courtesy of William L. Weston, MD.)

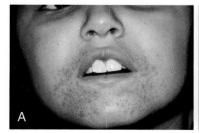
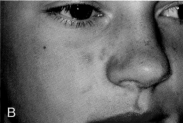

24. Mrs. Jones brings her 9-month-old infant with moderate atopic dermatitis to your office. What topical steroid do you prescribe?

Only low-potency steroids should be used in children under age 1. Once-daily application limited to areas of active inflammation after bathing is often sufficient, and the product should not be used more than twice daily. The treatment regimen should include skin lubrication to prevent rapid evaporation and transepidermal water loss. Oral antihistamines are often necessary for pruritus.

25. A 40-year-old woman presents with a 5-year history of chronic dermatitis on her palms. Lesions are plaques with abundant scale. What topical steroid do you prescribe?

Superpotent topical steroid is indicated because of the severity of disease. Additionally, the palmoplantar surfaces have reduced absorption when compared to other anatomic sites. The patient should be downgraded to a high- or midpotency topical when lesional thickness is improved. Proper lubrication and hand protection from irritants are also important for therapeutic success. If the patient requires prolonged treatment with high- or superpotency topical steroids, then alternating with nonsteroid therapies, such as topical tar or phototherapy, should be considered.

26. A 35-year-old woman with moderate psoriasis presents with scalp, facial, and body plaque lesions. What topical steroid do you prescribe?

Prescribe more than one topical steroid for this patient. A high-potency topical steroid lotion or solution would be recommended for the scalp, a low-potency cream for the face, and a high- or superpotency ointment for the trunk and extremities. When the psoriasis improves, the steroid can be downgraded to a lower-potency product or fewer applications. Topical steroid holidays or alternate treatments (i.e., anthralin, tar, vitamin D analog, phototherapy, methotrexate, biologics) should be considered for difficult chronic cases.

27. Mrs. Smith brings her 6-month-old infant with a 2-week history of diaper dermatitis to your office. What topical steroid do you prescribe? Would you recommend any other topical therapy?

For the diaper area, use only a low-potency topical steroid applied three times daily for no more than 7 to 10 days. The diaper area has air-tight occlusion, increasing the risk of local and systemic side effects (see Table 50-2). Any diaper dermatitis that has persisted for more than 3 days should be treated for secondary candidal infection. Avoid use of combination steroid/antifungal preparations.

Granuloma gluteale is a condition characterized by persistent reddish-purple nodules and plaques in the diaper area. Although the exact etiology of granuloma gluteale is debated, most agree that the inappropriate use of topical steroids and secondary candidiasis play important roles.

28. List some common mistakes that are made when prescribing a topical steroid.

- Incorrect diagnosis
- Failure to consider coexisting diseases
- Recommending a product that is either too potent or too weak
- Prescribing excessive or inadequate amount
- Recommending the wrong vehicle
- Failure to demonstrate proper application techniques
- Using the medication for too long or too short a period of time
- Use of air-tight occlusion
- Failure to recognize and monitor for topical steroid side effects
- Lack of timely follow-up to reassess disease and treatment regimen

FUNDAMENTALS OF CUTANEOUS SURGERY

Dieter K.T. Schmidt, MD, FAAD, FACMS

1. What does the term "dermatologic surgery" embrace?

Dermatologic surgery is a somewhat generic term, used to describe a variety of procedures, most commonly performed by dermatologists with specialized training in these procedures. This includes the surgical removal of tumors, both benign and malignant, with repair of the subsequent defects by simple side-to-side closure, flaps, or grafts; Mohs micrographic surgery (see Chapter 53); cryosurgery (see Chapter 52); laser treatment of vascular and pigmented skin lesions and tattoos (see Chapter 54); laser skin resurfacing for photodamaged skin; and techniques such as dermabrasion, chemical peeling, sclerotherapy, hair transplantation, liposuction, and soft tissue augmentation. Many of these procedures were pioneered by dermatologists. Several excellent textbooks have been devoted to dermatologic surgery.

Fewkes JL, Cheney ML, Pollack SV: *Illustrated atlas of cutaneous surgery*, New York, 1992, Gower Medical Publishing.
Lask GP, Moy RL: *Principles and techniques of cutaneous surgery*, New York, 1996, McGraw-Hill.
Lawrence C: *An introduction to dermatological surgery*, London, 1996, Blackwell Science.
Wheeland RG: *Cutaneous surgery*, Philadelphia, 1994, WB Saunders.

2. Local anesthetics can be broadly classified into one of two groups. Name these two groups and give a few examples of each.

The ester group of local anesthetics, which is seldom used in skin surgery, includes procaine (Novocaine), chloroprocaine (Nesacaine), tetracaine (Pontocaine), and cocaine hydrochloride. The amide group of local anesthetics, commonly used in skin surgery, includes lidocaine (Xylocaine), mepivacaine (Polocaine), bupivacaine (Sensorcaine, Marcaine), and prilocaine (Citanest).

3. How do the local anesthetics work?

Local anesthetics decrease the sodium permeability of the nerve fiber membrane, thereby lowering the action potential of the nerve fiber and preventing depolarization of the fiber.

4. What are the onset of action and the duration of action of the most commonly used local anesthetics in skin surgery?

The amides, especially lidocaine and bupivacaine, are the most commonly used local anesthetics in skin surgery. Lidocaine has an onset of action of approximately 5 minutes. Its potency and duration of action is significantly greater than that of procaine. When combined with epinephrine, it provides anesthesia for 60 to 400 minutes (average: 180 minutes), compared to 30 to 120 minutes (average: 90 minutes) without epinephrine. Bupivacaine, which is more potent than lidocaine, has an onset of action of approximately 8 minutes, and an average duration of action of 120 to 140 minutes without epinephrine, and 240 to 480 minutes with epinephrine. This makes it an ideal agent for regional nerve blocks and Mohs micrographic surgery.

5. How are the amide and ester anesthetics metabolized?

The amides are metabolized by hepatic microsomal enzymes. These drugs should therefore be used with great caution in patients with underlying liver disease. The esters are metabolized by plasma pseudocholinesterase, to form para-aminobenzoic acid (PABA) and diethylamino ethanol, both of which are excreted by the kidneys.

6. What is the greatest practical drawback of the ester anesthetics?

There is a relatively high incidence of allergic reactions in patients previously sensitized to PABA.

7. What are the maximum total dosages for 1% lidocaine (10 mg/mL) in adults and children?

See Table 51-1.

8. What are the symptoms and signs of lidocaine toxicity and how is it treated?

The effects on the central nervous system can be divided into early (serum lidocaine levels of 1 to 5 gm/mL), mid (5 to 12 gm/mL), and late (20 to 25 mg/kg) effects.

- **Early effects:** Talkativeness, metallic taste, diplopia, tinnitus, lightheadedness, nausea, circumoral pallor, and vomiting. Observation is the only treatment necessary. Recognition of early lidocaine toxicity is of paramount importance.
- **Mid effects:** Nystagmus, slurred speech, hallucinations, muscle twitching, facial/hand tremors, and seizures. Treatment includes observation, oxygen, and intravenous diazepam for seizures.

Table 51-1. Recommended Maximum Total Dosages for 1% Lidocaine (10 mg/mL) with and without Epinephrine in Adults and Children

ADULTS	CHILDREN
4.5 mg/kg (300 mg or 30 mL), without epinephrine	1.5–2.5 mg/kg, without epinephrine
7.0 mg/kg (500 mg or 50 mL), with epinephrine	3.0–4.0 mg/kg, with epinephrine

- **Late effects:** Apnea, coma. Cardiovascular effects include bradycardia, hypotension, atrioventricular block, ventricular arrhythmias, hypoxia, and acidosis. Treatment is directed accordingly, per advanced cardiac life support (ACLS) protocols.

9. **Do true allergic reactions to local anesthetics exist?**
Yes, but they are very uncommon. Usually, these reactions are seen with the ester anesthetics. These patients are either allergic to the paraben preservatives found in these preparations or to the ester metabolite, PABA. Parabens are known to cross react with PABA. Lidocaine is an excellent substitute in cases of true ester anesthetic allergy, as no cross-reactivity exists between the amide and ester groups of anesthetics. True allergic reactions to lidocaine are extremely rare. Most of the so-called allergic reactions to lidocaine are, in fact, due to vasovagal syncope or, less commonly, epinephrine side effects. However, patients may be allergic to the parabens and sodium metabisulfite preservatives. Preservative-free lidocaine is available.

10. **Describe the clinical features of true local anesthetic allergy. How is this best treated?**
Patients may present with urticaria, angioedema, anaphylactoid reactions, or even anaphylaxis. Treatment is directed accordingly, per ACLS protocols, using subcutaneous epinephrine (0.3 mL of a 1:1000 solution), intravenous antihistamines, intravenous dexamethasone (4 to 12 mg), and oxygen.

11. **What is the clinical presentation of patients with a vasovagal response to local anesthesia? How is this presentation best treated?**
Psychological factors, including needle phobia and altered pain perception, may induce a vasovagal response, the clinical features of which include pallor, diaphoresis, hyperventilation, nausea, vomiting, hypotension, and syncope. Usually, placing the patient in the Trendelenburg position (i.e., supine, with the head lower than the legs) and the application of moist towels to the patient's face is sufficient to reverse the condition. Aromatic spirits of ammonia may also be of benefit. For prolonged hypotension, an intravenous line must be established and vasopressors given, as needed. ACLS protocols should be followed.

12. **How does one manage the patient who refuses, or is truly allergic to, both the ester and the amide anesthetics?**
Normal saline (0.9%) may be an effective alternative to the ester and amide anesthetics for performing shave excisions and punch biopsies. "Anesthesia" is thought to result from the compression of nerve endings by the hydrostatic pressure of the injected saline. There may also be an added anesthetic effect from benzyl alcohol, a preservative in normal saline. Non-bacteriostatic saline should be used for patients sensitive to methylparaben. Diphenhydramine (10 to 25 mg/mL) is effective, but painful and sedating. It has a short duration of action and may induce tissue necrosis. Epinephrine, 1:200,000, can be added to prolong the anesthetic effect.

13. **What concentrations of epinephrine are the most effective for skin surgery? What is the safe maximum total dose?**
Epinephrine, 1:100,000 (1 mg/100 mL), is the most commonly used concentration in skin surgery, although a concentration of 1:200,000 is just as effective. Always try to use the lowest concentration possible. Dilutions of up to 1:500,000 are still effective. Concentrations of 1:50,000 or higher may induce tissue necrosis due to prolonged ischemia. The safe, maximum dose of epinephrine given at any one time is 0.2 mg for an adult. Onset of action may be as long as 15 minutes.

14. **What is the onset of action for epinephrine?**
Vasoconstriction starts to occur approximately 3 minutes after injection, but the full effect is not seen until 15 minutes have elapsed. Therefore, for procedures in which a relatively bloodless field is a priority, you should wait for 15 minutes before commencing surgery.

15. **What are the clinical features of epinephrine toxicity?**
Severe apprehension, restlessness, palpitations, headache, tachycardia, and hypertension.

16. **Are allergic reactions to epinephrine possible?**
Most authors doubt the existence of true allergic reactions to epinephrine. If they do occur, they are extremely rare.

17. When should epinephrine be used with great caution?

In patients with hypertension, ischemic heart disease, peripheral vascular occlusive disease, hyperthyroidism, or pheochromocytoma, epinephrine should either be avoided or diluted, and the patient must be carefully monitored. Epinephrine should either be avoided or diluted in patients taking beta-blocking drugs, especially propranolol, as they are at risk for developing paradoxical hypertension, reflex bradycardia, and cardiac arrest. Epinephrine is contraindicated in patients taking phenothiazines, tricyclic antidepressants, and monoamine oxidase (MAO) inhibitors. Epinephrine should also be avoided in pregnancy, especially during the first and third trimesters, and in patients with a history of psychiatric disease. Many authors also suggest avoiding epinephrine for the digits, especially if the patient is a heavy smoker or has peripheral arteriosclerosis, vasospastic disease, collagen vascular disease, or other peripheral vascular disease.

18. Which local anesthetics are "the safest" to use in pregnancy?

Bupivacaine and chloroprocaine. Both drugs are classified as Food and Drug Administration (FDA) pregnancy risk category C. However, it is preferable to avoid all local anesthetics, if possible. Epinephrine should not be used in pregnancy.

19. Describe measures that can be employed to diminish the pain associated with the injection of local anesthetics.

- **Antianxiety measures:** Explain the procedure in detail to the patient, and make sure they understand what you are about to do. Premedication with oral diazepam or similar drugs may be useful for extremely anxious patients.
- **Topical anesthetics**: These are especially useful in children. EMLA cream (2.5% lidocaine, 2.5% prilocaine), topical lidocaine creams and gels (2% to 30%), refrigerant spray, and ice blocks may all be useful. L-M-X-4 cream (4% lidocaine) has a more rapid onset than EMLA cream and does not require a prescription.
- **Increase pH of anesthetic solution:** Add 8.4% sodium bicarbonate to lidocaine, in a 1:10 ratio (1 part bicarbonate, 10 parts lidocaine). Buffering an anesthetic solution in this way may shorten its duration of action. Anesthesia can be reinforced using a nonbuffered or long-acting anesthetic.
- **Warm the anesthetic solution** before injection.

20. Discuss injection techniques that can be used to diminish pain.

- **Distractive measures:** These may include pinching or rubbing of the skin at the proposed needle entry site.
- **Small-diameter, long needles:** Half-inch, 30-gauge needles are a good choice for smaller areas. For larger areas, 1-inch, 30-gauge needles are best. Insert the needle through an accentuated skin pore, if present (e.g., the face).
- **Insert the needle quickly** with the bevel pointing upward; a slow insertion leads to greater discomfort. Inject a small aliquot of anesthetic, wait a minute, and then advance the needle slowly, before depositing further anesthetic. When anesthetizing large areas, needle reinsertion sites should be in skin that has already been anesthetized.
- **Limit the volume** of anesthetic and **inject it very slowly**. Rapid tissue distention is painful.

21. What are the two most commonly used skin preparation antiseptics in dermatologic surgery?

Povidone-iodine (Betadine) and chlorhexidine gluconate (Hibiclens).

22. Describe the mechanisms of action and spectra of coverage for these two preparations.

Povidone-iodine releases free iodine, which enters microbial cells through their cell membranes, causing cell death. Up to 5 minutes of contact time is required for microbial uptake of the free iodine and cell death. It should therefore be allowed to completely dry on the skin surface before starting surgery. The activity of povidone-iodine ends after it has dried. Povidone-iodine is microbicidal for gram-positive and gram-negative bacteria, fungi, viruses, protozoa, and yeasts. At lower concentrations, chlorhexidine gluconate is bacteriostatic, by binding to microbial cell walls with subsequent osmotic disequilibrium. At higher concentrations, it induces precipitation of intracytoplasmic organelles and cell death. Chlorhexidine gluconate is microbicidal for gram-positive and gram-negative bacteria, facultative anaerobes, aerobes, and yeast.

23. What are the most important advantages and disadvantages of povidone-iodine and chlorhexidine gluconate?

Povidone-iodine has a relatively slow onset of action, and its activity ends after it has dried. It is inactivated by contact with blood and other organic substances. It is also toxic to the cells within an open wound, with resultant delayed wound healing.

Chlorhexidine gluconate has a much faster onset of action and maintains its antimicrobial activity for up to 6 hours. It should not be used for preoperative skin preparation on the head and neck, due to possible ototoxicity and corneal erosions and opacifications with inadvertent exposure at these sites. Povidone-iodine is a better choice for the head and neck. However, chlorhexidine gluconate is preferable to povidone-iodine for the trunk and extremities, due to its more rapid onset of action, broader spectrum of antimicrobial coverage, and longer duration of activity.

24. What is meant by *absorbable* and *nonabsorbable* suture material?
The classification of suture material into absorbable or nonabsorbable is based on how quickly its tensile strength is lost. Most nonabsorbable sutures retain the majority of their tensile strength by day 60, and in fact, can, be completely absorbed over a prolonged period. Most absorbable sutures lose the majority of their tensile strength by day 60 and may be present for long periods before being absorbed.

25. How does multifilament suture differ from monofilament suture?
- **Multifilament suture** is usually in a braided configuration, and offers the advantages of improved ease of handling, low memory, and good knot security. Disadvantages include a supposed increase in the rate of associated wound infection, although this remains controversial. There is, however, increased tissue reaction to this type of suture material.
- **Monofilament suture** is associated with a lower rate of wound infection, and tissue reaction to the suture is generally much less than for braided sutures. Furthermore, this type of suture demonstrates improved ease of passage through tissue, making it ideal for subcuticular, running stitches. Disadvantages include increased memory with resultant poorer handling qualities and diminished knot security. Difficulties with handling are easily overcome with practice, and knot security can be greatly improved by an extra throw during knot tying.

26. Which types of suture material are best suited for subcutaneous stitches?
Generally, absorbable sutures are used for subcutaneous stitches.
- **Polyglactin 910 (Vicryl)** is a synthetic, absorbable, multifilament suture. It has a high tensile strength, 50% of which is lost by day 14, and is insignificant by day 30. Absorption occurs by enzymatic hydrolysis and is complete at approximately 90 to 120 days. Tissue reactivity is relatively low.
- **Polyglyconate (Maxon)** is a synthetic, absorbable, monofilament suture. It has a high tensile strength, 50% of which is lost by day 30, but may remain significant for 3 to 6 months. It is especially useful when prolonged wound support is needed. Complete absorption occurs after approximately 180 days. Tissue reactivity is similar to polyglactin 910 (Vicryl). It has a relatively low memory, very good handling characteristics, and good knot security.

27. Which types of suture material are best suited for cutaneous stitches?
Generally, nonabsorbable suture material is used for cutaneous stitches.
- **Nylon** is a synthetic, nonabsorbable suture, available in **monofilament (Ethilon)** and **braided (Nurolon)** forms. Nylon has high tensile strength and elicits very little tissue response as it is chemically inert. Monofilament nylon induces less of a tissue reaction than does braided nylon, but due to its greater memory, it is more difficult to handle and has lower knot security.
- **Polypropylene (Prolene, Surgilene)** is a synthetic, nonabsorbable, monofilament suture, characterized by very low tissue reactivity and great ease of tissue passage, making it an ideal choice for a running, subcuticular stitch. It has a high degree of memory, resulting in relatively poor handling and knot security.

28. Which sutures are good choices for mucosal surfaces, the vermilion lip, and intertriginous areas?
- **Silk** is a natural, nonabsorbable, braided suture with unsurpassed ease of handling and softness. It is an excellent choice for intertriginous areas, intraoral use, and the vermilion lip. It induces a significant tissue response and may be associated with an increased rate of wound infection. Suture removal may be relatively painful and more difficult than with other materials, as silk swells to almost double its original diameter by day 14.
- **Polyester** is a synthetic, nonabsorbable, braided suture available in uncoated (Mersilene) and coated (Ethibond) forms. The coated suture has improved handling characteristics and a softness similar to silk.

29. How is suture sized?
Suture size does not correspond to a specific diameter, but rather to a specific tensile strength. Thus, 4/0 polypropylene and 4/0 silk have different diameters. For any given suture type, the tensile strength (and diameter) of that suture decreases as the designated suture number (e.g., 4/0, 5/0, 6/0) increases.

30. Which suture needles are best suited to skin surgery?
A three-eighths (or half-circle) needle with a reverse cutting point is the preferred and most commonly used needle in cutaneous surgery. The point of the needle is triangular on cross section, with the apex of the triangle on the outside/convex side of the needle and the base of the needle on the inside/concave side. This decreases the tendency for the suture to cut inward toward the wound, thereby minimizing trauma.

31. What are the indications for a punch biopsy?
A punch biopsy may serve as an incisional or excisional skin biopsy, and is used to diagnose both inflammatory and neoplastic diseases. It provides a sample of tissue, which includes epidermis, dermis, and subcutaneous fat. When the pathology is thought to be localized to the epidermis and/or upper dermis, then a superficial shave biopsy may be more appropriate (Fig. 51-1). However, one should always try to completely remove pigmented lesions by conservative excisional or punch biopsy. When it is not possible to completely remove a pigmented lesion by excisional or punch biopsy, then the darkest and/or most elevated portion of the lesion should be biopsied, to achieve the highest

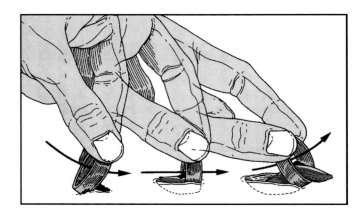

Figure 51-1. Schematic demonstrating the technique for a shave biopsy of skin. (From Fewkes JL, Cheney ML, Pollack SV: *Illustrated atlas of cutaneous surgery*, New York, 1992, Gower Medical Publishing, with permission.)

diagnostic yield. It may also be prudent in these cases to take multiple "scouting" biopsies from different areas of concern within the lesion, to increase your chances of an accurate diagnosis and, in the case of a melanoma, to obtain an accurate Breslow depth. Punches range in size from 2 to 8 mm, with 3- or 4-mm punches being the most commonly used sizes. Disposable punches are especially useful for patients with hepatitis B or C, or HIV disease.

32. Describe how a punch biopsy should be performed.

After anesthetizing and prepping the surgical site, the circular blade of the punch is placed over the lesion at 90 degrees to the skin surface. The handle of the punch is gently held between thumb and forefinger, and the blade is rotated in a fairly rapidly alternating clockwise, anticlockwise fashion, while maintaining skin tautness across the biopsy site using thumb and index finger. Initially, very little downward pressure should be applied to the punch while the punch's blade is still at the level of the epidermis, to prevent shearing of the epidermis from the dermis, which makes histologic examination difficult. Continue until the hub of the punch reaches the level of the skin. In certain anatomic sites with important superficial nerves and vessels, be careful not to hub the punch. Now remove the punch.

33. What is the preferred technique for removing the punch biopsy?

Gently grasp the biopsy specimen with a toothed forceps, preferably at the level of the subcutaneous fat. Be careful not to grasp the specimen with too much pressure as this may cause pressure artifacts, which will make histologic examination difficult. While pulling the specimen gently upward, carefully cut the specimen at the level of the deep subcutaneous fat. Hemostasis is usually achieved with suture closure of the defect. Alternatively, the defect may be allowed to heal by secondary intention.

34. What is meant by electrosurgery, electrocautery, and electrocoagulation?

- **Electrosurgery** is the use of an electric current in order to achieve hemostasis, tissue cutting, or the destruction of benign and malignant skin lesions.
- **Electrocautery** uses a low-voltage, high-amperage electric current to heat a filament tip, which transfers the heat to tissue, thereby inducing coagulation. No electric current is transferred to the tissue or patient, which makes this a good choice for cardiac pacemaker patients.
- **Electrocoagulation** uses a low-voltage, high-amperage current to coagulate blood vessels by generating heat in tissue. The patient forms part of the circuit by using a dispersive electrode, which allows for a greater degree of coagulation than either electrofulguration or electrodesiccation (see following text).

35. Describe what is meant by electrofulguration and electrodesiccation.

- **Electrofulguration** uses a high-voltage, low-amperage electric current to generate a spark that jumps from the electrode tip to the tissue, thereby achieving coagulation. There is no contact between the electrode and the tissue, resulting in little tissue damage.
- **Electrodesiccation**, like electrofulguration, uses a high-voltage, low-amperage electric current. However, unlike electrofulguration, there is contact between the electrode tip and the patient. Heat is thereby transferred to the tissue, resulting in desiccation. Tissue damage is typically greater than with electrofulguration.

36. What precautions need to be taken in patients with pacemakers who require electrosurgery?

Electrosurgery may cause a pacemaker to fire prematurely or not at all. Electrocautery is a safer alternative to electrosurgery in these patients. Consultation with the patient's cardiologist is imperative if electrosurgery is contemplated. Demand-type pacemakers are more sensitive to electrosurgery than are fixed-rate pacemakers. However, many newer pacemakers are protected from interference by electric currents. Demand pacemakers can be converted to fixed-rate pacemakers by placing a magnet over the pacemaker, thereby preventing interference from electrical current. The use of bipolar (biterminal) electrosurgery, with the dispersive electrode placed close to the treatment electrode and away from the pacemaker, and using short bursts of electricity will all reduce the chances of pacemaker interference.

37. Is it necessary to discontinue anticoagulant medications before elective surgery of the skin?

No. Most Mohs surgeons are comfortable performing surgery on patients who are on aspirin, clopidogrel, warfarin, or other anticoagulants. In fact, recent literature suggests that all patients should be kept on their anticoagulant therapy, so as to prevent acute cardiovascular events, including strokes. Meticulous intraoperative hemostasis is crucial to preventing hematoma formation. Consultation with the patient's internist or cardiologist is imperative if discontinuation of anticoagulant therapy is contemplated.

38. What are the so-called relaxed skin tension lines (RSTLs)? Why are they important?

The insertion of the underlying musculature into the skin results in a somewhat predictable pattern of skin creases, called RSTLs. Typically, these lines run perpendicular to the long axis of the underlying musculature (Fig. 51-2). Surgical incisions placed within or parallel to these lines will create the most favorable scar.

39. How does one determine the direction of the RSTLs in planning a surgical wound closure?

By simply pinching the skin in different directions around the proposed surgical excision site, the direction in which the closure will produce the least amount of tension across the wound (i.e., the direction of the RSTLs) is usually easily revealed. It is important to pinch the skin using the thumb and index finger of the *same* hand.

40. Which areas of the body typically scar worst?

The upper back, shoulders, upper arms, and central chest. Wounds at these sites are often under significant tension, which may be a contributing factor.

41. What is the superficial muscular aponeurotic system (SMAS)?

The SMAS may be defined as the combination of the muscles of facial expression and their enveloping fascia. The SMAS has its origin in the superficial cervical fascia, and allows the muscles of facial expression to act in a coordinated fashion. It is an important anatomic landmark in facial surgery.

Breisch EA, Greenway HT Jr: *Cutaneous surgical anatomy of the head and neck*, New York, 1992, Churchill Livingstone.

42. Describe the boundaries of the danger area for transecting the temporal branch of the facial nerve.

Consider the danger area to be a triangle, made up of a line drawn from a point 0.5 cm below the tragus to a point 2 cm above the lateral eyebrow, a line drawn along the zygoma to the lateral orbital rim, and a line drawn from the point above the lateral eyebrow down past the lateral eyebrow to the medial zygoma (Fig. 51-3). The temporal nerve lies just deep to the SMAS-temporoparietal fascia within this triangle.

Seckel BR: *Facial danger zones: avoiding nerve injury in facial plastic surgery*, St Louis, Quality Medical Publishing, 1994, Quality Medical Publishing.

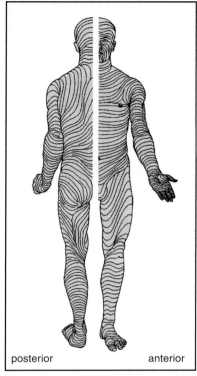

posterior   anterior

Figure 51-2. Schematic demonstrating the most likely direction of relaxed skin tension lines. (From Fewkes JL, Cheney ML, Pollack SV: *Illustrated atlas of cutaneous surgery*, New York, 1992, Gower Medical Publishing, with permission.)

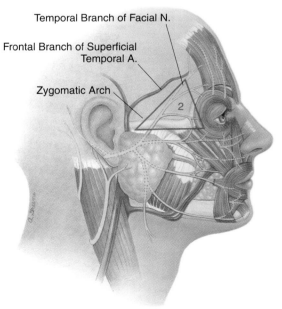

Temporal Branch of Facial N.

Frontal Branch of Superficial Temporal A.

Zygomatic Arch

2

Figure 51-3. Schematic demonstrating the danger zone for the temporal branch of the facial nerve (blue triangle). (From Seckel BR: *Facial danger zones: avoiding nerve injury in facial plastic surgery*, 2nd ed. St. Louis, Quality Medical Publishing, Inc., 2010, with permission.)

Key Points: Fundamentals of Cutaneous Surgery

1. Local anesthetics work by decreasing the sodium permeability of the nerve fiber membrane, thereby lowering the action potential and preventing depolarization.
2. Amide anesthetics are metabolized by hepatic microsomal enzymes, and ester anesthetics are metabolized by plasma pseudocholinesterase.
3. The safe total maximum dose of 1% lidocaine for adults is 7 mg/kg, if combined with epinephrine, and 4.5 mg/kg, if given without epinephrine.
4. The relaxed skin tension lines are a somewhat predictable pattern of skin creases, caused by the insertion of the underlying musculature into the skin.
5. Damage to the temporal branch of the facial nerve will result in an ipsilateral brow ptosis and ipsilateral lack of forehead animation.

43. Describe the clinical signs of damage to this nerve.

The temporal branch of the facial nerve supplies the frontalis muscle. Damage to this nerve will result in an ipsilateral brow ptosis and ipsilateral lack of forehead animation (Fig. 51-4).

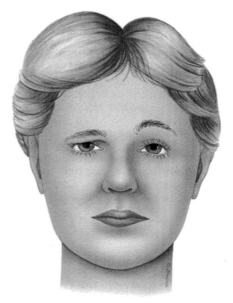

Figure 51-4. Schematic demonstrating ipsilateral brow ptosis as a result of damage to the right temporal branch of the facial nerve. (From Seckel BR: *Facial danger zones: avoiding nerve injury in facial plastic surgery*, 2nd ed. St. Louis, Quality Medical Publishing, Inc., 2010, with permission.)

CRYOSURGERY

Mariah Ruth Brown, MD, and Milton J. Schleve, MD

CHAPTER 52

1. What is cryosurgery?

Cryosurgery is the controlled application of cold to cause tissue damage. It can be used to treat both benign and malignant skin conditions. With cryosurgery, the degree of tissue damage is controlled in order to destroy the target lesion with minimal damage to normal surrounding tissue.

Gage AA: History of cryosurgery, *Semin Surg Oncol* 14:99–109, 1998.
Korpan N: *Atlas of cryosurgery*, Wien, Springer, 2001.

2. How does cryosurgery cause injury?

Freezing causes intracellular and extracellular ice crystals to form, and the subsequent vascular stasis causes tissue anoxia and necrosis. The most efficient technique employs a rapid freeze and slow thawing. Multiple short freezes produce more damage than a long freeze. Different cell types have variable susceptibility to the effects of freezing, with melanocytes being damaged at a much higher temperature than keratinocytes ($-5°$ C versus $-50°$ C). This differential freezing has implications for the treatment of melanocytic lesions, as well as the use of cryosurgery in patients with darkly pigmented skin.

Gage AA, Baust J: Mechanisms of tissue injury in cryosurgery, *Cryobiology* 37:171–186, 1998.

3. Which agents are used for cryosurgery?

Most cryosurgeons use liquid nitrogen. It is readily available, inexpensive, easy to store, easy to use, and it works quickly. Less commonly used cryogens are Freon 12, Freon 22, solid CO_2, liquid N_2O (nitrous oxide), and liquid helium (Table 52-1). Because a colder cryogen causes deeper destruction, the Freons, solid CO_2, and nitrous oxide are used only for topical anesthesia and superficial destruction. Liquid nitrogen is the only agent that is reliable for deeper destruction.

4. Do you need a lot of expensive equipment to use cryosurgery?

No. Compared to other surgical techniques, the amount of equipment needed is modest. First, you need a reservoir for the liquid nitrogen. This is normally a 20- to 30-liter thermos (Dewar flask). From here, the liquid nitrogen (LN_2) is transferred to smaller containers. For basic cryosurgery, most dermatologists use small, handheld thermoses that spray the LN_2 directly on the skin (Fig. 52-1). There are also various probes, neoprene cones, and thermocouple-pyrometer systems to treat malignant lesions.

Jackson A, Colver G, Dawber R: *Cutaneous cryosurgery: principles and clinical practice*, ed 3, New York, 2005, Taylor & Francis.

5. What types of skin conditions can be treated with cryosurgery?

Both benign (Table 52-2) and malignant (Table 52-3) lesions can be treated by cryosurgery. The most common lesions are warts, actinic keratoses, seborrheic keratoses, and molluscum contagiosum. Cryosurgery is one of the most common procedures performed by dermatologists.

Andrews MD: Cryosurgery for common skin conditions, *Am Fam Physician* 69:2365–2372, 2004.

6. How is cryosurgery performed?

There are several ways to apply cryogens. Various sizes of **swabs** can be dipped in LN_2 and touched to the lesion to freeze it. Due to the rapid dispersal of cold, swabs do not result in as much tissue cooling as the direct application of LN_2 to the skin. Swabs are not used to treat malignancies. Various surgical instruments, such as hemostats and pick-ups (tweezers), can be used for cryosurgery of raised or pedunculated lesions. The surgical instrument is submerged in LN_2

Table 52-1. Cryogens Used in Cryosurgery	
CRYOGEN	**BOILING POINT (°C)**
Liquid nitrogen	-195.8
Nitrous oxide, liquid	-89.5
Carbon dioxide, solid	-8.5
Chlorodifluoromethane (Freon 22)	-40.8
Dichlorofluoromethane (Freon 12)	-27.8

for 20 to 30 seconds and then the target lesion is grasped with the instrument. It is best to use a separate swab or surgical instrument and cup of cryogen for each patient to avoid cross-contamination

The **spray technique** uses modified thermoses that allow the LN_2 to spray out of a nozzle (see Fig. 52-1). The degree of freezing is changed by the nozzle size, the pressure in the thermos, the distance to the lesion, and the length of freeze. This apparatus can be used for several hours, and contamination is not an issue. It also can treat very large lesions. A modification of this technique is to use neoprene cones to confine the LN_2, causing a more concentrated freeze.

Some cryosurgeons use **probes** for freezing. A probe is a metal object that is cooled by the cryogen and applied to the lesion. The probe is usually the size of the lesion, but it can be applied multiple times for larger lesions. A probe can vary from a diameter of a few millimeters to a hollow brass doorknob. The disadvantages are that it is slower than the spray technique, a variety of sizes and shapes of probes are needed, and contamination can occur.

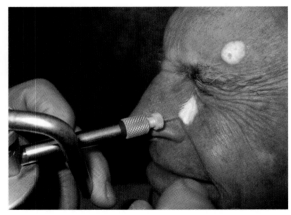

Figure 52-1. A handheld cryotherapy unit is being used to spray actinic keratoses with liquid nitrogen. Note the cutaneous ice ball that forms in the treated areas.

7. How are benign skin lesions treated?

The basic concept of all cryosurgery is that the depth of freezing is proportional to the width of the area frozen. When cryogen is applied, an ice ball forms in the skin for which the depth of freezing is equal to the radius of the surface freeze. Freezing 1 to 2 mm beyond the lesion with a single freeze-thaw cycle is adequate for most benign lesions. Warts can be deeper, so either a deeper freeze or multiple smaller freezes can be used. Thick seborrheic keratoses can be frozen lightly and quickly curetted. For benign lesions, you do not want to cause a scar, so it is always better to undertreat until you are experienced. When treating benign lesions, it is always important to be confident in your clinical diagnosis. If you have questions about whether or not a lesion is benign, or if a lesion does not resolve with cryosurgery, a biopsy should be performed to provide a histological diagnosis.

Jester DM: Office procedures: cryotherapy of dermal abnormalities, *Prim Care* 24:269–280, 1997.

Table 52-2. Benign Lesions Treatable by Cryosurgery	
Acne	Lentigo simplex
Acrochordon (skin tag)	Molluscum contagiosum
Actinic cheilitis	Myxoid cyst
Actinic keratosis	Pyogenic granuloma
Angioma	Sebaceous hyperplasia
Chondrodermatitis nodularis helicis	Seborrheic keratosis
Dermatofibroma	Warts
Genital warts	Keloid
Hypertrophic scar	

Table 52-3. Malignant Lesions Requiring Monitoring During Cryosurgery
Basal cell carcinoma
Squamous cell carcinoma in situ (Bowen's disease)
Kaposi's sarcoma
Squamous cell carcinoma
Keratoacanthoma
Lentigo maligna
Metastatic skin lesions (palliative)

8. How do you treat malignant lesions?

In treating cancers, we need to be very sure we treat them adequately. Most importantly, you should be able to clinically identify the margins of the lesion. Second, you must know the histology of the cancer to be sure cryosurgery is appropriate. Third, you must have equipment that ensures you reach a temperature of $-50°$ C to $-60°$ C beyond the peripheral extent and depth of the cancer. Malignant lesions require longer freeze times than benign lesions. Most malignant tumors require at least a 30-second freeze with two freeze-thaw cycles. Curetting or shaving tumors first to delineate and debulk the lesion prior to cryosurgery can permit more effective treatment. For large tumors, multiple treatments are often required. Repeat biopsies after cryosurgery can histologically confirm the resolution of the tumor.

Graham GF: Cryosurgery in the management of cutaneous malignancies, *Clin Dermatol* 19:321–327, 2001.

Key Points: Cryosurgery

1. Cryosurgery can be used for benign and malignant lesions.
2. Avoid scarring when treating benign lesions. Consider a biopsy, if no response.
3. When treating malignancies, choose the lesions carefully, document your treatment, and observe for recurrence.

9. Is cryosurgery a preferred method for the treatment of cutaneous malignancy?

The treatment of cutaneous cancers by cryosurgery is not accepted by all dermatologists. In general, surgically oriented dermatologists feel that the demonstration of negative surgical margins is preferable to cryosurgery for significant cancers. In addition, cryosurgery can have significant postoperative morbidity for patients and may result in less than ideal scars. As a result, many dermatologists reserve cryosurgery for malignant lesions to special circumstances. In particular, patients who cannot tolerate conventional surgery, due to other health concerns, are often ideal patients for cryosurgery. Cryosurgeons argue that the cure rates achieved by cryosurgery are comparable to those of other surgical modalities, especially when the margins of the tumor can be identified. They advocate that cryosurgery should be considered equivalent to surgical excision in the treatment of malignant cutaneous tumors.

Thissen M, Nieman F, Ideler A, et al: Cosmetic results of cryosurgery versus surgical excision for primary uncomplicated basal cell carcinomas of the head and neck, *Dermatol Surg* 26:759–764, 2000.

10. What are the cure rates of cryosurgery for malignant lesions?

Experienced cryosurgeons who treat many skin cancers report cure rates of 95% to 98% for primary basal cell carcinomas. These cure rates are comparable to those reported with surgery and radiation therapy. Similar rates are reported for the treatment of squamous cell carcinoma with cryosurgery. Lentigo maligna has also been successfully treated with cryosurgery due to its superficial nature and the sensitivity of melanocytes to freezing. Cure rates of great than 90% have been reported with cryosurgery in the treatment of lentigo maligna. However, cryosurgery is not an appropriate therapy for invasive melanoma. The cure rates using cryosurgery, radiation therapy, or excisional surgery for aggressive or recurrent skin cancers are significantly lower than those reported for simple, primary tumors. In these cases, Mohs micrographic surgery is often recommended.

Neville J, Welch E, Leffell D: Management of nonmelanoma skin cancer in 2007, *Nat Clin Pract Oncol* 4:462–469, 2007.
Stevenson O, Ahmed I: Lentigo maligna: prognosis and treatment options, *Am J Clin Dermatol* 6:151–164, 2005.

11. Are there contraindications to cryosurgery?

People with cold-related conditions, such as cryoglobulinemia, cryofibrinogenemia, cold urticaria, and Raynaud's disease, should not be treated with cryosurgery. Patients with heavily pigmented skin should be treated with caution because they are more likely to heal with hyperpigmented or hypopigmented scars, due to the sensitivity of melanocytes to freezing. In addition, the use of cryosurgery in hair-bearing areas may result in alopecia.

12. For which patients is cryosurgery better than other methods?

Cryosurgery can be used for patients with bleeding disorders and in elderly patients in nursing homes. It avoids cross-contamination in patients with warts, hepatitis, and HIV.

13. What are the complications of cryosurgery?

After using cryosurgery, the wound is allowed to heal by itself (second intention). A normal cryosurgery wound can blister, ooze, form an eschar, and take 1 to 6 weeks to heal. Complications are uncommon and include infection, hypertrophic scars, nerve damage, and unacceptable scars. Before performing cryosurgery, the normal course of healing and the potential risks of the procedure should be discussed with the patient.

MOHS SURGERY

Mariah Ruth Brown, MD, and J. Ramsey Mellette Jr., MD

1. What is Mohs surgery?

In 1936, Dr. Frederic Mohs, of the University of Wisconsin, developed a precise tumor extirpation technique that involved the controlled, serial, microscopic examination of tissue that had been chemically fixed with zinc chloride paste. The excised tissue was systematically mapped, frozen sections were examined, and the process was then repeated at foci of residual malignancy until a completely tumor-free plane was reached. The goals of Mohs surgery are to completely remove the tumor and to maximize tissue conservation.

2. Is Mohs surgery still performed with the zinc chloride chemical paste?

Very rarely. The technique has evolved to use fresh frozen tissue methods. In the 1970s, the use of frozen sections alone in Mohs surgery was shown to have comparable cure rates to the use of zinc chloride paste. The elimination of zinc chloride paste allowed Mohs surgery to take place in a single day and avoided the pain associated with paste application. In addition, the use of frozen sections made it possible for reconstruction of the Mohs defect to occur the same day as tumor removal.

3. When is Mohs surgery indicated for basal cell and squamous cell carcinoma?

Mohs micrographic surgery is especially effective in treating basal cell carcinomas (BCC) and squamous cell carcinomas (SCC) of the face and other cosmetically sensitive areas, because it can eliminate the cancer while sparing surrounding normal skin. It is also ideal for the removal of recurrent skin cancers. In these tumors, cancer cells persist in areas of scar tissue, and the clinical margins of the recurrent tumor are often indistinct. Cure rates are 99% for primary basal cell cancers and 95% for recurrent tumors. Other indications for Mohs' surgery include

- BCC with aggressive histopathologic features, such as morpheaform or sclerotic (desmoplastic), micronodular, superficial spreading, and infiltrative growth patterns, subtypes which often extend beyond visualized margins
- Excessively large or deeply invasive cancers
- Primary BCC or SCC with poorly defined borders, especially those present in locations known to have high recurrence rates (nasolabial fold, nasal ala, medial canthus, pinna, and postauricular sulcus)
- Any BCC or SCC adjacent to or within an orifice, such as nostrils or ear canals
- Any location where maximum preservation of normal tissue is paramount (e.g., nasal tip, nasal ala, lips, eyelids, ears, genitalia, fingers)
- Tumors with positive margins after standard excision
- Tumors in immunosuppressed patients

Otley CC, Salasche SJ: Mohs' surgery: efficient and effective, *Br J Ophthalmol* 88:985–988, 2004.

4. Is Mohs surgery appropriate for all basal and squamous cell carcinomas?

BCC and SCC are epidemic in the United States. Standard treatments, including excisional surgery, electrodesiccation and curettage, cryosurgery, and radiation therapy, have cure rates in selected series near 90%. Mohs surgery should usually be limited to indications outlined in Question 3, due to the time and expense required by the procedure.

5. In addition to basal cell and squamous cell carcinoma, what other cutaneous tumors can be treated with Mohs surgery?

Almost any type of cutaneous tumor that grows in a contiguous fashion can be treated with Mohs surgery. The technique has been found to be particularly effective for aggressive cutaneous tumors that often recur after conventional excision. Cutaneous tumors that have been demonstrated to have high cure rates with Mohs surgery (90% to 100%) include

- Dermatofibrosarcoma protuberans (DFSP)
- Microcystic adnexal carcinoma
- Sebaceous carcinoma
- Merkel cell carcinoma
- Extramammary Paget's disease

Thomas C, Woods G, Marks V: Mohs micrographic surgery in the treatment of rare aggressive cutaneous tumors: the Geisinger experience, *Derm Surg* 33:333–339, 2007.

6. Is Mohs surgery appropriate therapy for malignant melanoma?

The use of Mohs surgery for melanoma varies between practitioners. Many dermatologic surgeons perform Mohs surgery on lentigo maligna, as the poorly defined margins of the tumor make it a good candidate for the technique. Some surgeons perform Mohs surgery on melanocytic tumors with fresh frozen sections alone, while others perform special stains such as Melan-A (MART-1) to better highlight the atypical melanocytes. The use of Mohs for invasive melanoma remains more controversial. Multiple studies have reported 5-year cure rates with Mohs surgery for invasive melanoma as being equivalent or better than those seen with standard wide local excision. However, some practitioners feel that fresh frozen tissue does not allow adequate assessment of melanocytic tumors. Modifications of the Mohs technique, such as "slow Mohs" with rush permanent paraffin sections, has been advocated as a way to perform tissue sparing surgery without fresh frozen sections.

Whalen J, Leone D: Mohs micrographic surgery for the treatment of malignant melanoma, *Clin Dermatol* 27:597–602, 2009.

7. How is Mohs micrographic surgery performed today?

Mohs surgery is performed in the outpatient setting. Patients are instructed to plan for the procedure to last an entire day. After informed consent is obtained, the tumor site is identified, measured, and photographed. Local anesthetic is then infiltrated into the tumor. Prior to taking the Mohs layer, many surgeons will debulk the cancer with curette or scalpel to better delineate its dimensions. A saucer-shaped piece of tissue is then excised from the cancerous area by beveling the surgical blade at about a 45-degree angle (in contrast to traditional surgical techniques, where the incision is made perpendicular to the skin).

The specimen is then sectioned into manageable pieces, if needed, and these slices are color coded with ink. Using an anatomic cartoon representation of the site, a map is drawn to precisely label the area from which the tumor is taken. The tissue is then submitted to the Mohs histotechnician, who prepares frozen tissue sections under the supervision of the Mohs surgeon. These sections are obtained by cutting the undersurface in a horizontal plane so that the depth and most peripheral skin edge will be available for microscopic examination. Theoretically, 100% of the margin is examined, in contrast to routine histologic processes. If tumor is identified, the map is used as a guide to obtain additional tissue layers only from the areas of positivity until a tumor-free plane is reached. Between stages of Mohs surgery, the wound is covered with a temporary dressing, and the patients wait in a comfortable area. Various steps of the procedure are illustrated in Fig. 53-1 using an apple model.

Davis DA, Pellowski DM, Hanke WC: Preparation of frozen sections, *Dermatol Surg* 30:1479–1485, 2004.

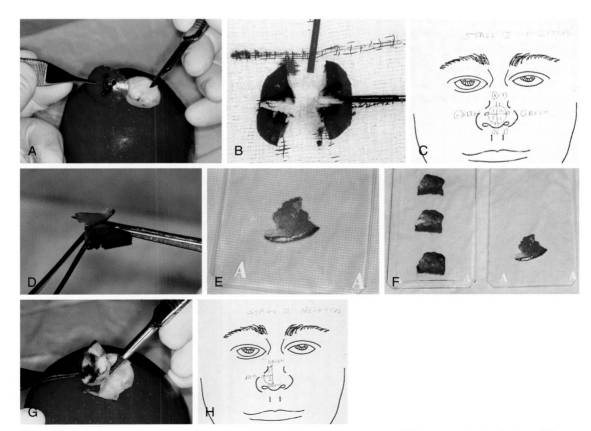

Figure 53-1. Apple model with tumor. **A,** Cancerous tissue is excised with the blade beveled. **B,** Tissue is sectioned and color coded. **C,** Anatomic map is labeled. **D to F,** Horizontal frozen sections are obtained to allow examination of the entire excision margin. **G to H,** Residual tumor is excised until the margins are clear.

8. What histologic stains are used in Mohs surgery?

The majority of Mohs surgeons stain their fresh frozen tissue with hematoxylin and eosin (H&E), the most common stain used in paraffin fixed sections. Some Mohs surgeons use toluidine blue, a stain that is particularly useful for highlighting basal cell carcinoma, but this has become less common. The most common immunohistochemical stain used by Mohs surgeons is a Melan-A (MART-1) stain used to highlight melanocytic cells in lentigo maligna and other melanocytic tumors. Other immunohistochemical stains that can be used for more rare tumors include CD-34 for dermatofibrosarcoma protuberans and cytokeratin-7 for squamous cell carcinoma. However, the majority of Mohs surgeons use only H&E staining in their day to day practice.

Stranahan D, Cherpelis B, Glass L, et al: Immunohistochemical stains in Mohs surgery: a review, *Dermatol Surg* 35:1023–1034, 2009.

9. How are the defects created in Mohs surgery repaired?

The precision of Mohs surgery allows for maximum preservation of normal tissue. However, the surgical defect created during Mohs surgery must be repaired in most cases. Some tumors can be allowed to heal in by themselves (second intention healing), but this should be limited to smaller, shallow defects on concave surfaces. The majority of Mohs defects will need to be reconstructed, using elliptical (primary) closures, flaps, or skin grafts (Fig. 53-2). Mohs surgeons, especially those who have completed fellowships, are well trained and experienced in aesthetic reconstruction.

Key Points: Mohs Surgery

1. Mohs micrographic surgery is the controlled, serial, microscopic examination of skin cancers.
2. Mohs micrographic surgery allows maximum preservation of uninvolved tissue and, consequently, results in smaller defects compared to conventional tumor excision protocols.
3. Mohs micrographic surgery is indicated for basal cell and squamous cell carcinomas arising on the face and other sites where the maximal preservation of normal skin and cosmesis are important goals.
4. Mohs micrographic surgery is also indicated for skin cancers that are large, recurrent, and those with an infiltrative histologic growth pattern, as well as for rare skin cancers, such as dermatofibrosarcoma protuberans and microcystic adnexal carcinoma.
5. Mohs micrographic surgery is well suited for the removal of tumors from sites where tissue sparing is essential (such as the nasal tip, nasal ala, lips, eyelids, ears, genitalia, or fingers).

10. Who performs Mohs surgery?

The American College of Mohs Micrographic Surgery currently recognizes about 50 training centers in the United States where qualified applicants receive comprehensive training in Mohs micrographic surgery. The period of training is 1 to 2 years, during which time the dermatologist acquires extensive experience with all aspects of the technique. Once training is completed, the physician becomes eligible for membership in the College.

Many dermatologists know the basic techniques and employ them in their practices. However, when patients require more extensive surgery, they usually are referred to a member of the College.

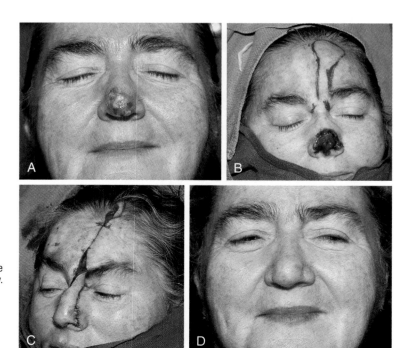

Figure 53-2. A, Preoperative basal cell carcinoma of the nasal tip. **B,** Defect of the nose following Mohs micrographic surgery. Paramedian forehead flap is designed. Note preservation of cartilaginous skeleton. **C,** Paramedian forehead flap is attached to reconstruct the nose. The forehead defect is closed. The pedicle is divided at 2 weeks. **D,** Long-term results.

11. What are the advantages and disadvantages of Mohs surgery?

Mohs surgery allows for the targeted removal of tumor, while sparing the greatest amount of normal tissue. The technique allows for the visualization of 100% of the margin of the specimen, while traditional sectioning allows for the examination of <0.1% of the margin. Mohs surgery has the highest cure rate of any technique to treat skin cancer. It also spares the patient the risks of general surgery and allows the removal of tumor and reconstruction to occur in a single day. One disadvantage of the procedure is that it can be time consuming, and the long days can be hard for patients. Additionally, Mohs surgery can be more expensive than other modalities for treating skin cancer.

CHAPTER 54

LASERS IN DERMATOLOGY

Stephen W. Eubanks, MD

1. What does the term "laser" stand for?

Laser is an acronym for "light amplification by stimulated emission of radiation."

Herd RM, Dover JS, Arndt KA: Basic laser principles, *Dermatol Clin* 15:355–372, 1997.

2. What does "stimulated emission of radiation" mean?

Stimulated emission is a complicated phenomenon of physics, first described by Albert Einstein. Atoms must be in an excited state (an electron is in an elevated orbit). Normally, adding a photon with energy equal to the energy between orbits would raise this electron to a higher orbit. Instead, in special circumstances found in laser systems, two photons are released from the atom, and the electron returns to its lower, resting state. These two photons are then able to enter two other atoms with excited electrons, allowing rapid multiplication of photons in a process similar to a chain reaction. This process accounts for the stimulated emission of radiation used in the acronym *laser*.

3. How is the light amplified in the laser system?

The laser system uses an optical resonator to amplify and orient the light. This is a cylindrical chamber filled with the laser medium. There are mirrors on each end and an absorptive lining. The photons of light are reflected between the mirrors. The lining will absorb any light that is not perfectly parallel. These parallel photons continue to enter additional atoms, producing more photons by stimulated emission. By this process, the laser light is amplified. One end of the optical resonator has a mechanism to release the light periodically from the chamber.

4. What types of medium are used in laser systems?

The ability of an atom to be used in a laser system is a complicated function of quantum mechanics and the physical characteristics of the lattice in which it is constructed. The basic requirement of any medium is to be able to support a population inversion so that there may be stimulated emission. Some types of lasers include the following:

- **Solids:** Ruby crystal: composed of aluminum oxide (Al_3O_2) with scattered atoms of chromium (Cr) replacing some aluminum atoms in the crystal lattice
- **Gases:** Carbon dioxide (CO_2)
- **Dyes:** Fluorescent liquid dye (often rhodamine)
- **Other:** Electrical diodes

5. What are the special features of laser light?

Laser light is unique because of three inherent features:

- **Coherence:** Coherence is the property that represents a uniform wave front, that is, the peaks and valleys of the waves are aligned as the light exits the laser, which allows the light to be in phase and focused to very small areas. This also allows the energies to be additive.
- **Monochromaticity:** This means all light waves have the same wavelength. Some lasers produce more than one wavelength of light, but these are predictable and the laser still produces only those specific wavelengths of light expected by the laser medium used.
- **Collimation:** This means that all of the light exiting the laser is parallel and will not diffuse over distances.

6. Why is monochromatic light useful?

Many lasers target specific chromophores, which are biologic structures with a specific absorption spectrum. Two common chromophores are hemoglobin within the red blood cell and melanin within melanosomes. The absorption spectrum is the amount of light absorbed at various wavelengths. The idea is to match a peak absorption wavelength with the wavelength of the laser.

7. What is selective photothermolysis?

The theory of selective photothermolysis assumes the laser light will pass through tissue until it targets a specific chromophore with an absorption spectrum corresponding to the wavelength of the laser. The target then absorbs the light, generating heat in the target tissue. The spread of heat is determined by the thermal relaxation time (TRT) of the tissue. This is the amount of time necessary for 50% of the peak heat to diffuse out of the target. It is important for the laser pulse duration not to exceed the thermal relaxation time of the target or the heat will diffuse into surrounding tissue, causing damage and possibly scarring. Thus, the TRT depends on the actual size of the target. The smaller the target, the shorter the TRT, and thus the need for shorter laser pulse durations.

Anderson RR, Parrish JA: Selective photothermolysis: precise microsurgery by selective absorption of pulsed radiation, *Science* 220:524–527, 1983.

8. What is an ablative laser?

An ablative laser vaporizes tissue. Different lasers cause different types of ablative reactions. Er:YAG lasers, due to their very high water absorption, cause almost pure ablation with very little collateral thermal heating. CO_2 lasers have less water absorption and therefore deliver less pure ablation and have more collateral heating. This heat causes thermal damage in a positive and negative manner. An example of a positive effect is collagen contraction and new collagen stimulation. Other positive effects of CO_2 lasers are sealing of blood vessels leading to less bleeding and sealing of nerve endings leading to less pain. An example of a negative effect is hypopigmentation due to inadvertent melanocyte damage. Scarring from laser procedures is usually due to excessive collateral heating.

9. What is a nonablative laser?

Most lasers are capable of delivering laser energy in a nonablative or nonvaporizing manner. Pulsed dye lasers, long-pulsed alexandrite, and Nd:YAG and many diode lasers deliver energy so as not to ablate tissue. The only lasers that truly ablate are those listed above and are used to remove tissue in a physical manner. The entire concept of selective photothermolysis is the ability to deliver energy in a nonablative manner.

Alexiades-Armenakas MR, Dover JS, Arndt KA: The spectrum of laser skin resurfacing: nonablative, fractional, and ablative laser resurfacing, *J Amer Acad Dermatol* 58:719–737, 2008.

10. What is Q-switching?

Q-switching is a way of obtaining short, powerful pulses of laser radiation. The "Q" stands for the "quality" factor of the optical resonator. There are many electrical, mechanical, or optical methods to Q-switch. The pulses generated by Q-switching are in the nanosecond (10^{-9}) range.

11. What is a fractional laser?

Fractional lasers deliver short pulses of laser that are separated by space on the surface of the skin. These lasers may either by nonablative, leaving a column of heat-damaged skin, or ablative, leaving a column of true ablation. This will be discussed in detail in a later question. The concept of fractional lasers was first proposed by Dr. Rox Anderson.

Manstein D, Herron GS, Sink RK, et al: Fractional photothermolysis: a new concept for cutaneous remodeling using microscopic patterns of thermal injury, *Lasers Surg Med* 34(5):426–438, 2004.

12. How are the types of dermatologic lasers classified?

The lasers are usually classified by the laser medium that generates the light, the specific wavelength of laser light, the length of the laser pulse, and the uses of the laser (Table 54-1).

13. What lasers have historic interest but are seldom used?

The argon laser (488 nm, 514 nm), was one of the first dermatologic lasers. This is seldom used because of scarring issues. The krypton laser generates dual wavelengths: 520-nm (green) and 568-nm (yellow) light. The continuous-wave thermal nature of the laser caused too much surface heating. Copper vapor lasers generate dual wavelengths of 511 nm (green light) and 578 nm (yellow light). These lasers are not currently used. There was a pulsed dye pigment lesion laser with a wavelength of 504 nm. This laser effectively treated surface pigmentation but was mechanically unsound and is no longer available (Table 54-2).

14. What are the basic features of the carbon dioxide (CO_2) laser?

The CO_2 laser emits radiation at 10,600 nm, in the far-infrared region. All water in tissue absorbs this wavelength of light, and this absorption is not dependent on selective absorption by any biologic tissue. As the water absorbs energy, the temperature rapidly rises, vaporizing the tissue. The amount of tissue damage is related to the energy setting and the amount of time the laser impacts on the target. There is some true ablation of tissue and this is surrounded by a zone of thermal damage. This area of thermal damage is used in resurfacing by causing immediate collagen contraction and later collagen remodeling.

The standard delivery system for the CO_2 laser is an articulated arm, which comprises a series of rigid tubes with mirrored joints capable of rotating in all directions. The CO_2 laser light is invisible and therefore must use a helium-neon laser as an aiming beam. The CO_2 laser operates in a range between 1 W and 30 W of power. The mechanical pulses are set between 0.01 sec and 0.1 sec, but the laser may also operate in a continuous-wave mode. CO_2 lasers are usually used in a focused or defocused mode, the former for high intensity use, such as cutting, and the latter for low-power destructive uses.

The new superpulsed and ultrapulsed CO_2 lasers have powers up to 60 W and pulse duration in the range of 250 μsec to 1 msec. There are now many fractional CO_2 lasers designed to reduce the side effects of CO_2 laser ablation (Table 54-3).

Table 54-1. Types of Lasers

LASER MEDIUM	WAVELENGTH	PULSE DURATION	USES
Carbon dioxide	10,600 nm	msec	Destruction of benign growths Ablative skin resurfacing
Pulsed dye	577–600 nm	msec	Vascular lesion removal Nonablative skin resurfacing Scar improvement Lentigines Wart removal Treatment of rosacea Reduction of poikiloderma of Civatte
Nd:YAG laser (Q-switched)	1064 nm	nsec	Black, blue tattoos Lentigines Nonablative laser resurfacing
Nd:YAG laser (long-pulsed)	1064 nm	msec	Hair removal Vascular lesions Skin tightening
KTP laser (Q-switched)	532 nm	nsec	Red tattoos
KTP laser (long-pulsed)	532 nm	msec	Vascular lesions Lentigines
Alexandrite laser (Q-switched)	755 nm	nsec	Green tattoos Lentigines
Alexandrite laser (long-pulsed)	755 nm	msec	Hair removal Lentigines Vascular lesions
Ruby laser (Q-switched)	694 nm	nsec	Black, blue tattoos
Ruby laser (long-pulsed)	694 nm	msec	Hair removal
Diode laser	810 nm	msec	Hair removal
Diode laser	1350–1450 nm	msec	Nonablative skin resurfacing

Table 54-2. Lasers of Historic Interest Only

LASER MEDIUM	WAVELENGTH	PROBLEMS
Argon	488 nm, 512 nm	Scarring
Krypton	520 nm, 568 nm	Scarring
Copper vapor	511 nm, 578 nm	Ineffective
Pulsed pigment	504 nm	Mechanical nightmare

Table 54-3. Carbon Dioxide Lasers

10,600-nm light
Energy absorbed by water
Nonspecific vaporization of tissue
Used for tissue destruction
Used for laser resurfacing of moderate wrinkles
May be used for surgical cutting

15. What are some uses for the standard carbon dioxide laser?

Treatment of warts has been the hallmark of CO_2 laser therapy. Large plantar and periungual warts are effectively treated. The main advantage of CO_2 laser treatment in these larger warts is the ability to decrease the bleeding during the laser excision and a slight decrease in scarring. Any benign lesion may be removed using CO_2 laser but this is not a common method used in dermatology. CO_2 lasers in a high-power focused mode are very effective at surgical cutting, especially in patients on anticoagulants or those with other bleeding disorders.

Olbricht SM: Use of the CO_2 laser in dermatologic surgery, *J Dermatol Surg Oncol* 19:364–369, 1993.

16. How is the CO₂ laser used for resurfacing?

Historically, the ultrapulsed CO_2 laser effectively removed the top layers of the epidermis and caused collagen contraction in the superficial dermis. This combination of effects allows the treatment of moderate facial wrinkles and sun damage. This procedure is seldom used at this time because of very prolonged healing and many side effects.

At this point, most CO_2 laser resurfacing is performed using fractional laser devices that dramatically reduce the healing time and side effects.

17. What precautions must be used with the CO₂ laser?

The main precaution with the CO_2 laser is smoke evacuation. During the procedure, the laser generates a large amount of smoke that may harbor viral particles. Studies have suggested the presence of live viral particles or genetic material of human papillomavirus (HPV), hepatitis viruses, and human immunodeficiency virus (HIV). Adequate vacuum devices and surgical masks are a must for use with this laser. The CO_2 laser will also burn any cloth or paper that it contacts; therefore, appropriate fire precautions must be observed. Clear plastic or glass eyewear is adequate to protect the eyes from this wavelength of laser light. Patients having skin resurfacing with CO_2 laser must be treated both before and immediately after the laser treatment with antiherpes simplex medication.

18. What are the basic features of the erbium:YAG laser?

YAG crystals are composed of **y**ttrium and **a**luminum in a **g**arnet crystal matrix. The Erbium:YAG crystal has some of the atoms of yttrium replaced with erbium atoms. The laser output is at 2490 nm. This wavelength is absorbed by water 10 times better than the 10,600-nm light of CO_2 lasers. This more efficient effect leads to little collateral damage to surrounding collagen and more efficient ablation of tissue. The clinical result is less effect on wrinkles but a smoother, faster-healing resurfacing procedure. By itself, the erbium:YAG laser has been used to treat mild facial sun damage, some sun damage on necks and hands, and acne scarring. In treating scars, the laser has the ability to plane down the edges of acne scars. Er:YAG lasers are also often used as a fractional device to decrease the healing time and side effects (Table 54-4).

Goldberg DJ, Cutler KB: The use of the erbium:YAG laser for the treatment of class III rhytids, *Dermatol Surg* 25:713–715, 1999.
McDaniel DH, Lord J, Ash K, Newman J: Combined CO_2/erbium:YAG laser resurfacing of perioral rhytides and side-by-side comparison with carbon dioxide laser alone, *Dermatol Surg* 25:285–293, 1999.

19. What are pulsed dye lasers?

The most common pulsed dye lasers use a flashlamp to energize the laser. The active medium is a fluorescent dye, often rhodamine. This will generate a wavelength between 200 and 700 nm. The older vascular lesion pulsed dye lasers used either 577 nm or 585 nm as the preferred wavelength, corresponding to a small peak in the oxyhemoglobin absorption spectrum in an area that does not have much competition from melanin. Newer pulsed dye lasers offer wavelengths that range from 585 to 600 nm. The flashlamp generates pulses with a duration of 300 to 500 msec in older lasers and up to 40 msec in newer lasers.

20. What is the flashlamp pulsed dye vascular lesion laser used to treat?

The pulsed dye lasers may be the most effective lasers in treating the thin, lightly colored port wine stains, especially those in children. These lesions have been treated without scarring in children as young as 1 week of age. Increasing the wavelength to 595 nm theoretically allows the treatment of many port wine stains that were resistant to treatment with the shorter wavelengths. Pulsed dye laser treatment is effective for facial telangiectasias, cherry angiomas, childhood hemangiomas, poikiloderma of Civatte (a mottled vascular condition on the necks of adults), warts, scars, and possibly stretch marks. Leg veins less than 1 mm in diameter are also effectively treated with pulsed dye lasers using 595- to 600-nm light and a pulse duration of up to 20 msec. One of the newer pulsed dye lasers even has a handpiece to treat pigmented lesions. This is a compression handpiece designed to physically compress out the blood, thereby removing one of the competing chromophores of this wavelength. This leaves the laser energy able to treat the remaining melanin targets.

Fitzpatrick RE, Lowe NJ, Goldman MP, et al: Flashlamp-pumped pulsed dye laser treatment of port-wine stains, *J Dermatol Surg Oncol* 20:743–748, 1994.
Hsia J, Lowery JA, Zelickson B: Treatment of leg telangiectasia using a long-pulse dye laser at 595 nm, *Lasers Surg Med* 20:1–5, 1997.

21. What is nonablative resurfacing and how does a pulsed dye laser accomplish this?

Theoretically, gentle heating of the superficial dermal layer will stimulate the production of new collagen. This helps to fill in fine wrinkles on the face. There is some controversy about this procedure, but most patients think it is helpful.

Table 54-4. Er:YAG Lasers
2094-nm light
Energy absorbed by water (10 times CO_2)
Used for pure tissue ablation (no collateral heating)
Treatment of fine wrinkles and acne scars

Pulsed dye lasers at low to moderate fluences (nonpurpuric settings) are used for this nonablative resurfacing. The low fluences help to stimulate collagen production. Many other lasers and intense pulsed light (IPL) machines are also purported to be effective.

Goldberg DJ: Nonablative resurfacing, *Clin Plastic Surg* 27:287–292, 2000.

22. What are the disadvantages of the pulsed dye laser?

The pulsed dye lasers are not very useful in treating thicker vascular lesions, because the short pulse duration is not usually sufficient to damage the target vessels without increasing the power to a level that could lead to generalized damage and scarring. There may be significant posttreatment purpura that takes 7 to 10 days to resolve. This purpura results from the explosive opticoacoustic pulse generated by the pulsed dye lasers. This is a cosmetic problem that limits the use of the laser in some patients. The newer pulsed dye lasers are able to treat lesions without purpura by using longer pulse durations in the range of 10 msec (Table 54-5).

23. What is an Nd:YAG laser?

The Nd:YAG laser uses an yttrium-aluminum-garnet crystal in which neodymium has been dispersed into the crystal. The standard wavelength of light emitted is 1064 nm, which is in the near-infrared spectrum. The light from these lasers may be passed through a potassium-titanyl-phosphate (KTP) crystal to double the frequency, halving the wavelength to 532 nm, in the green spectral region. These lasers are usually referred to as KTP lasers. Nd:YAG lasers may be long-pulsed in the 3- to 100-msec pulse duration range or Q-switched with pulses in the 5- to 50-nsec pulse range.

24. How are the long-pulsed Nd:YAG (1064-nm) lasers used?

The long-pulsed Nd:YAG laser (at 1064 nm) has been used for hair removal in dark-skinned patients (Fitzpatrick types IV to VI). This laser has also been used for hair removal in tanned patients, but I would recommend avoiding laser treatments with recently tanned skin. These long-pulsed lasers are also very useful for treating vascular lesions including leg veins and larger vessels on the nose. Long-pulsed Nd:YAG lasers have also been reported to help with skin tightening.

25. How are the long-pulsed KTP lasers used?

This laser is primarily used to treat vascular lesions. Red vessels on the face respond the best. Leg veins do not appear to respond well to these lasers. The primary advantage over pulsed dye lasers is the lack of purpura after treatment. These lasers are seldom used today.

Goldberg DJ, Meine JG: A comparison of four frequency-doubled Nd:YAG (532 nm) laser systems for treatment of facial telangiectases, *Dermatol Surg* 25:463–467, 1999.

Massey RA, Katz BE: Successful treatment of spider leg veins with a high-energy, long-pulse, frequency-doubled neodymium:YAG laser (HELP-G), *Dermatol Surg* 25:677–680, 1999.

26. How are the Q-switched Nd:YAG lasers used?

The Q-switched Nd:YAG lasers are primarily used to remove tattoos. The 1064-nm laser effectively removes black, blue-black, and blue tattoo pigment. This laser has also been useful in treating dermal pigmented lesions such as nevus of Ota and nevus of Ito. The 532-nm laser effectively removes red tattoo pigment. The 532 Q-switched Nd:YAG laser is also used for removal of brown lesions such as lentigines, nevus of Ota, and café-au-lait spots (Table 54-6).

27. What is the alexandrite laser?

Alexandrite crystal, a rare gemstone, is named after the Russian tsar Alexander II. The most sensational feature about this stone, however, is its surprising ability to change its color. Green or bluish-green in daylight, alexandrite turns a soft shade of red, purplish-red, or raspberry red in incandescent light. An alexandrite laser is a solid state laser in which chromium ions (Cr^{+3}), at the amount of 0.01% to 0.4%, are embedded in a $BeAl_2O_4$ crystal. Ions of chromium are contaminants in the crystal. Both Q-switched and flashlamp-pumped alexandrite lasers are available. These lasers deliver a wavelength of 755-nm light.

28. How are the alexandrite lasers used?

The Q-switched alexandrite laser is effective in removing green and black tattoo pigment. This laser has also been used to remove brown macules. The long-pulsed alexandrite laser is the gold standard for laser hair removal.

Table 54-5. Pulsed Dye Lasers
585–600 nm
Main target, oxyhemoglobin
Alternative target, epidermal melanin
Alternative target, dermal collagen
Used to treat vascular lesions
Used to treat scars, warts, sebaceous hyperplasia
Nonablative wrinkle removal

Table 54-6. Nd:YAG Lasers

LASER	MODE	USES
Nd:YAG, 1064 nm	Long-pulsed	Hair removal Blood vessels, nose Leg veins Skin tightening
Nd:YAG, 1064 nm	Q-switched	Black, blue tattoos Nevus of Ota
KTP, 532 nm	Long-pulsed	Facial telangiectasias
KTP, 532 nm	Q-switched	Red tattoos Epidermal pigmentation

Dark hair in Fitzpatrick types I to IV skin is very effectively removed. The long-pulsed laser has been reported to effectively remove leg veins that are 1 to 2 mm in diameter and blue in color. This laser has recently also been reported to effectively treat brown lentigines on the face and hands (Table 54-7).

Alster TS: Q-switched alexandrite laser treatment (755 nm) of professional and amateur tattoos, *J Am Acad Dermatol* 33:69–73, 1995.
Ash K, Lord J, McDaniel DH, et al: Hair removal using a long-pulsed alexandrite laser, *Dermatol Clin* 17:387–399, 1999.

29. What is the ruby laser?
The ruby laser has an active medium of aluminum oxide (Al_2O_3) that has been chromium-doped. Some of the aluminum (Al^{+3}) atoms have been replaced with chromium (Cr^{+3}) atoms. This laser emits a wavelength of 694 nm that is in the red visible light spectrum. These lasers may be Q-switched or long-pulsed.

30. How are the ruby lasers used?
The Q-switched ruby laser light is well absorbed by black, blue, and occasionally green tattoo pigment. The Q-switched ruby lasers have also been used in treating some dermal pigmentation abnormalities such as nevus of Ota. The long-pulsed ruby laser has been used primarily for laser hair removal (Table 54-8).

Taylor CR, Gange RW, Dover JS, et al: Treatment of tattoos by Q-switched ruby laser, *Arch Dermatol* 126:893–899, 1990.
Williams RM, Christian MM, Moy RL: Hair removal using the long-pulsed ruby laser, *Dermatol Clin* 17:367–372, 1999.

31. What is a diode laser?
Diode lasers use microscopic chips of gallium-arsenide or other semiconductors to generate coherent light. The energy of the light is generated by the differences between energy levels within the semiconductor. The wavelength may be varied to a wide spectral range. The high energy of medical lasers is generated by stacking arrays of the diodes. The advantage of the diode lasers is lower cost, a wide range of wavelengths, and smaller lasers.

32. How are the diode lasers used?
The 810-nm diode lasers are primarily used for hair removal and, occasionally, for treatment of vascular lesions. The 1320-nm diode lasers have been used for nonablative laser resurfacing and treatment of acne scarring. The 1450-nm diode lasers have been used for nonablative laser resurfacing, treatment of acne scarring, and the treatment of active acne (Table 54-9).

Table 54-7. Alexandrite Lasers

LASER	MODE	USES
755 nm	Q-switched	Tattoos (green, black) Brown spots
755 nm	Long-pulsed	Hair removal Leg veins (1–2 mm blue) Brown spots

Table 54-8. Ruby Lasers

LASER	MODE	USES
694 nm	Q-switched	Tattoos (black) Nevus of Ota
694 nm	Long-pulsed	Hair removal

Table 54-9. Diode Lasers

WAVELENGTH	PULSE DURATION	USES
532 nm	10–150 msec	Vascular lesions
810 nm	10–1000 msec	Hair removal Vascular lesions
1320 nm	20 msec	Nonablative resurfacing Acne scarring
1450 nm	3 msec	Nonablative resurfacing Acne scarring Acne treatment

33. What are nonablative fractional lasers, and for what are they used?

The Fraxel (Reliant Technologies, Palo Alto, CA) was the first fractional laser. This was a nonablative 1550-nm erbium-doped fiber laser that generated what was termed microscopic treatment zones (MTZ). Being nonablative, the epidermis is thought to remain intact. Within the area of the thermal damage, there is heat-coagulated tissue termed microepidermal necrotic debris (MEND) that is exfoliated through the intact epidermis. The theory is that there will be melanin and elastic tissue removed, and the thermal injury will lead to collagen stimulation.

Since this first laser, there have been many nonablative lasers with a variety of wavelengths and theoretical mechanisms. These include 1410-nm, 1540-nm, and a combination of 1440- and 1320-nm light. These lasers are purported to treat acne scars, surgical scars, and facial photodamage, including fine rhytids and dyschromia, melasma, and striae distensae. Table 54-10 lists the nonablative fractional lasers.

Narurkar VA: Nonablative fractional laser resurfacing, *Dermatol Clin* 27:473–478, 2009.

34. What are ablative fractional lasers, and how are they used?

Ablative fractional lasers fire a vaporizing pulse into the skin. There is a column of tissue ablation formed. The fractional lasers spread the pulses out using a variety of scanning devices. The theory of these fractional ablative lasers is to markedly reduce the healing time by spreading the pulses out, leaving normal epidermis between the pulses. As with nonfractional laser pulses, Er:YAG is more purely ablative than CO_2. The latter uses the surrounding tissue heating to help collagen contraction and remodeling. The first ablative fractional laser used was a 2940-nm (Er:YAG) laser called PIXEL. This has been joined by other Er:YAG fractional devices and many CO_2 10,600-nm fractional lasers. There is even a diode 532-nm ablative fractional laser.

Fractional lasers are primarily used for cosmetic purposes. They help with mild to moderate facial rhytids, hyperpigmentation, and lentigines, and are very effective in helping acne scarring. Table 54-11 lists the ablative fractional lasers.

Brightman LA, Brauer JA, Anolik R, et al: Ablative and fractional ablative lasers, *Dermatol Clin* 27:479–489, 2009.

35. What is an intense pulse light machine?

Intense pulse light (IPL) is a system that uses a flashlamp to generate a high-energy pulse of noncoherent light. The spectrum usually runs from about 550 nm up to 1200 nm. This light, having a wide spectrum, is then subjected to "cutoff" blocking filters to give specific starting wavelengths to each handpiece.

Raulin C, Greve B, Grema H: IPL technology: a review, *Lasers Surg Med* 32:78–87, 2003.

Key Points: Lasers in Dermatology

1. The wavelengths of common lasers are as follows: KTP, 532 nm; pulsed dye, 585 nm; ruby, 684 nm; alexandrite, 755 nm; diode, 810 to 1450 nm; Nd:YAG, 1064 nm; erbium:YAG, 2490 nm; and carbon dioxide, 10,600 nm.
2. The carbon dioxide and the erbium:YAG lasers are used for tissue ablation.
3. The pulsed dye laser is the gold standard for treatment of vascular lesions, but the KTP, Nd:YAG, and alexandrite lasers are also useful.
4. The long-pulsed alexandrite laser is the gold standard for laser hair removal, but the long-pulsed Nd:YAG and the long-pulsed ruby lasers are also used.
5. The Q-switched alexandrite and the Q-switched 532-nm Nd:YAG lasers are the gold standards for treatment of brown spots. The long-pulsed alexandrite is becoming very popular for this purpose.
6. Black tattoos are removed with the Q-switched 1064-nm Nd:YAG, the Q-switched alexandrite, and the Q-switched ruby lasers. Green tattoo pigment is removed only by the Q-switched alexandrite laser. Red tattoo pigment is removed only with the Q-switched 532-nm Nd:YAG laser.

---

36. What are IPL machines used to treat?

The wide range of available wavelengths allows the IPLs to be very versatile. They have been used for hair removal, treatment of vascular lesions, treatment of pigmented lesions, and nonablative resurfacing. IPL machines have a base

Table 54-10. Nonablative Fractional Lasers

NAME	TYPE	WAVELENGTH
Fraxel re:fine	Single-mode fiber	1410 nm
Affirm	Nd:YAG	1320 nm/1440 nm
Lux1440 Fractional	Nd:YAG	1440 nm
Lux1540 Fractional	Er:glass	1540 nm
Fraxel re:store	Erbium fiber	1550 nm

Table 54-11. Ablative Fractional Lasers

WAVELENGTH	TYPE	COMPANY	NAME
2940 nm	Er:YAG	Alma	PIXEL
2940 nm	Er:YAG	Cynosure	Affirm
2940 nm	Er:YAG	Focus Medical	NaturaLase Er
2940 nm	Er:YAG	Fotona	XS Dualis
2940 nm	Er:YAG	Fotona	Venus-i
2940 nm	Er:YAG	Palomar	Lux2940 Fractional
2940 nm	Er:YAG	Sciton	ProFractional
2790 nm	Er:YSGG	Cutera	Pearl Fractional
10600 nm	CO_2	Alma	Pixel CO2
10600 nm	CO_2	Candela	Quadralase
10600 nm	CO_2	Cynosure	Afirm CO2
10600 nm	CO_2	Eclipse	SmartXide DOT
10600 nm	CO_2	LaseringUSA	MiXto XS
10600 nm	CO_2	Lumenis	Ultrapulse
10600 nm	CO_2	Lutronics	eCO2
10600 nm	CO_2	Solta Medical	Fraxel re:pair

platform that delivers the energy to the handpiece. These handpieces now have not only pure IPL but have a variety of laser handpieces. These deliver many different wavelengths based on the different handpieces.

37. Are there any risks for IPL use?

As with all of the lasers that have been discussed, there may be risks of hypopigmentation and hyperpigmentation with the IPL machines. Any delivery of high energy may rarely be associated with scarring.

38. What is radiofrequency resurfacing?

These machines deliver radiofrequency to the skin at a frequency of about 6 megahertz. This energy heats the dermal layer and stimulates collagen formation. The end result is similar to many of the other lasers and IPLs that accomplish nonablative resurfacing. The difference with radiofrequency is that some collagen denatures and thereby contracts immediately. This allows rapid apparent changes in the superficial wrinkles.

Fitzpatrick RE, Geronemus R, Goldberg D, et al: Multicenter study of noninvasive radiofrequency for periorbital tissue tightening, *Lasers Surg Med* 33:232–242, 2003.

39. Are there any risks with radiofrequency treatments?

There is a moderate amount of discomfort associated with this treatment. There have been some preliminary reports of scarring and loss of underlying subcutaneous fat after treatment with radiofrequency.

40. What new technologies will soon be available?

There are now radiofrequency machines that do what is called sublative resurfacing. The machines focus the radiofrequency energy just below the epidermis and cause some coagulative ablation. The newest technology is that of intense focused ultrasound for sublative resurfacing. Here, the ultrasound energy is focused just below the epidermis for ablation similar to that above.

Hruza GJ, Taub AF, Collier SL, et al: Skin rejuvenation and wrinkle reduction using a fractional radiofrequency system, *J Drugs Dermatol* 8:259–265, 2009.

Laubach HJ, Makin AR, Barthe PG, et al: Intense focused ultrasound: evaluation of a new treatment modality for precise microcoagulation within skin, *Dermatol Surg* 34:727–734, 2008.

THERAPEUTIC PHOTOMEDICINE

Todd T. Kobayashi, MD, Lt Col, USAF, MC, and Paul B. Thompson, MD

1. What is phototherapy?

Phototherapy is the use of nonionizing electromagnetic radiation (usually in the ultraviolet [UV] range, but also extending into the visible light range) to treat cutaneous disease (Fig. 55-1).

- Broadband UVB (BBUVB): 290 to 320 nm
- Narrowband UVB (NBUVB): 311 nm
- Xenon chloride (excimer) laser: 308 nm
- UVA: 320 to 400 nm
- UVA1: 340 to 400 nm
- PUVA: Psoralen plus UVA light: 320 to 400 nm
- Blue light in Soret band: Approximately 400 to 410 nm
- Pulsed dye laser: 585 to 595 nm
- Intense pulsed light and broadband light: 300 to >2000 nm

2. What diseases can be treated with phototherapy?

See Table 55-1.

Gambichler, T, Breuckmann F, Borns S, et al: Narrowband UVB phototherapy in skin conditions beyond psoriasis, *J Am Acad Dermatol* 52:660–670, 2005.

3. How does traditional phototherapy work?

Immunomodulation locally, and possibly systemically, is the primary mechanism of action of phototherapy. Effects on keratinocyte proliferation and differentiation are likely secondary to the immunomodulatory effects. Immunomodulatory effects include: T-cell apoptosis (CD8+ in epidermis, CD4+ in dermis, CD25+ in both epidermis and dermis), inhibition and depletion of antigen-presenting cells (Langerhans cells in epidermis, dermal dendritic cells in dermis), release of immunosuppressive cytokines (interleukin [IL]-10 and IL-4, reduced expression of tumor necrosis factor–α [TNF-α]), interferon (IFN)-γ, and IL-12 locally, photoisomerization of trans-urocanic acid to cis-uracanic acid (which suppresses cellular immune responses, such as antigen presentation by Langerhans cells), and upregulation of CD95L (Fas ligand that binds to the Fas receptor on T cells inducing apoptosis).

Ozawa M, Ferenczi K, Kikuchi T, et al: 312-nanometer ultraviolet B light (narrow-band UVB) induces apoptosis of T cells within psoriatic lesions, *J Exp Med* 89:711–718, 1999.

Walters IB, Ozawa M, Cardinale I, et al: Narrowband (312-nm) UV-B suppresses interferon gamma and interleukin (IL) 12 and increases IL-4 transcripts: differential regulation of cytokines at the single-cell level: *Arch Dermatol* 139:155–161, 2003.

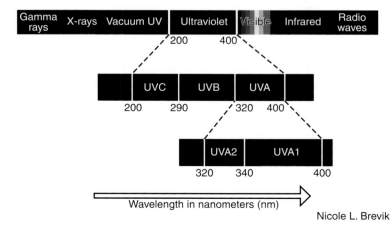

Figure 55-1. Electromagnetic spectrum.
(Courtesy of Nicole L. Brevik.)

Table 55-1. Diseases Treated with Phototherapy

DISEASE	PHOTOTHERAPY TYPE	EFFECTIVENESS	EVIDENCE
Psoriasis	Broadband UVB	++	+++
	Narrowband UVB	+++	+++
	PUVA	+++	+++
	308-nm laser	+++	++
	595-nm laser	+	+
Vitiligo	Broadband UVB	++	++
	Narrowband UVB	+++	+++
	PUVA	+++	+++
	308-nm laser	+++	++
Cutaneous T-cell lymphoma (mycosis fungoides)	Broadband UVB	+	+
	Narrowband UVB	+++	++
	PUVA	+++	+++
Parapsoriasis	Broadband UVB	+	−
	Narrowband UVB	+++	+
	PUVA	+++	++
Atopic dermatitis	UVA	++	++
	Broadband UVB	+	+
	Narrowband UVB	++	+
	PUVA	++	+
Polymorphous light eruption	Broadband UVB	+	+
	Narrowband UVB	++	+
	PUVA	+++	++
	UVA	+	+
Actinic prurigo	Broadband UVB	+	+
	Narrowband UVB	++	+
	PUVA	++	+
Chronic actinic dermatitis/actinic reticuloid	Narrowband UVB	+	+
	PUVA	+	+
Pityriasis rosea	Broadband UVB	+	+
	Narrowband UVB	++	+
	PUVA	++	′″
Pityriasis lichenoides	Broadband UVB	++	+
	Narrowband UVB	++	+
Nummular dermatitis	Broadband UVB	+	′″
	Narrowband UVB	++	′″
	PUVA	++	′″
Lichen planus	Broadband UVB	+	+
	Narrowband UVB	+	+
	PUVA	+	+
HIV-associated pruritus	UVB	+	+
	UVA	+	+
Pruritus associated with renal failure	Broadband UVB	++	+
	Narrowband UVB	−	−
	PUVA	−	−
Pruritus associated with polycythemia vera	UVA/B	+	+
	Narrowband UVB	+	+
	PUVA	+	+
Seborrheic dermatitis	Narrowband UVB	+	+
	PUVA	+	+
Acquired perforating disorders	UVB	+	+
	Narrowband UVB	+	+
Morphea/scleroderma	UVA1	++	++
	PUVA	++	+
	Narrowband UVB	+	+

Continued

Table 55-1. Diseases Treated with Phototherapy—cont'd

DISEASE	PHOTOTHERAPY TYPE	EFFECTIVENESS	EVIDENCE
Solar urticaria	Broadband UVB	+	+
	Narrowband UVB	+	+
	UVA	+	+
	PUVA	++	+
Cutaneous mastocytosis	PUVA	++	+
	UVA1	+	+
	Narrowband UVB	+	+

−, Not effective or not studied; +, case reports; ++, small studies; +++, controlled studies or strong evidence.

4. How is phototherapy administered?

It is usually administered in a physician's office or treatment center. Less commonly, patients purchase UVB phototherapy units and treat themselves at home. Patients receive a controlled dose of ultraviolet light while standing in a booth lined with high-output ultraviolet light bulbs (Fig. 55-2). The initial ultraviolet light exposure is determined by assessing the patient's skin type and history of burning or by establishing the minimal erythema dose (MED).

5. Compare the induction phase, maintenance phase, and tapering phase for various forms of phototherapy.

Induction phase:

- BBUVB: Daily treatments, increasing approximately 10% each treatment until pink or therapeutic level reached
- NBUVB: 3 times weekly, increasing approximately 10% each treatment until pink or therapeutic level reached
- UVA1: Daily or 3 times weekly, starting at 5 to 10 J/cm^2, usually set at a standard dose depending on condition being treated. In general, high-dose regimens (130 J/cm^2), medium-dose regimens (30 to 50 J/cm^2) and low-dose regimens (20 J/cm^2) have been used.
- PUVA: 3 times weekly, increasing 0.5 J/cm^2 each treatment until pink or therapeutic level reached

The induction phase is continued until clearing of skin lesions is noted or end point is reached. Periods of remission with NBUVB and PUVA may last for months.

Maintenance phase:

- BBUVB: Ranges from 2 to 3 times weekly to once every other week
- NBUVB: Typically once weekly to once every other week
- UVA1: Once weekly to once every other week
- PUVA: Once every other week to once monthly

Tapering phase: Decreasing frequency of treatments over a period of 1 to 2 months until patient is completely tapered off therapy or enters maintenance therapy. If flaring of disease occurs after discontinuing therapy or during maintenance therapy, the induction phase is restarted.

Note: The tanning effect may significantly decrease after 2 weeks, and the potential for burning patients with treatments spaced greater than every 2 weeks is much higher. Therefore, exercise caution and consider decreasing dose if greater than 2 weeks have elapsed since the last treatment.

6. What advantages does narrowband UVB have over broadband UVB?

Narrowband UVB utilizes a TL-01 light source emitting UV light almost exclusively at 311 nm, which is near the most effective action spectrum for induction of T-cell apoptosis in inflammatory skin diseases such as psoriasis. The absence of other wavelengths of UV light decreases side effects (erythema, carcinogenesis, photoaging) without sacrificing efficacy. Unlike broadband UVB, suberythemogenic doses are effective.

7. What advantages does narrowband UVB have over PUVA?

Narrowband UVB does not have the risks, side effects, and inconvenience of taking oral psoralens, including nausea, vomiting, dizziness, headache, insomnia, depression and anxiety, hepatotoxicity, drug interactions, allergic reactions, photoallergic reactions, PUVA keratoses, PUVA lentigines, PUVA pain, transient nail

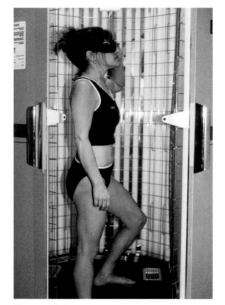

Figure 55-2. Typical ultraviolet booth demonstrating banks of bulbs. Most modern ultraviolet booths deliver either both UVB and UVA, or deliver narrow band UVB. Note that the patient is wearing sunglasses with wraparound eye protection.

pigmentation, photoonycholysis, facial hypertrichosis, licheoid eruptions, photosensitivity for 24 hours (even through windows), risk of cataracts, increased risk of melanoma and other skin cancers including genital skin cancers, narrow window of treatment after taking medication (1 to 2 hours), variability of tissue response depending on medication absorption and distribution (which is time sensitive), and need to wear sunglasses and avoid natural sunlight after taking medication for 24 hours. Narrowband UVB has not demonstrated increased carcinogenicity, thus far in humans, and the efficacy is similar. However, increased carcinogenicity has been noted in rats, and long-term follow-up is not yet available.

Laube S, George SA: Adverse effects with PUVA and UVB phototherapy, *J Dermatol Treat* 12:101–105, 2001.

8. What is targeted laser phototherapy?

An excimer (XeCl) laser, which emits a wavelength of 308 nm (near the narrowband UVB wavelength of 311 nm) is effective in treating individual psoriatic plaques. Supererythemogenic doses, from 6 to 8 MEDs, are used on individual plaques for 8 to 12 treatments and may induce months of remission. This localized form of UVB phototherapy is also an effective treatment for patches of vitiligo. It is advantageous in that it avoids irradiating healthy, nonlesional skin. It more effectively induces T-cell apoptosis, as well. In psoriasis, it is able to target individual plaques with higher fluences and reaches deeper T cells within the dermis. The pulsed dye laser at 585 to 595 nm has also been shown to be efficacious in treating individual psoriatic plaques, but appears less effective than the 308 nm excimer laser.

Nicolaidou E, Antoniou C, Stratigos A, Katsambas AD: Narrowband ultraviolet B phototherapy and 308-nm excimer laser in the treatment of vitiligo: a review, *J Am Acad Dermatol* 60:470–477, 2009.

Zakarian K, Nguyen A, Letsinger J, Koo J: Excimer laser for psoriasis: a review of theories regarding enhanced efficacy over traditional UVB phototherapy, *J Drugs Dermatol* 6:794–798, 2007.

9. What is UVA1 phototherapy and why is it used?

UVA1 is 340 to 400 nm UV light used mainly to treat atopic dermatitis and scleroderma/morphea, but it is less effective than UVB in treating psoriasis, mycosis fungoides, and other inflammatory skin disorders. It has different mechanism of action: It induces singlet oxygen–induced T-cell apoptosis, reduces Langerhans cell ability to migrate out of the epidermis, decreases the number of IgE-bearing Langerhans cells and dendritic cells in the epidermis and dermis, decreases collagen synthesis, and increases collagenase I and matrix metalloproteinases in sclerosing disorders of the skin. It penetrates deeper than UVB and appears more effective in cutaneous mastocytosis compared to UVB in depleting mast cells from the skin. UVA1 does not increase viral load in HIV-positive patients, unlike UVB, which has shown a 6- to 10-fold increase of cutaneous viral load.

Beissert S, Schwarz T: Role of immunomodulation in diseases responsive to phototherapy, *Methods* 28:138–144, 2002.

10. What is the Soret band?

A 400- to 410-nm blue light, which is the absorption spectrum of porphyrins. It is an important spectrum in photodynamic therapy. It is named after Jacques-Louis Soret, who discovered this band in 1883.

11. What is balneophototherapy?

Salt water bathing in combination with UV phototherapy. Potential mechanisms of action include the following: Magnesium salts may decrease antigen presentation in the skin, water-soaked skin allows more UV light to penetrate the skin due to decreased reflectance, and perhaps there is a neuropsychiatric influence (relaxation, vacation, decreased stress).

12. What do MED and MPD mean and why are they important?

Minimal erythema dose (UVB and UVA) and minimal phototoxic dose (PUVA), which represent the lowest dose that produces erythema (sunburn reaction) of the skin. The MED varies depending on skin type.

- UVA: 20 to 40 J/cm^2 (maximum erythema noted within 12 hours of treatment)
- BBUVB: 20 to 40 mJ/cm^2 (within 24 hours)
- NBUVB: 200 to 400 mJ/cm^2 (48 to 72 hours)
- PUVA: 4 to 15 J/cm^2 (48 to 72 hours)
- BBUVB is approximately 1000 times more erythemogenic than is UVA. Note that UVA is measured in Joules/cm^2 and UVB is measured in mJ/cm^2.

The MED/MPD testing is important because it allows the clinician to start phototherapy at a higher dose, achieving quicker responses with fewer treatments.

13. What is Goeckerman therapy?

Goeckerman therapy, named in honor of Dr. William H. Goeckerman, who developed it in 1925, is UVB phototherapy used in combination with topical coal tar to treat psoriasis. The therapy is administered by having patients apply crude coal tar or tar derivatives to the skin and removing the excess tar before exposure to UVB. After treatment, the patient takes a bath or shower to remove any remaining tar or scale. With each visit, the dose of UVB administered is gradually increased, with the treatment being administered three or more times per week for 3 to 4 weeks or longer. This extremely safe treatment can be supplemented with topical corticosteroid preparations or descaling agents. Once remission is achieved, patients may stay in remission for 12 to 18 months or longer. Long remission rates and relative safety have made this the therapy of choice in many psoriasis treatment centers. Disadvantages include its inconvenience, messiness of the tar, and need for numerous office visits.

14. What are the most common acute UVB phototherapy side effects?

The most common acute side effect is a sunburn-like effect within 24 hours of treatment manifested by erythema and tenderness of the skin. When this occurs, therapy is usually withheld until the erythema fades, and the amount of UVB administered is usually reduced at the next treatment session. Patients who fail to wear eye protection that blocks UVB may develop corneal burns. Occasionally, patients with psoriasis may experience temporary pustular flares of psoriasis during treatment. Topical preparations used in conjunction with UVB phototherapy, such as emollients and tar, may produce a folliculitis. This complication can be prevented by instructing the patient to apply topical preparations in a downward fashion to prevent follicular irritation. A severe blistering burn is rare when UVB is properly administered, and may be associated with Koebner's isomorphic phenomenon resulting in psoriatic plaques in the burned area of skin.

15. What are the most common long-term UVB phototherapy side effects?

Long-term side effects include skin cancer and skin aging (dermatoheliosis). The exact risk of skin cancer has not been determined, but it is greater in patients with fair skin, with a family history of skin cancer, or who use other therapies associated with a risk of producing skin cancer (i.e., PUVA). Patients with prolonged UVB therapy and other risk factors should have periodic skin examinations to detect early skin cancers.

16. What is PUVA phototherapy?

PUVA is an acronym for psoralen and ultraviolet light, type A. It involves the combined use of a prescription psoralen (methoxsalen or trioxsalen) and long-wave ultraviolet light (UVA). PUVA therapy for psoriasis was approved by the Food and Drug Administration in 1982 and has since become one of the treatments of choice for many adult patients with extensive patch and plaque-type psoriasis and mycosis fungoides. The psoralen usually is administered orally (sometimes topically) and followed by exposure to UVA light. While UVA is most commonly delivered in booths, special portable units are also available to treat the hands, feet, and scalp (Fig. 55-3).

17. What are psoralens?

Psoralens are a subclass of drugs that belong to a group of compounds called furocoumarins, which are derived from the fusion of a furan with coumarin (Fig. 55-4). Psoralens are natural constituents in a large variety of medicinal plants (e.g., limes, lemons, figs, parsnips). The two psoralens that are used therapeutically in the United States are methoxsalen and trioxsalen. Methoxsalen (8-methoxpsoralen, 8-MOP) is a naturally occurring photoactive plant substance found in the seeds of *Amnii majus*, a plant that grows wild along the Nile delta. Methoxsalen is absorbed from the upper gastrointestinal tract and metabolized by the intestine and liver. Ninety percent is excreted within 24 hours, with the major portion being excreted in the urine. Trioxsalen is a synthetic psoralen usually reserved for the treatment of vitiligo.

18. How do the psoralens work?

Psoralen compounds by themselves do not affect the skin in the absence of UVA, but in the presence of UVA (320 to 400 nm), they are potent photosensitizers. Ninety minutes after oral ingestion, absorption of UVA photons

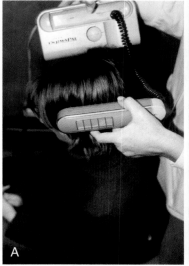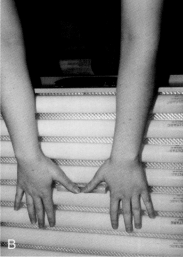

Figure 55-3. Portable UVA units for treating the scalp **(A)** or the hands and feet **(B)**.

photochemically links the DNA by forming cycloadditive products between the intercalated psoralen and the pyrimidine bases of cellular DNA. These psoralen-DNA cross-links cause a decrease in the rate of epidermal DNA synthesis, which some authorities believe to be the primary mechanism of action of these agents. Irradiation of psoralens also induces the formation of reactive oxygen species that can damage both cell membranes and organelles, as well as activate arachidonic acid metabolism. There is considerable evidence that PUVA therapy has a direct effect on the cutaneous immune system, and some authorities feel that this may be more important in terms of the therapeutic effect. The induction of T-cell apoptosis, decreased function of antigen-presenting cells, and altered cytokine profile is likely the most important component of PUVA therapy in most modern views.

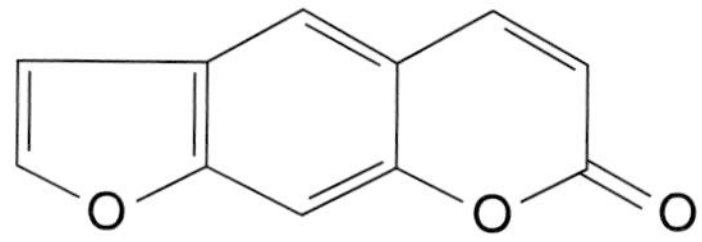

Figure 55-4. Molecular structure of furo-coumarin from plants of the *Psoralea* genus.

19. Are there contraindications to using PUVA?

Contraindications include a history of psoralen hypersensitivity reactions; photosensitive diseases including lupus erythematosus, porphyria, xeroderma pigmentosum, and albinism; malignant melanoma; pregnancy; and aphakia (absence of a lens may produce retinal damage). PUVA photochemotherapy should be used with caution in patients with fair skin, a history of previous ionizing radiation, history of multiple skin cancers, cataracts, immunosuppression, uremia, or renal failure. Patients with severe myocardial or other diseases that may disallow standing for prolonged periods in the treatment cabinet may not be able to receive photochemotherapy.

20. What is bath PUVA?

The patient is immersed for 15 minutes in a bathtub containing five 10-mg capsules of methoxsalen dissolved in the water. Topical methoxsalen gradually loses its photoactivity, and the patient should ideally be treated with the standard UVA light treatments within 15 minutes after immersion. Bath PUVA therapy using trimethylpsoralen (TMP), which is more hydrophobic than 8-methoxypsoralen (8-MOP), has been used for more than 30 years in Sweden and Finland, with no observed increase in the number of skin cancers. It is also useful for patients who are not able to tolerate oral methoxsalen because of nausea, and for children under 15 years of age. This technique also may be adapted for use on the palms and soles for hand and foot dermatoses.

Coven TR, Murphy FP, Gilleaudeau P, et al: Trimethylpsoralen bath PUVA is a remittive treatment for psoriasis vulgaris. Evidence that epidermal immunocytes are direct therapeutic targets, *Arch Dermatol* 134:1263–1268, 1998.

Key Points: Therapeutic Photomedicine

1. Phototherapy is used to treat many inflammatory skin diseases, is safe and effective, has relatively low cost, and provides another tool for the dermatologist to treat patients.
2. Narrowband UVB is now the phototherapy treatment of choice for psoriasis, vitiligo, and possibly mycosis fungoides (patch stage) and atopic dermatitis (in some experts' opinions) given its superior efficacy to broadband UVB and decreased side effects compared to oral PUVA.
3. Phototherapy exerts its effects primarily through immunomodulation (T-cell apoptosis within the epidermis and dermis, and suppression/depletion of Langerhans cells within the epidermis).
4. Photodynamic therapy utilizes aminolevulinic acid, which is converted to protoporphyrin IX in keratinocytes, and when illuminated with blue or red light is activated, producing phototoxic products and free radicals that induce cellular apoptosis.
5. PUVA is the acronym for psoralen and ultraviolet light, type A (UVA).
6. Treatment with PUVA is associated with an increased risk of skin cancer, including squamous cell carcinoma and malignant melanoma.
7. RePUVA is the combination of a retinoid (e.g., acitretin) and PUVA.

---

21. What is RePUVA?

RePUVA treatment uses an oral retinoid (usually acitretin) and PUVA in combination. Studies suggest that this therapeutic combination offers a practical way to clear psoriasis (with an overall response rate of 73%) with less cumulative UVA exposure than PUVA alone. Additionally, RePUVA can be successfully applied in patients resistant to standard PUVA. Patients receiving acitretin plus PUVA clear 40% faster than those treated with PUVA alone, even though the UVA dose is reduced by 50%. Most commonly, the oral acitretin is begun 7 to 10 days before the first PUVA treatment, and the two therapies are given concurrently until 100% clearing occurs. The acitretin is usually discontinued, and the patient is maintained on PUVA for about 2 months. Retinoids may also be used in combination with BBUVB and NBUVB.

22. What is photopheresis?

Photopheresis, also known as extracorporeal photochemotherapy (ECP), is a form of apheresis therapy. First introduced for the treatment of cutaneous T-cell lymphoma (CTCL), it has since been evaluated in studies and randomized trials as a potential treatment for autoimmune diseases, solid organ transplant rejection, and graft-versus-host disease. ECP is a relatively new procedure that involves discontinuous leukapheresis by centrifugation, followed by exposure of the buffy coat lymphocytes to UVA light in a special unit about 2 hours after the administration of methoxsalen. Following exposure of the lymphocytes to UVA, the photoirradiated cells are reinfused into the patient. The procedure is done on two consecutive days at 4-week intervals. The adverse side effects are minimal; patients may experience nausea and about 10% develop a transient fever after reinfusion.

23. Which diseases have been treated with extracorporeal photopheresis?

Photopheresis is approved for the treatment of cutaneous T-cell lymphoma (mycosis fungoides). It is most effective in the erythrodermic variants (Sézary syndrome) that involve >25% of the body surface. The response rate in this group of patients is about 64%. Photopheresis, as a form of immunotherapy, has also been tried on other T cell–mediated diseases, such as pemphigus vulgaris, chronic Lyme arthritis, psoriatic arthritis, and progressive systemic sclerosis.

Armus S, Keyes B, Cahill C, et al: Photophoresis for the treatment of cutaneous T-cell lymphoma, *J Am Acad Dermatol* 23:898–902, 1990.

24. How is photodynamic therapy used in dermatology?

Photodynamic therapy is a two-step process. A photosensitizing agent is topically applied to the patient's skin, followed by illumination with a light source of the proper wavelength. Aminolevulinic acid (ALA) is used most often in the United States and is converted to protoporphyrin IX by keratinocytes. Keratinocytes lack the final enzyme in the heme synthesis pathway, and the process ends with protoporphyrin IX, which is photosensitizing, particularly in the Soret band (400 to 410 nm). Porphyrins used in combination with blue (415 to 425 nm) or red light (600 to 700 nm) are the most common forms of photodynamic therapy. Smaller absorption peaks are also noted around 585 to 595 nm, which correlates with the pulsed dye laser absorption spectrum. Cancer cells and precancerous cells derived from keratinocytes (actinic keratoses, squamous cell carcinomas, basal cell carcinomas) accumulate porphyrins at higher concentrations than normal keratinocytes and are more susceptible to the phototoxic effects of the treatment. In acne, *P. acnes* is susceptible to both blue light alone and to porphyrin-induced injury. The sebaceous glands in the skin accumulate significant amounts of porphyrin and are very susceptible to injury by photodynamic therapy (PDT). When used in combination with the pulsed dye laser at 585 to 595 nm, deeper penetration into the sebaceous gland is achieved and a better therapeutic outcome is noted when treating acne. After 3 monthly treatments, acne may stay in remission for up to a year.

25. What is blue-light phototherapy?

Some degree of jaundice is common in newborns and is seen in up to 50% of infants between the second and fourth day of life. Before birth, bilirubin is conjugated and excreted chiefly by the placenta; however, after birth, this function shifts to the neonatal liver. Transient neonatal hyperbilirubinemia is the result of insufficient activity of the conjugative hepatic enzyme glucuronyl transferase. Phototherapy with blue light (460 nm) is an effective means of preventing hyperbilirubinemia by producing a photoproduct called photobilirubin, which is nontoxic. In the treatment of hyperbilirubinemia, phototherapy should be considered at serum bilirubin levels of 222 to 260 mmol/L, taking into account other clinical factors. Blue light phototherapy alone is also used to treat acne vulgaris. *P. acnes* is susceptible to blue light (415 to 425 nm) and is significantly reduced in number within the pilosebaceous unit. Improvement in acne is well documented.

CHAPTER 56

RETINOIDS

James E. Fitzpatrick, MD

1. What are retinoids?

Retinoids are structural analogs of vitamin A (retinol). Vitamin A is a fat-soluble vitamin that was first extracted from egg yolk in 1909. It can be obtained directly from the diet (e.g., liver) or produced from carotenoids, a pigmented precursor that is found in abundance in yellow vegetables such as carrots. Beta-carotene, the primary carotenoid found in carrots, is particularly efficient in its ability to be converted to vitamin A. The physiologic effects of vitamin A are broad, but the most important functions include tissue differentiation (especially epithelial tissues), general growth, visual function, and reproduction. Retinoids may be produced naturally during vitamin A metabolism, but most retinoids used in the treatment of skin diseases are synthetic. Synthetic retinoids are produced by changing either the polar end group, polyene side chain, or cyclic group of vitamin A. More than 1500 retinoids have been synthesized and tested for their biologic properties since 1968.

2. How do vitamin A and retinoids exert their effect at a molecular level?

Vitamin A exerts its effect on cells by a mechanism similar to that of corticosteroids; some authorities have suggested that it should be classified as a hormone. Vitamin A acts on cells by binding to nuclear retinoic acid receptors (RAR) and/ or other retinoid X receptors (RXR) that are closely related to the steroid and thyroid hormone receptors. Each of these receptors demonstrates three distinct receptor subtypes, which have been named α, β, and γ. Retinoids vary in their affinity for these six receptors, which partially accounts for the different pharmacologic effects produced by different retinoids. Another important factor is that different tissues appear to vary in the expression of receptor subtypes. In human keratinocytes, RAR-γ is the major retinoid receptor expressed. Tissues appear to regulate their requirement for vitamin A and retinoids by changing the concentration of the binding proteins.

3. Which retinoids are prescribed for the treatment of skin diseases?

Retinoids may be used topically or orally. Topical retinoids approved for use in the United States include tretinoin (all-trans retinoic acid), a naturally occurring metabolite of vitamin A; tazarotene, a synthetic retinoid; and alitretinoin (9-cis-retinoic acid). Adapalene is a retinoid-like drug that is also available topically. The three oral synthetic retinoids available in the United States are isotretinoin, acitretin, and bexarotene. Etretinate was formerly available, but it has been pulled from the market and replaced by acitretin. Prescription retinoids are summarized in Table 56-1.

4. Are there any retinoids found in topical over-the-counter (OTC) products?

Yes. Numerous OTC topical products, especially antiwrinkle and skin rejunuvation products, contain **retinol** or, less commonly, **retinyl palmitate** or **retinaldehyde**. These OTC retinoids do not bind to retinoid receptors and do not exert a biologic effect until they have been enzymatically converted in the skin into the active form, retinoic acid. Retinyl palmitate is first converted to retinol, which is then converted to retinaldehyde before being finally converted to the

---

Table 56-1. Prescription Retinoids

TOPICAL PREPARATIONS	ORAL PREPARATIONS
Tretinoin (all-trans retinoic acid)	**Isotretinoin (13-cis-retinoic acid)**
Retin-A (0.025%, 0.05%, 0.1% cream;	Multiple brands (10-, 20-, 30-, and 40-mg capsules)
0.025% gel; 0.05% liquid)	**Acitretin**
Retin-A Micro (0.04%, 0.1% gel microsphere)	Soriatane (10- and 25-mg capsules)
Renova (0.02%, 0.05% emollient cream)	**Bexarotene**
Avita (0.025% cream and gel)	Targretin (75-mg capsules)
Atralin (0.05% gel)	
Refissa (0.05% cream)	
Tazarotene	
Avage (0.1% cream)	
Tazorac (0.05%, 0.1% gel)	
Alitretinoin (9-cis-retinoic acid)	
Panretin (0.1% gel)	
Adapalene (retinoid-like drug)	
Differin (0.1% gel, solution, cream, pledgets)	
Epiduo (also contains benzoyl peroxide)	

Generic drugs appear as bold terms in the list.

biologically active retinoic acid. Because the conversion is incomplete, and these topical retinoids are easily oxidized and degraded, they are less effective than prescription retinoids.

5. What are the clinical indications for using topical tretinoin?

Topical tretinoin has received Food and Drug Administration (FDA) approval only for treatment of acne, mottled facial pigmentation, and dermatoheliosis (sun-induced skin aging); however, it has been used in many other dermatologic conditions (Table 56-2).

6. What is the mechanism of action of tretinoin in acne vulgaris?

The precise mechanism of action is not proved, but tretinoin is believed to exert its therapeutic effect by decreasing the cohesiveness of follicular epithelial cells that are responsible for producing microcomedones. Microcomedones are the earliest recognizable abnormality in acne vulgaris. Tretinoin also stimulates mitotic activity of follicular keratinocytes, promotes extrusion of comedones by rapid cell turnover, and decreases the production of sebum, although this effect is minimal.

Bikowski JB: Mechanisms of the comedolytic and anti-inflammatory properties of topical retinoids, *J Drugs Dermatol* 4:41–47, 2005.

7. How should topical tretinoin be used to treat acne vulgaris?

Tretinoin is applied once per day to affected areas. It should be applied in the evening to minimize photodegradation. The strength and formulation depend on the severity of the acne and the tolerance of the individual patient. After washing the face, the patient should wait 20 to 30 minutes before applying the medication, or use a hair dryer to blow-dry the face before application. The periocular skin, mouth, and angles of the nose should be avoided, because these are more susceptible to irritant reactions. The medication should be applied sparingly to dry skin. Care should be taken when using other topical preparations, such as benzoyl peroxide or antibiotics in conjunction with tretinoin, because the irritant effect of these medications is additive.

8. After starting topical tretinoin for acne vulgaris, the patient reports that her acne is worse. Should she immediately discontinue the drug?

No. While many textbooks state that acne vulgaris may flare during initiation of topical treatment; current evidence suggests that this most likely represents normal fluctuation in the intensity of disease. Patients should not discontinue therapy and should understand that beneficial effects may not be seen for 6 weeks. Maximum improvement may take up to 6 months or more with continued therapy. The most common reasons for tretinoin failures are failure of the health care provider to instruct patients thoroughly about proper application and failure to provide an accurate assessment about expected results. Patients often discontinue therapy after failing to see improvement during the first month.

Yentzer BA, McClain RW, Feldman SR: Do topical retinoids cause acne to "flare"? *J Drugs Dermatol* 8:799–801, 2009.

9. Is topical tretinoin cream really useful in treating photoinduced wrinkles?

Yes. Several vehicle-controlled studies have clearly demonstrated that topical tretinoin improves the wrinkling and irregular pigmentation of photoaged skin. It does not make the skin normal but it does increase both the thickness of the epidermis and the synthesis of anchoring fibrils and collagen. New blood vessels form, and cutaneous blood flow also increases. Topical tretinoin is not a panacea; prevention of dermatoheliosis by reducing sun exposure and using sunscreens is still preferable.

Kockaert M, Neumann M: Systemic and topical drugs for aging skin, *J Drugs Dermatol* 2:435–441, 2003.

Table 56-2. Therapeutic Applications of Topical Tretinoin

FDA-APPROVED INDICATIONS	SELECTED NONAPPROVED APPLICATIONS
Acne vulgaris	Acanthosis nigricans
Dermatoheliosis (photodamaged skin)	Actinic keratoses
Mottled facial hyperpigmentation	Fox-Fordyce disease
	Ichthyoses (e.g., ichthyosis vulgaris, lamellar ichthyosis)
	Keloids and hypertrophic scars
	Keratosis follicularis (Darier's disease)
	Keratosis pilaris
	Lichen planus (cutaneous and oral)
	Linear epidermal nevus
	Melasma (chloasma)
	Nevus comedonicus
	Porokeratosis
	Postinflammatory hyperpigmentation
	Psoriasis
	Reactive perforating collagenosis
	Striae distensae (stretch marks)
	Verruca plana (flat warts)

10. Is there clinical evidence that topical retinoids improve melasma?

Yes. Topical retinoids have been used in the treatment of many pigmentary disorders including melasma, solar lentigines, and postinflammatory hyperpigmentation. An evidence-based review found fair evidence to support the use of topical tretinoin as a monotherapy in the treatment of both melasma and solar lentigines. This study also found evidence to support clinical efficacy of topical tretinoin in a fixed, triple-combination therapy (hydroquinone 4%/tretinoin 0.05%/fluocinolone acetonide 0.01%) for the treatment of melasma.

Kang HY, Valerio L, Bahadoran P, Ortonne JP: The role of topical retinoids in the treatment of pigmentary disorders: an evidence-based review, *Am J Clin Dermatol* 10:251–260, 2009.

11. What are the side effects of topical tretinoin?

The most common side effect is an irritant reaction that manifests as erythema and scaling. Severe irritant reactions may require decreasing the concentration or frequency of application. True allergic contact dermatitis to topical tretinoin preparations has been reported but is rare. An unusual potential problem is that the topical tretinoin gels are flammable. At least one dermatologist has reported that it is useful during hunting trips for starting campfires! Patients who are not able to tolerate tretinoin gel or cream may be able to tolerate tretinoin gel with microspheres and adapalene gel, because they are less irritating.

12. Is topical tretinoin safe to use during pregnancy or when nursing?

Topical tretinoin is classified as a pregnancy category C drug, which means that a risk to the fetus cannot be ruled out. Prospective human studies are lacking, but studies on animals using doses up to 320 times those used in humans did not produce teratogenic effects. A retrospective British study on pregnant women who had received topical tretinoin did not demonstrate teratogenic effects. However, because high-dose (1000 times the topical human dose) oral tretinoin has been demonstrated to be teratogenic in rats, many dermatologists do not use this drug in pregnant women to avoid litigation in the event congenital abnormality occurs. Birth defects have been reported in rare patients receiving topical tretinoin or topical adapalene; however, it is unknown whether these birth defects were due to the topical retinoids. Because of the lack of data, it is probably prudent to not use topical retinoids in pregnant patients if possible. It is not known whether topical tretinoin is secreted in human milk, but the manufacturers recommend that caution be exercised when this drug is administered to nursing mothers.

Akhavan A, Bershad S: Topical acne drugs: review of clinical properties, systemic exposure, and safety, *Am J Clin Dermatol* 4:473–492, 2003.

13. What are the clinical indications for tazarotene?

Tazarotene is a recently introduced synthetic retinoid. It is a prodrug that is rapidly converted in vitro by skin esterases to tazarotenic acid. Tazarotenic acid has a high affinity for RAR-γ, which is the primary retinoid receptor in keratinocytes. Tazarotene is approved for the treatment of psoriasis and acne vulgaris. Dermatologists typically use a topical corticosteroid in conjunction with tazarotene when treating psoriasis.

Yamauchi PS, Rizk D, Lowe NJ: Retinoid therapy for psoriasis, *Dermatol Clin* 22:467–476, 2004.

14. What are the clinical indications for alitretinoin?

Alitretinoin (9-cis-retinoic acid) is a retinoid that binds to all six retinoid receptors. It is indicated for the topical treatment of Kaposi's sarcoma. It is formulated in a 0.1% gel that is applied to individual lesions. Irritant dermatitis is seen in approximately 75% of patients and severe irritant dermatitis is seen in about 10% of patients. In two different studies, 35% and 36% of patients, respectively, demonstrated significant responses. A recent double-blind, placebo-controlled, multicenter trial has also demonstrated efficacy of oral alitretinoin in the treatment of chronic hand dermatitis that is refractory to standard treatments.

Ruzicka T, Larsen FG, Galeeicz D, et al: Oral alitretinoin (9-cis-retinoic acid) therapy for chronic hand dermatitis in patients refractory to standard therapy: results of a randomized, double-blind, placebo-controlled, multicenter trial, *Arch Dermatol* 140:1453–1459, 2004.

15. Do retinoids have any role in the treatment or prevention of cancer?

Oral isotretinoin, etretinate, acitretin, and bexarotene have all been used as monotherapy or in combination with other drugs for a variety of cutaneous and internal malignancies. Oral retinoids have been used in experimental studies for the treatment of myelocytic leukemias, head and neck squamous cell carcinoma, breast carcinoma, cervical intraepithelial dysplasia, cervical cancer, and renal cell carcinoma. Bexarotene, which is a highly selective retinoid-X receptor retinoid, induces apoptosis of malignant cells in mycosis fungoides and has received FDA approval for use in this disease. Retinoids, particularly acitretin, have also achieved modest success in preventing squamous cell carcinomas in solid organ transplant patients.

Chen K, Craig JC, Shumack S: Oral retinoids for the prevention of skin cancers in solid organ transplant recipients: a systematic review of randomized controlled trials, *Br J Dermatol* 152:518–523, 2005.

Zhang C, Duvic M: Retinoids: Therapeutic implications and mechanisms of action in cutaneous T-cell lymphoma, *Dermatol Therap* 16:322–330, 2003.

16. What are the clinical indications for oral isotretinoin?

Oral isotretinoin is FDA-approved for the treatment of severe recalcitrant cystic or nodular acne vulgaris and disorders of keratinization. It is the most effective form of therapy for acne vulgaris; however, it is not a first-line drug and should

Table 56-3. Therapeutic Applications of Oral Tretinoin

FDA-APPROVED INDICATIONS	SELECTED NONAPPROVED APPLICATIONS
Severe recalcitrant acne vulgaris	Dissecting cellulitis of the scalp Hidradenitis suppurativa Ichthyoses Keratosis follicularis (Darier's disease) Lichen planus Lupus erythematosus, cutaneous Mycosis fungoides (cutaneous T-cell lymphoma) Nevoid basal cell carcinoma—prevention of basal cell carcinomas Pityriasis rubra pilaris Rosacea Xeroderma pigmentosum—prevention of skin cancers

be reserved for patients with cystic acne who are not responsive to conventional therapies such as oral antibiotics. Isotretinoin produces wide-ranging biologic effects and is used in many other diseases. Many authorities consider it to be the drug of choice for pityriasis rubra pilaris, severe lichen planus, Darier's disease, and the ichthyoses. A partial list of clinical indications is presented in Table 56-3.

17. What is the mechanism of action of oral isotretinoin in acne vulgaris?

Like tretinoin, the mechanism of action has not been precisely determined. Isotretinoin is the most effective known inhibitor of sebum production (up to 90% inhibition). Because clinical improvement in acne vulgaris appears to correlate with a reduction of sebum production, this is believed to be the most important mechanism of action. Isotretinoin also markedly affects keratinization and probably exerts an effect on the cohesiveness of the follicular keratinocytes, thus reducing microcomedone formation. Less important actions include antiinflammatory effects, antibacterial effects, and inhibition of microbial enzyme activity.

18. Are there any contraindications to the use of oral isotretinoin?

Isotretinoin is classified as a pregnancy category X drug, which means that it is absolutely contraindicated for patients who are pregnant. Between 1982 and 1989, the manufacturer received 151 reports of patients who carried their fetuses to term. In 47% there were significant congenital malformations, with most being cardiovascular, craniofacial, or central nervous system in nature.

In 2002, an intensive program (System to Manage Accutane-Related Teratogenicity, or SMART) consisting of counseling, consent forms, videotapes, written information, utilization of two forms of effective contraception, and two negative urine or serum pregnancy tests (to include one within the first 5 days of the menstrual period before implementing therapy) was undertaken. The program was not successful in preventing pregnancies while on therapy. In 2006, the FDA has implemented a very controlled restrictive program called **iPledge** to reduce the access of this drug. In this new program, both doctors and pharmacists are required to register and use a website to prescribe this drug. This new program is so restrictive that it is actually easier to buy a firearm in most states than it is to prescribe oral isotretinoin.

Patients who become pregnant while taking the drug should consider the desirability of continuing the pregnancy. Health care providers who are not knowledgeable about the proper way to administer and monitor oral retinoids should never use this class of drugs. Relative contraindications for oral retinoid therapy include patients with pseudotumor cerebri, inflammatory bowel disease, hyperlipidemia, hepatitis, and those who are children.

19. How is oral isotretinoin administered for the treatment of acne vulgaris?

Patients should initially have comprehensive counseling about the potential side effects of this drug. Under the iPledge program, they must register online and answer a series of questions regarding their menstrual periods, method of birth control, and other mandatory information before they can enter the program. At a minimum, all patients should have pretreatment blood lipid and liver function studies. Some dermatologists also obtain complete blood counts. An initial pregnancy test is required to enter the iPledge program, followed by a second pregnancy test at an approved laboratory before actually receiving the drug.

Oral isotretinoin is taken with food in a dose range of 0.5 to 2.0 mg/kg given in two divided doses for 15 to 20 weeks. It is better absorbed if taken with a fatty meal. Women of childbearing age should start therapy on the second or third day of their next normal menstrual period after having had a negative serum pregnancy test. After 20 to 24 weeks, therapy should be stopped. If significant acne is still present after a 2-month period, a second course of isotretinoin therapy may be considered.

20. What are the side effects of oral retinoid therapy?

More than 50 different acute and chronic adverse reactions of oral retinoid therapy have been documented in the literature (Table 56-4). More than 90% of patients receiving oral isotretinoin at therapeutic levels demonstrate cheilitis

Table 56-4. Oral Retinoid Toxicity

ACUTE ADVERSE REACTIONS	CHRONIC ADVERSE REACTIONS
Mucocutaneous	Mucocutaneous
Alopecia (<10%)	Alopecia, persistent (rare)
Cheilitis (>90%)	Dry eyes (rare)
Dermatitis (50%)	Systemic
Pruritus (<20%)	Osteoporosis
Pyogenic granuloma-like lesions in acne vulgaris (rare)	Premature epiphyseal closure
Xerosis (>50%)	Skeletal hyperostosis
Laboratory	
Elevated liver function tests (<10%)	
Hyperlipidemia (25%)	
Leukopenia (<10%)	
Systemic	
Arthralgias (16%)	
Impaired night vision	
Mental depression (uncommon)	
Pancreatitis (rare)	
Pseudotumor cerebri (rare)	
Spontaneous abortion	
Teratogenicity (cardiac, head and neck, CNS)	

or xerosis to some degree. A very controversial side effect is the association of inflammatory bowel disease (Crohn's disease, ulcerative colitis) with oral isotretinoin. There are numerous recent law suits and pending litigation regarding this alleged and controversial association. While one recent study concluded that isotretinoin is not associated with the induction of inflammatory bowel disease, a second study found a weak link between isotretinoin use and the development of ulcerative colitis.

Bernstein CN, Nugent Z, Longobardi T, Blanchard JF: Isotretinoin is not associated with inflammatory bowel disease: a population-based case-control study, *Am J Gastroenterol* 104:2774–2778, 2009.

Crocket SD, Porter CQ, Martin CF, et al: Isotretinoin use and the risk of inflammatory bowel disease: A case-control study. *Am J Gastroenterol* Mar 30, 2010. [Epub ahead of print.]

21. **Are there any strategies or treatments that reduce the dry skin and lips associated with retinoid therapy?**

Yes. The most common adjunctive treatment is lip balm for the lips and moisturizers for the skin. Preliminary reports suggested that taking 800 IU of vitamin E (α-tocopherol) was effective in reducing the cheilitis and, to a lesser extent, the dry skin. A subsequent investigator-blinded, randomized study could not demonstrate any benefit of vitamin E in ameliorating the side effects of isotretinoin.

Kus S, Gun D, Demircay Z, Sur H: Vitamin E does not reduce the side-effects of isotretinoin in the treatment of acne vulgaris, *Int J Dermatol* 44:248–251, 2005.

22. **Are the clinical indications for acitretin the same as for isotretinoin?**

No. While both drugs are orally administered retinoids, and they have many of the same therapeutic effects, they also demonstrate significant differences. As a general rule, isotretinoin is more effective in follicular disorders (e.g., acne vulgaris, rosacea, gram-negative folliculitis), and acitretin is more effective in pustular psoriasis and chronic pustular eruptions of the palms and soles. They appear to be of equal efficacy in disorders of keratinization, such as the ichthyoses and pityriasis rubra pilaris, although good comparative studies are lacking.

Acitretin is FDA-approved only for the treatment of severe recalcitrant psoriasis. It is especially effective for pustular and erythrodermic psoriasis. It is often used as monotherapy in these variants but also may be used in conjunction with other forms of therapy such as psoralen plus ultraviolet light, type A (PUVA) in plaque-type psoriasis. Like isotretinoin, acitretin has been used in many other cutaneous diseases (Table 56-5).

Table 56-5. Therapeutic Applications of Oral Acitretin

FDA-APPROVED INDICATION	SELECTED NONAPPROVED APPLICATIONS
Severe recalcitrant psoriasis	Granuloma annulare, generalized
	Ichthyoses (e.g., ichthyosis vulgaris)
	Keratosis follicularis (Darier's disease)
	Mycosis fungoides (cutaneous T-cell lymphoma)
	Palmar/plantar pustulosis
	Pityriasis rubra pilaris
	Porokeratosis
	Subcorneal pustular dermatosis

23. What is the mechanism of action of acitretin?

As with the other retinoids, the mechanism of action is not known. Acitretin's clinical and histologic effect on psoriasis and disorders of keratinization suggests normalization of keratinization. The therapeutic response of pustular psoriasis, pustular eruptions of the palms and soles, and subcorneal pustular dermatosis, suggest that this drug also modifies neutrophil function.

24. How is acitretin administered for the treatment of psoriasis?

After appropriate counseling and laboratory tests (liver function tests, serum lipid tests, pregnancy tests), oral acitretin is initially taken with food twice per day in a dosage range of 25 to 50 mg/day. Studies have shown that higher doses are only marginally more effective, but the dose-related side effects are much more common and severe. After the initial response to therapy, which usually takes 8 to 16 weeks, the maintenance dose can often be lowered to 25 mg/day or every other day.

Key Points: Retinoids

1. Retinoids are structural analogs of vitamin A (retinol).
2. The physiologic effects of vitamin A and retinoids are broad, but the most important functions include tissue differentiation (especially epithelial tissues), general growth, visual function, and reproduction.
3. Vitamin A and retinoids act on cells by binding to retinoic acid receptors (RAR) and/or other retinoid X receptors (RXR) that are found in the nucleus.
4. In human keratinocytes, RAR-γ is the major retinoid receptor expressed.
5. Systemic retinoids are potent teratogenic drugs.

---

25. What are the contraindications for using oral acitretin?

The contraindications are the same as for oral isotretinoin (previously discussed). As for isotretinoin, acitretin is a pregnancy category X drug and is absolutely contraindicated in pregnant patients. In contrast to isotretinoin, which has a terminal elimination half-life of 10 to 20 hours, acitretin has a longer half-life of 2 to 4 days. Acitretin should not be taken with alcohol, because the alcohol induces esterification of acitretin to etretinate, which has a terminal half-life of 120 days. Women of childbearing age should begin effective contraception for at least 1 month before starting therapy and continue for at least 3 years after discontinuation of therapy.

CHAPTER

NEONATAL INFECTIONS

Elizabeth R. Shurnas, MD

1. What are the TORCHES infections in a neonate?

This acronym stands for several etiologic agents of congenital infections:

- **T**oxoplasmosis
- **O**ther (varicella-zoster virus, parvovirus B19)
- **R**ubella
- **C**ytomegalovirus (causes most morbidity and mortality)
- **H**erpes simplex virus, **H**uman immunodeficiency virus (HIV)
- **E**nteroviruses, **E**pstein-Barr virus
- **S**yphilis

Boyer S, Boyer K: Update on TORCH infections in the newborn infant, *Newborn Infant Nurs Rev* 4:70–80, 2004.

2. Describe the cutaneous findings in neonatal herpes simplex viral (HSV) infections.

HSV infection usually presents as grouped vesicles on an erythematous base. These lesions can be present on any part of the skin but are more common on the face, scalp, or buttocks (Fig. 57-1). They may also be generalized or disseminated or occur in the perianal region in a breech-delivered baby. In the intrauterine-exposed baby, they may present as atrophic areas with scarring.

Corey L, Wald A: Maternal and neonatal herpes simplex virus infections, *N Engl J Med* 361:1376–1385, 2009.

3. Is neonatal herpes simplex dangerous?

Neonatal herpetic infections are usually severe (especially if lesions are disseminated or the central nervous system [CNS] is involved) and require immediate diagnosis and treatment. The majority of infants with HSV infection acquire it in the intrapartum period or postnatally. Even with adequate treatment, the mortality rate approaches 50% in infants with disseminated disease, and the incidence of long-term morbidity is significant.

Kohl S: Herpes simplex virus. In Behrman R, Kliegman R, Jenson H, editors: *Nelson textbook of pediatrics.* Philadelphia, 2004, WB Saunders, pp 1051–1057.

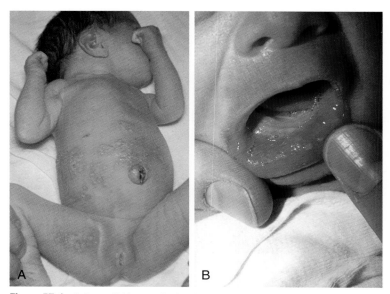

Figure 57-1. A, Congenital herpes simplex virus infection. **B,** Congenital mucosal herpes simplex virus infection. (Courtesy of William L. Weston, MD.)

4. What percentage of herpes-infected neonates display skin or mucosal lesions?

About 65% of infected infants display lesions shortly after birth, with disseminated disease occurring during the first 2 weeks of life. This includes infants with skin, eye, and mouth lesions (40%) as well as those with disseminated disease (25%) that includes the skin. If intrauterine exposure has occurred, lesions are usually present at birth. Fortunately, intrauterine transmission of HSV occurs in fewer than 5% of cases.

Jacobs RF: Neonatal herpes simplex virus infections, *Semin Perinatol* 22:64–71, 1998.

5. What percentage of these lesions are HSV-1, as opposed to HSV-2?

The majority of neonatal infections are due to perinatally acquired HSV-2 infection.

Fitzpatrick T, Wolff K, Johnson RA, Suurmond D: *Fitzpatrick's color atlas and synopsis of clinical dermatology*, ed 5, New York, 2005, McGraw-Hill.

6. What tests can be done to diagnose herpes infections? How should material be obtained for these tests?

To obtain specimens for diagnostic testing, scrape the base of a blister and smear the material on a microscope slide. Stain (e.g., Wright's stain) and look for multinucleated giant cells. If available, send another slide for a HSV-fluorescein antibody test. Confirmation of a cytopathic effect can be made by immunofluorescence using antibodies specific to HSV-1 and HSV-2. Material from the blister base can be sent for viral culture. The sensitivity of performing a culture is best for a vesicular lesion. It is also advisable to culture urine, nasopharynx, conjunctiva, and cerebrospinal fluid, if indicated. The polymerase chain reaction (PCR) detects viral DNA and can be important in diagnosing HSV encephalitis.

Boyer S, Boyer K: Update on TORCH infections in the newborn infant, *Newborn Infant Nurs Rev* 4:70–80, 2004.

7. What is congenital varicella syndrome?

Intrauterine infection with varicella virus that occurs in the first trimester may result in congenital varicella syndrome. These infants are born with hypoplasia of the limbs and exhibit cutaneous zosteriform scars and atrophy. Interestingly, there have been reports of neonates developing herpes zoster, which implies that they must have had chickenpox in utero. The future of varicella disease may be altered by the continued use of the varicella vaccine.

Seward J, Watson B, Peterson C, et al: Varicella disease after introduction of varicella vaccine in the United States: 1995–2000, *JAMA* 287:606–611, 2002.

8. What is the average age of onset of lesions in a neonate exposed to varicella perinatally? When is there an increased risk of mortality?

The age of onset of varicella lesions is usually within the first 10 days of life. Neonatal varicella is fatal in about 30% of patients whose mothers developed lesions from 5 days before to 2 days after delivery.

Smith CK, Arvin AM: Varicella in the fetus and newborn, *Semin Fetal Neonatal Med* 14:209–217, 2009.

9. What is the treatment of neonatal HSV and varicella infection?

Early identification of infection and initiation of therapy are the most important aspects of treatment. Intravenous acyclovir or vidarabine is recommended for either infection. The usual course is 14 to 21 days. Ophthalmologic examination may be necessary and adequate isolation precautions must be instituted. For varicella infection, varicella-zoster immune globulin (VZIG) is recommended for cases with evidence of maternal infection 5 days before to 2 days after delivery (given within 48 to 96 hours after exposure). VZIG is not indicated for infants born to mothers with herpes zoster.

Arvin A: Varicella-zoster virus. In Long SS, Pickering LK, Prober CG, editors. *Principles and practice of pediatric infectious diseases*, New York, 2003, Churchill-Livingstone, pp 1041–1049.

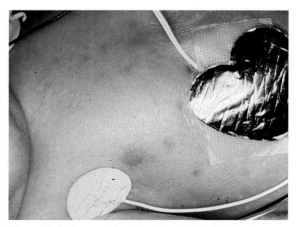

10. What is a "blueberry muffin baby"? What is the significance of this diagnosis?

This term applies to babies exhibiting blue-red or red indurated macules or papules on the face, trunk, or scalp present at birth, or within the first 2 days of life (Fig. 57-2). These lesions represent extramedullary dermal erythropoiesis and are seen in congenital rubella syndrome, toxoplasmosis, cytomegalovirus infection, neuroblastoma, leukemia, erythroblastosis fetalis, and twin transfusion syndrome.

Figure 57-2. Extramedullary dermal erythropoiesis. Although described as "blueberry muffin" babies, because of the bluish tint in some cases, they can also have red indurated nodules, as seen in this patient. (Courtesy of the Fitzsimons Army Medical Center teaching files.)

Holland KE, Galbraith SS, Drolet BA: Neonatal violaceous skin lesions: expanding the differential of the "blueberry muffin baby," *Adv Dermatol* 21:153–192, 2005.

11. At what time during pregnancy is there the highest risk of congenital rubella following maternal infection?

The risk is highest if maternal exposure occurs during the first 20 weeks of pregnancy. The risk of fetal infection is 90% during the first trimester; the majority of these infants suffer from congenital defects. Between the 12th and 20th weeks of gestation, the infection risk drops to 50%, and about one third of these infants have sequelae.

Fitzpatrick T, Wolff K, Johnson RA, Suurmond D: *Fitzpatrick's color atlas and synopsis of clinical dermatology*, ed 5, New York, 2005, McGraw-Hill.

12. List the classic triad of congenital rubella syndrome (CRS).

- Congenital cataracts
- Deafness
- Congenital heart malformations

The syndrome also includes microcephaly, microphthalmia, and intrauterine growth retardation. It is important to follow at-risk infants as two thirds of infants with CRS may be asymptomatic at birth. Most will develop sequelae within the first 5 years of life.

Maldonado Y: Rubella. In Behrman R, Kliegman R, Jenson H, editors: *Nelson textbook of pediatrics*, Philadelphia, 2004, WB Saunders, pp 1032–1034.

13. Are any precautions necessary for infants with congenital rubella syndrome at the time of hospital discharge?

Yes. These infants represent potential risks to other pregnant women, as 5% to 10% of affected infants may shed virus for 12 to 18 months.

Fitzpatrick T, Wolff K, Johnson RA, Suurmond D: *Fitzpatrick's color atlas and synopsis of clinical dermatology*, ed 5, New York, 2005, McGraw-Hill.

14. Why is human parvovirus infection important to a pregnant woman?

Human parvovirus B19, the etiologic agent of erythema infectiosum, readily infects erythroblasts and may, therefore, result in hydrops fetalis and fetal death. This risk is small, with current studies showing a 2% to 9% risk after infection during the first 16 to 28 weeks of pregnancy. Fortunately, about 50% of pregnant women have serologic evidence of prior exposure to parvovirus B19.

Tolfvenstam T, Broliden K: Parvovirus B19 infection, *Semin Fetal Neonatal Med* 14:218–221, 2009.

Key Points: Neonatal Infection

1. The **TORCHES** infections are **t**oxoplasmosis; **o**ther (varicella-zoster virus, parvovirus B19); **r**ubella; **c**ytomegalovirus; **h**erpes simplex virus and **H**IV; **e**nteroviruses and **E**pstein-Barr virus; and **s**yphilis.
2. Only 65% of neonates with HSV infection will have cutaneous disease.
3. The classic triad of congenital rubella syndrome (CRS) consists of congenital cataracts, deafness, and congenital heart malformations.
4. Ninety percent of congenital cytomegalovirus (CMV)-infected infants are asymptomatic.
5. Hoarse voice changes in infants might signify HPV laryngeal infection.
6. Infected and uninfected HIV infants usually cannot be clinically distinguished at birth.

---

15. Are most infants with congenital cytomegalovirus (CMV) infection symptomatic?

No. Ninety percent of congenitally CMV-infected infants are asymptomatic. The other 5% to 10% usually have disease manifested by hepatosplenomegaly, hemorrhagic diatheses, and jaundice. The mortality rate in overtly symptomatic infants is almost 30%.

DeVries J: The ABC's of CMV, *Adv Neonatal Care* 7:248–255, 2007.

16. What cutaneous findings are seen in congenital CMV infection?

- Petechiae
- Purpura
- Maculopapular rash
- Papulonodular eruptions (with blueberry muffin lesions)
- Vesicular eruption (rarely)

Hicks T, Fowler K, Richardson M, et al: Congenital cytomegalovirus infection and neonatal auditory screening, *J Pediatr* 123:779–782, 1993.

17. What clinical findings are seen in congenital Epstein-Barr virus infection?

- Micrognathia
- Cryptorchidism
- Cataracts
- Hypotonia
- Hemolytic anemia

- Scaly erythematous rash
- Hepatosplenomegaly
- Persistent atypical lymphocytosis

Hurwitz S: *Clinical pediatric dermatology*, Philadelphia, 1993, WB Saunders.

18. Describe a clinical presentation of congenital human papillomavirus infection.

The infant can present with voice changes or a persistent abnormal hoarse cry, due to laryngeal papillomas thought to be acquired during passage through the infected birth canal. The time between rupture of the amnion and delivery seems to be a critical factor in vertical transmission rate. These signs of infection may not be evident for several months to several years of age.

Anogenital warts in young children can also be acquired as a congenital infection, through sexual abuse, or by other postnatal, nonsexual contact with affected adults (Fig. 57-3).

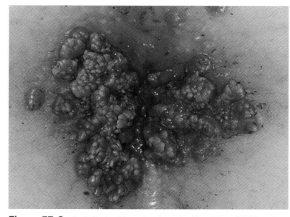

Figure 57-3. An infant with perianal warts. (Courtesy of William L. Weston, MD.)

Tenti P, Zappatore R, Migliora P, et al: Perinatal transmission of human papillomavirus from gravidas with latent infections, *Obstet Gynecol* 93:475–479, 1999.

19. What is the risk of HIV infection transmission to an infant born from an HIV-positive mother?

The risk of transmission ranges from 2% for HIV-infected mothers receiving multidrug antiretroviral therapies up to 30% for mothers with no previous preventative treatment during pregnancy. By 2005, in the United States, almost 8500 children had been diagnosed with acquired immunodeficiency syndrome (AIDS) who were infected perinatally. Since 1994, studies show the risk of perinatal transmission to be even less than 2% (as published by the Pediatric AIDS Clinical Trials Group 076). Most often, infected and uninfected infants cannot be clinically distinguished at birth.

CDC: HIV/AIDS surveillance report, 2005, vol 17, revised ed, Atlanta, 2007, US Department of Health and Human Services, CDC, pp 1–54.
Goldschmidt RH, Fogler JA: Opportunities to prevent HIV transmission in newborns, *Pediatrics* 117:208–209, 2006.

20. What is Hutchinson's triad?

Interstitial keratitis, Hutchinson's teeth, and eighth nerve deafness. These are common findings in late congenital syphilis. Interstitial keratitis is the most common lesion in this triad. It is rare before age 8 and after age 40. Both eyes are usually affected, and the corneal clouding may be spotty or diffuse. Hutchinson's teeth are due to deficient development of the permanent teeth buds and are characterized by conical central incisors with notching of the distal free margin. Eighth nerve deafness usually occurs after interstitial keratitis, is usually bilateral, and is often preceded by tinnitus and vertigo.

Azimi P: Syphilis. In Behrman R, Kliegman R, Jenson H, editors: *Nelson textbook of pediatrics*, Philadelphia, 2004, WB Saunders, pp 978–982.

21. Are there any other stigmata of late congenital syphilis?

Bone involvement is common with periostitis of long bones, resulting in thickened and bent tibias (saber shins) and other bony abnormalities. Other stigmata include scarring and wrinkling at the corners of the mouth (rhagades), saddle nose, dish facies, Parrot's nodes on the skull, and salt-and-pepper fundi.

Weston WL, Lane AT, Morelli JG: *Color textbook of pediatric dermatology*, St Louis, 2002, Mosby.

22. What are the physical findings of early congenital syphilis?

Syphilitic rhinitis is the most important and frequent physical finding in early congenital syphilis. It is characterized by a profuse serous nasal discharge (snuffles) that is teeming with spirochetes. The inflammatory process leads to eventual cartilage and bone deformity. Other findings include papulosquamous skin lesions, perianal erosions (Fig. 57-4), blistering of the hands and feet, hepatosplenomegaly, meningitis, meningoencephalitis, and osteochondritis. Congenital syphilis is a serious infection that, if untreated, has significant mortality.

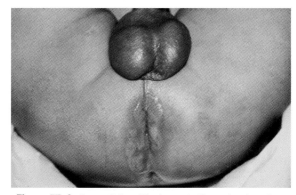

Figure 57-4. Congenital syphilis demonstrating perianal erosions.

PEDIATRIC DERMATOLOGY

Joseph G. Morelli, MD

1. **What is the most common skin disease seen in children?**

   Acne vulgaris is the most prevalent skin condition observed in the pediatric age group, with two peaks of onset. The first is in the neonatal period, and the second is during adolescence.

2. **Name the papulopustular facial eruption often associated with inappropriate topical steroid use.**

   Periorificial dermatitis is a perioral, periorbital, and perinasal, erythematous, slightly scaling papulopustular eruption seen most commonly in preschool children. Treatment of this condition is the discontinuation of topical steroids and the use of the same oral or topical antibiotics that are used for acne vulgaris. Tetracycline and derivatives should not be used in children under 8 years of age.

   Nguyen V, Eichenfield LF: Periorificial dermatitis in children and adolescents, *J Am Acad Dermatol* 55:781–785, 2006.

3. **At what age does atopic dermatitis typically begin?**

   Atopic dermatitis generally first appears between 1 and 4 months of age. By adolescence, over 90% of people who get atopic dermatitis will have manifested the disease.

4. **What is the natural history of atopic dermatitis?**

   By grade school, only one third of children who had atopic dermatitis will continue to have difficulties with the disease. By adolescence, 90% will no longer have symptoms of atopic dermatitis.

5. **What organism commonly complicates irritant diaper dermatitis?**

   Candida albicans. It can be expected to superinfect any diaper dermatitis that has been present for 3 or more days.

6. **Red, scaly, itchy, weight-bearing skin surfaces of the feet in children are usually not due to tinea pedis, but to what?**

   Juvenile plantar dermatosis. This is a nonspecific dermatitis with a debatable relationship to atopic dermatitis. The disorder may persist for months or years but ultimately clears spontaneously during childhood or adolescence (Fig. 58-1).

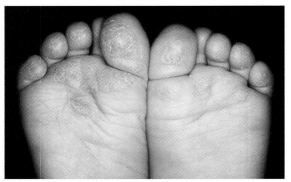

Figure 58-1. Juvenile plantar dermatosis. Characteristic hyperkeratosis and shiny appearance, with tendency to affect the ball of the foot and the toe pads. (Courtesy of the Fitzsimons Army Medical Center teaching files.)

7. **Plant dermatitis, such as poison ivy, is the most prevalent cause of allergic contact dermatitis in children. What are some others?**

   Neomycin, nickel, and potassium dichromate.

8. **One- to 2-mm keratotic papules located on the face, outer upper arms, and thighs are frequently misdiagnosed as folliculitis. What are they really?**

   Keratosis pilaris. It may be inherited as an autosomal dominant disease or be associated with xerosis and/or atopy. The keratotic plugs are composed of corneocytes and sebum. Keratosis pilaris often spontaneously clears in adulthood.

9. **What is the most common cutaneous bacterial infection in children?**

   Impetigo. This common, contagious, superficial infection is due to streptococci, staphylococci, or a combination of the two organisms.

10. **What two organisms are most often responsible for tinea capitis?**

    Trichophyton tonsurans and *Microsporum canis*.

11. How is tinea capitis treated?

Oral griseofulvin is the treatment of choice. Oral terbinafine and itraconazole are also used. Topical antifungals have no role in the treatment of tinea capitis. Some authorities recommend twice-weekly shampooing with 2% selenium sulfide or ketoconazole shampoos as a useful adjunctive therapy to griseofulvin, because it is sporicidal and may prevent spread to other children and family members.

Trovato MJ, Schwartz RA, Janniger CK: Tinea capitis: current concepts in clinical practice, *Cutis* 77:93–99, 2006.

12. What is the hypersensitivity reaction to tinea capitis that is commonly mistaken for a bacterial superinfection?

This very inflammatory condition is called a kerion.

13. Name the three conditions most often misdiagnosed as tinea corporis.

The herald patch of pityriasis rosea, nummular dermatitis, and granuloma annulare.

14. What percentage of children with psoriasis will have guttate psoriasis?

Although psoriasis vulgaris is still the most common type of psoriasis in childhood, up to one third of children with psoriasis will have guttate flares. Guttate psoriasis is most often associated with streptococcal pharyngitis but may also be seen following perianal streptococcal infections.

Tollefson MM, Crowson CS, McEvoy MT, Maradit Kremers HM: Incidence of psoriasis in children: a population-based study, *J Am Acad Dermatol* 62:979–987, 2010. [Epub ahead of print.]

15. Describe the rash associated with childhood dermatomyositis.

A malar photosensitive rash, with red flat-topped papules on the knuckles (Gottron's papules) and edematous plaques on the elbows and knees, is often seen in childhood dermatomyositis (Fig. 58-2). Unlike adult disease, childhood dermatomyositis is not related to internal malignancies.

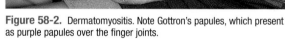

Figure 58-2. Dermatomyositis. Note Gottron's papules, which present as purple papules over the finger joints.

16. A child's mother tells you that the rash started at one end of her child's extremity and has now progressed to form a line the entire length of the limb. What is your diagnosis?

Lichen striatus. It occurs in children aged 2 to 12 years and characteristically begins at one end of an extremity and slowly progresses the length of the extremity. The nature of the rash may vary from hypopigmented and macular to thickened and scaly (Fig. 58-3). No treatment is effective, and the lesions disappear spontaneously. The pathogenesis of this unusual dermatosis is unknown.

17. Name the most common sun-induced disease of childhood.

Sunburn. Excessive exposure to ultraviolet radiation causes sunburn. It is now known that excessive sun exposure and frequent sunburns in childhood are important in the development of skin cancers in adulthood.

18. If it is not sunburn but a photosensitive eruption is suspected, what is it?

Polymorphous light eruption (Fig. 58-4), erythropoietic protoporphyria, and systemic lupus erythematosus are the three most common causes of a nonsunburn photoeruption in childhood.

19. Name the mildly inflammatory tongue eruption with day-to-day changes in appearance.

Geographic tongue (Fig. 58-5) is the name given to this usually asymptomatic childhood disorder.

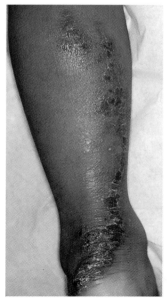

Figure 58-3. Lichen striatus presenting as hyperkeratotic linear plaque on the lower leg of a child.

20. Which disease should be considered in a child with easy blistering of the skin?

A child with skin that blisters with minimal trauma should be evaluated for one of the mechanobullous diseases, also known as epidermolysis bullosa. There are multiple subtypes, but clinically there are three important variants: epidermal and junctional, which are both nonscarring, and dermal, which is scarring (see Chapter 6).

21. Two common nodules are seen in childhood. Name them.

Epithelial (epidermoid) cysts comprise 60% of the nodules seen in children, and pilomatricomas (Fig. 58-6) account for another 10%. The other 30% of nodules in children are caused by many relatively uncommon problems.

22. Crusted purpuric papules and a scaly seborrheic-like eruption in the scalp and groin are seen in what serious disease of childhood?

This constellation of findings should suggest Langerhans cell histiocytosis (formerly called histiocytosis-X) (Fig. 58-7). The disease can vary from a mild cutaneous-only eruption to a severe, life-threatening, systemic disease. Traditionally, this disease has been treated by pediatric oncologists.

Windebank K, Nanduri V: Langerhans cell histiocytosis, *Arch Dis Child* 94:904–908, 2009.

23. Name the skin nodule in childhood that is characterized by frequent bleeding.

Pyogenic granulomas (lobular capillary hemangiomas) are <1-cm, dull-red, firm nodules that bleed easily when traumatized. They are neither pyogenic nor granulomatous, but are thought to be the result of excessive blood vessel formation in response to minor trauma. Treatment is either pulsed dye laser or curettage followed by electrocautery.

Lin RL, Janniger CK: Pyogenic granuloma, *Cutis* 74:229–233, 2004.

24. Flesh-colored to brown macules and papules that hive when stroked (Darier's sign) are diagnostic of what eruption?

Mastocytosis. Mastocytosis is due to an excess of normal-appearing mast cells in the skin. There are four forms, with solitary mastocytomas and urticaria pigmentosa (Fig. 58-8) being the most common. Diffuse cutaneous mastocytosis

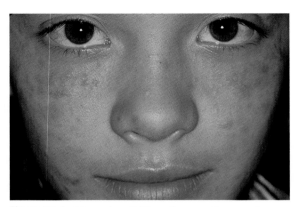

Figure 58-4. Polymorphous light eruption presenting as erythematous photodistributed papules.

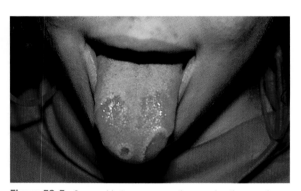

Figure 58-5. Geographic tongue presenting as migrating annular lesions on the tongue.

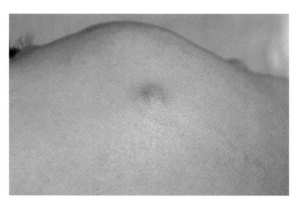

Figure 58-6. Pilomatricoma presenting as a firm nodule on the cheek of a child.

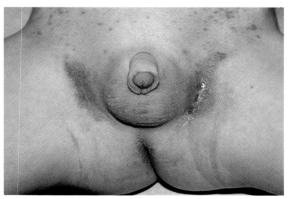

Figure 58-7. Langerhans cell histiocytosis demonstrating erythematous scale and crusted papule in the groin of a child.

and telangiectasia macularis eruptival perstans are the other types.

Bunimovich O, Grassi M, Baer MR: Systemic mastocytosis: classification, pathogenesis, diagnosis, and treatment, *Cutis* 83:29–36, 2009.

25. The onset of annular erythema in sun-exposed areas in children less than 6 months of age should make you want to do what test on the infant's mother?

This eruption is consistent with neonatal lupus erythematosus and is associated with maternal autoantibodies to SS-A/Ro and/or SS-B/La. The mothers are often asymptomatic or have only mild symptoms of Sjögren's syndrome at the time of delivery. Neonatal lupus can also cause complete heart block.

Lee LA: The clinical spectrum of neonatal lupus, *Arch Dermatol Res* 30:107–110, 2009.

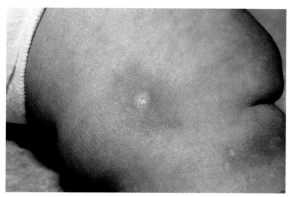

Figure 58-8. Urticaria pigmentosa demonstrating positive Darier's sign (wheal and flare of a brown papule after stroking) in a child with multiple lesions.

26. Which is the most common type of vasculitis seen in children?

Henoch-Schönlein or anaphylactoid purpura. This type of vasculitis frequently follows upper respiratory tract infections and is characterized by the finding of IgA depositions in the blood vessels. The disease may affect only skin, but arthritis, gastrointestinal pain and bleeding, and kidney and central nervous system (CNS) disease may occur.

Roberts PF, Waller TA, Brinker TM, et al: Henoch-Schönlein purpura: a review article, *South Med J* 100:821–824, 2007.

Key Points: Pediatric Dermatology

1. Acne vulgaris is the most common skin condition in childhood.
2. Many children with perioral dermatitis will have been previously treated with topical steroids.
3. Tinea capitis requires oral antifungal therapy.
4. Guttate psoriasis is more common in childhood than in later life.
5. Pyogenic granulomas are neither pyogenic nor granulomatous; they are neovascularizations.
6. The three common causes of acquired circumscribed hair loss are alopecia areata, tinea capitis, and trichotillomania.
7. Tuberous sclerosis and neurofibromatosis are two important genetic disorders in which skin findings are often the presenting feature.

---

27. What is a spider telangiectasia (nevus araneus)?

It is a small telangiectatic macule radiating from a central arteriole. They are commonly seen on the faces of children aged 2 to 10 years. Pulsed dye laser treatment is simple and very effective.

28. Outline the major classes of hair loss in children.

A simple classification of hair loss makes it easier for one to reach a diagnosis:
- Congenital circumscribed
- Acquired circumscribed
- Congenital diffuse
- Acquired diffuse

29. List the three most common types of acquired circumscribed hair loss in children.

Alopecia areata, tinea capitis, and trichotillomania. Alopecia areata is thought to be an autoimmune disorder, whereas tinea capitis is a fungal infection of the scalp hairs. Trichotillomania is self-inflicted and shows an irregular pattern of hair loss. Scalp appearance is normal in alopecia areata and scaly in tinea capitis; trichotillomania is associated with petechiae.

30. What are the two most common causes of congenital circumscribed hair loss?

Sebaceus nevus (organoid nevus) and aplasia cutis congenita. **Sebaceus nevus** is a birthmark of sebaceous glands. It presents as a yellow-orange plaque on the scalp, face, and upper chest. **Aplasia cutis congenita** is a localized absence of skin. It presents as either an open ulceration or a scar. The scalp is the most common location, but areas of aplasia cutis congenita may be seen anywhere on the body. When either of these lesions is present on the scalp, no hair grows in the affected area.

31. What should you think of in a 3-year-old who has never required a haircut?

Such a child is likely to have either a hair shaft defect or a type of ectodermal dysplasia. Hair shaft defects are structural abnormalities that cause hair to be fragile and easily breakable. The defects can be recognized by microscopic evaluation. The ectodermal dysplasias may affect not only hair but also nails, teeth, and sweat glands.

32. What are the cutaneous findings seen in tuberous sclerosis complex?

Two congenital lesions may be seen: hypopigmented macules and connective tissue nevi (shagreen patch). The acquired lesions are facial angiofibromas, fibrous forehead plaque, and periungual fibromas.

Napolioni V, Curatolo P: Genetics and molecular biology of tuberous sclerosis complex, *Curr Genomics* 9:475–487, 2008.

33. How many café-au-lait macules must be present on a child to make you worry about neurofibromatosis type 1 (von Recklinghausen's disease)?

Six or more café-au-lait macules >5 mm in diameter in a prepubertal child are one of the major diagnostic criteria for neurofibromatosis type 1.

Lu-Emerson C, Plotkin SR: The neurofibromatoses. Part 1: NF-1, *Rev Neurol Dis* 6:47–53, 2009.

34. What is a Mongolian spot (middermal melanocytosis)?

This is a blue-black macule found in up to 90% of black and Asian newborns. The most common location is the sacral region (Fig. 58-9), but they may be seen on any portion of the body.

35. What are congenital pigmented nevi, and who cares?

Congenital pigmented nevi (see Fig. 58-9) are developmental errors of pigment cells (melanocytes). They should be defined as small (<1.5 cm), medium (1.5 to 20 cm), and large (>20 cm) in their largest diameter at birth. Some authorities define large as covering >5% of the body surface. Small/medium congenital pigmented nevi are quite common (1/100), whereas large congenital pigmented nevi are rare (1/20,000). The controversy surrounding these lesions concerns their malignant potential. Lifetime risk for the development of melanoma in large congenital pigmented nevi is 1% to 2%.

Kinsler VA, Birley J, Atherton DJ: Great Ormond Street Hospital for Children Registry for Congenital Melanocytic Naevi: prospective study 1988–2007. Part 1—epidemiology, phenotype and outcomes, *Br J Dermatol* 160:143–150, 2009.

36. Child abuse is often incorrectly suspected when a young girl presents with what disease?

Lichen sclerosus. This problem frequently presents as hypopigmented perianal and perivaginal plaques. The epidermis is thinned, and the dermis is sclerotic. Purpura, telangiectasias, ulcerations, and excoriations may also be present. Itching and burning of the genital area are often the complaints that bring the child to the physician. Treatment is with superpotent topical steroids.

Smith SD, Fischer G: Paediatric vulval lichen sclerosus, *Australas J Dermatol* 50:243–248, 2009.

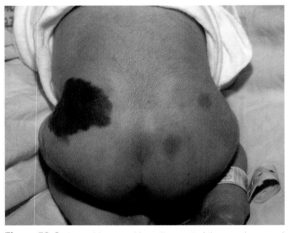

Figure 58-9. Large blue-gray Mongolian spot of the sacral area and dark brown congenital nevus. (Courtesy of the William L. Weston, M.D. Collection.)

GERIATRIC DERMATOLOGY

James E. Fitzpatrick, MD

CHAPTER 59

"Old age isn't so bad when you consider the alternative."

—Maurice Chevalier, *New York Times*

1. How common are skin disorders in the elderly population?
Survey studies have demonstrated that skin diseases are more common in the geriatric population than in the general population. One study revealed that 40% of Americans between the ages of 65 and 74 years had a cutaneous disease significant enough to warrant treatment by a physician. Patients older than 74 years are even more likely to develop significant skin diseases.

Beauregard SA, Gilchrest BA: Survey of skin problems and skin care regimens in the elderly, *Arch Dermotol* 123:1638–1643, 1987.

2. What is intrinsic aging of the skin?
Aging of the skin may be divided into that due to intrinsic aging and that secondary to extrinsic aging (Table 59-1). Intrinsic aging includes those changes that are due to normal maturity and senescence and thus occurs in all individuals. Classically, intrinsic aging has not been considered to be preventable, but there is renewed interest in the role of antioxidants, such as vitamins C and E, in preventing intrinsic aging. Despite numerous articles in the lay literature, there is no proof that these treatments are effective.

3. What is extrinsic aging of the skin?
Extrinsic aging of the skin consists of those changes produced by external agents. The most important extrinsic factor is cumulative ultraviolet (UV) light exposure. The cutaneous changes produced by sunlight are collectively referred to as **dermatoheliosis**. Most of the changes associated with aging of the skin, such as wrinkles, yellow leathery skin, thin skin, hyperpigmentation, hypopigmentation, lentigo senilis (liver spots), telangiectasias, and senile (solar) purpura, are all secondary to damage from the sun or other UV light sources such as tanning booths. Less important extrinsic agents that accelerate aging of the skin include smoking and possibly environmental pollutants.

Fitzpatrick JE, Schleve MJ: Geriatric dermatology. In Jahnigen DW, Schrier RW, editors: *Geriatric medicine*, ed 2, Cambridge, 1996, Blackwell Science, pp 823–836.

4. How does intrinsically aging human skin vary from young skin under the microscope?
Microscopically, the epidermis in aged skin demonstrates flattening of the dermoepidermal junction with loss of the normal rete ridge pattern (see Fig. 59-2A) with fewer melanocytes and Langerhans cells. The dermis demonstrates atrophy with fewer fibroblasts, mast cells, and blood vessels associated with depigmentation of hair, loss of hair follicles, and fewer sweat glands. The amount of collagen, elastin, and ground substance also decreases.

Table 59-1. Age-Related Changes in the Skin

INTRINSIC AGING	EXTRINSIC AGING (PRIMARILY UV LIGHT)
Decrease in corneocyte adhesion	Altered keratinocyte maturation (xerosis)
Slight decrease in epidermal thickness with flattening of rete pegs	Freckles (ephelides)
Decreased number of eccrine sweat glands	Solar lentigo
Decreased numbers of hair follicles	Guttate hypomelanosis
Canities (gray hair)	Wrinkling
Thinning and ridging of nails	Elastosis (yellowish skin)
Decreased dermal collagen (decreases 1% per year)	Telangiectasia
Decreased number of dermal elastic fibers	Senile purpura
Decreased dermal ground substance	Venous lakes
Loss or increase in subcutaneous fat (site-dependent)	Comedones

5. Why does skin wrinkle as we age?

The answer is complicated, because some authorities recognize as many as five different subtypes of wrinkles. The most common type of wrinkles on non–sun-exposed skin are fine wrinkles (glyphic wrinkles) that represent accentuation of normal skin markings. Microscopically, this is due to focal thinning and decreased numbers of keratinocytes. This appears to be intrinsic to aging (Fig. 59-1). The deeper wrinkles in photodamaged skin demonstrate a groove in the epidermis associated with solar elastosis that protrudes on both sides of the groove. These deeper wrinkles are due to extrinsic aging, primarily resulting from ultraviolet light.

6. Does smoking cigarettes accelerate skin aging?

Yes. Epidemiologic studies clearly indicate that smoking is an important extrinsic factor in accelerating aging of the skin. This is also support by animal studies and in vitro studies that have demonstrated that smoking increases the production of tropoelastin and matrix metalloproteinases, resulting in increased degradation of matrix proteins (e.g., collagen, elastic fibers) and abnormal production of abnormal elastotic material. Just another reason not to smoke!

Morita A: Tobacco smoke causes premature skin aging, *J Dermatol Sci* 48:169–175, 2007.

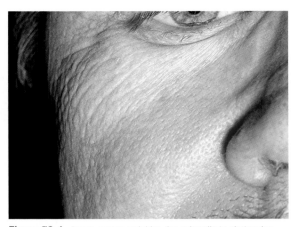

Figure 59-1. Large, coarse wrinkles due primarily to photoaging. Some of the fine wrinkles near the eye are glyphic wrinkles and are intrinsic to aging.

7. What is solar elastosis?

Solar (actinic) elastosis refers to the changes due to abnormal elastotic fibers (Fig. 59-2A) produced by fibroblasts in the papillary and superficial reticular dermis in response to UV light exposure. These abnormal elastotic fibers stain with elastic tissue stains; electron microscopy demonstrates that these fibers are similar, but not identical, to normal elastic fibers. Recent research suggests that they are the result of UVA damage to fibroblasts that results in the over-production and accumulation of elafin, which binds to elastic fibers making them resistant to normal degradation by elastase. Large aggregates of these fibers impart a yellowish color and account for the yellow leathery appearance of sun-exposed skin in geriatric individuals. Solar elastosis is often most easily appreciated in the posterior neck, where it is termed *cutis rhomboidalis nuchae* (Fig. 59-2B).

Muto J, Kurodo K, Wachi H, et al: Accumulation of elafin in actinic elastosis of sun-damaged skin: elafin binds to elastin and prevents elastolytic degradation, *J Invest Dermatol* 127:1358–1366, 2007.

8. What is nodular elastosis with cysts and comedones?

Nodular elastosis with cysts and comedones, also known as Favre-Racouchot syndrome, is characterized by the presence of marked solar elastosis and comedones on the lateral and inferior periorbital areas (Fig. 59-3). Severe cases may demonstrate cysts. The reason for this regional presentation is not understood, but it has been suggested that the fibroblasts around the hair follicles are damaged by UV light and no longer produce normal elastic tissue. This predisposes to dilatation of the hair follicles, resulting in comedones and cysts. Most cases can be successfully treated with topical tretinoin cream and comedonal extraction.

Patterson WM, Fox MD, Schwartz RA: Favre-Racouchot disease, *Int J Dermatol* 43:167–169, 2004.

Figure 59-2. A, Severe solar elastosis. The pale, light blue-gray material in the superficial dermis has largely replaced the normal highly eosinophilic collagen bundles. Also note the loss of the normal rete pegs in the epidermis (hematoxylin and eosin [H&E]). **B,** Cutis rhomboidalis nuchae. Severe solar elastosis and wrinkling of the posterior neck secondary to sun exposure that clearly demarcates from more–normal-appearing skin that is less sun-damaged.

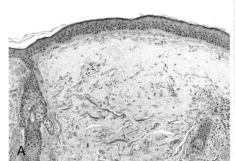
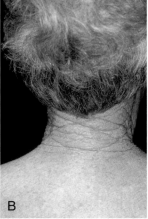

9. How do liver spots, solar lentigo, and lentigo senilis differ?

Liver spots, age spots, and the more proper dermatologic terms solar lentigo and lentigo senilis all refer to the same entity. More than one half of all patients over age 64 will have at least one solar lentigo, and most patients have more than one. Clinically, they are flat to slightly raised, tan to brown lesions on sun-exposed skin, most commonly on the dorsum of the hands, forearms, and face, where they are the result of excessive cumulative UV light exposure. Microscopically, solar lentigos demonstrate elongation of the rete ridges (lentiginous hyperplasia) and increased numbers of melanocytes that produce more than the normal amount of melanin. They may be removed with a light freeze of liquid nitrogen, various types of chemical peels, 2% mequinol/0.01% tretinoin, or special lasers. They may also be temporarily bleached with over-the-counter (1% to 2% concentration) or prescription (3% to 4% concentration) hydroquinone creams.

Farris PK: Combination therapy for solar lentigines, *J Drugs Dermatol* 3:S23–S26, 2004.

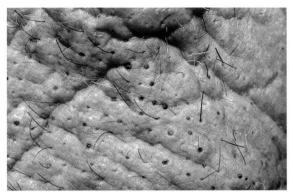

Figure 59-3. Nodular elastosis with comedones. Numerous comedones in characteristic location associated with background of solar elastotic skin.

10. Why do elderly patients frequently develop bleeding into the skin on the dorsum of their hands and arms?

These lesions, referred to as senile purpura (solar purpura, Bateman's purpura, purpura senilis), are common. One study of patients over age 64 years found them in 9% of those examined. The lesions are characterized by sharply demarcated areas of purpura that typically measure 1 to 5 cm (Fig. 59-4). The associated skin is atrophic and inelastic. Patients typically report that these lesions are brought on by minor trauma. It is believed that they are secondary to UV damage to the fibroblasts surrounding the blood vessels, which results in the

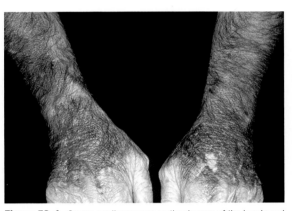

Figure 59-4. Severe senile purpura on the dorsum of the hands and forearms of an elderly patient.

loss of normal supporting collagen. The role of solar damage is supported by case reports of lateralization of solar purpura to one arm that receives more sunlight (e.g., left arm of a taxicab driver).

Joshi RS, Phadke VA, Khopar US, Wadhwa SL: Unilateral solar purpura as a manifestation of asymmetrical photodamage in taxi drivers, *Arch Dermatol* 132:715–716, 1996.

11. Advertisements in newspapers and magazines frequently tout products that "rejuvenate" the skin or make the skin younger. Is there truth to these claims?

No. There are no known therapies or products that rejuvenate the skin or make it younger. There are therapies that make the skin appear less wrinkled and thus appear younger. Topical applications of isotretinoin cream and α-hydroxy acids, such as lactic acid-containing moisturizers, both have been shown in controlled scientific studies to thicken the skin and make wrinkles less noticeable, but the results of these topical treatments vary from almost imperceptible to, at most, moderate. More dramatic results can be achieved by chemical facial peels, laser therapy (laser skin resurfacing), injection of bovine collagen into wrinkles, and facelifts. The best treatment for extrinsic aging of the skin is prevention, by minimizing sun exposure with avoidance, appropriate clothing, and sunscreens. Abstinence from the use of tobacco products also helps.

12. What is the difference between superficial, medium, and deep chemical peels?

As the names imply, it is related to the depth of injury produced. There are many variations and different techniques, but the most commonly used peels and their depth of injury are listed below:
Superficial peel (stratum granulosum to superficial papillary dermis)
- Trichloroacetic acid (TCA) 10% to 30%
- α-hydroxy acid 30% to 70%
Medium peel (papillary to upper reticular dermis)
- Trichloroacetic acid 35% to 50%
- Trichloroacetic acid "combination peels" (e.g., TCA + dry ice)
Deep peel (midreticular dermis)
- Phenol peels

13. Are some sunscreens better than others in preventing wrinkles due to photodamage?

Probably. The definitive study has not been done, but most of the UV-induced deep wrinkles are believed to be attributable to both UVA and UVB. Based on this, sunscreens with both UVB and UVA protection should be the most efficient in preventing wrinkling.

14. Which are the most common inflammatory skin diseases in the elderly?

- Xerosis (dry skin)
- Dermatophytosis (see Chapter 31)
- Contact dermatitis (see Chapter 9)
- Stasis dermatitis
- Seborrheic dermatitis (see Chapter 8)
- Rosacea

Farage MA, Miller KW, Berardesca E, Maibach HI: Clinical implications of aging skin: cutaneous disorders in the elderly, *Am J Clin Dermatol* 10:73–86, 2009.

15. Why are elderly patients prone to develop xerosis?

Xerosis (dry skin, asteatosis, dermatitis hiemalis) is the most common geriatric dermatosis and the most frequent cause of pruritus. Xerosis is believed to be more common in the elderly because of abnormal maturation and adhesion of keratinocytes, which results in rough skin characterized by fine white scale. Diminished eccrine function and sebaceous gland lipids may also play a role but do not represent the primary defect. Asteatosis, which means "without oil," is really a misnomer because this is not the primary cause of dry skin.

16. What is the best way to treat xerosis?

Xerosis is aggravated by low ambient humidity, especially in dry climates and heated homes, and irritants such as soaps. Xerosis can be improved by increasing the ambient humidity (with a humidifier) and by using soaps that are mild, such as Dove or Oil of Olay. Most patients also require treatment with an emollient. The most effective emollients contain lactic acid or a lactate salt, but these are expensive, and the best ones require a prescription. The effectiveness of all emollients is improved by applying them immediately to the skin after bathing, when the skin is hydrated.

Norman RA: Xerosis and pruritus in the elderly: recognition and management, *Dermatol Ther* 16:254–259, 2003.

17. How common is chronic venous insufficiency in the geriatric population?

Epidemiologic studies show an incidence in the geriatric population that approaches 6%. The economic impact of this condition is enormous; the estimated total cost in the United States for the treatment of venous ulcers is more than 1 billion dollars per year in the United States and between 400 and 600 million pounds in the United Kingdom.

Simka M, Majewski E: The social and economic burden of venous leg ulcers: focus on the role of micronized purified flavonoid fraction adjuvant therapy, *Am J Clin Dermatol* 4:573–581, 2003.

18. Explain the pathogenesis of chronic venous insufficiency.

Chronic venous insufficiency is due to venous hypertension secondary to valvular incompetence in the superficial, perforator, or deep veins, with many patients having defects in two or more valve systems. The most severe disease is produced by deep valvular insufficiency. Valvular insufficiency may be the consequence of hereditary factors (absent or congenitally incompetent valves), prolonged standing, and venous thrombosis that may damage valves. Chronic venous hypertension, depending on the degree of severity, may manifest as edema, varicosities, brown pigmentation secondary to hemosiderin, superficial neovascularization, dermatitis, and venous ulcers (Fig. 59-5). Studies have also shown that obesity is a separate risk factor for the development of chronic venous insufficiency.

19. How should you manage chronic venous insufficiency?

Treatment is directed primarily toward reducing venous pressure. This end can be achieved with elevation of the legs, active exercise, supportive stockings, sclerotherapy of selected perforator veins, or surgical treatment. Surgical options are dependent on the site involved but include ligation and stripping of the saphenous vein, ligation of incompetent perforators, or valve replacement. Dermatitis (stasis dermatitis), if present, may be treated with mild to moderate

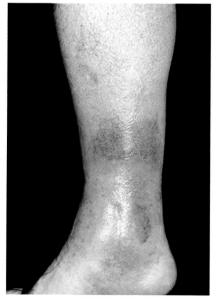

Figure 59-5. Chronic venous insufficiency manifesting as marked erythema and edema, often called stasis dermatitis.

corticosteroids, and oral antibiotics may be used if secondary infection is present. Venous ulcers are treated with these options but also require wound management.

Sieggreen MY, Kline RA: Recognizing and managing venous leg ulcers, *Adv Skin Wound Care* 17:302–311, 2004.

20. What is rosacea? How does it present?

Rosacea, or acne rosacea, is a common skin condition that may affect up to 12% of the geriatric population. The pathogenesis is not understood, but it is known that patients with rosacea have increased blood flow to the skin and are more likely to demonstrate infestation with *Demodex folliculorum*, the human hair follicle mite (although its relevance to the pathogenesis of rosacea is unclear). Rosacea primarily affects the forehead, cheeks, nose, and chin. The three primary lesions are telangiectasis, sebaceous gland hyperplasia, and acneiform papules and pustules (see Chapter 21). One or more of these primary lesions may predominate in a particular patient.

Key Points: Geriatric Dermatology

1. Forty percent of Americans between the ages of 65 and 74 years have had a cutaneous disease significant enough to warrant treatment by a physician.
2. Aging of the skin may be divided into that due to intrinsic aging (normal maturity and senescence) and that secondary to extrinsic aging (external factors such as ultraviolet light).
3. There are no known therapies or products that rejuvenate the skin or make it younger.
4. Xerosis (dry skin, asteatosis, dermatitis hiemalis) is the most common geriatric dermatosis and the most frequent cause of pruritus.

---

21. Is rhinophyma related to alcohol abuse?

Rhinophyma is a clinical variant of rosacea that presents as severe sebaceous gland hyperplasia of the nose, which may distort its contour. The most famous example of rhinophyma is the actor W.C. Fields. The lay public often assumes that people with rhinophyma are alcohol abusers. Studies have not been able to demonstrate increased alcohol use in patients with rhinophyma. Patients with rosacea and rhinophyma demonstrate prominent flushing following the consumption of alcohol. This flushing has been incorrectly perceived as being the cause of rhinophyma.

Curnier A, Choudhary S: Rhinophyma: dispelling the myths, *Plast Reconstr Surg* 114:351–354, 2004.

22. Name the most common types of skin tumors seen in the elderly.

- **Benign tumors:** Seborrheic keratoses, cherry hemangiomas, nevi, acrochordons, sebaceous hyperplasia
- **Premalignant tumors:** Actinic keratoses, Bowen's disease
- **Malignancies:** Basal cell carcinoma, squamous cell carcinoma

Dewberry C, Norman RA: Skin cancer in elderly patients, *Dermatol Clin* 22:93–96, 2004.

23. What are seborrheic keratoses?

Seborrheic keratoses are common, benign epidermal growths of the skin. In patients over age 64 years, the incidence of these growths is 88%. The pathogenesis is uncertain, but the most recent evidence suggests that they are derived from keratinocytes of the most superficial part of the hair follicle and are not derived from the epidermis, as previously thought. They typically begin appearing during middle age or later. They may be located on any cutaneous surface other than the palms and soles but are most commonly found on the face and trunk. Clinically, they present as tan, brown, gray, or black, sharply demarcated, exophytic papules that appear to be "stuck on" the skin. The surface often has an irregular contour or pebbly surface but may be verrucous or smooth (Fig. 59-6).

24. What are stucco keratoses?

Stucco keratoses are a variant of seborrheic keratoses that present as 1- to 4-mm gray to white scaly papules. These are most commonly located on the arms and lower legs (Fig. 59-7).

25. What is sebaceous hyperplasia?

Sebaceous hyperplasia is the most common benign sebaceous neoplasm. The lesions present in middle age and increase in number in the elderly. They present as asymptomatic, solitary or multiple yellow or yellowish-white papules that frequently demonstrate a central dell (Fig. 59-8). Increased numbers of lesions are seen in patients with *Muir-Torre syndrome* (sebaceous gland tumors associated with internal malignancy) and in transplant patients.

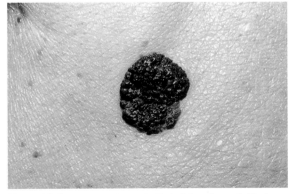

Figure 59-6. Seborrheic keratosis. Typical deep-brown to black exophytic seborrheic keratosis with a "stuck-on" appearance. This is the most common benign cutaneous growth of the elderly.

Treatment options include no treatment, intralesional electrodesiccation, pulse dye laser, and shave removal.

Bader RS, Scarborough DA: Surgical pearl: intralesional electrodesiccation of sebaceous hyperplasia, *J Am Acad Dermatol* 42:127–128, 2000.

26. A 70-year-old man presents to your clinic with the sudden onset of hundreds of seborrheic keratoses. Is there any reason for concern?

Yes. This patient may have the sign of Leser-Trélat, which is characterized by the sudden appearance of numerous seborrheic keratoses associated with an underlying malignancy. About one third of patients with this sign may also present with acanthosis nigricans, another potential cutaneous marker of internal malignancy. The most common associated malignancy is an abdominal adenocarcinoma.

Ceylan C, Alper S, Kiline I: Leser-Trélat sign, *Int J Dermatol* 41:687–688, 2002.

27. Describe the methods for treating seborrheic keratoses.

First of all, not all seborrheic keratoses need to be treated, and many health plans do not pay for their treatment because they are benign lesions. Patients frequently want them removed for cosmetic reasons or because they are pruritic. The most common treatment is cryotherapy with liquid nitrogen, because it is quick and effective. Seborrheic keratoses can also be removed by curetting or shave biopsy. Shave biopsies are usually done when the lesion has an atypical clinical appearance and a malignancy, such as squamous cell or basal cell carcinoma, is in the differential diagnosis. Seborrheic keratoses can also be treated with the topical application of α-hydroxy acids.

28. An elderly man presents with a soft blue papule on the helix of his cheek and is concerned about malignant melanoma. What is the most likely diagnosis?

The differential diagnosis includes a blue nevus, malignant melanoma, tattoo, and venous lake. In this case, the diagnosis of a venous lake can be established by compression of the papule, which will cause collapse of the lesion (Fig. 59-9). Venous lakes, like hemorrhoids, are dilated veins that have lost elasticity of their walls. They are usually 1 to 5 mm in diameter and are typically located on sun-exposed surfaces, such as the lips, ears, and face of

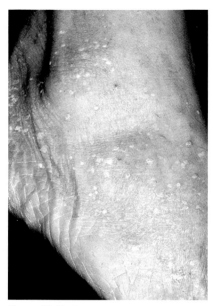

Figure 59-7. Typical stucco keratosis manifesting as small white or white-gray scaly papules with "stuck-on" appearance.

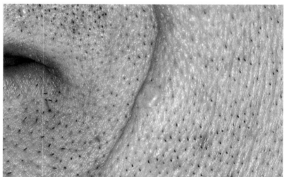

Figure 59-8. Sebaceous hyperplasia. Typical, small, yellowish-white, symmetrical papule with central depression. (Courtesy of the Fitzsimons Army Medical Center teaching files.)

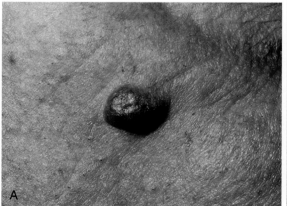
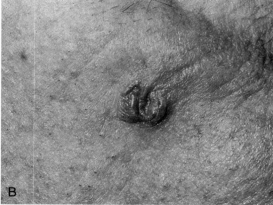

Figure 59-9. A, Venous lake presenting as dark blue-violaceous papule on the cheek. **B,** Same venous lake demonstrating collapse after compression.

the elderly. They are very common, with one epidemiologic study of elderly patients finding venous lakes in 12% of those examined. They are of no clinical significance, except that they may mimic malignant melanoma and occasionally become painful or thrombosed. They can be treated by excision, carbon dioxide laser, infrared coagulation, or by the injection of sclerosing agents such as polidocanol.

Kuo HW, Yang CH: Venous lake of the lip treated with a sclerosing agent: report of two cases, *Dermatol Surg* 29:425–428, 2003.

29. Is there a future in geriatric dermatology?

One hundred years ago, only 2% of the U.S. population was over 65 years old. By 1980, this percentage was 11%, and, by the year 2030, it will be 20%. Given the high incidence of significant dermatologic diseases in the elderly, it is clear that all health care providers need to familiarize themselves with the diagnosis, prevention, and treatment of skin diseases seen in this population.

DERMATOSES OF PREGNANCY

Misha D. Miller, MD, FACOG

SPECIFIC DERMATOSES OF PREGNANCY

1. Name four pregnancy-specific dermatological disorders
- Pruritic urticarial papules and plaques of pregnancy
- Pemphigoid gestationis
- Atopic eruption of pregnancy
- Intrahepatic cholestasis of pregnancy

Ambros-Rudolph CM, Müllegger RR, Vaughan-Jones SA, et al: The specific dermatoses of pregnancy revisited and reclassified: results of a retrospective two-center study on 505 pregnant patients, *J AM Acad Dermatol* 54(3):395–404, 2006.

2. What is pruritic urticarial papules and plaques of pregnancy?
Pruritic urticarial papules and plaques of pregnancy (also known as polymorphic eruption of pregnancy, or PUPPP) has an incidence of 1/200 pregnancies. The onset of PUPPP is usually in the third trimester. The pruritic, erythematous, papules and plaques are usually first seen in the abdominal striae (stretch marks) and then spread to the chest, trunk, and extremities. The papules and plaques typically spare the palms, soles, face, and mucous membranes. Large vesicles or bullae are uncommon, though pinpoint vesicles may be seen (Fig. 60-1).

Ahmadi S, Powell FC: Pruritic urticarial papules and plaques of pregnancy: current status, *Austr J Dermatol* 46:53–60, 2005.
Matz H, Orion E, Wolf R: Pruritic urticarial papules and plaques of pregnancy: polymorphic eruption of pregnancy (PUPPP), *Clin Dermatol* 24(2):105–108, 2006.

3. Does PUPPP have any associated morbidity?
The pruritis associated with PUPPP can be very uncomfortable for the mother. There are no fetal sequelae. The skin lesions and pruritus associated with PUPPP usually spontaneously resolve within 1 or 2 weeks after delivery.

4. How is PUPPP treated?
Topical corticosteroids and oral antihistamines are the most common methods of treatment. However, the efficacy of oral antihistamines in treating the pruritus of PUPPP is questionable. The use of oral corticosteroids is rare.

Matz H, Orion E, Wolf R: Pruritic urticarial papules and plaques of pregnancy: polymorphic eruption of pregnancy (PUPPP), *Clin Dermatol* 24(2):105–108, 2006.

5. From which dermatosis of pregnancy must PUPPP be differentiated?
Pemphigoid gestationis. It may be difficult to clinically differentiate PUPPP from pemphigoid gestationis.

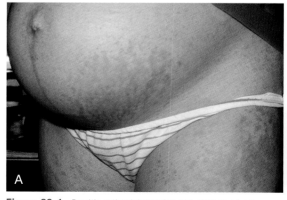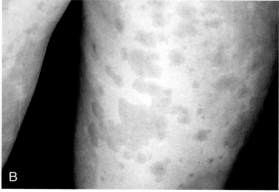

Figure 60-1. Pruritic urticarial papules and plaques of pregnancy (PUPPP). **A,** Erythematous papules in the striae of a 21-year-old primigravida woman. **B,** Urticarial papules and plaques that are not associated with striae on the thighs of a woman with PUPPP.

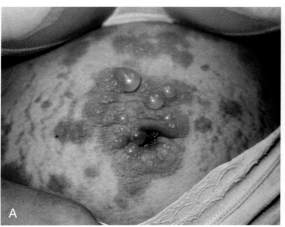 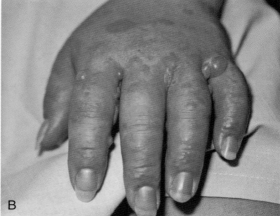

Figure 60-2. Pemphigoid gestationis. **A,** Umbilical urticarial plaques and tense blisters in a woman with pemphigoid gestationis. **B,** Intertriginous area between fingers demonstrating tense blisters. This is another commonly affected site in pemphigoid gestationis. (Courtesy of the Fitzsimons Army Medical Center teaching files.)

6. What is pemphigoid gestationis?

Pemphigoid gestationis (also called herpes gestationis or gestational pemphigoid) is an autoimmune subepidermal bullous disorder of pregnancy that may start in the 2nd trimester, the 3rd trimester, or in the postpartum period. The skin lesions are characterized by urticarial papules and plaques, which then progress into painful bullae. The lesions of pemphigoid gestationis initially present periumbilically (Fig. 60-2A), and then spread to involve the trunk and extremities (Fig. 60-2B), usually sparing the face.

Semkova K, Black M: Pemphigoid gestationis: current insights into pathogenesis and treatment, *Eur J Obstete Gynecol Reprod Biol* 145(2):138–144, 2009.

7. What are the antigens associated with the development on pemphigoid gestationis?

Bullous pemphigoid antigen 2 (BPAG2) is a 180 kDal transcellular glycoprotein that is part of the hemidesmosome (a structure that binds epithelial cells to the basement membrane of the epidermis). IgG binds to BPAG2 and triggers the classic complement pathway leading to a deposition of C3 along the basement membrane zone (Fig. 60-3). Deposition of complement along the basement membrane zone leads to a recruitment of inflammatory cells, particularly eosinophils. This cascade ultimately leads to a release of proteolytic enzymes that cleave portions of the epidermis from the dermis.

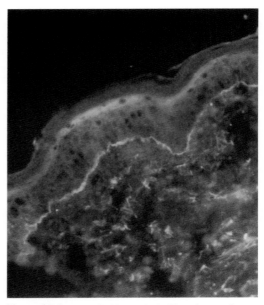

Figure 60-3. Pemphigoid gestationis. Direct immunofluorescent study demonstrating linear C3 along the basement membrane zone. Less commonly, linear IgG is also seen.

Key Points: Pemphigoid Gestationis

1. Pemphigoid gestationis is an autoimmune disease that occurs during pregnancy, and it is characterized by IgG_1 antibodies directed at bullous pemphigoid antigen–1 in the basement membrane zone.
2. Direct immunofluorescent study demonstrates linear C3 and/or IgG along the basement membrane zone and is the diagnostic test of choice to establish the diagnosis.
3. The primary lesions of pemphigoid gestationis consist of urticarial plaques and/or blisters.
4. The umbilical area is preferentially affected in pemphigoid gestationis and can be a clue to the diagnosis.
5. Neonates of mothers with pemphigoid gestationis may demonstrate a lower birth weight and may occasionally demonstrate transient blisters, but are otherwise healthy.

8. **Which histocompatibility leukocyte antigen (HLA) types have been associated with pemphigoid gestationis?**
   HLA-DR3 and HLA-DR4.

   Powell AM, Sakuam-OyamaY, Oyama N, et al: Usefulness of BP180 NC16a enzyme-linked immunosorbent assay in the serodiagnosis of pemphigoid gestationis and in differentiating between pemphigoid gestationis and pruritic urticarial papules and plaques of pregnancy, *Arch Dermatol* 141(6):705–710, 2005.

9. **Compare PUPPP and pemphigoid gestationis.**
   See Table 60-1.

   High W, Hoang MP, Miller MD: Pruritic urticarial papules and plaques of pregnancy with unusual and extensive palmoplantar involvement, *Obstet Gynecol* 105(5):1261–1264, 2005.

10. **What is atopic eruption of pregnancy?**
    Atopic eruption of pregnancy is classified to include eczema of pregnancy, prurigo gestationis, and folliculitis of pregnancy. According to the retrospective study by Ambros-Rudolph et al, it is the most common dermatoses of pregnancy, with a prevalence of 50.7%. In this study 20% of the patients were known to have preexisting atopic dermatitis, but 80% of the patients reviewed experienced symptoms de novo during pregnancy. It is known to start early in pregnancy, before the third trimester. The skin lesions are erythematous, excoriated papules, plaques, or nodules on the extensor surfaces of the limbs and on the trunk, and may appear crusted and eczematous. The treatment involves topical corticosteroids, and the disease usually resolves in the postpartum period.

    Ambros-Rudolph CM, Müllegger RR, Vaughan-Jones SA, et al: The specific dermatoses of pregnancy revisited and reclassified: results of a retrospective two-center study on 505 pregnant patients, *J Am Acad Dermatol* 54(3):395–404, 2006.

11. **What is intrahepatic cholestasis of pregnancy?**
    Intrahepatic cholestasis of pregnancy (ICP) is characterized symptomatically by an intense pruritus, most often starting on the palms and soles, and then becoming generalized. There are no other dermatologic findings except excoriations. ICP usually occurs in the third trimester of pregnancy. The etiology of intrahepatic cholestasis of pregnancy is not completely understood, but there is a strong indication that there is interplay between a rise in pregnancy hormones (estrogen and progesterone), accumulation of bile acids secondary to liver dysfunction, and genetic susceptibility contributing to development of this disease.

    Geenes V, Williamson C: Intrahepatic cholestasis of pregnancy, *World J Gastroenterol* 15(17):2049–2066, 2009.

12. **What is the epidemiology of ICP?**
    In South America, where it is most common, the incidence has been reported as high as 10%. The incidence of cholestasis of pregnancy in Western countries is ~1%. It is more common in the winter months.

13. **Are there specific laboratory findings to establish the diagnosis?**
    Yes. The most specific laboratory derangements are found when measuring bile acids, specifically cholic acid and deoxycholic acid, which may be elevated more than 100 times (upper end of normal: 10 μmol/L). Liver transaminases

Table 60-1. Compare and Contrast PUPPP and Pemphigoid Gestationis

	PUPPP	PEMPHIGOID GESTATIONIS
Clinical presentation	Pruritic erythematous papules and plaques Initial lesions present in the abdominal striae, spreading to the trunk and extremities; vesicles may be present Usually spares the palms and soles	Urticarial papules, plaques, and blisters Initial lesions start periumbilically and spread to the trunk and extremities The palms and soles are commonly involved
Direct immunofluorescence	Occasional complement deposition in a perivascular location or in a granular formation along the dermal–epidermal junction	Linear deposition of IgG (25% of the time) and complement (C3) at the dermal–epidermal junction. (see Fig. 60-3)
Fetal sequelae	None	Increased risk of intrauterine growth restriction and prematurity 3%–10% of newborns have lesions of neonatal pemphigus
Treatment	Topical corticosteroids Oral antihistamines	Topical or oral corticosteroids (prednisone 0.5 mg/kg/day) Oral antihistamines Dapsone, cyclosporine (results are mixed)
Recurrence in future pregnancies	Usually does not recur	Usually recurs at an earlier gestation and is typically more severe

Table 60-2. Treatment Regimens of ICP

Ursodeoxycholic acid 15 mg/kg/day	Decreases bile acid concentration Aids in transplacental transport of bile acids
S-adenosyl-methionine	Reverses estrogen induced cholestasis in experimental animals Minimally improves bile acid laboratory values and pruritus Studies show conflicting evidence regarding the efficacy of this drug
Cholestyramine	Generally not shown to be effective
Dexamethasone	Inhibits placental estrogen synthesis Does not improve pruritus or transaminase levels Repeated doses may be associated with decreased birth weight and other fetal complications
Delivery	Delivery is the cure for ICP Most authors recommend early delivery by 38 weeks (~36 weeks for severe laboratory derangements)

(aspartate transaminase [AST], alanine transaminase [ALT]) may also be elevated, but ALT is thought to be the more sensitive marker, with an increase of 2 to 10 times the upper limit of normal. Bilirubin levels may be elevated, but total bilirubin levels do not often exceed 6 mg/dL.

14. What risks and outcomes are associated with intrahepatic cholestasis of pregnancy?

The main risks are to the fetus; the fetus is unable to excrete cholic acid, resulting in toxicity. Sudden intrauterine fetal death occurs in 1% to 2% of pregnancies affected by ICP. Other complications include respiratory distress syndrome, meconium staining of amniotic fluid membranes, and premature delivery. The risk of fetal complications increases with bile acids levels >40 µM/L. There are not usually any long-term maternal sequelae. The pruritus associated with ICP usually resolves within 48 hours to 2 weeks, after delivery.

Hepburn I: Pregnancy-associated liver disorders, *Dig Dis Sci* (53):2334–2358, 2008.

15. How is cholestasis of pregnancy treated?

See Table 60-2.

Hepburn I: Pregnancy-associated liver disorders, *Dig Dis Sci* (53):2334–2358, 2008.

16. Is impetigo herpetiformis a distinct clinical disease?

Impetigo herpetiformis is a rare disorder that typically presents in the third trimester. This disease is characterized by sterile pustules on an erythematous plaque initially presenting on the flexural and intertriginous areas, and then progressing to involve the trunk and remaining surfaces of the extremities. Impetigo herpetiformis can involve the mucous membranes. There also can be nail involvement, as well as systemic symptoms such as fever and malaise. It is associated with an increased risk of intrauterine growth restriction and stillbirth. Clinically and histologically, impetigo herpetiformis resembles pustular psoriasis, and it is debated whether or not impetigo herpetiformis is a distinct disease.

Lim KS, Tang MB, Nq PP: Impetigo herpetiformis—a rare dermatosis of pregnancy associated with prenatal complications, *Ann Acad Med Singapore* 34(9):565-568, 2005.

17. Are there lab findings associated with impetigo herpetiformis?

Yes. Associated lab findings include leukocytosis, elevated erythrocyte sedimentation rate, and occasionally hypocalcemia.

18. What is the treatment for impetigo herpetiformis?

Systemic corticosteroids are the first-line treatment. Some studies have reported good outcomes with cyclosporine. The condition resolves with delivery. It is important to be aware of secondary infections of the lesions, and then to treat with appropriate antimicrobial medications.

Brightman, L, Stefanato CM, Bhawan J, et al: Third-trimester impetigo herpetiformis treated with cyclosporine, *J Am Acad Dermatol* 56(Suppl 2)S62–S64, 2005.

PHYSIOLOGIC SKIN CHANGES IN PREGNANCY

19. List the physiologic skin changes that can occur as a normal part of pregnancy.

- Pigmentary changes
- Hair changes
- Vascular changes

- Connective tissue changes (striae distensae)
- Cutaneous tumors

Muallem MM, Rubeiz NG: Physiological and biological skin changes in pregnancy, *Clin Dermatol* 24(2):80–83, 2006.

20. What are some of the normal pigmentary changes that can be associated with pregnancy?

- Darkening of the nipples, areola, genitalia, axilla, inner thighs, and periumbilical area
- Darkening of the linea alba, which is then is referred to as the linea nigra
- Darkening of recent scars
- Melanonychia
- Melasma, which is hyperpigmentation of the face involving the cheeks, nose, or the chin (Fig. 60-4)
- Darkening of ephelides and nevi

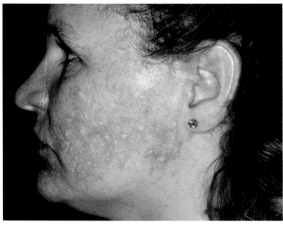

Figure 60-4. Photodistributed macular hyperpigmentation typical of melasma.

21. Why do these pigmentary changes occur?

The exact mechanism is not known, but it is thought that an increase in estrogen, progesterone, and melanocyte-stimulating hormone stimulates melanogenesis.

Barankin B, Silver SG, Carruthers A: The skin in pregnancy, *J Cutan Med Surg* 6(3):236–240, 2002.

22. How does pregnancy affect patients with melanoma?

Melanoma accounts for 8% of malignancies in pregnancy. Pregnancy is no longer thought to worsen the prognosis of melanoma, and the survival rates for similarly staged pregnant and nonpregnant individuals are not statistically significant.

Pagés C, Robert C, Thomas L, et al: Management and outcome of metastatic melanoma during pregnancy, *Br J Dermatol* 162:274–281, 2009. [Epub ahead of print.]

23. Is pregnancy associated with changes in hair growth?

In pregnancy, women experience a prolonged anagen phase, which leads to clinical thickening of the hair. The hairs shift into a telogen phase 1 to 5 months following delivery, and these patients then experience a telogen effluvium. Hirsutism (male pattern facial and body terminal hair growth) may also increase in pregnancy, and usually resolves 6 months postpartum.

24. List the vascular changes that can occur in pregnancy.

- Palmer erythema (Fig. 60-5)
- Spider angiomas
- Varicose veins
- Hemorrhoids

Muallem MM, Rubeiz NG: Physiological and biological skin changes in pregnancy, *Clin Dermatol* 24(2):80–83, 2006.

25. What factors influence the development of striae distensae (commonly known as "stretch marks")?

- Greater degrees of abdominal distention (such as in multiple gestation)
- High degree of weight gain
- Genetic predisposition
- Estrogen, adrenocortical hormone, and relaxin, all of which play a role in connective tissue formation.

26. Discuss two cutaneous tumors often associated with pregnancy.

1. **Pyogenic granuloma of pregnancy** (granuloma gravidarum) is a cutaneous tumor consisting of a vascular proliferation, most often of the gingival tissue in pregnant women. These tumors may ulcerate and become painful. Pyogenic granuloma usually spontaneously regresses after pregnancy, and if not, can be treated with an ND:YAG laser.
2. **Molluscum fibrosum gravidarum** are skin tags that develop on the face, neck, chest, axilla, and inframammary areas of pregnant women. They may regress spontaneously postpartum, and, if not, are easily treated through surgical removal.

Muallem MM, Rubeiz NG: Physiological and biological skin changes in pregnancy, *Clin Dermatol* 24(2):80–83, 2006.

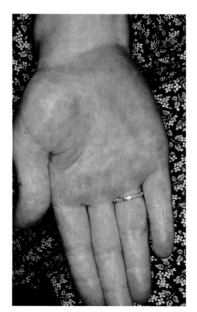

Figure 60-5. Marked palmar erythema in a pregnant woman.

27. Do some diseases improve with pregnancy?

Yes. Examples of such diseases include

- Psoriasis
- Rheumatoid arthritis
- Systemic lupus erythematosus
- Hidradenitis suppurativa
- Fox-Fordyce disease

The regression of psoriasis, rheumatoid arthritis, and systemic lupus erythematosus is thought to be related to the suppressed maternal immunity of pregnancy. Improvement of hidradenitis suppurativa and Fox-Fordyce disease is possibly secondary to the decreased apocrine gland activity in pregnancy.

Oumeish OY, Al-Fouzan AW: Miscellaneous diseases affected by pregnancy, *Clin Dermatol* 24(2):113–117, 2006.
Raychaudhuri SP, Navare T, Gross J, et al: Clinical course of psoriasis during pregnancy, *Int J Dermatol* 42(7):518–520, 2003.

28. Do some mucocutaneous diseases worsen in pregnancy?

Yes. See Table 60-3.

Winton GB: Skin diseases aggravated by pregnancy, *J Am Acad Dermatol* 20:1–13, 1989.

Table 60-3. Mucocutaneous Diseases Exacerbated by Pregnancy

Infections
Candidal vaginitis
Trichomoniasis
Condyloma acuminata
Pityrosporum folliculitis
Herpes simplex
Varicella-zoster
Leprosy

Diseases of altered immunity
Lupus erythematosus
Systemic sclerosis (renal)
Polymyositis/dermatomyositis
Pemphigus

Metabolic diseases
Porphyria cutanea tarda
Acrodermatitis enteropathica

Connective tissue disorders
Ehlers-Danlos syndrome (laceration, postpartum hemorrhage)
Pseudoxanthoma elasticum

Miscellaneous conditions
Erythrokeratodermia variabilis
Mycosis fungoides
Neurofibromatosis
Acquired immunodeficiency syndrome
Hereditary hemorrhagic telangiectasia

DISORDERS OF THE FEMALE GENITALIA

Misha D. Miller, MD, FACOG

NONNEOPLASTIC EPITHELIAL DISORDERS OF THE VULVA

1. What is lichen sclerosus (also known as lichen sclerosus et atrophicus)?
Lichen sclerosus (LS) (Fig. 61-1) is an inflammatory condition that primarily affects the superficial dermis. The disease process results in thinned or atrophic white papules and plaques of the skin. LS primarily affects the anogenital region, but it can also present on the trunk or extremities. Lichen sclerosus of the vulva most commonly affects postmenopausal women, but it can also develop in 7% to 15% of prepubertal females.

2. Describe the clinical signs of lichen sclerosus of the vulva.
The characteristic findings associated with lichen sclerosus include white, thinned, crinkled skin (it is frequently described as "cigarette paper" atrophy). Often there are areas of ecchymoses in the involved skin. The majority of the vagina is usually unaffected; however, a patient may have involvement of the vaginal introitus, leading to stenosis. One also may find fusion of the labia minora, phimosis of the clitoral hood, and fissures. LS can also simultaneously involve the perianal area, which then forms a "figure-of-eight" pattern.

Val I, Almeida G: An overview of lichen sclerosus, *Clin Obstet Gynecol* 48(4):808–817, 2005.

3. What are the symptoms of lichen sclerosus?
The most common symptom associated with lichen sclerosus is pruritus. Patients may also report burning, bleeding, and tearing of the vulva or vaginal introitus. If stenosis of the vaginal introitus is present, dyspareunia is often reported.

4. Is there a need to biopsy lichen sclerosus of the vulva?
Yes. Biopsy of the affected site can aid in differentiating lichen sclerosus from other disorders, such as vitiligo (Fig. 61-2) and lichen planus. Hyperkeratotic, ulcerated, or nodular lesions should be sampled to rule out vulvar intraepithelial neoplasia (VIN) or squamous cell carcinoma of the vulva. The risk of LS becoming malignant is 4% to 6%.

5. How does one treat lichen sclerosus?
The most widely accepted first-line treatment is use of a high-potency topical corticosteroid, most commonly clobetasol proprionate. Other less common therapies used for recalcitrant LS include intralesional corticosteroids, retinoids, oral potassium para-aminobenzoate, chloroquine, tacrolimus/pimecrolimus, cyclosporine, and photodynamic therapy with topical 5-aminolevulinic acid. LS in children often will resolve at the time of puberty.

Smith YR, Haefner HK: Vulvar lichen sclerosus: pathophysiology and treatment, *Am J Clin Dermatol* 5:105–125, 2004.

6. What is the differential diagnosis of lichen sclerosus of the vulva?
- Lichen planus
- Vitiligo
- VIN
- Sexual abuse (children)
- Inverse psoriasis

7. What is lichen planus?
Lichen planus is an autoimmune inflammatory disorder. The exact pathogenesis is not completely understood, but it is thought to be a T-cell–mediated disorder that results from damage to the epidermal basement membrane secondary to antibodies directed against components of the basal keratinocytes.

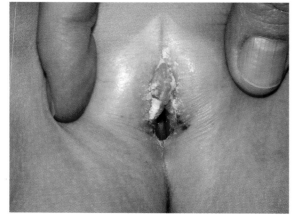

Figure 61-1. Lichen sclerosus demonstrating typical ill-defined hypopigmentation with wrinkled atrophic appearance that is best visualized near the bottom of the lesion. (Courtesy of James E. Fitzpatrick, MD.)

8. Are there different variants of lichen planus that affect the vulva?

Yes. Variants that affect the vulva include erosive lichen planus, papulosquamous lichen planus, and hypertrophic lichen planus. The most common variant found in the vulva is erosive lichen planus. This variant is characterized by erosions on a background of violaceous papules and plaques. The skin of the vulva may also appear shiny, reticulated and white. Rarely, oral-vulval-vaginal lichen planus may also be seen. Of the approximate 1% of the population with oral lichen planus, 25% have vulvovaginal disease.

ACOG Practice Bulletin No. 93: Diagnosis and management of vulvar skin disorders, *Obstet Gynecol* 93:1243–1253, 2008.

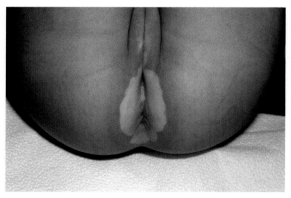

Figure 61-2. Vitiligo showing characteristic total depigmentation with evidence of atrophy. Notice the typical scalloped margins. (Courtesy of Fitzsimons Army Medical Center teaching files.)

9. What are the clinical symptoms of vulval lichen planus?

Patients most commonly present with complaints of vulvovaginal burning, pruritus, postcoital bleeding, and dyspareunia. Up to 70% of patients also have vaginal lesions. There may be an associated purulent vaginal discharge and chronic erosions of the vaginal epithelium can lead to the development of extensive adhesions leading to vaginal narrowing and obliteration.

Lewis FM: Vulval lichen planus, *Br J Dermatol* 138(4):569–575, 1998.

10. Is lichen planus associated with malignancy?

Vulvar malignancy developing in patients with lichen planus has been reported, but it is rare.

Kennedy CM, Peterson LB, Galask RP: Erosive vulvar lichen planus: a cohort at risk for cancer? *J Reprod Med* 53:781–784, 2008.

11. How do you treat lichen planus of the vulva?

Treatment of lichen planus of the mucosal surfaces, such as the vulvovaginal areas, is very difficult. Potent topical steroids are commonly used, but have mixed results. Other therapies that have been reported include pimecrolimus, tacrolimus, hydroxychloroquine, cyclosporine, and methotrexate.

Cooper SM, Haefner HK, Abrahams-Gessel S, et al: Vulvovaginal lichen planus treatment: a survey of current practices, *Arch Dermatol* 144:1520–1521, 2008.

12. Describe lichen simplex chronicus of the vulva.

Lichen simplex chronicus is an end-stage response that results from chronic scratching or rubbing of the skin. The skin becomes thickened, lichenified (exaggeration of the normal skin lines), and will often show excoriations. Any condition that causes pruritus of the skin, in combination with the patient scratching the involved area, will ultimately result in the development of lichen simplex chronicus. The primary skin condition is most commonly eczema.

13. Psoriasis can be present on the vulva. How does it present?

Psoriasis of the vulva presents as beefy red symmetrical plaques. The silvery scale associated with psoriatic lesions on other areas of the body is typically absent. A patient may have inverse psoriasis of the inguinal creases, referred to as inverse psoriasis. Skin lesion of psoriasis in this area may be more inflamed and have undergone maceration secondary to friction and moisture. Vulvar pruritus and burning may be prominent symptoms.

14. How is psoriasis of the vulva treated?

Low-potency topical steroids are generally the first line of treatment. Calcipotriene, pimecrolimus, and tacrolimus, though less efficacious, are also used to avoid steroid affects such as atrophy of the more delicate genital skin.

Kalb RE, Bagel J, Korman NJ, et al: Treatment of intertriginous psoriasis: from the Medical Board of the National Psoriasis Foundation, *J Am Acad Dermatol* 60:120–124, 2009.

15. What are other common causes of vulvar pruritus?

- Vulvar contact dermatitis (Table 61-1)
- Vulvovaginal infections
- Vulvar malignancy

16. Name some common vulvovaginal infections associated with pruritus?

- Fungal (candidiasis, tinea cruris)
- Bacterial vaginosis

Table 61-1. Common Causes of Vulvar Contact Dermatitis

- Bath soaps
- Feminine hygiene sprays, deodorant sprays
- Fragrance
- Lubricants
- Spermicides
- Semen
- Condoms
- Clothing dyes
- Sanitary pads
- Benzocaine
- Neomycin
- Antifungal creams
- Urine

- Trichomoniasis
- Infestations such as scabies
- Condyloma accuminta (genital warts)
- Molluscum contagiosum

17. Compare and contrast condyloma accuminatum and molluscum contagiosum.
See Table 61-2.

VASCULITIC DISEASE OF THE VULVA

18. What is Behçet's disease?
Behçet's disease (Fig. 61-3) is a chronic relapsing vasculitis of unknown etiology that results in ocular, mucocutaneous, genital, pulmonary, neurologic, gastrointestinal, and articular involvement. Oral and genital lesions are manifested as painful aphthous-like ulcers, and may be the earliest signs of this disease. Behçet's disease is most prevalent along the "silk road," which spans from Japan and China to the Mediterranean Sea (countries such as Turkey), but it is also seen in the Unites States, though uncommonly. The disease usually presents in the third decade of life.

Table 61-2. Condyloma Accuminatum versus Molluscum Contagiosum

	CONDYLOMA ACCUMINATA	MOLLUSCUM CONTAGIOSUM
Clinical appearance	Soft fleshy cauliflower-like papules. Can be very small with a dome shape and thus difficult to differentiate from molluscum contagiosum	Small, dome-shaped, typically flesh-colored papules with a central umbilication when squeezed on the lateral edges
Etiology	Human papilloma virus (HPV) HPV 6 and 11 are responsible for 90% of these lesions	DNA poxvirus—molluscum contagiosum virus (MCV). MCV-1 is most prevalent, MCV-2 is most commonly associated with sexually transmitted molluscum contagiosum
Transmission	Sexually transmitted Highly contagious	Sexually transmitted in adults (this disease is common in children on non-genital skin, and is not thought to be sexually transmitted) Highly contagious; known to be spread through fomites (e.g., wet towels, etc.)
Autoinoculation	Yes	Yes
Treatment	Imiquimod Podophyllin Trichloroacetic acid Laser ablation Cryosurgery	Imiquimod Cantharidin Trichloroacetic acid Curettage Laser ablation Cryosurgery Expectant management (many lesions will spontaneously resolve within two years)
Vaccine?	Quadrivalent vaccine for immunity against HPV 6, 11, 16, and 18	None

19. What is the treatment for Behçet's disease?

- Topical corticosteroids
- Antibiotic solutions
- Topical anesthetics
- Silver nitrate

For more severe disease:

- Oral corticosteroids
- Colchicine
- Oral antibiotics (benzathine penicillin)
- Immunosuppressive agents (azathioprine, cyclosporin)
- Biologic agents (antitumor necrosis factor–α agents, interferon)

Alpsoy E, Akman A: Behçet's disease: an algorithmic approach to its treatment, *Arch Dermatol Res* 301:693–702, 2009

NEOPLASTIC DISORDERS OF THE VULVA

20. What is the most common cancer of the vulva?

Ninety percent of vulval cancer is squamous cell carcinoma (SCC). The remaining 10% of malignancies involving the vulva include melanoma, basal cell carcinoma, Paget's disease, and other rare cancers.

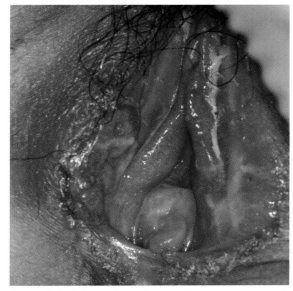

Figure 61-3. Behçet's disease demonstrating a nonspecific vaginal ulcer. (Courtesy of the William L. Weston, M.D. collection.)

Key Points: Disorders of the Female Genitalia

1. Lichen sclerosus commonly involves the anogenital area, forming a "figure-of-eight" pattern on the skin.
2. There is a low but present risk (4% to 6%), of squamous cell carcinoma arising in lichen sclerosus.
3. Patients with vulvar lichen planus also commonly have vaginal lesions that may lead to significant morbidity secondary to vaginal adhesions and obliteration.
4. Lichen simplex chronicus is the end-stage result (thickened, lichenified skin) from chronic scratching or rubbing of the skin.
5. The majority of vulvar carcinoma is squamous cell carcinoma.

---

21. Is squamous cell carcinoma of the vulva associated with a precancerous state?

Yes. Vulvar intraepithelial neoplasia (VIN) is the term used to describe dysplasia of vulvar epithelial cells. VIN is further divided into VIN usual type, which is associated with high-risk human papilloma virus (HPV) strains, such as HPV 16 and HPV 18, and differentiated VIN, which is associated with chronic vulvar dermatoses, particularly lichen sclerosus. VIN is associated with vulvar pruritus and burning. The lesion may be described as a raised papule or nodule that is erythematous or white.

Maclean AB, Jones RW, Scurry J, Neill S: Vulvar cancer and the need for awareness of precursor lesions, *J Low Genit Tract Dis* 13:115–117, 2009.

22. How long does it take VIN to progress to squamous cell carcinoma of the vulva?

The mean time from the initial diagnosis of VIN to the diagnosis of SCC of the vulva is 4 to 8 years.

23. How does one treat VIN/SCC of the vulva?

VIN is treated mostly with surgical excision. Using topical imiquimod is also becoming more common. SCC of the vulva is treated surgically, usually by a gynecologic oncologist. Adjuvant therapy may include regional lymphadenectomy, chemotherapy, and radiation.

24. What is the second most common vulvar malignancy?

Malignant melanoma. It is most common in elderly women in the seventh or eighth decade of life. Unlike other cutaneous melanomas that develop in sun-exposed areas, and are thus thought to be related to ultraviolet light exposure, melanomas of the vulva are thought, possibly, to be associated with chronic inflammatory disease, chemical irritants, viral infections (including HPV), and genetic susceptibility.

De Simone P, Silipo V, Buccini P, et al: Vulvar melanoma: a report of 10 cases and review of the literature, *Melanoma Res* 18:127–133, 2008.

25. How does melanoma of the vulva present?

Patients with melanoma of the vulva present with a pigmented mass of the labia majora, labia minora, or clitoris. Most patients will complain of bleeding or pruritus and, less often, discharge or ulceration.

26. Are melanomas of the vulva more aggressive than other cutaneous melanomas?

No. Melanomas found in the vulvar area do not behave differently than melanomas on other areas of the body. Vulvar melanomas tend to be diagnosed at a later stage than other cutaneous melanomas that are on skin that is more visible and examined more frequently than the vulva. The 5-year survival rate is between 36% and 60%.

Nasu K, Kai Y, Ohishi M, et al: Conservative surgical treatment for early-stage vulvar malignant melanoma, *Arch Gynecol Obstet* 281:335–338, 2010.

27. What is the treatment of melanoma of the vulva?

Traditionally, treatment of vulvar melanoma involves surgical management in the form of a radical vulvectomy with bilateral inguinal–femoral lymph node dissection. However, this disfiguring therapy, which leads to a high rate of morbidity, has not been shown to increase the survival rates or lower the recurrence rate over more conservative management. More conservative surgical treatment includes wide local excision for early stage disease. The use of adjuvant chemotherapy varies according to the institution.

28. What is Paget's disease of the vulva?

Paget's disease (Fig. 61-4) is a neoplasia of the vulva that consists of adenocarcinoma-type cells that invade the epidermis, the appendages of the skin, and occasionally the dermis. It represents 1% of vulvar neoplasms. However, 25% of the time that extramammary Paget's disease is present, it is associated with an underlying adenocarcinoma (most commonly of the skin adnexa or Bartholin gland) or at a distant site (e.g., the breast, genitourinary system, or the intestinal tract). Thus, it is prudent to search for other possible malignancies if Paget's disease of the vulva is diagnosed.

Shaco-Levy R, Bean SM, Vollmer RT, et al: Paget disease of the vulva: a histologic study of 56 cases correlating pathologic features and disease course, *Int J Gynecol Pathol* 29:69–78, 2010.

29. How does Paget's disease of the vulva present?

The most common symptom is pruritus. On examination, there are usually erythematous plaques with white hyperkeratotic areas. Over time, these areas may desquamate.

30. What is the differential diagnosis of Paget's disease?

- Seborrheic dermatitis
- Psoriasis
- Atopic dermatitis
- Tinea cruris
- Candidiasis

31. How does one treat Paget's disease of the vulva?

Surgical excision is the gold standard of treatment. However, clear margins are difficult to obtain. Moreover, recurrence rates after surgical excision are high (up to 58%) in some studies. Other nonsurgical treatments that have been reported include imiquimod, 5-fluorouracil, and laser ablation.

Geisler JP, Manahan KJ: Imiquimod in vulvar Paget's disease: a case report, *J Reprod Med* 53:811–812, 2008.

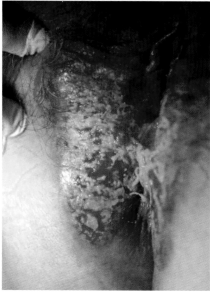

Figure 61-4. Genital extramammary Paget's disease demonstrating marked erythema with superficial erosions. (Courtesy of Whitney A. High, MD.)

CHAPTER 62

SPECIAL CONSIDERATIONS IN SKIN OF COLOR

Whitney A. High, MD, JD, MEng, and Nadja Y. Grammer-West, MD, COL, MC, USA

1. What is "skin of color"?

There are many ways to subcategorize human beings. Widely recognized racial groups include Africans, African-Americans, Asians, Middle Easterners, Northern Europeans, Native Americans, Pacific Islanders, and Hispanics, to name a few. Even within a racial group gradations exist with regard to skin pigmentation. Simply put, people with "skin of color" have darker skin tones than those of typical white skin. The term may be used also to reference other shared cutaneous characteristics, such as hair color or quality, or a common reaction pattern to skin insults, all of which may be clinically relevant. By 2050, about 54% of the United States population will be composed of people with skin of color. Accordingly, a solid understanding of the myriad differences in diagnosing and treating persons with skin of color is essential to the competent practice of dermatology.

Taylor SC, Cook-Bolden F: Defining skin of color, *Cutis* 69:435–437, 2002.

U.S. Census Bureau: 2008 national population projections: tables and charts. Available at: http://www.census.gov/population/www/projections/tablesandcharts.html. Accessed March 13, 2010.

2. What accounts for differences in color between ethnic and racial groups?

Although the number of melanocytes varies within anatomic regions of the body, interestingly, among different races and ethnicities, the actual number of melanocytes in the skin does not vary with skin color. Instead, among variations, it is the amount and distribution of melanin produced that changes. In mammals, two types of melanin are produced by melanocytes, eumelanin and pheomelanin. Eumelanin is a tyrosine-derived, dark brown or black pigment. Pheomelanin, derived from a biochemical shunt in the normal melanin production pathway, has a yellow to red-brown hue. Pheomelanin is the predominant pigment produced by those with freckles and red hair. It is also increased in Asian skin, and in women when compared to men. Melanin is packaged in melanosomes, which are membrane-bound vesicles containing a unique scaffolding of matrix proteins. Melanosomes within keratinocytes of white skin are distributed as membrane-bound clusters. In black skin, melanosomes tend to be larger and more diffusely located in the cell. Therefore, the quantity and composition of melanin, as well as melanosome size and distribution, vary considerably within the epidermis, both with ethnicity and with chronic sun exposure, yielding various degrees and hues of pigmentation.

Thong HY, Jee SH, Sun CC, Boissy RE: The patterns of melanosome distribution in keratinocytes of human skin as one determining factor of skin colour, *Br J Dermatol* 149:498–505, 2003.

3. Do any physiologic differences exist between black skin and that of other racial/ethnic groups?

Yes. In truth, the color of "black" skin ranges from light brown to very dark brown/black, and it is difficult to generalize given this tremendous variability. Nevertheless, studies have demonstrated that the stratum corneum of most black skin maintains more layers and is more compact and cohesive than white skin. This finding may explain why black skin tends to manifest a decreased susceptibility to cutaneous irritants. One study demonstrated that black skin had a spontaneous desquamation rate 2.5 times that of white skin, and this may explain why some blacks experience a particular type of xerosis commonly referred to as *ashy skin*. Ashy skin consists of fine white flakes yielding a dry appearance. Other differences in black skin include an increased transepidermal water loss (TEWL), lower pH, and larger mast cell granules compared with white skin. Black skin also produces less vitamin D3 in response to equivalent sunlight, and this has been postulated to possibly represent the driving evolutionary force in development of paler skin as early humans migrated away from the equator. Conflicting data exist regarding differences in resistance, capacitance, conductance, impedance, and skin microflora.

Jablonski NG, Chaplin G: The evolution of human skin coloration, *J Hum Evol* 39:57–106, 2000.

Wesley NO, Maibach HI: Racial (ethnic) differences in skin properties: the objective data, *Am J Clin Dermatol* 4:843–860, 2003.

4. Are the brown streaks on the nails of people with skin of color always a cause for concern?

No. Pigmented streaks of the nail may be a normal variant in people with skin of color. The condition is called *melanonychia striata,* and it is characterized by longitudinal bands of pigmentation that may vary from light brown to dark black. Multiple bands may be seen within the same nail or, alternatively, several nails may be involved. The cause is unknown, but the rarity of bands in children may indicate that they are a sequela of accumulated trauma. Some studies have revealed that such bands are present in >75% of blacks older than 20 years. Another recent study found that simple racial variation was the most common cause of nail pigmentation in Hispanics as well, although malignancy was a cause in about 6% of cases. In general, solitary bands are of greater concern than are multiple lesions. Close examination of the nail fold may be helpful, assessing for diffusion of pigment into the surrounding skin; however, the absence of this sign does not rule out a more serious condition, such as nail unit melanoma. Other causes of nail pigmentation include drugs such as actinomycin, antimalarials, bleomycin, cyclophosphamide, doxorubicin, 5-fluorouracil, melphalan, methotrexate, minocycline, nitrogen mustard, and zidovudine, to name a few. Laugier-Hunziker syndrome, Addison's disease, hemochromatosis, Peutz-Jegher syndrome, and vitamin B12 deficiency may also cause nail pigmentation.

Dominguez-Cherit J, Roldan-Marin R, Pichardo-Velazquez P, et al: Melanonychia, melanocytic hyperplasia, and nail melanoma in a Hispanic population, *J Am Acad Dermatol* 59:785–791, 2008.
Pappert AS, Scher RK, Cohen JL: Longitudinal pigmented nail bands, *Dermatol Clin* 9:703–716, 1991.

5. Is pigmentation of the oral mucosa in people with skin of color invariably concerning?

No. Pigmentation of the oral mucosa is often subdivided into conditions related to melanin (including racial differences in pigmentation), and non–melanin-associated conditions, such as metabolic conditions or pigmentation related to drugs. Therefore, oral pigmentation in people with skin of color is neither uncommon, nor necessarily indicative of a serious condition. Idiopathic, racially related pigmentation of the oral mucosa often involves the gingiva, hard palate, buccal mucosa, or tongue. The color may vary, but it often has a blue or gray appearance. Symmetry is frequently observed. As always, obtaining an appropriate medical history is important, particularly with respect to the length of time present and any associated symptoms.

Meleti M, Vescovi P, Mooi WJ, van der Waal I: Pigmented lesions of the oral mucosa and perioral tissues: a flow-chart for the diagnosis and some recommendations for the management, *Oral Surg Oral Med Oral Pathol Oral Radiol Endod* 105:606–616, 2008.

6. Are there other areas of the body where hyperpigmentation represents a normal racial variant?

Hyperpigmented macules of the palms and soles occur in people with skin of color, particularly in those with darker skin types. Such lesions may vary in color from light tan to dark brown. The number of lesions may range from one or two lesions to dozens or more. This potential for natural racial variation must be kept in mind, particularly when one considers other diseases associated with palmoplantar lesions, such as erythema multiforme and secondary syphilis. As acral lentiginous melanoma is the most common form of melanoma occurring in blacks, Asians, and Hispanics, this potentially life-threatening diagnosis must always be considered, and excluded by biopsy where indicated. Other areas with possible increased pigmentation among persons with skin of color include the sclera, the labia and vaginal mucosa, and the glans penis.

Coleman WP III, Gately LE III, Krementz AB, et al: Nevi, lentigines, and melanomas in blacks., *Arch Dermatol* 116:548–555, 1980.

7. What are Futcher's lines?

Futcher's lines, also known as *Voigt's lines* or *Futcher-Voigt lines* or *Ito's lines*, are areas of abrupt demarcation between lighter and darker pigmented skin. Common locations include the anterior arms, the sternum, and the posterior thighs and legs (Fig. 62-1). There appears to be no appreciable difference in melanin concentration between the adjacent darker and lighter areas when examined by light microscopy. The distribution and symmetry of the lines allows differentiation from other diagnoses, such as hypomelanosis of Ito, incontinentia pigmenti, linear epidermal nevus, or lichen striatus.

Interestingly, drug eruptions have, on occasion, affected preferentially the skin on one side of the line, suggesting the skin in these areas has slightly different embryologic origin, at least with regard to a susceptibility to metabolic insult.

James WD, Carter JM, Rodman OG: Pigmentary demarcation lines: a population survey, *J Am Acad Dermatol* 16:584–590, 1987.
Shelley ED, Shelley WB, Pansky B: The drug line: the clinical expression of the pigmentary Voigt-Futcher line in turn derived from the embryonic ventral axial line, *J Am Acad Dermatol* 40:736–740, 1999.

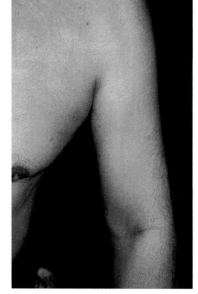

Figure 62-1. Futcher's (Voigt's) line of the upper arm. (Courtesy of James E. Fitzpatrick, MD.)

8. What causes postinflammatory hyperpigmentation?

Postinflammatory hyperpigmentation represents a residual darkening of the skin as a result of an inflammatory insult, such as lichen planus, lupus erythematosus (Fig. 62-2), or atopic dermatitis (Fig. 62-3). It is most severe in those diseases that result in significant disruption of the basal layer, which allows melanin to escape into the upper dermis where it is engulfed by macrophages. The resultant hyperpigmentation requires months to years for fading. Treatment includes bleaching creams, such as hydroquinone, tretinoin, and azelaic acid; however, if the pigmentation is significantly deep, topical management does not often augment the body's normal, albeit slow, corrective mechanisms. Bleaching agents containing >4% hydroquinone may cause exogenous ochronosis, with a resultant blue-gray discoloration of the skin. Patients from countries in Africa and Europe may have access to harsh bleaching agents without prescription, and should be warned against such use. Disorders such as inflammatory acne, occurring in dark skin types, should be treated early and aggressively, to prevent pigmentary alterations.

Olumide YM, Akinkugbe AO, Altraide D, et al: Complications of chronic use of skin lightening cosmetics, *Int J Dermatol* 47:344–353, 2008.

9. What causes postinflammatory hypopigmentation?

Postinflammatory hypopigmentation, another sequela of inflammatory skin disorders in dark skin, is thought to result from impaired transfer of melanosomes from melanocytes to keratinocytes. This occurs in many diseases, such as atopic dermatitis (see Fig. 62-3) and psoriasis. The increased mitotic rate of keratinocytes, and the decreased transit time of cells within the epidermis, does not allow sufficient pigment transfer. After the inflammatory process resolves, pigment typically normalizes over weeks to months.

Nordlund JJ, Abdel-Malek ZA: Mechanisms for post-inflammatory hyperpigmentation and hypopigmentation, *Prog Clin Biol Res* 256:219–236, 1988.

10. Is pityriasis alba the same thing as postinflammatory hypopigmentation?

Pityriasis alba is seen primarily in children with darker skin types, and it manifests as hypopigmented macules on the face and/or upper arms (Fig. 62-4). The lesions lack a distinct border and may have overlying fine scale. Patients often report a history of atopic dermatitis. Some studies show boys may be preferentially affected. While many consider pityriasis alba to be a mild form of postinflammatory hypopigmentation, it is often considered a separate entity. Although the condition typically resolves with time, brief treatment with low-potency topical corticosteroids and/or generous emollients may be helpful.

Blessmann Weber M, Sponchiado de Avila LG, Albaneze R, et al: Pityriasis alba: a study of pathogenic factors, *J Eur Acad Dermatol Venereol* 16:463–468, 2002.

11. Is vitiligo more common in patients with darker skin?

Vitiligo is a common disorder, affecting 1% to 2% of the world's population. There is no clear racial predisposition for vitiligo; however, the condition is more readily apparent in darker skin. Consequently, people with darker skin types may seek medical attention or manifest with more cosmetically debilitating disease. Also, the tendency for familial inheritance of vitiligo must be considered when conducting prevalence studies.

In some societies, particularly Indian culture, there is a social stigma associated with vitiligo that pertains to a historic overlap with the appearance of cutaneous leprosy. In these cultures, patients with the condition, especially young women, may be considered "unfit for marriage," and the sociodynamic aspects of vitiligo must always be carefully considered by the clinician.

Shah H, Mehta A, Astik B: Clinical and sociodemographic study of vitiligo, *Indian J Dermatol Venereol Leprol* 74:701, 2008.
Nordlund JJ: The epidemiology and genetics of vitiligo, *Clin Dermatol* 15:875–878, 1997.

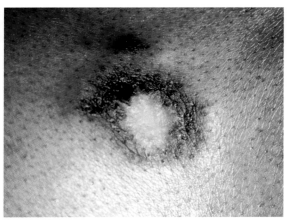

Figure 62-2. Postinflammatory hyperpigmentation in a patient with lupus erythematosus. (Courtesy of James E. Fitzpatrick, MD.)

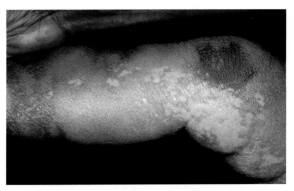

Figure 62-3. Postinflammatory hyperpigmentation and hypopigmentation in a child with atopic dermatitis. (Courtesy of James E. Fitzpatrick, MD.)

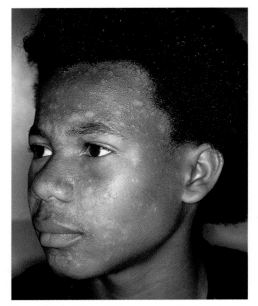

Figure 62-4. Pityriasis alba, demonstrating hypopigmented macules of the face. (Courtesy of James E. Fitzpatrick, MD.)

12. Why does tinea versicolor cause hypopigmented spots on dark skin?

Tinea versicolor, also known as *pityriasis versicolor*, is a common superficial yeast infection caused by the lipophilic organism *Malassezia furfur* and other species in this genus. The typical presentation in darker skin types is that of multiple hypopigmented thin plaques with fine scale distributed over the densely seborrheic skin of the chest, upper back, and proximal upper extremities. The cause of the hypopigmentation is not completely understood; however, extracts from cultured organisms contain dicarboxylic acids that may competitively inhibit tyrosinase, an enzyme important in melanin production. Production of other indoles or tryptophan-based metabolites may also be involved in the resultant hypopigmentation.

Thoma W, Kramer HJ, Mayser P: Pityriasis versicolor alba, *J Eur Acad Dermatol Venereol* 19:147–152, 2005.

13. Why is it more difficult to appreciate erythema in darker skin?

Erythema, or the amount of visible redness in the skin, is caused by increased blood flow and/or blood vessel engorgement in the dermis with the presence of oxyhemoglobin. If the epidermis is deeply pigmented, the red hues of oxyhemoglobin may be difficult to visualize. For this reason, the interpretation of patch testing for sensitivity to cutaneous allergens in black patients is challenging. This is an important point to remember, as many diseases that have erythema as a hallmark, such as seborrheic dermatitis or atopic dermatitis, may present more subtly in a black patient. Cyanosis is also difficult to perceive in a dark-skinned patient for similar reasons.

Ben-Gashir MA, Hay RJ: Reliance on erythema scores may mask severe atopic dermatitis in black children compared with their white counterparts, *Br J Dermatol* 147:920–925, 2002.

14. Can any other generalizations be made about common cutaneous reaction patterns in skin of color?

In addition to the difficulty in perceiving erythema, there exist other cutaneous reaction patterns more prevalent in darker skin. Papulosquamous diseases, such as psoriasis and nummular eczema, tend to exhibit a more violaceous color, leading to possible confusion with lichenoid conditions. Certain diseases, such as atopic dermatitis or tinea versicolor, may demonstrate a follicular accentuation (Fig. 62-5). Pityriasis rosea may present atypically, with either papular or vesiculobullous forms, in black skin. In addition, some disorders, such as lichen planus and seborrheic dermatitis, have an increased propensity toward formation of annular lesions (Fig. 62-6). The reasons for these observations remain largely unknown.

McLaurin CI: Unusual patterns of common dermatoses in blacks, *Cutis* 32:352–355, 358-360, 1983.

15. What is the significance of multiple brown papules often seen on the periorbital area, cheeks, and nose?

The condition described is dermatosis papulosa nigra, and it is commonly seen in blacks, particularly black women. They are often referred to colloquially as "flesh moles." In truth, they are not "moles" (nevi) at all and represent a variant of seborrheic keratoses. The lesions tend to increase in number over time and do not typically resolve on their own. They have no malignant potential and are largely a cosmetic concern. Removal may be accomplished by light electrodesiccation (a personal favorite) and/or curettage. Alternatively, lesions may be treated with light application of liquid nitrogen, but care must be taken to avoid permanent hypopigmentation, a sequela of increased risk in persons with dark skin.

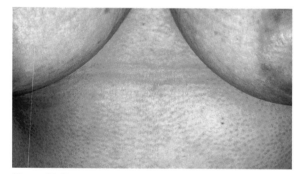

Figure 62-5. Tinea versicolor with follicular accentuation. (Courtesy of James E. Fitzpatrick, MD.)

16. What is cutaneous sarcoidosis?

Cutaneous sarcoidosis is a granulomatous process of unknown etiology that is more prevalent among blacks, particularly among those in the southern United States, where the incidence is 3 to 4 times that of appropriately matched white patients. The cause of the disease is unknown. Cutaneous lesions may occur in association with pulmonary disease, or may be present in isolation. Diverse patterns of skin lesions occurring in black patients with sarcoidosis have been observed. Shiny, somewhat waxy papular lesions are the most frequent cutaneous manifestation of sarcoidosis in blacks. When such

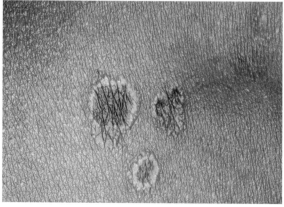

Figure 62-6. Annular lichen planus, demonstrating central postinflammatory hypopigmentation. (Courtesy of James E. Fitzpatrick, MD.)

dermal granulomatous papules are located near the nose, the condition has been referred to as *lupus pernio* (Fig. 62-7), and it may be indicative of a higher association with pulmonary disease (for photos, *see interactive reference*). Because of its protean cutaneous manifestations, sarcoidosis should be included in the differential diagnosis of nearly all chronic dermatoses in black patients.

High WA: A woman with "keloids" on the nose and restrictive pulmonary disease, *Medscape Dermatol Clin*, September 7, 2004. Available at: http://www.medscape.com/viewarticle/488343. Accessed March 13, 2010.

17. What are keloids?

Keloids are benign dermal neoplasms composed of broad collagen bundles (Fig. 62-8). It is believed they represent an aberrant healing process. In distinction from hypertrophic scars, keloids extend beyond the bounds of the original wound. There exists a distinct tendency toward keloid formation in persons of color. Sites of predilection include the shoulders, mandible, earlobes, presternal area, and deltoid region. Any form of trauma can induce keloids, including thermal injuries, insect bites, acne scars, injection sites, or cosmetic piercings and surgical incisions. Keloids may occur spontaneously, particularly in the central chest area. It is quite possible that such a "spontaneous" keloid represents a reaction to unrecognized trauma. The causal abnormality in the normal healing process is not known with certainty. It appears, however, that genetically predisposed fibroblasts are stimulated to produce abnormally high levels of procollagen messenger RNA, leading to excessive collagen production and secretion.

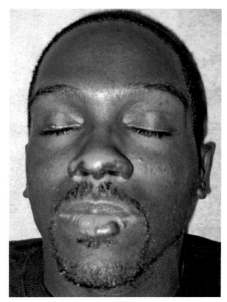

Figure 62-7. Multiple sarcoidal granulomas along the right eyelid, nasal margin, and lower lip in a patient with sarcoidosis. (Courtesy of Whitney A. High, MD)

Treatment options have included radiation or pressure therapy, cryotherapy, intralesional corticosteroids or verapamil, interferon, fluorouracil, topical silicone dressings, and laser treatment (either pulsed dye or Nd:YAG). Surgical excision is typically followed by recurrence unless adjunct preventive therapies are employed.

Kelly AP: Update on the management of keloids, *Semin Cutan Med Surg* 28:71–76, 2009.

18. What are "razor bumps"?

The hair follicles of blacks and many other people of color, such as Puerto Ricans, are elliptical, leading to development of tightly curled hair. After shaving, as the hairs regrow, there is a tendency for the sharp end of the curled hair to curve back into the skin. When the hair pierces the skin, it causes an inflammatory reaction, just as one might see with a splinter. This inflammatory reaction leads to the development of pseudofolliculitis barbae. This condition is not normally seen in men who grow beards, because after attainment of a certain length, usually 3 to 6 mm, the hair does not curve back into the skin. Accordingly, the condition is most common among populations required to be clean-shaven, such as black men in the military. Acne keloidalis nuchae represents a similar condition arising on the occipital scalp and/or nuchal area of those with shaved or very tightly cropped haircuts.

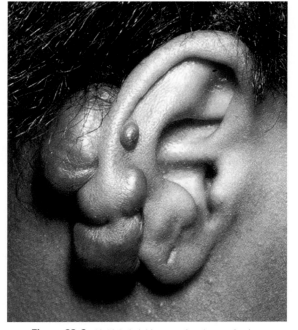

Figure 62-8. Multiple keloids secondary to ear piercing.

Kelly AP: Pseudofolliculitis barbae and acne keloidalis nuchae, *Dermatol Clin* 21:645–653, 2003.

19. How is pseudofolliculitis barbae treated?

Clearly, the definitive treatment is growth of a beard; however, if this is not an option, several techniques may decrease the number of inflamed papules. The beard should be shaved in the direction of growth with a single-edged razor. The skin should *not* be stretched while shaving. Hairs that have clearly recurved into the skin should be released with a sterile needle, but such hairs should *not* be plucked. Some men with this condition may use clippers that purposefully leave short stubble. Others may obtain good results with chemical depilatories. If inflammation is severe, short-term treatment with a low-potency topical corticosteroid may be effective. Laser hair removal or topical eflornithine represent emerging treatment options for those with intractable disease and a requisite need to maintain a clean shaven appearance.

Schulze R, Meehan KJ, Lopez A, et al: Low-fluence 1,064-nm laser hair reduction for pseudofolliculitis barbae in skin types IV, V, VI, *Dermatol Surg* 34:98–107, 2009.
Garcia-Zuazaga J: Pseudofolliculitis barbae: review and update on new treatment modalities, *Mil Med* 168:561–564, 2003.

20. Are there other racial differences that may affect the treatment of hair or scalp conditions in blacks?

Blacks have elliptical follicular ostia and tightly curled hair with a small mean cross-sectional area. Asians have round ostia and straight hair with a large mean cross-sectional area. Whites have round to slightly ovoid follicles with an intermediate mean cross-sectional area. Nevertheless, these remain broad generalizations, and the entire racial and genetic makeup of the individual must be considered. The angles of curvature in the spiral structure of black hair yields multiple vulnerable points along the hair shaft, making it relatively fragile and prone to breakage. This structural arrangement also inhibits effective transmission of secreted sebum down the shaft, making the hair drier and

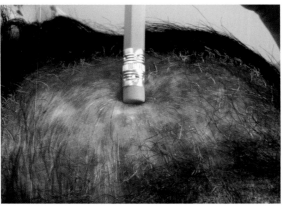

Figure 62-9. Lipedematous scalp in an elderly black woman, indicated by pressure applied using a pencil, yielding remarkable induration of the skin. (Courtesy of Whitney A. High, MD)

less manageable relative to other hair types. For these reasons, the hair of blacks cannot be shampooed as often as that of other racial groups. Daily washing would lead to excessive dryness and hair breakage. A moisturizing conditioner should be used after shampooing. Such differences in hair care must be considered when prescribing treatment for scalp conditions that involve medicated shampoos. When evaluating alopecia, a thorough history of hair grooming techniques used should be obtained. Specifically, questions about the use of chemical relaxers, permanent hair dyes, curling irons, hot combs, blow dryers, braids, or weaves should be inquired of, because many of these modalities cause damage to the hair shaft or the scalp. Finally, some unusual forms of alopecia, such as lipedematous alopecia (Fig. 62-9), with associated cotton-batting textural changes of the scalp, are associated nearly exclusively with black women.

High WA, Hoang MP: Lipedematous alopecia, *J Am Acad Dermatol* 53:S157–S161, 2005.
McMichael AJ: Ethnic hair update: past and present, *J Am Acad Dermatol* 48:S127–S133, 2003.

Key Points: Skin of Color

1. Skin of color, particularly black skin, manifests minor physiologic differences, including a stratum corneum with increased layers and cohesiveness and a decreased ability to synthesize vitamin D3.
2. Erythema may be more difficult to appreciate on darkly pigmented skin, and this must be considered during clinical examination.
3. Pigmentation of the oral mucosa, benign-appearing palmoplantar macules, or multiple longitudinal pigmented streaks of the nails, may represent normal variants in persons with darker skin types.
4. Many cutaneous diseases may present with follicular accentuation or other unusual clinical aspects in persons with darker skin types.
5. Ethnic and cultural differences in skin and hair must be considered in the examination and treatment of persons with skin of color.

---

21. Are patients with skin of color particularly susceptible to any life-threatening illnesses?

Coccidioidomycosis, also known as San Joaquin Valley fever, is a deep fungal infection caused by *Coccidioides immitis*. It is typically acquired via inhalation of arthrospores and demonstrates occasional hematogenous dissemination to subcutaneous tissues, bone, or skin. Endemic areas include the Sonoran life zone of southern California, Arizona, New Mexico, southwestern Texas, and northern Mexico. It has also been reported in certain areas of South America. Infection occurs equally in both sexes, and in all races and ages. For reasons that are not entirely clear, black persons are 14 times more likely to have severe disseminated disease than are caucasians (Fig. 62-10), and individuals of Filipino descent are 10 times more likely to develop coccidioidomycosis-related meninigitis than caucasians. Further investigation has revealed that certain host genetics, in particular the human leukocyte antigen (HLA) class II and ABO blood group genes, influence susceptibility to severe coccidioidomycosis.

Untreated, nonmeningeal coccidioidomycosis has a 50% mortality rate; therefore, early aggressive treatment with systemic antifungal agents is essential.

Louie L, Ng S, Hajjeh R, et al: Influence of host genetics on the severity of coccidioidomycosis, *Emerg Infect Dis* 5:672–680, 1999.

Pappagianis D: Epidemiology of coccidioidomycosis, *Curr Top Med Mycol* 2:199–238, 1988.

22. Do any special considerations exist when performing skin surgery on patients with skin of color?

Due to the increased risk of pigmentary alterations, hypertrophic scars, and keloids among black patients, any surgical undertaking should be carefully considered with respect to the risks and benefits of the procedure. Because melanocytes are more sensitive to cold injury than keratinocytes, liquid nitrogen can cause permanent loss of pigmentation, and this is generally more noticeable in darker skin types. Treatment of benign growths, such as warts or seborrheic keratoses, with cryotherapy can result, therefore, in permanent loss of pigment, and this modality must be judiciously implemented.

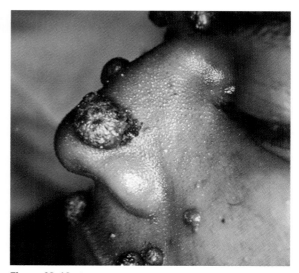

Figure 62-10. Coccidioidomycosis. Disseminated coccidioidomycosis in a young black soldier. (Courtesy of the Fitzsimons Army Medical Center teaching files.)

Grimes PE, Hunt SG: Considerations for cosmetic surgery in the black population, *Clin Plast Surg* 20:27–34, 1993.

23. Why is skin cancer less common in skin of color?

Ultraviolet (UV) radiation-induced damage to the DNA of cells in the lower epidermis, including keratinocyte stem cells and melanocytes, is prevented to a greater degree in darker skin, suggesting that the pigmented epidermis serves as an efficient UV filter. In addition, UV radiation-induced apoptosis (programmed cell death) is significantly greater in darker skin, indicating that any damaged cells may be removed more efficiently from the epidermis in skin of color. Together, the combination of decreased DNA damage due to ultraviolet radiation and the more efficient removal of damaged cells likely play a critical role in the decreased photocarcinogenesis seen in individuals with skin of color.

Yuji Y, Takahashi K, Zmudska BZ, et al: Human skin responses to UV radiation: pigment in the upper epidermis protects against DNA damage in the lower epidermis and facilitates apoptosis, *FASEB J* 20:E630–E639, 2006.

24. Are there any unique presentations of skin cancer when it does occur in patients with darker skin?

Although skin cancer is decidedly less common in people with skin of color, it is often associated with greater morbidity and mortality. Squamous cell carcinoma (SCC) is the most common skin cancer in blacks and Asian Indians, and it is the second-most common cancer in Chinese and Japanese. Also, in skin of color, malignancies occur more often upon non–sun-exposed surfaces and the lower extremities. In fact, the most important risk factors for developing SCC in blacks are chronic scarring processes and areas of chronic inflammation. Acral lentiginous melanoma presents more often in persons with skin of color. Other reported risk factors for melanoma in blacks include albinism, burn scars, radiation therapy, trauma, immunosuppression, and preexisting pigmented lesions. Mycosis fungoides (MF), a type of cutaneous T-cell lymphoma (CTCL), occurs more often in persons with skin of color (see Chapter 46). Because many individuals with dark skin do not believe that they are susceptible to skin cancers, they may delay seeking care for a suspicious lesion, thereby leading to a less favorable prognosis. Public education in ethnic communities regarding the performance of self-skin examination, and the utility of regular visits to a dermatologist when skin conditions exist may lessen the associated morbidity and mortality of skin cancer in these populations.

Gloster HM, Neal K: Skin cancer in skin of color, *J Am Acad Dermatol* 55:741–760, 2006.

Hinds GA, Herald P: Cutaneous T-cell lymphoma in skin of color, *J Am Acad Dermatol* 60:359–375, 2009.

25. List skin diseases or conditions that are often considered more common in persons with skin of color.

The diseases listed in Table 62-1, while not all-inclusive, represent many skin conditions thought to be seen with higher frequency in blacks. Some diseases, particularly the tropical infections, may be more common in blacks living outside of the United States. The perception of these diseases being more common in blacks may be related purely to this geographic distribution. Furthermore, such entities may be rarely encountered within the United States but are listed here for completeness.

Table 62-1. Dermatologic Conditions More Common in Skin of Color

Acne keloidalis nuchae	Lichen nitidus
Acral lentiginous melanoma	Lichen simplex chronicus
Acropustulosis of infancy	Loiasis
African histoplasmosis	Madura foot
Ainhum	Melanonychia striata
Buruli ulcer	Mongolian spots
Chancroid	Nevus of Ito
Dermatitis cruris pustulosa et atrophicans	Nevus of Ota
Dermatosis papulosa nigra	Onchocerciasis
Dissecting cellulitis of the scalp	Papular eruption of blacks
Dracunculiasis (guinea worm)	Pityriasis rotunda
Filariasis	Pomade acne
Granuloma inguinale	Porphyria cutanea tarda (South African Bantus)
Granuloma multiforme	Pseudofolliculitis barbae
Hamartoma moniliformis	*Pseudomonas* toe web infection
Infundibulofolliculitis	Sarcoidosis
Juxtaclavicular beaded lines	Sickle cell ulceration
Kaposi's sarcoma (endemic)	Traction alopecia
Keloids	Transient neonatal pustular melanosis
Leishmaniasis	Tropical ulcer
Leprosy	Trypanosomiasis

CULTURAL DERMATOLOGY

Scott A. Norton, MD, MPH, COL, MC, USA, and James E. Fitzpatrick, MD

CHAPTER 63

1. A child from southern India has had a recent decline in school performance and is noted to be anemic. On examination, the child has adorable, dark, mascara-like makeup around her eyes. As an astute cultural dermatologist, you suspect that the makeup is the cause of the difficulties in school and the hematologic profile. What is the name for the traditional Indian eye makeup?

Surma. This is the Punjabi name for the eye makeup and the name that appears most frequently in the medical literature. It is also called *kajal* or *kohl* in other Indian dialects.

2. What is surma made from? How did it affect the child?

Surma (kohl) is a fine powder resembling mascara that is applied to the margins of the palpebral conjunctiva. It was originally made from antimony sulfide or from carbon soot, but now it is often adulterated with lead sulfide.

This child has chronic lead toxicity caused by absorption of the lead-based pigments related to her surma-cosmetic plumbism. Surma usually has lead-based pigments and has created problems with lead toxicity in several Asian communities in the United Kingdom. For that reason, surma is now banned in England. In the Middle East, a similar traditional eye cosmetic has also been demonstrated to frequently contain high levels of lead.

Al-Ashban RM, Aslam M, Shah AH: Kohl (surma): a toxic traditional eye cosmetic study in Saudi Arabia, *Public Health* 118:292–298, 2004.

Mojdehi GM, Gurtner J: Childhood lead poisoning through kohl, *Am J Public Health* 86:578–587, 1996.

3. A Vietnamese child is seen in the emergency department with an earache and, on examination, is noted to have several linear ecchymoses on her back. The physician suspects child abuse as the cause of the bruises, but the interpreter says it is not. What caused the marks on the child?

Cao gió (phonetically pronounced gow yaw), or coin rubbing. This is a traditional Vietnamese medical practice. The traditional healer massages the patient's skin with a liniment and then rubs a metal object, usually a coin, forcefully over the area. Petechiae and linear ecchymoses often develop. These have been mistaken many times for stigmata of battering by Western providers who are unfamiliar with *cao gió*.

Davis RE: Cultural health care or child abuse? The Southeast Asian practice of cao gió, *J Am Acad Nurse Pract* 12:89–95, 2000.

Yeatman GW, Dang VV: Cao gió (coin rubbing), *JAMA* 244:2748–2749, 1980.

4. An older Chinese man is noted to have dozens of fairly uniform round scars on his back. They resemble self-inflicted cigarette burns, only much larger. The patient is unconcerned about the lesions and indicates that someone like you, a doctor perhaps, did this to him. What ancient Chinese medical practice produces burn scars?

Moxibustion.

5. What is moxibustion?

It is derived from the words moxa and combustion. Moxa is from mokusa, the Japanese word for wormwood (*Artemisia moxa* of the sagebrush and absinthe genus), is a commonly used combustible medicinal herb. Moxibustion is the ancient oriental medical practice of igniting medicinal herbs on the skin. When the healer extinguishes the flame, the herb's therapeutic properties supposedly enter the body. A burn scar is the necessary sequela of properly conducted moxibustion. The sites on which moxibustion is performed are often the same as those used in acupuncture, and it, along with cupping and acupressure, is considered to be a nonneedle forms of acupuncture. The practice is still taught in Chinese colleges of traditional medicine.

Note that moxibustion was introduced into Europe by the end of the 17th century. In the movie *The Madness of King George*, there is a scene in which his physicians are treating him with moxibustion to cure his "madness." In actuality, he is believed to have had variegate porphyria.

Look KM, Look RM: Skin scraping, cupping, and moxibustion that may mimic physical abuse, *J Forens Sci* 42:103–105, 1997.

6. Can acupuncture cause dermatologic problems?

Yes. In a large survey of more than 6300 acupuncture patients in the United Kingdom, patients reported at least one adverse event in about 10% of cases; however, only 3 patients had a serious adverse event. There have been reports of abundant petechiae (in one case, resembling meningococcemia) caused by acupuncture needles. Hematomas and ecchymoses occur frequently. Pyoderma, prolonged anesthesia, needle breakage, burns, itching, foreign body granuloma, "carcinoma of the skin," and the Koebner phenomenon have been reported. Transmission of HIV and hepatitis virus has occurred via acupuncture needles.

Macpherson H, Scullion A, Thomas KJ, Walters S: Patient reports of adverse events associated with acupuncture treatment: a prospective national survey. *Qual Saf Health Care* 13:349–355, 2004.

Yamashita H, Tsukayama H, Taanno Y, Nishijo K: Adverse events in acupuncture and moxibustion treatment: a six-year survey at a national clinic in Japan, *J Altern Complement Med* 5:229–236, 1999.

7. Do any Western medical practices cause permanent changes in the skin?

Of course, both intentionally and unintentionally. Think of surgical scars and keloids, radiation-port tattoos, radiation dermatitis, amniocentesis pits, hair transplants, ad infinitum.

8. Where did the practice of tattooing start?

Archaeologic evidence, such as human remains, shows that tattooing was part of indigenous cultures worldwide. For whatever reasons, tattoos were used in ancient Europe, the Mediterranean region and Middle East, southern Asia, northern Japan, the Americas, and throughout the Pacific islands.

Levy J, Sewell M, Goldstein N: A short history of tattooing, *J Dermatol Surg Oncol* 5:851–856, 1979.

9. What does the word *tattoo* mean?

Tattoo comes from the pan-Polynesian word *tatau* meaning "to mark." Polynesian tataus were, and still are, richly symbolic, revealing heritage and status.

10. What culture has the most elaborate tattoos?

The Marquesan Islanders of French Polynesia once applied tattoos to almost the entire body. Hawaiians, Samoans (Fig. 63-1), and New Zealand Maoris also had extensive tattoos. The practice is experiencing a cultural resurgence in many Polynesian groups today. Japanese tattoos (horimono) are often regarded as the most skillful and artistically prepared.

11. Why do sailors have tattoos?

European sailors adopted the habit during voyages to the Polynesian islands in the 18th century. The practice is still associated with the occupation of working at sea.

12. Sailors sometimes have rooster and pig tattoos on their lower legs. Does this have a meaning?

Yes, many ethnic groups, cultures, and even subcultures, including sailors, have tattoos with specific meanings. For example, the reason that sailors tattoo a rooster and pig on their lower legs (Fig. 63-2) or feet is that these barnyard animals do not swim, and they believe that if the ship sinks, or they are thrown overboard, having the tattoo will get them to land quickly. Other examples of tattoos with specific meanings include an **anchor,** meaning that the sailor had sailed the Atlantic Ocean, or a **fully-rigged sail ship,** indicating that the sailor had sailed around Cape Horn.

13. Who is the Ice Man? Why are his tattoos so important?

The Ice Man is the name given to the 5200-year-old frozen corpse of a Bronze Age hunter found preserved in the ice of a Tyrolean glacier on the border of Austria and Italy. He had 15 groups of tattoos that are noteworthy because they are neither decorative nor on exposed surfaces. Most of the Ice Man's tattoos are on standard acupuncture sites. Subsequent radiographic examinations of the body revealed old traumas at appropriate sites and strengthen the notion that the Ice Man's tattoos served as a form of therapy, akin to acupuncture.

Dorfer L, Moser M, Bahr F, et al: A medical report from the Stone Age? *Lancet* 354:1023–1025, 1999.

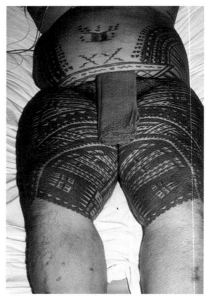

Figure 63-1. Samoan man with extensive and elaborate cultural tattoo. The traditional patterns of Polynesian tattoos are distinctive for each island or island group. (Courtesy of the Fitzsimons Army Medical Center teaching files.)

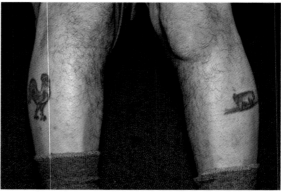

Figure 63-2. Sailor with tattoos of a rooster and pig on his leg. (Courtesy of the Fitzsimons Army Medical Center teaching files.)

14. **A man from rural Nigeria has several sets of small parallel scars on his face. He says that his village doctor made these with a sharp stone when the man was young. What are ritually placed incisions called?**
Scarification.

15. **Scarification is performed in a number of societies. Why?**
Ornamentation and beautification, group identification, protection (from illness or evil), and therapy.

16. **What is an omega brand?**
It symbolizes the rite of passage by initiates entering the American college fraternity Omega Psi Phi. Although not officially sanctioned by the fraternity's national office, tens of thousands of men (and many "little sisters") have voluntarily permitted themselves to be branded on the deltoid or pectoral region with hot metal in the shape of the Greek letter O.

17. **Name the familiar dark-red spot placed on the central forehead of Hindu women.**
Bindi, kumkum, or tilak.

Kumar AS, Pandhi RK, Bhutani LK: Bindi dermatoses, *Int J Dermatol* 25:434–435, 1986.

18. **What dermatologic problems can bindi cause?**
Allergic contact dermatitis caused by the pigments (mercuric or lead compounds, turmeric), hyperpigmentation that is either postinflammatory or due to a lichenoid eruption, and contact leukoderma.

19. **While on a surfing trip to an outer island of Fiji, you notice that many of the men have dry, scaly skin. You guess there must be a hyperendemic focus of X-linked ichthyosis. The villagers laugh when you ask if the men are born that way and explain that the skin problem is called kani and is caused by drinking too much yanggona. What is this?**
Kani is the Fijian word for kava dermopathy, which is an acquired ichthyosiform disorder caused by excessive consumption of kava (called yanggona in Fiji). The mechanism for the skin disorder is unknown.

Norton SA, Ruze P: Kava dermopathy, *J Am Acad Dermatol* 31:89–97, 1994.

20. **What is kava?**
Kava is a beverage made from the roots of *Piper methysticum*, a true pepper found on many tropical Pacific islands. Kava has psychoactive properties and is used socially and ceremonially throughout Micronesia, Melanesia, and Polynesia.

21. **Your favorite professor has invited you to accompany her on an assessment of a refugee camp in southern Africa. In the camp, you see hundreds of children and adults with a strikingly similar shiny, slightly erosive eruption along exposed areas of their clavicular regions and forearms. What is this eruption?**
Pellagra.

22. **Why is pellagra abundant in the refugee camps?**
The inadequate food supplies available in the camps are often heavily reliant on corn-based products that have insufficient levels of nicotinic acid (niacin). This explanation also accounts for the pellagra outbreaks in the southern United States in orphanages and prisons, and among sharecroppers in the early 20th century, where the diet was based almost exclusively on corn.

Centers for Disease Control and Prevention: Outbreak of pellagra among Mozambican refugees-Malawi, 1990, *MMWR* 40:209–213, 1991.

23. **What is betel nut? Who chews it?**
Betel nut refers to the fruit of the areca palm *(Areca catechu)* that is typically chewed when wrapped in betel leaves (Piper betle). It is chewed extensively in many cultures from Pakistan to Micronesia. It has been estimated that 0% to 20% of the world chews betel nut. There are many variations with some cultures adding lime, clove, cardamom, catechu, or even tobacco. This compound is chewed by men and women alike, presumably for the mild psychoactive muscarinic properties of the alkaloids found in the areca nut and the eugenol found in the betel leaf. Asian and Pacific island immigrants to the United States often continue this practice. Technically, there is no betel nut; "betel" refers to the leaves and the "nut" is actually the areca nut which is technically a drupe. Betel leaves have been reported to cause mottled dyschromia of the skin, perhaps as a chemical contact dermatitis.

24. **What dermatologic changes are associated with chewing betel nut?**
Betel nut chewing stains the teeth, gingiva, and oral mucosa. The color ranges from red to black, depending on the preparation used. Chewers regard the color change as cosmetically appealing. More worrisome, however, is the greatly increased risk of oral squamous cell carcinomas in chewers, attributable to both the areca nut and the lime.

Norton SA: Betel: consumption and consequences, *J Am Acad Dermatol* 38:81–88, 1998.

25. The visa of a Somali family living in your town has expired. The mother is fighting deportation because she fears that her daughters will be compelled to undergo circumcision if they return to Mogadishu. What is female circumcision?

Female circumcision is the encompassing term that Westerners use for several forms of culturally sanctioned surgical procedures on the female genitalia. It is most commonly performed in the predominantly Muslim nations of North Africa, where perhaps 100 million women have had the procedure.

There are several forms of female circumcision, ranging from partial clitoridectomy (Sunna circumcision) to total infibulation (or pharaonic circumcision), the removal of the clitoris, labia minora, incisions of the labia majora, and suturing that partially closes the vaginal orifice.

Dare FO, Oboro VO, Fadiora SO, et al: Female genital mutilation: an analysis of 522 cases in South-Western Nigeria, *J Obstet Gynaecol* 24:281–283, 2004.

Horowitz CR, Jackson JC: Female "circumcision": African women confront American medicine, *J Gen Intern Med* 12:491–499, 1997.

26. What are the complications of female circumcision?

There can be medical (infections), surgical (hemorrhage), reproductive (fetal death), sexual (dyspareunia), psychological (chronic anxiety), social (peer pressures), and legal (immigration status) complications to the procedure. On the other hand, failure to perform the procedure may also have adverse cultural consequences. An interesting aside is the unsupported hypothesis that infibulation has hastened the spread of HIV infection in Africa by promoting exposure to blood during intercourse.

Hardy DB: Cultural practices contributing to the transmission of human immunodeficiency virus in Africa, *Rev Infect Dis* 9:1109–1119, 1987.

Key Points: Cultural Dermatology

1. There is an increased mobility and immigration of different cultures and ethnic groups into Western countries, and health care providers are increasingly exposed to different changes in the skin related to different cultural practices.
2. Western health care providers who are not aware of these differences may mistake cultural health care for child or spouse abuse (e.g., *cao gió*).
3. Western "cosmetic" procedures (e.g., breast augmentation, circumcision, liposuction) and non-Western cultural practices (e.g., voluntary female circumcision, scarification) are very similar in that they are approved by the culture that utilizes the practice and are often viewed with distaste from the perspective of a different culture.

---

27. What is the most common culturally sanctioned mutilation in the United States?

Ah, mutilation is such a pejorative term. Let's use "surgical alteration" instead. After all, piercing one's ears is the answer, and we do not want to tag these persons as mutilated.

28. What about culturally sanctioned surgical alterations of male genitalia?

Dozens of these exist, including the religion-associated ritual circumcisions of Judaism, Islam, and the Seventh Day Adventist faith. Many Western societies practice widespread routine circumcision of neonates. Australian aborigines practiced subincision, an incision of the distal ventral penis exposing the urethra. Ancient Pompeians practiced hemicastration (removal of one testicle) as a manhood rite. Many cultures practice the simple release of the ventral frenulum. Occupational castration (eunuchs of the seraglio), punitive castrations, and gender-altering surgery among transsexuals have also received varying degrees of cultural acceptance throughout history.

29. What are artificial penile nodules?

Objects placed permanently under the skin of the prepuce or penile shaft, purportedly to enhance the partner's pleasure during intercourse. Other names include *tancho nodules* and *bulleetus*. It is most commonly practiced in East Asian nations (e.g., Thailand and Philippines). In Japan, members of the yakuza, or Japanese criminal underground, often have artificial penis nodules.

Norton SA: Fijian penis marbles: an example of artificial penile nodules, *Cutis* 51:295–297, 1993.

30. Your cousin is marrying a woman from Mumbai (Bombay). On the wedding day, the bride's hands are painted with an intricate filigree-like pattern of reddish-brown pigment. What is this form of ornamentation called?

The Indian name for this is *mehndi*. It is produced by a semipermanent dye called henna.

31. Describe the use of henna on the skin.

Henna is a natural red-brown pigment obtained from the plant *Lawsonia inermis*. It is used to prepare ceremonial body paint used in many Middle Eastern and South Asian societies. It is most commonly used by women on the palms and soles, especially for celebrations such as weddings. Henna is now commonly used in a deritualized fashion by Western women.

32. Are there any medical problems associated with henna?

Yes, but they are rare. Some people develop irritant contact dermatitis using henna. Henna may also cause hemolysis in G6PD-deficient individuals after percutaneous absorption. Also, some henna preparations contain para-phenylenediamine additives that can induce cutaneous and pulmonary allergic reactions (Fig. 63-3).

Lestringant GG, Bener A, Frossard PM: Cutaneous reactions to henna and associated additives, *Br J Dermatol* 141:498–500, 1999.

33. A patient with a referral to the otolaryngology clinic mistakenly arrives in the dermatology clinic. You see that the consultation is to "rule out congenital absence of the uvula." Sure enough, on your examination, there is no uvula. What gives?

Your patient is missing the uvula due not to a congenital absence but due, instead, to a perinatal uvulectomy. This procedure is performed in many societies from West Africa to the Middle East. The usual explanation is that uvulectomy alleviates problems associated with vomiting or cough. It is performed by nonphysicians on infants or toddlers. Uvulectomy is also performed by Western physicians as a treatment for obstructive sleep apnea. The name of this procedure, uvulopalatopharyngoplasty, is bigger than the tissue that is removed. (Avoid confusing UPPP with PUPPP, which is a skin disease.)

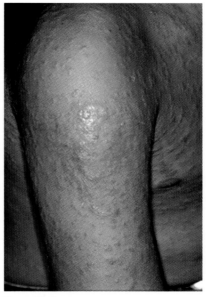

Figure 63-3. Allergic contact dermatitis to henna tattoo on the arm. The outline of the tattoo is clearly visible. The other skin lesions represent an id reaction (autoeczematization) to the allergic contact dermatitis. (Courtesy of the William L. Weston, M.D. Collection.)

34. A 51-year-old Muslim woman from Saudi Arabia is noted to have asymptomatic thickening and hyperpigmentation on the forehead, knees, ankles, and on the dorsa of her feet. What does she have?

She has "prayer marks." Prayer marks with this distribution are most common in Muslims who pray for prolonged periods. The changes are due to the repeated prolonged friction and pressure associated with praying. Prayer marks are not confined to Muslims and may be seen in any religious person who prays for prolonged periods.

Abanmii AA, Al Zouman AY, Al Hussaini H, Al-Asmari A: Prayer marks, *Int J Dermatol* 43:985–986, 2002.

35. A 22-year-old man from India presents with tinea cruris that involves the penis. What most likely accounts for this highly atypical clinical distribution of infection?

The man most likely wears a langota, which is a semiocclusive undergarment that is associated with increased involvement of the penis in patients with tinea cruris. At one time, in some parts of India, it was the only type of underwear that many men used; it is still used by some men. In some parts of India, it is still considered to be the garment of choice for various athletic endeavors such as traditional wrestling, martial arts training, and gymnastics. A very similar garment called the *fundoshi* is worn in Japan.

Pandey SS, Chandra S, Guha PK, et al: Dermatophyte infection of the penis. Association with a particular undergarment, *Int J Dermatol* 20:112–114, 1981.

EMERGENCIES AND MISCELLANEOUS PROBLEMS

1. "Dermatologic emergencies" sounds like an oxymoron. Are there dermatologic emergencies?

Yes. Several groups of diseases in dermatology are emergencies. In some, the skin is the primary organ affected (e.g., pemphigus vulgaris) and, in others, the cutaneous manifestations are an important diagnostic finding of a severe underlying condition (e.g., meningococcemia). Rapid recognition and diagnosis of dermatologic emergencies are important because these conditions are often acutely lethal but can be treated successfully if the diagnosis is made early in the disease course.

2. What are the major groups of dermatologic emergencies?

- Vesiculobullous disorders and drug reactions (e.g., Stevens-Johnson syndrome, toxic epidermal necrolysis, pemphigus vulgaris)
- Infections
- Autoimmune disorders (e.g., acute cutaneous eruption of systemic lupus erythematosus, juvenile rheumatoid arthritis)
- Inflammatory cutaneous disorders (e.g., desquamative erythroderma, acute pustular psoriasis, acute drug eruptions)
- Environmental disorders (e.g., child abuse, heatstroke, electrical burns)

VESICULOBULLOUS DISORDERS AND DRUG REACTIONS

3. How does toxic epidermal necrolysis differ from the Stevens-Johnson syndrome or erythema multiforme major?

Toxic epidermal necrolysis (TEN) and Stevens-Johnson syndrome are commonly confused entities, in part because many clinicians use the two terms interchangeably. Because these two diseases have significantly different prognoses and treatments, it is important to differentiate between them (Table 64-1). The diseases can usually be distinguished by their clinical presentation (Fig. 64-1), histologic findings, and course.

The relationship between TEN and Stevens-Johnson syndrome is one of the great controversies in dermatology. Some in vitro research suggests that they are different diseases based on pathogenic mechanisms, but some authorities regard TEN as a more severe form of Stevens-Johnson syndrome. It is universally accepted that Stevens-Johnson syndrome is a more severe form of erythema multiforme.

Wolf R, Orion E, Marcos B, Matz H: Life-threatening acute adverse cutaneous drug reactions, *Clin Dermatol* 23:171–181, 2005.

4. How do you treat TEN?

Patients with TEN should be treated as burn patients, with supportive care to maintain fluid balance, avoid infection, and prevent adult respiratory distress syndrome (ARDS). In essence, TEN patients should be treated as severe burn victims. There are in vitro data to suggest that this entity may be the result of direct toxicity of drugs, or their metabolites, to skin cells. Anecdotal reports suggest that systemic corticosteroids are actually detrimental to TEN patients, although others continue to advocate their use. Initial anecdotal reports suggested that intravenous immunoglobulin therapy improved survival; however, this is controversial because other reports have not demonstrated efficacy.

Table 64-1. Clinicopathologic Features of Toxic Epidermal Necrolysis (TEN) versus Stevens-Johnson Syndrome (SJS)

	TEN	SJS
Maximal intensity	1–3 days	7–15 days
Skin pain	Severe	Minimal
Mucosal involvement	Mild	Severe
Lesional pattern	Diffuse erythema, desquamation	Annular and targetoid lesions
Skin histology	Few inflammatory cells	Numerous inflammatory cells
Prognosis	Poor	Excellent

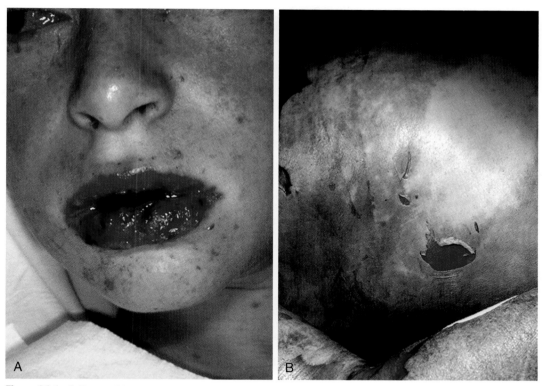

Figure 64-1. A, Stevens-Johnson syndrome demonstrating typical mucosal inflammation of the mouth, lips, and conjunctiva. **B,** Fatal case of captopril-induced toxic epidermal necrolysis showing violaceous discoloration with sheets of epidermis peeling away from the skin. (Courtesy of James E. Fitzpatrick, MD.)

5. How do you treat Stevens-Johnson syndrome?

Stevens-Johnson syndrome appears to be immunologically mediated and responds to systemic corticosteroids. Patients with severe symptoms, especially involvement of the oral mucosa, which interferes with eating and fluid intake, may be treated with a short trial of systemic corticosteroids. Stevens-Johnson syndrome is usually a self-limited disease with a 3-week course, and milder cases may not require systemic corticosteroids. Some authorities consider the use of systemic corticosteroids in this condition as controversial, because there are no good prospective, controlled studies evaluating this treatment. Therefore, an empirical 3- to 4-day trial of high-dose systemic steroids should be considered. If there is no clinical improvement at that time, the treatment should be discontinued.

6. What is pemphigus vulgaris?

Pemphigus vulgaris is a superficial blistering disease that typically affects middle-aged individuals (Fig. 64-2). It often presents initially with mouth ulcerations (60% of cases) but can involve blistering on areas above the waist. Pemphigus vulgaris may present acutely and, in severe cases, may resemble TEN or Stevens-Johnson syndrome. Early diagnosis is important because this condition is usually fatal if untreated, and current therapies are effective.

Groves RW: Pemphigus: a brief review, *Clin Med* 9: 371–375, 2009.

7. Describe Nikolsky's sign and its relationship to pemphigus vulgaris.

Pemphigus vulgaris involves only the upper layers of the epidermis; therefore, the blisters are very fragile, and typically patients present with only superficial ulcerations. Because of the fragility of the skin, one can apply lateral pressure with a finger to the intact

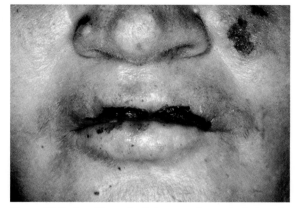

Figure 64-2. Pemphigus vulgaris demonstrating erosive lesions of the lips and left cheek. (Courtesy of James E. Fitzpatrick, MD.)

skin around a lesion, causing the upper layer of the skin to become detached. This is called the Nikolsky's sign, and it occurs in pemphigus and other superficial blistering diseases. This clinical sign can be helpful in differentiating superficial from deeper blistering diseases (e.g., bullous pemphigoid, bullous lupus erythematosus), in which Nikolsky's sign is usually absent.

8. How is pemphigus vulgaris treated?
Therapy is designed to decrease the production of the antidesmosomal antibodies or to reduce the inflammatory response. Because pemphigus can be deadly, corticosteroids in high doses are used initially, despite their serious side effects. Prednisone is given in daily oral doses of 120 mg as an initial dose, which is then adjusted lower or higher depending on the patient response. Other immunosuppressive drugs, such as azathioprine and cyclophosphamide, have been used in conjunction with corticosteroids because of their steroid-sparing effect.

9. What is the DRESS syndrome?
DRESS stands for **d**rug **r**ash with **e**osinophilia and **s**ystemic **s**ymptoms, and it is a life-threatening reaction. It is characterized by a papulosquamous eruption, fever, enlarged lymph nodes, leukocytosis with eosinophilia, and liver or kidney involvement. Typical drugs that induce this reaction include anticonvulsants, allopurinol, and other sulfa drugs. The syndrome develops several weeks after drug initiation and can persist and recur for prolonged periods after the drug has been stopped. Therapy includes high-dose steroids and cyclophosphamide.

INFECTIOUS DISEASES

10. Are any dermatologic emergencies infectious in origin?
Yes. These are most commonly bacterial (e.g., necrotizing fasciitis, tularemia, meningococcemia, subacute and acute bacterial endocarditis) but also include viral infections (e.g., hemorrhagic fevers, neonatal herpes simplex infection), rickettsial infections (e.g., Rocky Mountain spotted fever), and fungal infections (e.g., mucormycosis).

11. Can emergent infections be differentiated by their cutaneous presentations?
Yes, although few cutaneous findings in emergent infections are pathognomonic. Infections that involve the skin can be organized generally by the appearance of the primary lesion (Table 64-2). Major cutaneous patterns of presentation include
- **Petechial/purpuric papules** (e.g., chronic gonococcal septicemia, meningococcemia, subacute/acute bacterial endocarditis, and Rocky Mountain spotted fever) (Fig. 64-3)
- **Vesicular** (e.g., neonatal herpes simplex, Kaposi's varicelliform eruption)
- **Pustular** (e.g., disseminated candidiasis)
- **Maculopapular** (e.g., hepatitis B, Lyme disease)
- **Diffusely erythematous** (e.g., staphylococcal scalded skin syndrome)

12. What is the differential to consider in hemorrhagic lesions other than infection?
- Coagulation abnormalities, such as idiopathic thrombocytopenia, disseminated intravascular coagulation, and clotting factor deficiencies
- Toxic epidermal necrolysis, which initially can present with petechial lesions
- Vasculitides, such as leukocytoclastic vasculitis secondary to an underlying collagen vascular disease, or periarteritis nodosa
- Raynaud's syndrome or disease
- Ergot poisoning

13. What causes necrotizing fasciitis?
Necrotizing fasciitis has been well described for years but has recently received much attention in the lay press as the "flesh-eating bacteria." It is a bacterial infection that is rapidly progressive, often over hours, destroying muscle and subcutaneous tissues. Death or loss of a limb may occur, if it is not diagnosed and treated early in its course. It is most commonly associated with β-hemolytic streptococci but may also be due to other gram-positive or gram-negative organisms, or it may be polymicrobial.

Sarani B, Strong M, Pascual J, Schwab CW: Necrotizing fasciitis: current concepts and review of the literature, *J Am Coll Surg* 208:279–288, 2009.

14. Describe the clinical presentation of necrotizing fasciitis.
The bacteria usually enter through a surgical or traumatic wound and quickly move along fascial planes destroying vessels and tissue. Within the first 48 hours, the involved area that is initially erythematous, indurated, and painful becomes a dusky blue, indicating lack of circulation in the area (Fig. 64-4). Because there is significant vessel thrombosis, a biopsy usually results in little or no bleeding, and this is a useful diagnostic sign if present. Surgical debridement in addition to systemic antibiotics is necessary and often reveals extensive covert tissue necrosis.

Table 64-2. Diagnostic Signs in Dermatologic Infectious Emergencies

Petechial/Palpable Purpura
Neisseria gonorrhoeae septicemia
Neisseria meningitidis septicemia
Acute/subacute bacterial endocarditis (*Staphylococcus aureus*, streptococci)
Rickettsia rickettsii (Rocky Mountain spotted fever)
Rickettsia prowazekii (louse-borne typhus)
Borrelia sp. (relapsing fever)
Hemorrhagic fevers (dengue, Rift Valley, Congo-Crimean, Korean)
Cytomegalovirus (viral hepatitis)
Hepatitis B virus
Yellow fever
Rubella
Plasmodium falciparum (malaria)
Trichinosis

Violaceous Skin Discoloration
Infectious gangrene
Necrotizing fasciitis
Mucormycosis

Purpura Fulminans (Purpura Secondary to Disseminated Intravascular Coagulation)
Neisseria meningitidis
Streptococcus spp.
Escherichia coli
Salmonella typhi
Bacteroides fragilis
Other enteric gram-negative organisms
Hemorrhagic fevers
Vibrio vulnificus

Vesicular
Neonatal herpes simplex virus
Disseminated vaccinia

Pustular
Staphylococcal endocarditis/sepsis
Disseminated candidiasis
Herpes simplex virus
Corynebacterium diphtheriae

Diffuse Erythema
Toxic shock syndrome

Maculopapular Eruptions
Viral infections
Rickettsial infections
Spirillum minor (rat-bite fever)
Disseminated fungal infections
Toxoplasma gondii
Tularemia
Leptospirosis

Annular Erythema
Lyme disease (*Borrelia burgdorferi*)

15. Can other cutaneous infections look like necrotizing fasciitis?
Actually, necrotizing fasciitis is a type of infectious gangrene or cellulitis that rapidly progresses to destroy skin, subcutaneous tissue, and muscle. There are other types of gangrene, all of which have cutaneous findings similar to those of necrotizing fasciitis:

- *Staphylococcus aureus* and, occasionally, gram-negative organisms can cause progressive bacterial synergistic gangrene. This disease presents with a dusky erythematous discoloration of the skin followed by deep ulceration.
- In gas gangrene or clostridial gangrene, caused by the anaerobe *Clostridium perfringens*, patients typically present after a penetrating or crush wound with a tender, painful, edematous, white area that often becomes bronze with cutaneous blistering. Occasionally, when one palpates the area, crepitation or a crackling sensation is noted secondary to

gas formation in the tissue. As with necrotizing fasciitis, timely diagnosis and treatment are necessary to
minimize morbidity and mortality.

16. Are there any parasitic disease "emergencies" that have cutaneous manifestations?

Trichinosis is caused by the small parasitic worm
Trichinella spiralis, which is ingested in inadequately
cooked meat containing its cysts. Common sources
of encysted meat include bears and other carnivores
or omnivores. Ingestion of pork, once a common
source of trichinosis, is an extremely rare source
today. The cutaneous signs include a macular or
petechial eruption, splinter hemorrhages, periorbital
edema, and conjunctivitis. The systemic signs and
symptoms begin 1 to 4 weeks after ingestion and
consist of eosinophilia, fever, headache, myalgias,
and brain hemorrhage, which can lead to death.

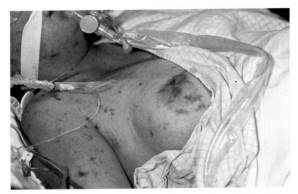

Figure 64-3. Palpable purpura and ecchymoses in a patient with meningococcemia. (Courtesy of the William L. Weston, M.D. Collection.)

17. Are there any other parasitic disease emergencies?

Yes. Another is cysticercosis cutis, which is a
cestoidal infection due to the larval form of the pork
tapeworm, *Taenia solium*. Typically, *Taenia* eggs
enter the stomach from the intestine via reverse
peristalsis, and they develop into oncospheres that
penetrate the stomach wall and enter the circulation.
They become lodged in internal organs, such as the
heart, brain, muscles, lungs, and eye. They also
move to the subcutaneous tissues and develop into
cysts that contain cysticercus larvae. They are
usually numerous and can become calcified as
evidenced by x-ray. With the presentation of multiple
subcutaneous cysts in a patient with unexplained
neurologic signs or symptoms, one must keep this
diagnosis in mind.

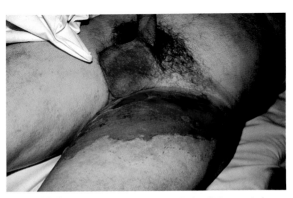

Figure 64-4. Necrotizing fasciitis. The typical well-demarcated, dusky purpuric lesion is caused by thrombosis of the involved vessels.

Miura H, Itoh Y, Kozuka T: A case of subcutaneous cysticercosis (cysticercus cellulosae cutis), *J Am Acad Dermatol* 43:538–540, 2000.

18. Do mycobacterial infections cause any dermatologic emergencies?

Most mycobacterial infections are relatively chronic and do not constitute emergencies. However, when patients with
Hansen's disease (leprosy) are treated, they may undergo a "reversal reaction" that is secondary to a change in their
immune status, resulting in acute inflammation of the involved areas. This may produce mild erythema and swelling of
the skin and subcutaneous tissue. The apparent benignity of the situation belies its seriousness. The involved nerves
are completely destroyed, resulting in permanent motor and sensory damage to the area. The lack of sensory input and
resultant trauma over years lead to severe disfigurement of the extremities. Treatment consists of high-dose
prednisone tapered over weeks.

AUTOIMMUNE DISORDERS

19. What collagen vascular diseases may become dermatologic emergencies?

- Acute cutaneous and bullous systemic lupus erythematosus (SLE)
- Dermatomyositis
- Leukocytoclastic vasculitis (necrotizing venulitis)
- Still's disease
- Neonatal lupus erythematosus

20. What are the cutaneous findings in acute and bullous SLE?

The cutaneous findings of acute SLE are most common on the sun-exposed areas of the skin. The eruption consists of
an evanescent erythema that is especially evident over the malar area of the face, producing the characteristic
"butterfly rash." The erythema lasts hours to days and can resolve without residua. In a significant number of patients,
the acute erythema can evolve into discoid lupus erythematosus, which is a chronic scaling eruption with scarring.

In bullous SLE, the patients present with tense vesicles or bullae, usually in sun-exposed sites. These are important
presentations, because both may be associated with severe internal disease.

21. How does neonatal lupus erythematosus (NLE) present?

It is an acute self-limited disease that gradually improves over 1 to 2 months. The cutaneous findings include diffuse superficial erythema and scaling that are often most apparent in the malar area of the face but can occur anywhere. Neonates frequently have other systemic findings, such as those seen in SLE: anemia, thrombocytopenia, jaundice, and hepatosplenomegaly with abnormal liver function tests. Another prevalent finding is atrioventricular heart block, which is permanent.

22. Why are prompt recognition and treatment of NLE important?

Frequently, NLE eruptions are misdiagnosed as infectious in origin. This subjects the infant to the unnecessary risks of systemic antibiotics, while the presence of heart block may be missed, and appropriate systemic treatment (steroids) for the other NLE problems is delayed.

Key Points: Dermatologic Emergencies

1. Dermatologic emergencies do exist, and some, such as toxic epidermal necrolysis and necrotizing fasciitis, have characteristic skin signs.
2. Recognition of specific skin signs and the early diagnosis of emergent skin disorders can be lifesaving.
3. Skin signs of TEN include diffuse and severe skin tenderness and "cayenne pepper" nonblanching erythema that evolves into widespread blistering and superficial ulcers.
4. Recognition of the skin signs of necrotizing fasciitis is crucial to patient survival. These signs include systemic toxicity; localized painful induration; well-defined, dusky blue coloration; and lack of bleeding in the area when incised.

---

23. Why is dermatomyositis considered an emergency?

Dermatomyositis can develop rapidly with significant mortality. Skin findings in this disease can predate significant muscle involvement and be quite helpful in early diagnosis and treatment, especially in children. The skin findings that are helpful in diagnosis are

- **Gottron's papules,** occurring over the dorsa of the distal interphalangeal (DIP) and proximal interphalangeal (PIP) joints of the hands
- **Swelling and "heliotrope" erythema** of the eyelids
- **Periungual erythema** (erythema around the proximal nail fold)

24. What is leukocytoclastic vasculitis?

This term is histologically descriptive of a group of diseases that cause acute neutrophilic inflammation and damage to the small vessels of the dermis. This damage can occur without apparent underlying etiology or as a cutaneous manifestation of a systemic disease, such as Henoch-Schönlein purpura, SLE, or cryoglobulinemia. The eruption typically consists of "palpable purpura," varying in size from a few millimeters to several centimeters, mainly on the lower extremities. The cutaneous lesions of this group of diseases usually resolve without sequelae, but the internal organ involvement can be severe. The differential diagnosis of leukocytoclastic vasculitis should include infections that cause palpable purpura, such as meningococcemia.

25. What are the skin signs of Still's disease?

The diagnosis of Still's disease (juvenile rheumatoid arthritis) can be perplexing because a significant number of these patients (25% to 30%) do not present with arthritis but with an evanescent eruption, spiking fever, leukocytosis, lymphadenopathy, and splenomegaly. The disease can be rapidly progressive, with severe bone and joint destruction and growth retardation. The rash, which occurs in 25% to 40% of patients, can be present for months to years before the arthritis. The eruption is typically but not always fleeting, lasting up to 24 hours, and usually occurs in conjunction with fever. The rash may be diffuse with truncal accentuation and consists of coral-salmon red, flat macules to slightly elevated papules. Treatment for this disease usually consists of locally injected or systemic steroids. Other immunosuppressive drugs have also been used successfully.

INFLAMMATORY CUTANEOUS DISORDERS

26. Why is pyoderma gangrenosum a dermatologic emergency?

Pyoderma gangrenosum is one of a group of inflammatory skin diseases called *neutrophilic dermatoses* because, histologically, they have dermal infiltrates of neutrophils. It is a dermatologic emergency because it is often rapidly progressive, causing severe local tissue destruction. Pyoderma gangrenosum is frequently misdiagnosed as an infectious process or a brown recluse spider bite and is then treated by debridement. However, surgical procedures or any mechanical manipulation of acute lesions induces progression of disease to the normal surrounding skin, enlargement of the lesion, and further tissue destruction. Therefore, it is imperative to recognize and treat these lesions correctly early to avoid massive tissue destruction and loss.

27. How does pyoderma gangrenosum present?

Clinically, the lesions begin as a small papule/pustule that enlarges to form an ulcer. The ulcer has a necrotic center that typically involves the skin and subcutaneous tissues down to muscle, tendons, and fascia (Fig. 64-5). In older lesions, the intact epidermis at the borders of the lesion is erythematous with a purple hue and has a characteristic undermined edge. Another helpful clinical feature is the extreme pain and tenderness of these lesions. There are few cutaneous diseases that approach pyoderma gangrenosum in the severity of lesional pain and tenderness.

Most cases of pyoderma gangrenosum occur without an underlying disease (50%), but this condition has been associated with several systemic diseases, most notably Crohn's disease (1% to 5%), ulcerative colitis (30% to 60%), leukemias, rheumatoid arthritis, and other collagen vascular disease.

28. Under what circumstances do childhood vascular anomalies become dermatologic emergencies?

The most common vascular anomalies (about 3% of births) that have the potential to become dermatologic emergencies are infantile capillary hemangiomas. These lesions can be present at birth (approximately 20%) but more often develop over the first several weeks of life. Infantile hemangiomas have a rapid growth phase, during which they rapidly enlarge, and then they regress.

Most commonly, these tumors are only a cosmetic problem, but if they occur around the eyes or in the oral cavity (Fig. 64-6), they can cause significant morbidity and mortality. Some ophthalmologists suggest that even a few days of obstructed vision in a newborn can inhibit normal visual development. Therefore, an infantile hemangioma that may block an infant's visual fields should be treated aggressively. Likewise, enlarging infantile hemangiomas of the upper respiratory tract and oral cavity can result in acute emergent situations and must be treated early in their course. In rare cases, large hemangiomas can also produce high-output cardiac failure.

29. How are hemangiomas treated?

Hemangiomas can be treated with intralesional steroids, but in lesions involving the facial area, this treatment should be avoided because there have been reports of steroid suspension embolism of the central nervous system (CNS) and retinal vessels. In these cases, systemic steroids should be utilized. Recombinant interferon-α and porpranolol have also been used to treat infantile hemangiomas that have not responded to corticosteroid therapy. Rarely, large, rapidly growing hemangiomas have been associated with platelet trapping and acute thrombocytopenia.

Fledelius HC, Illum N, Jensen H, Prause JU: Interferon-alfa treatment of facial infantile hemangiomas: with emphasis on the sight-threatening varieties. A clinical series, *Acta Ophthalmol Scand* 79:370–373, 2001.

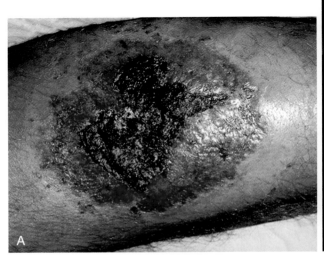
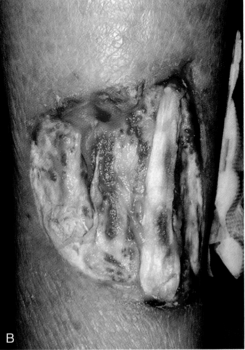

Figure 64-5. Pyoderma gangrenosum. **A,** Rapidly expanding classic lesion demonstrating characteristic undermined border. **B,** Older lesion without an active edge. Note that the depth of the ulcer exposes underlying tendons. (Courtesy of James E. Fitzpatrick, MD.)

30. Is acne fulminans a dermatologic emergency?
Although acne is not usually considered an emergency, this condition, if not treated acutely, can lead to severe cutaneous scarring and its attendant psychological problems. This type of acne usually occurs in teenage males, but there are cases reported in females. The eruption is characterized by rapid suppuration of large, highly inflamed nodules and plaques, resulting in ragged ulcerations and scarring of the chest, back, and, less commonly, face. Often attendant with the cutaneous symptoms are fever, leukocytosis, arthralgias, and myalgias, suggesting a systemic upregulation of the immune system.

31. What is the treatment for acne fulminans?
The treatment for this condition is high-dose oral steroids (e.g., prednisone) and early institution of oral retinoids such as 13-cis-retinoic acid. Paradoxically, oral retinoic acid can also induce acne fulminans in the first month of treatment. Physicians who use this medication should be aware of this potential side effect.

32. Are there drug eruptions that are dermatologic emergencies?
Most drug eruptions are relatively benign and consist of a morbilliform or macular erythema that occurs without other signs or symptoms. On occasion, drug eruptions can present as diffuse exfoliative erythroderma, or red man syndrome. In these cases, patients develop a total body erythroderma with pruritus and scaling. In addition to drugs, other causes of exfoliative erythroderma that must be ruled out include psoriasis, lymphoma, and flares of seborrheic or atopic dermatitis. Other types of drug eruptions that can be dermatologic emergencies include toxic epidermal necrolysis, leukocytoclastic vasculitis, and severe urticaria or angioedema.

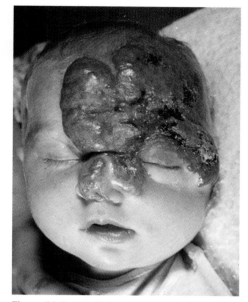

Figure 64-6. Infantile hemangioma. Rapidly growing infantile hemangioma occluding the orbital space and nasal cavity. (Courtesy of the Fitzsimons Army Medical Center teaching files.)

33. What are the mucocutaneous findings in Kawasaki's disease?
- Conjunctival congestion
- Oropharyngeal lesions (mucosal injection, strawberry tongue, fissured lips)
- Hand and foot erythema
- Exanthem

These findings, along with lymphadenopathy, constitute the minor criteria for Kawasaki disease. Four of the five minor plus the major criterion of fever >38.38° C are necessary for the diagnosis. The hand and foot erythema may demonstrate variable edema followed by acral desquamation about 2 weeks after the onset. The exanthem is a generalized macular erythema.

Newburger JW, Fulton DR: Kawasaki disease, *Curr Opin Pediatr* 16:508–514, 2004.

34. How do you treat Kawasaki's syndrome?
High-dose aspirin during the febrile phase (100 mg/kg/day), in addition to intravenous gammaglobulin (400 mg/kg/day for 3 to 4 days).

ENVIRONMENTAL DISORDERS

35. Is heatstroke considered a dermatologic emergency?
Although heatstroke is not typically considered a "dermatologic problem," it does have characteristic skin findings that are helpful in making a quick diagnosis. In a heatstroke victim, the skin is erythematous, hot, and dry. These findings in association with unconsciousness should alert one to the diagnosis. Therapy needs to be instituted promptly to prevent death or severe CNS damage.

36. What are the cutaneous signs of child abuse?
Because child abuse can lead to acute morbidity and mortality, its recognition should be of paramount importance when evaluating pediatric patients. Cutaneous signs of abuse include:
- **Bruising and abrasions:** These lesions are usually present in patterns or in areas not consistent with the history or trauma from common childhood accidents (Fig. 64-7).
- **Burns with unusual patterns:** Some examples are cigarette burns that appear randomly over the body or dunking scald injuries, which have distinct borders and, occasionally, have a "doughnut" pattern around the buttock area when the buttock is pressed against the cooler tub surface.

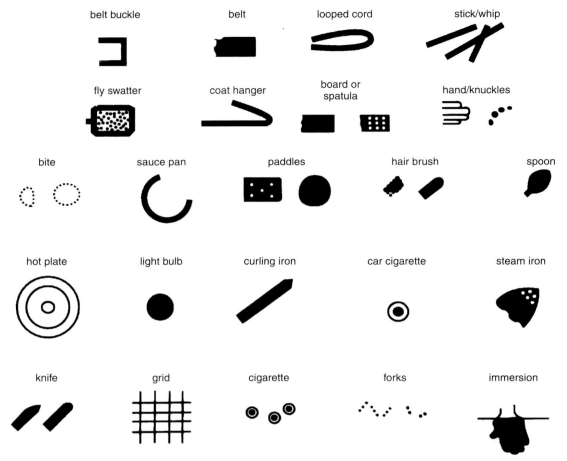

belt buckle · belt · looped cord · stick/whip

fly swatter · coat hanger · board or spatula · hand/knuckles

bite · sauce pan · paddles · hair brush · spoon

hot plate · light bulb · curling iron · car cigarette · steam iron

knife · grid · cigarette · forks · immersion

Figure 64-7. Various cutaneous patterns of child abuse.

- **Generalized wastage and dermatitis:** These are due to neglect and malnutrition.
- **Traumatic alopecia:** This alopecia demonstrates hemorrhage, irregular outlines, or hematoma formation.
- **Bite marks of adults** can be distinguished from a child's by the width, which in adults is >4 cm.

Mudd SS, Findlay JS: The cutaneous manifestations and common mimickers of physical child abuse, *J Pediatr Health Care* 18:123–129, 2004.

37. What are the skin signs of a lightning strike?

Lightning strike patients often have very characteristic skin findings. In addition to entry and exit burn wounds, the skin of these patients can often exhibit a swirled or fernlike erythema of the involved area (Fig. 64-8). If there is any doubt of the etiology, the biopsy findings in the skin are pathognomonic. It is important to diagnose this injury, because significant covert injury to the underlying fascia and muscles can occur. The degree of damage must be assessed and the patient treated for arrhythmias, shock, fluid and electrolyte imbalances, peripheral and central neural damage, and covert tissue damage to optimize recovery.

38. What is scleredema neonatorum?

It is typically seen in newborns but has been reported in infants up to 3 months of age. Clinically, it presents as a hardening of the skin with decreased temperature, vascular mottling, and a yellow-white

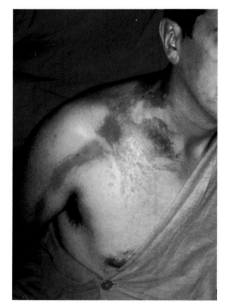

Figure 64-8. Lightning strike skin burn. Note the whorled fernlike pattern characteristic of this type of burn injury.

discoloration in a symmetrical distribution, usually over the thighs and trunk. It usually occurs in the setting of an underlying severe illness and is associated with a 50% mortality rate.

The pathophysiology of this sign probably is initiated by decreased body temperature that results in the hardening and solidification of the subcutaneous fat. This occurs in newborns because they have increased amounts of saturated lipids in their fatty tissue that solidify at higher temperatures than normal fat. Because this clinical condition often heralds death, it is important to recognize this entity early and aggressively treat the underlying illness.

39. What are the cutaneous findings in cholesterol emboli?

Cholesterol emboli can present anywhere in the body, but cutaneous manifestations most commonly occur on the lower extremities. This condition can occur spontaneously, but often cholesterol emboli to the skin present after angiography when trauma to aortic plaques dislodges cholesterol into the circulation. Clinically, the patient presents acutely with fairly well-demarcated areas of cyanosis or livedo reticularis on the feet and lower legs as a result of emboli blocking arterial circulation. These areas can undergo necrotic changes, resulting in painful ulcers.

40. How are cholesterol emboli diagnosed?

Cholesterol crystals within the lumina of the vessels on biopsy are diagnostic. The skin biopsy should ideally be an excision, and step sections should be examined because the atheromatous emboli are often focal. It is helpful to auscultate carefully over the major vessels of the abdomen and lower extremities after the patient has exercised to increase the pulse rate. This presentation is important because patients often have involvement of other organ systems, especially the kidneys. Further angiographic studies should be limited and treatment of the underlying hyperlipidemia initiated.

Manganoni AM, Venturini M, Scolari F, et al: The importance of skin biopsy in the diverse clinical manifestations of cholesterol embolism, *Br J Dermatol* 150:1230–1231, 2004.

OCCUPATIONAL DERMATOLOGY

Leslie A. Stewart, MD

1. What is the most common type of skin disease due to workplace exposures?

Contact dermatitis accounts for >90% of occupational skin disease (OSD) cases. The most common location of job-related contact dermatitis is workers' hands. It is generally accepted that 80% of the contact dermatitis cases are irritant (Fig. 65-1), while 20% are allergic (Fig. 65-2). Recent studies have challenged those figures, demonstrating that up to 40% of work-related skin diseases were from allergic contact dermatitis (ACD). Pure allergic contact dermatitis in the occupational setting is uncommon because a component of irritant contact dermatitis (ICD) is frequently present. Bureau of Labor and Statistics data show that OSD accounted for 16.5% of all occupational illnesses in 2005. Some have estimated the true number of cases to be 10 to 50 times higher than that due to underreporting and underdiagnosis. The "standard" allergens patch test screens for only approximately 75% of common allergens, so additional specialized testing with industrial chemicals to which the worker is exposed is frequently warranted. Testing should only be done with known materials in accepted concentrations.

Lushniak, BD: Occupational contact dermatitis, *Dermatol Ther* 17:272–277, 2004.

2. List some other types of OSDs and give examples of their causes.

- Folliculitis or acne (e.g., due to greases and oils)
- Chemical-related depigmentation (e.g., due to germicidal phenolic detergents)
- Lichen planus (e.g., from photographic developing agents)
- Granulomas (e.g., due to silica or beryllium dust)
- Infections (e.g., a dentist contracting herpetic whitlow from a patient with oral herpes)
- Photodermatoses (e.g., due to celery psoralens in agricultural workers)
- Contact urticaria (e.g., due to latex gloves in hospital workers)

Adams R: *Occupational skin disease*, ed 3, Philadelphia, 1999, WB Saunders.

3. Are there any risk factors for the development of an OSD?

Various investigators have found a personal history of atopic dermatitis to be a significant risk factor. Other preexisting skin diseases with compromised epidermal barriers, such as xerosis or nummular eczema, can predispose a person to contact dermatitis because of enhanced absorption of irritants and allergens through the skin. Poor personal hygiene plays a role in patients who neglect to wash off irritating and sensitizing chemicals, thereby prolonging contact time. However, overwashing is actually the more common problem. The use of harsh soaps and frequent wetting/drying cycles induce chapping and desiccation, which compromises the skin barrier. Environmental factors are also important. If it is hot and humid, workers may perspire, which can solubilize particulate matter, enhancing its penetration into the skin. Sweat can also leach out allergens, such as chromates from leather shoes, inducing an allergic contact dermatitis. Conversely, low temperature and humidity causes chapping of the skin, which can lead to irritant contact dermatitis. Certain jobs also are more likely to be associated with OSD, such as nursing and health care aides.

Belsito D: Occupational contact dermatitis: etiology, prevalence, and resultant impairment/disability, *J Am Acad Dermatol* 53:303–313, 2005.

Rietschel RL, Mathias CG, Fowler JF Jr, et al: A preliminary report of the occupation of patients evaluated in patch test clinics, *Am J Contact Dermat* 12:72–76, 2001.

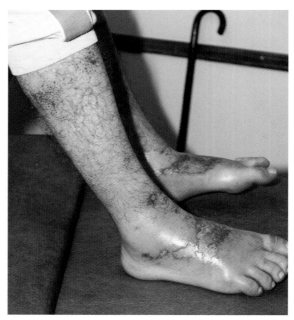

Figure 65-1. Acute toxic insult–form of irritant contact dermatitis in a cement worker who developed cement burns from fresh cement getting into his boots.

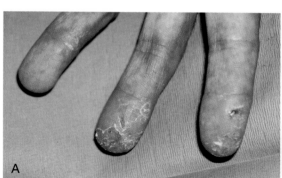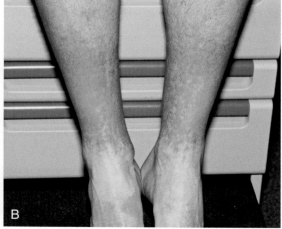

Figure 65-2. Chronic allergic contact dermatitis. **A,** A case in an orthodontist who was allergic to nickel and to the glutaraldehyde used to sterilize his instruments. Note how the scaling dermatitis can mimic irritation. **B,** This patient developed sensitization to chromium, which was used to tan the leather in his work boots. The dorsal foot distribution is typical for a shoe contact dermatitis.

4. My patient has a hand dermatitis that appeared to begin at his job. Does this mean he has an occupationally related skin disease?

Not necessarily. Just because a patient has a rash, and he or she works, does not mean it is job-related. To help make that determination, investigators have outlined seven criteria to be assessed. Four out of the seven should be present for reasonable medical probability:

1. Is the eruption consistent with a contact dermatitis? It should look like an eczematous dermatitis and not like other disorders (i.e., vasculitis).
2. Are there occupational exposures to possible irritants or allergens? There should be known documented irritating or sensitizing compounds to which the patient has been exposed at work.
3. Is the anatomic location of the eruption consistent with the exposure a worker would obtain on the job? For example, a worker may handle a chemical daily and break out with dermatitis only on his back. This is not consistent with an OSD because he should have developed an eruption where he contacted the compound the most, namely, his hands.
4. Is the onset and time course of the eruption consistent with contact dermatitis? Allergic contact dermatitis is a delayed reaction (occurring 48 to 72 hours after exposure), while irritant reactions may be immediate or delayed. Contact dermatitis is not, for example, consistent with a worker's one-time exposure to a chemical when a rash occurs 3 months after that one incident.
5. Are nonoccupational exposures excluded as a possible cause of the dermatitis? Hobbies, second jobs, and household contactants should be pursued as possible sources of contact dermatitis.
6. Does the eruption improve away from work? Work-related eruptions tend to improve when a worker is away from his job, although sometimes the same allergens and irritants may be found at home. Also, approximately 25% of workers with an OSD have a chronic and persistent dermatitis despite leaving their job and therapeutic intervention, and improvement does not occur when the worker is away from his place of employment.
7. Does patch testing reveal a likely causative agent? If a positive patch test reveals a likely allergen source with which the worker had contact, it is useful for pointing to the job exposure as the problem. However, patch tests must be interpreted within the context of the patient's history and physical examination. A positive test does not necessarily mean the allergen is responsible for the patient's current dermatitis, because it could be unrelated sensitization. The patch test reaction must always be assessed for its relevance to the present eruption.

Mathias CGT: Contact dermatitis and workers' compensation: criteria for establishing occupational causation and aggravation, *J Am Acad Dermatol* 20:842–848, 1989.

5. How do I find out what a worker is exposed to on his job?

By law, employers must provide their employees information regarding all possible workplace exposures. Each of these information sheets, known as Material Safety Data Sheets, has information about a particular compound, including hazardous ingredients that it contains in concentrations >1%. They also list the manufacturer's name and phone number, which is useful for the dermatologist to check on other ingredients, because many cutaneous allergens are present in the final product in concentrations <1%. Dermatology and occupational medicine textbooks also provide general lists of allergens and irritants that may be specific to a particular occupation. On occasion, a more in-depth investigation may require a visit to the patient's place of employment. It is a unique opportunity to observe the worker performing his duties, the general working conditions, protective measures used, and other contactants that the patient might have overlooked.

Adams R: *Occupational skin disease*, ed 3, Philadelphia, 1999, WB Saunders.

Key Points: Occupational Dermatology

1. Contact dermatitis is the most common form of OSD.
2. Irritants cause 75% of occupationally induced contact dermatitis, while allergens are responsible for 25%.
3. Hands are the most frequent site of OSD.
4. OSD can be chronic, but early diagnosis and treatment improve prognosis.
5. Treatment includes allergen and irritant avoidance, protective clothing, moisturizers, and topical steroids.

6. What are some typical workplace irritants and allergens?

- **Irritants:** Water, soaps and detergents, solvents, particulate dusts, food products, fiberglass, plastics, resins, oils, greases, agricultural chemicals, and metals. Of note, irritating compounds can be allergenic, and allergenic compounds can be irritating.
- **Allergens:** Metals (e.g., nickel), germicides (e.g., formaldehyde, glutaraldehyde), plants (e.g., poison ivy), rubber additives (e.g., thiurams), organic dyes (e.g., para-phenylenediamine in hair dye), plastic resins (e.g., acrylics and epoxies), and first-aid medications containing neomycin.

    Table 65-1 summarizes possible contactants associated with common occupations.

Elsner P: Occupational dermatoses. In Burgdorf WH, Plewig G, editors: *Braun-Falco's dermatology*, ed 3, Berlin, Heidelberg, 2009, Springer, pp 402–408.

7. What is the prognosis of an OSD?

In general, workers with occupational hand dermatitis do not fare well. Approximately 25% have complete remission, 50% have periodic recurrences, and 25% have chronic persistent dermatitis, despite a change in jobs and therapeutic intervention. Some remediable reasons for persistent dermatitis include failure to diagnose and remove the sensitizer responsible for allergic contact dermatitis, continued exposure to nonspecific irritants at home and work, continued inadvertent allergen exposure, and secondary sensitization (e.g., to preservatives contained in moisturizers and topical steroids that physicians give as treatment). Early diagnosis can be important in preventing chronic OSD. Studies have shown that delay of diagnosis for more than 1 year and continual exposure are crucial factors for chronicity.

Belsito, D: Occupational contact dermatitis: etiology, prevalence, and resultant impairment /disability, *J Am Acad Dermatol* 53:303–313, 2005.
Warshaw E, Lee G, Storrs FJ: Hand dermatitis: a review of clinical features, therapeutic options, and long-term outcomes, *Am J Contact Dermat* 14:119–137, 2003.

8. Aren't gloves enough protection for preventing OSD?

No. There is a widespread misconception that gloves guarantee safety. Although gloves are recommended on a routine basis to protect against environmental insults, they are also the cause of a great deal of contact dermatitis themselves. Irritant dermatitis occurs because patients sweat underneath their gloves. Allergic contact dermatitis occurs commonly with rubber gloves containing the chemicals thiuram, mercaptobenzothiazole, and carbamates, which are "rubber accelerator" chemicals used to speed up the vulcanization process. Some allergens can penetrate various glove materials and become trapped against the skin. For example, acrylics, formaldehyde, glutaraldehyde, and epoxy resins all penetrate latex gloves (Fig. 65-3).

9. How do you treat an occupationally related skin disease?

Remove the allergen and as many irritants as possible from both work and home. Allergens must be substituted with less sensitizing alternatives. For example, vinyl gloves can be used in place of rubber gloves. Patients must be instructed

Table 65-1. Selected Occupations and Their Possible Contactants

OCCUPATIONS	IRRITANTS	ALLERGENS
Construction workers	Cleansers, solvents, cement, dirt	Chromium (cement, leather boots), rubber chemicals (gloves), epoxy resin (adhesives)
Hairdressers	Shampoo, water, permanent wave solutions	Para-phenylenediamine (hair dyes), formaldehyde (shampoos), fragrances (shampoos and cosmetics), glyceryl monothioglycolate (permanent hair wave solutions)
Housekeepers	Cleansers, disinfectants, water	Rubber chemicals (gloves), fragrances and preservatives (cleaning and disinfectant solutions)
Health care workers	Soap, water, gloves, disinfectants	Rubber chemicals (gloves), glutaraldehyde (cold sterilizer for instruments), preservatives (skin care products)
Photographers	Water, developers, fixers, bleaches	Color developers, black and white developers

to avoid both excessive water exposure and frequent hand washing. The constant wetting and drying can lead to chapping, which makes all hand dermatitis worse. Hands can be protected from the elements by using cotton glove liners to absorb perspiration inside a proper protective glove for the job. Moisturizers should be used immediately after wetting the hands or whenever they appear dry and scaling. Topical corticosteroids are the mainstay of therapy for occupational contact dermatitis, with systemic steroids reserved for acute, severe situations. Other treatments for severe chronic OSD have included cyclosporine, methotrexate, topical tacrolimus, and phototherapy. With treatment and hand protection, many workers can and do continue to work despite a hand dermatitis. Job change should only be considered in patients whose inadvertent and direct exposure to irritants or an allergen cannot be eliminated adequately. Most workers suffer financial and social consequences from changing occupations and do best with environmental modifications that allow them to remain on their job.

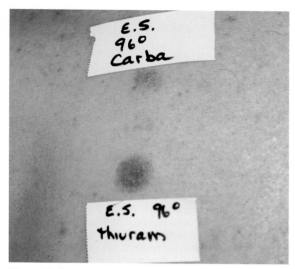

Figure 65-3. Positive patch test reactions to the rubber accelerators thiuram and carbamates found in rubber gloves in a health care worker.

CHAPTER 66

PSYCHOCUTANEOUS DISEASES

Margaret E. Muldrow, MD, and James E. Fitzpatrick, MD

1. How do the fields of psychiatry and dermatology overlap?

Many studies confirm that a high percentage of dermatology patients have coexistent psychiatric morbidity. Our understanding of this phenomenon remains limited. We do know that the skin and nervous system have the same embryologic origin, and that tactile stimulation is critical for full neuropsychological development, but many questions remain.

Recent biomedical advances have begun to take psychocutaneous disease out of the realm of speculation and myth. As we examine shared symptom complexes and responses to pharmacologic intervention, many psychocutaneous disorders can now be thought of in terms of neurotransmitters and their receptors, with all the inherent implications for treatment. This does not negate a role for various modalities of psychotherapy. Instead, our deeper understanding of psychocutaneous disease can only lead to improved patient care.

2. What types of psychocutaneous disease are encountered in dermatology?

Psychocutaneous disease can be classified into three major categories:
- Primary psychiatric disorders with dermatologic manifestations
- Primary dermatologic disorders that result in secondary psychiatric problems
- Primary dermatologic disorders exacerbated by stress

3. How often do patients with dermatologic disorders have associated psychologic morbidity?

This figure is difficult to assess; however, some studies have reported that more than 40% of all dermatologic patients have associated psychologic morbidity. Although many skin conditions are trivial, they are usually visible to the patient and often to the public. Healthy-appearing skin is a reflection of health and well-being, and abnormalities can seriously affect the patient's happiness.

Gupta MA: Psychosomatic dermatology: is it relevant? *Arch Dermatol* 126:90–93, 1990.

4. What is the differential diagnosis of patients who complain that they are infested with parasites?

- True parasitic infestation
- Intoxication or withdrawal from alcohol, amphetamines or cocaine
- Drugs such as corticosteroids and methylphenidate
- Organic brain syndromes
- Systemic disease such as diabetes, renal or hepatic failure, endocrinopathies, multiple sclerosis, and lymphoma
- Pellagra
- Vitamin B12 or folate deficiency
- Obsessions, phobias, delusions, and hallucinations

5. Define obsession or compulsion, phobia, delusion, and hallucination.

- **Obsession:** A persistent preoccupation with an idea or impulse
- **Compulsion:** A persistent, repetitive behavior performed in response to an obsession
- **Phobia:** An overwhelming fear that motivates individuals to avoid others or particular situations
- **Delusion:** A fixed, false idiosyncratic belief
- **Hallucination:** A perception without a stimulus

6. What is "delusions of parasitosis"?

These patients falsely believe that their skin is infested with parasites. They often describe insects mating, laying eggs, and crawling around in their skin. They do not admit to actually seeing the insects themselves, as they are not hallucinating. On presentation, patients may bring in specimens containing hair, lint, and even living organisms for examination (Fig. 66-1). They develop elaborate purification rituals and are often well known to pest control organizations. It is not uncommon for the delusion to be shared by other family members. This is called *folie à deux*.

Of note is the fact that the delusion is often referred to as a monosymptomatic hypochondriacal psychosis. It is "circumscribed," and patients tend to function well in other aspects of their lives; however, their delusional behavior is not corrected by either argument or evidence that they do not have an infestation.

Edlich RF, Cross CL, Wack CA, Long WB 3rd: Delusions of parasitosis, *Ann J Emerg Med* 27:997–999, 2009.

7. How do you diagnose this disorder?

Delusions of parasitosis is a diagnosis of exclusion. One must rule out all other possible reasons that a patient might complain that he or she is infested with parasites.

8. How do you treat this problem?

Delusions, like hallucinations, are psychotic symptoms that are theorized to result from increased levels of dopamine in parts of the brain. Patients with delusions of parasitosis have been shown to respond to neuroleptics; in particular, the dopamine antagonist pimozide (Orap) is, historically, the commonly used treatment. However, more recent anecdotal success has been reported with other agents having fewer side effects, including risperidone, olanzapine, and escitalopram. Although, large, well-controlled, randomized trials comparing the efficacy of these drugs are lacking, these drugs are now probably the drugs of choice.

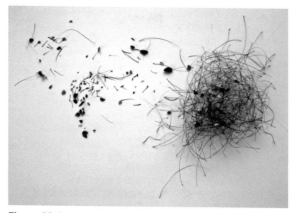

Figure 66-1. Scale, scabs, and hair brought in by a patient with delusions of parasitosis who insists that these are parasites.

Fellner MJ, Majeed MH: Tales of bugs, delusions of parasitosis, and what to do, *Clin Dermatol* 27:135–136, 2009.

9. What are the major side effects of pimozide?

- **Anticholinergic effects:** Dry eyes, dry mouth, constipation, urinary retention
- **Extrapyramidal symptoms:** Dystonia (muscle spasm), akathisia (motor restlessness), Parkinsonian-like syndrome (characterized by a pill-rolling tremor, rigidity, stiffened gait, and flattened facial expression)
- **Antiadrenergic effects:** Orthostatic hypotension
- **Tardive dyskinesia:** Less common

In addition to having these side effects, pimozide is a calcium channel blocker with the potential to alter cardiac conduction and prolong the QT interval. Although the medication is usually used only in small doses, patients should be followed closely for any adverse effects. A baseline electrocardiogram (ECG) should be obtained and repeated after initiation of therapy and periodically with dose increases.

Lorenzo CR, Koo J: Pimozide in dermatologic practice: a comprehensive review, *Am J Clin Dermatol* 5:339–349, 2004.

10. What if the patient is noncompliant with pimozide treatment?

It is often difficult to convince a patient with delusions of parasitosis to take medication. Diphenhydramine (Benadryl) is very helpful in relieving extrapyramidal symptoms and often helps prevent patients from discontinuing their medication.

11. What is Ekbom syndrome?

Ekbom syndrome is a relatively obscure name that is synonymous with delusions of parasitosis.

Hinkle NC: Ekbom syndrome: the challenge of the "invisible bug" infestations, *Annu Rev Entomol* 55:77–84, 2010.

12. What is dysmorphophobia?

In syndromes of dysmorphophobia, patients hold delusional beliefs about the structure or function of their skin. Symptoms range from complaints of excessive facial redness, scarring, or large pores, to olfactory delusions in which patients feel they are passing excessively smelly flatus or emitting body odor that drives people away. Diagnosis and treatment are similar to those for delusions of parasitosis. Prognosis is poor, especially in women with facial symptoms, who tend to be severely depressed and even suicidal. Patients with olfactory delusions can be driven to homicide.

13. Name the three major categories of self-inflicted skin lesions. What differentiates them?

- **Obsessive-compulsive disorders:** Patients acknowledge being driven to self-inflict skin lesions through conscious repetitive action.
- **Dermatitis artefacta, or factitious dermatitis:** Patients self-inflict skin lesions but adamantly deny doing so. The motive for their actions remains unclear. Although they are conscious of what they are doing, patients are unable to change their behavior easily.
- **Malingering:** Patients consciously and deceitfully self-inflict skin lesions for a goal that is recognizable when circumstances are known. The behavior may or may not eventually be acknowledged, but patients can stop producing the symptoms when they are no longer useful to them.

14. What are the clinical manifestations of dermatitis artefacta?

The self-inflicted lesions vary widely in morphology and distribution. Depending on the method used, it is possible to see blisters from suction cups, burns from caustic chemicals or cigarettes, edema and ulcerations from the use of elastic bands, or deep scars from the use of glass or knives. Lesions are often bizarre and irregularly rectilinear

(Figs. 66-2 and 66-3). They are necessarily within reach. Dermatitis artefacta is more common in women.

Koblenzer CS: Dermatitis artefacta: clinical features and approaches to treatment, *Am J Clin Dermatol* 1:47–55, 2000.

15. How should patients with dermatitis artefacta be treated?

In most patients, the creation of the skin lesions satisfies an internal psychological need. In some cases, the disease is transient and triggered by a recent event or stress; however, in many cases, the disease is chronic or recurrent, and it is best evaluated by a qualified psychiatrist or psychologist with expertise in this area. In patients who refuse psychiatric referral, some success has been reported with atypical antipsychotic agents and selective serotonin reuptake inhibitors at higher doses.

16. What is the Gardner-Diamond syndrome?

Also known as *autoerythrocyte sensitization syndrome* or *psychogenic purpura*, this disorder is characterized by the sudden unexplained appearance of purpura in young and middle-aged women. Skin lesions are associated with times of stress and are often preceded by burning pain. Permanent damage is rare. The exact etiology of the purpura remains controversial. Patients usually deny a history of trauma. Some individuals have been reported to have a positive skin test to their own red blood cell membranes, but laboratory evaluation is usually otherwise unremarkable. Interestingly, similar lesions have been produced by suggestion under hypnosis. Most authors believe that the disorder represents a factitious dermatitis.

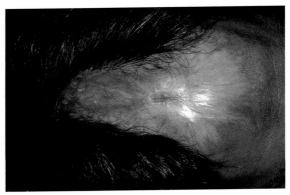

Figure 66-2. Patient-induced ulceration and scars of the scalp.

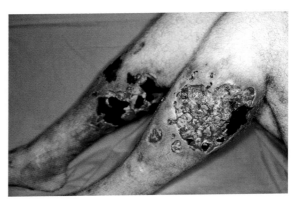

Figure 66-3. Young man with factitial panniculitis. The patient was injecting unknown substances into his legs in an attempt to get doctors to provide him with narcotic agents. (Courtesy of James E. Fitzpatrick, MD.)

Archer-Dubon C, Orozco-Topete R, Reyes-Gutierrez E: Two cases of psychogenic purpura, *Rev Invest Clin* 50:145–148, 1998.

17. How do Munchausen syndrome and Munchausen syndrome by proxy differ?

Munchausen syndrome is a chronic factitious disorder in which patients totally fabricate their symptoms, self-inflict lesions, or exaggerate or exacerbate a preexisting physical condition. The motive for the behavior remains unclear. Unfortunately, the disorder often leads to multiple hospital admissions and unnecessary procedures, surgery, and laboratory studies. When confronted with evidence that the symptoms are factitious, patients usually deny the allegations and leave against medical advice, only to repeat their actions in another hospital, city, state, or country.

In Munchausen syndrome by proxy, a third party facilitates an illness in another individual, usually a child, and receives some vague secondary gain from the behavior.

Falagas ME, Christopoulou M, Rosmarakis ES, Vlastou C: Munchausen's syndrome presenting as severe panniculitis, *Int J Clin Pract* 59:504–505, 2005.

18. What is the differential diagnosis of patchy nonscarring alopecia?

- Alopecia areata
- Tinea capitis
- Traction alopecia
- Trichotillomania

19. What is the psychiatric diagnosis associated with trichotillomania?

Trichotillomania is an obsessive-compulsive disorder in which patients are driven to pull out their own scalp hair or, less commonly, their eyebrows, eyelashes, and even pubic hair.

Duke DC, Keeley ML, Geffken GR, Storch EA: Trichotillomania: a current review, *Clin Psychol Rev* 30:181–193, 2010.

20. How do you differentiate among the different forms of nonscarring alopecia?

In alopecia areata, there usually are circular areas of noninflammatory, nonscarring alopecia with "exclamation point" hairs at the margins, and there may be associated nail pitting. Tinea capitis is characterized by patchy alopecia with varying degrees of erythema and scale that is KOH and/or fungal culture positive. In patient with traction alopecia, a distinct pattern that corresponds to a hair style is present (e.g., corn rows).

In trichotillomania, irregular patches of nonscarring, noninflammatory alopecia are covered with broken-off hairs of variable lengths that are scattered randomly between empty hair follicles (Fig. 66-4). Patients with trichotillomania often pull out their upper lid eyelashes but leave the lower lid eyelashes, as these are more difficult to grasp. Patients with alopecia areata may have eyelash loss on both the upper and lower lids.

21. Can a biopsy help in the differential diagnosis of patchy nonscarring alopecia?

Yes. A biopsy would reveal nonscarring alopecia with hemorrhage, and pigmented follicular casts in trichotillomania. Alopecia areata shows a perifollicular lymphocytic infiltrate and small anagen hairs. Tinea capitis shows fungal elements within hair follicles.

22. What is trichotemnomania?

Trichotemnomania is an obsessive-compulsive disorder characterized by the compulsion to cut or shave the hair. This is in contrast to trichotillomania, where the hair is pulled out.

Happle K: Trichotemnomania: obsessive-compulsive habit of cutting or shaving hair, *J Am Acad Dermatol* 52:157–159, 2005.

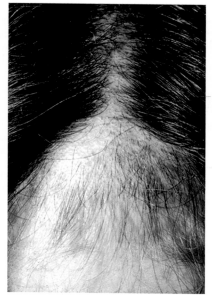

Figure 66-4. A young girl with trichotillomania. Note hairs of varying length. (Courtesy of John L. Aeling, MD.)

23. What are neurotic excoriations?

In this disorder, patients compulsively pick at their skin. Lesions may be preceded by focal pruritus or insect bites, or they may be generated de novo by rubbing. Once initiated, ritualized picking of all lesions occurs when they catch the patient's attention, or at a particular hour or location. On exam, lesions are found in all stages of development, ranging from ulcerations with hyperpigmented or hypopigmented margins to hypertrophic nodules and atrophic scars. They are usually found within easy reach of the dominant hand (Fig. 66-5).

24. How do you treat this disorder?

Obsessive-compulsive disorders have been theorized to be associated with a deficiency of the neurotransmitter serotonin in the brain. Not surprisingly, patients with neurotic excoriations and trichotillomania who have an underlying obsessive-compulsive disorder have been shown to respond to serotonin reuptake inhibitors such as fluoxetine (Prozac). Isolated case reports have also reported

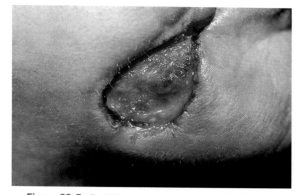

Figure 66-5. Factitial ulcer. (Courtesy of John L. Aeling, MD.)

success with various other medications including doxepin, pimozide, and olanzapine. Hypnosis and behavioral modification treatment has also been used with anecdotal success.

Arnold LM, Auchenbach MB, McElroy SL: Psychogenic excoriation. Clinical features, proposed diagnostic criteria, epidemiology, and approaches to treatment, *CNS Drugs* 15:351–359, 2001.

Key Points: Psychocutaneous Diseases

1. Forty percent of all dermatologic patients have associated psychologic morbidity.
2. Patients with delusions of parasitosis have monosymptomatic hypochondriacal psychosis; the remainder of their mental functions are typically normal.
3. Munchausen syndrome is a chronic factitious disorder in which patients totally fabricate their symptoms, self-inflict lesions, or exaggerate or exacerbate a preexisting physical condition.
4. Trichotillomania is most common in young girls and, in most cases, has an excellent prognosis.
5. Adults who develop trichotillomania are more likely to have a prolonged course.

---

25. What are the side effects of fluoxetine?

The major side effects include anxiety, insomnia, headache, tremor, dizziness, sweating, and gastrointestinal complaints, such as nausea and diarrhea. Although a relatively safe medication, this drug should not be administered to patients on monoamine oxidase inhibitors or to those individuals with a bipolar disorder.

26. What is glossodynia?

Glossodynia, or painful tongue, is one of the many atypical pain syndromes encountered in dermatology. Others include burning mouth syndrome (diffuse burning of the oral mucosa), vulvodynia, burning feet syndrome, and atypical facial pain. Patients with these disorders often have underlying depression and often respond to antidepressants, such as amitriptyline or doxepin. Isolated cases have also responded to antipsychotic agents, such as olanzapine or anticonvulsants such as gabapentin.

Gick CL, Mirowki GW, Kennedy JS, Bymaster FP: Treatment of glossodynia with olanzapine, *J Am Acad Dermatol* 51:463–465, 2004.

Klasser GD, Fischer DJ, Epstein JB: Burning mouth syndrome: recognition, understanding, and management, *Oral Maxillofac Surg Clin North Am* 20:255–271, 2008.

27. Name some primary dermatologic disorders that might result in secondary psychiatric problems. What sorts of problems might these patients have?

As an organ of self-expression, the skin plays a key role in emotional development and often defines interaction with others. Major disfiguring conditions, such as cystic acne, can result in a poor self-image and feelings of isolation and anger. Studies reveal that these individuals also suffer from higher rates of substance abuse, unemployment, and mental illness than the general population.

28. Can stress exacerbate a primary dermatologic disorder?

Yes. Psoriasis and atopic dermatitis are two dermatologic disorders that are classically exacerbated by stress. Also, all psychiatric conditions associated with dermatologic disorders will be exacerbated by stress.

Farber EM, Nickoloff BJ, Recht B, Fraki JE: Stress, symmetry, and psoriasis: possible role of neuropeptides, *J Am Acad Dermatol* 14:305–311, 1986.

APPROACHING THE PRURITIC PATIENT

Theresa R. Pacheco, MD

CHAPTER 67

1. What is the most common symptom of dermatologic disease?
Pruritus, or "itching."

2. What is an "itch"?
It is an unpleasant sensation of the skin leading to the desire to scratch.

3. Is an itch a separate modality of pain or a submodality of pain?
Cutaneous nerve fibers arranged in an arborizing plexus immediately below the epidermis receive itch impulses. Unmyelinated C fibers conduct itch impulses from the skin to the ipsilateral dorsal root ganglia, ascend in the opposite anterolateral spinothalamic tract (closely associated with pain fibers), continue to the thalamus, and proceed through the internal capsule to the sensory cortex.

Although controversial, the general consensus views an itch as a separate modality of pain. Though distinguishing between the sensations of pain and pruritus is easy, distinguishing between the neurophysiology of pruritus and pain is not. Pruritus and pain share many neurophysiologic features and pathways. The following factors support that pain and itch are separate and distinct sensations: Itch leads to the reflex or urge to scratch; pain leads to withdrawal. Itch occurs only in the skin; pain arises from deeper structures as well. Heat may stop itch; heat usually increases pain. Removal of the epidermis eliminates itch; removal of the epidermis causes pain.

4. What causes an itch?
Itch is mediated by a number of local and central substances. Histamine, produced by skin mast cells, is the classical pruritus mediator. Pricking the skin with histamine produces pruritus in most individuals; however, histamine does not account for all pruritus. Other pruritus mediators include prostaglandin, serotonin, tachykinins, cytokines, and opioid receptors. Prostaglandin E_1 lowers the threshold of the skin to itching provoked by histamine. Serotonin, 5-hydroxytryptamine (5-HT), may regulate itch by acting on $5-HT_3$ receptors. Tachykinins, such as the neuropeptide substance P, cause pruritus for reasons attributable to histamine release from mast cells. Cytokine interleukin-2 may be an important peripheral mediator of itching. Opioid receptors in the central nervous system regulate the intensity and quality of perceived itch.

Understanding pruritus mediators can help classify itch accordingly to origin. The classification of itch includes: a) pruritoceptive—cutaneous nerves are activated by pruritogens at sensory endings, b) neuropathic—diseased or lesion pruritic neurons generate itch, c) neurogenic—itch caused by mediators acting centrally, and d) psychogenic. Although classifications are important, there are limitations as itch can have more than one origin.

Bernard JD, editor: Itch: mechanisms and management of pruritus, New York, 1994, McGraw-Hill.
Buddenkotte J, Steinhoff M: Pathophysiology and therapy of pruritus in allergic and atopic diseases. *Allergy* 65:805-821, 2010.
Fazio SB: Pruritus, UpToDate 2000, 2005. Available at: http://www.uptodate.com.
Greaves MW, Wall PD: Pathophysiology of itching, *Lancet* 348:938–940, 1996.

5. Describe the difference between localized and generalized pruritus.
Pruritus occurs with a host of dermatologic conditions, or it can mark systemic disease. Some dermatologic conditions that cause pruritus are inconspicuous or nonspecific. Other dermatologic conditions are apparent on physical exam. A physician must differentiate between localized and generalized pruritus and know a variety of skin diseases that cause pruritus.

Localized pruritus is defined as itching focused to certain regions. Localized pruritus usually results from a regional infection or dermatosis. **Generalized pruritus** typically appears as itching that affects the entire body surface. It implies a dermatologic or systemic disorder. Generalized pruritus can be distinguished as acute or chronic. Chronic pruritus is defined as lasting 6 or more weeks.

6. What is the best approach to evaluation of a patient with localized pruritus?
The most important diagnostic tools are the history and physical exam. After obtaining a thorough history, the best clinical approach is to organize the patient regionally. The physician should ask the patient if there are any lesions associated with pruritus. The patient's physical exam should focus on identifying a primary skin lesion or disorder in the affected region. After identifying a primary lesion, the physician can categorize the skin disease based on the lesion's morphology.

7. What are the common causes of localized pruritus?
The differential diagnosis of localized pruritus should include dermatoses that are limited to certain parts of the body and those that are diffuse but have a predilection for these sites (Table 67-1).

Table 67-1. Differential Diagnosis of Localized Pruritus

LOCATION	DISEASES
Scalp	Psoriasis, seborrheic dermatitis
Trunk	Contact dermatitis (axillae, waistline), erythrasma (axillae), psoriasis (periumbilical), notalgia paresthetica, scabies, seborrheic dermatitis, urticaria
Inguinal region	*Candida*, contact dermatitis, erythrasma, overuse of topical steroids, pediculosis, scabies, tinea cruris
Anal region	*Candida*, contact dermatitis, gonorrhea, hemorrhoids, pinworm, psoriasis, tinea cruris
Hands	Contact dermatitis, scabies, eczema
Legs	Atopic dermatitis (popliteal fossae), dermatitis herpetiformis (knees), lichen simplex chronicus (malleoli), neurotic excoriations, nummular eczema, stasis dermatitis
Feet	Contact dermatitis, pitted keratolysis, tinea pedis

8. What is notalgia paresthetica?

Notalgia paresthetica is an acquired unilateral localized form of pruritus that develops near the inferomedial border of either scapula. The skin typically appears normal, although some patients demonstrate subtle hyperpigmentation secondary to repeated rubbing or excoriation. The cause is not understood, although there is substantial evidence to suggest that it is due to spinal nerve impingement. Occasional cases have been familial, and the term "hereditary localized pruritus" has been applied to this variant. The management typically consists of topical capsaicin cream or topical preparations containing lidocaine.

Savk O, Savk E: Investigation of spinal pathology in notalgia paresthetica, *J Am Acad Dermatol* 52:1085–1087, 2005.

9. What is the physician's best approach when seeing a patient with generalized pruritus?

The physician's most important diagnostic tools are a thorough and systematic history and physical exam. Laboratory testing for systemic disease may be necessary. Common questions include the following:

- What are the extent, severity, and quality of the itch?
- When does the pruritus occur, and what is its duration?
- Are there provocative factors, such as change in temperature or climate?
- Does the patient have a history of previous skin disorders or allergies?
- What are the patient's current medications?
- Has the patient taken any new oral medications or ingested any new foods?
- How often does the patient bathe?
- What products does the patient use on his/her skin?
- Has the patient used any new skin products?
- Is there a history of systemic illness?
- Is health maintenance up to date?
- Is there a history of psychiatric illness?
- What is the home environment?
- Are there pets at home?
- Does any other family member experience itching?
- Has there been any recent travel?
- Is there any emotional stress?

In examining the skin, the physician should focus on whether it is normal or abnormal. Care should be made to differentiate between primary and secondary skin lesions. The primary skin lesion can identify the causal disease, whereas secondary skin lesions are usually reactive from the pruritus itself. Pruritus can occur in the setting of normal skin.

10. After obtaining a complete history and physical examination, what clinically oriented classification scheme should be followed?

New diagnostic tools are evolving to better evaluate patients with pruritus. The International Forum for the Study of Itch has published a clinical classification utilizing the physician exam to provide physicians with a framework for improving the care of the pruritic patient.

Patient can be classified as group I, patient with pruritus on diseased inflamed skin; group II, patients with pruritus on normal noninflamed skin; and group III, patients with pruritus on chronic secondary reactive lesions such as scratching/rubbing (Table 67-2).

Diagnostic tests for group I include a skin biopsy and laboratory investigation, such as IgE or indirect immunofluorescence. Diagnostic tests for group II include a laboratory and radiologic investigation based on the patient's history. Diagnostic tests for group III include a skin biopsy and laboratory and radiologic investigation based on patient's history.

Table 67-2. Classification of Generalized Pruritus

CATEGORY	DISEASES
I. Dermatologic (arising from diseases of the skin)	Xerosis (dry skin), atopic dermatitis, contact dermatitis, urticaria, bullous pemphigoid, dermatitis herpetiformis, lichen planus, mastocytosis, polymorphic eruption of pregnancy, prurigo gestationis, cutaneous T-cell lymphoma, other leukemic infiltrates
II. Systemic (arising from diseases of organs other than the skin, such as liver, kidney, blood, and drugs)	Uremia, cholestasis, primary biliary cirrhosis, chronic renal failure, HIV infection, dermatophysis, drugs, polycythemia rubra vera, Hodgkin's lymphoma, iron-deficiency anemia, carcinoid syndrome, drug-induced pruritus, solid tumor (such as colon, prostate), perimenopausal pruritus
III. Neurologic (arising from disease of the central nervous system or peripheral nervous system	Multiple sclerosis, neoplasms, cerebral or spinal infarcts, brachioradial pruritus, notalgia paresthetica, postherpetic neuralgia, vulvodynia
IV. Psychogenic/psychosomatic (somatoform pruritus)	Depression, anxiety disorders, obsessive-compulsive disorders, schizophrenia
V. Mixed (overlapping and coexistence of several diseases)	
VI. Other	

Initial tests include
- Skin biopsy
- Complete blood count and differential
- Liver function tests, including alkaline phosphatase for obstructive liver disease
- Renal function testing, including blood urea nitrogen, creatinine, and urinalysis
- Optional tests including thyroid function tests and chest x-ray

Other tests based on patient's history and preexisitng diseases include a fasting glucose, stool exams for occult blood, Papanicolaou smear, serum iron, serum protein electrophoresis, urine for 5-hydroxyindoleacetic acid (5-HIAA), urine for mast cell metabolites, skin biopsy with direct immunofluorescence (to exclude dermatitis herpetiformis and bullous pemphigoid), and biopsy with special stains (to exclude mastocytosis).

Stander S, Weisshaar E, Mettang T, et al: Clinical classification of itch: a position paper of the International Forum for the Study of Itch, *Acta Derm Venereol* 87:291–294, 2007.

11. What are common causes of generalized pruritus?

The numerous causes of generalized pruritus are numerous but can be classified as category I, dermatologic origin of pruritus; category II, systemic origin of chronic pruritus; and category III/IV, neurologic and psychiatric/psychosomatic origin of pruritus.

Stander S, Weisshaar E, Mettang T, et al: Clinical classification of itch: a position paper of the International Forum for the Study of Itch, *Acta Derm Venereol* 87:291–294, 2007.

12. How prevalent is an underlying systemic disease in a patient who seeks medical attention for pruritus?

Medical literature reports suggest that the prevalence of an underlying systemic disease in a patient who seeks medical attention for pruritus has been reported to be between 10% and 50%. Therefore, most causes of pruritus are secondary to a dermatologic disease. The following dermatoses are among the most severely pruritic: xerosis, atopic dermatitis, contact dermatitis, urticaria, pediculosis, scabies, bullous pemphigoid, and dermatitis herpetiformis.

13. What is "winter itch"? In which patient population is it common?

Winter itch is the term applied to xerosis (dry skin), which is aggravated by the low ambient humidity that occurs in many homes during the winter months. Xerosis occurs with great frequency in elderly patients and is the most common cause of pruritus for this age group. Xerosis is also aggravated by repeated water exposure due to excessive bathing, swimming, or hot tub use, and strong soaps. The physical exam often shows dry, cracked, scaly skin on the lower legs. Treatment includes limiting frequency, duration, and water temperature of bathing; use of superfatted soaps; and use of emollients immediately after bath or shower. Use of oral antihistamines may help treat "winter itch."

14. The patient complains that "wool makes me itch" or "I am allergic to wool." What disease does this patient probably have?

Pruritus is such an integral part of atopic dermatitis that no diagnosis of active atopic dermatitis can be made without a history of itching. External factors, such as irritating clothing (e.g., wool), dry air, and emotional stress, exacerbate atopic dermatitis. Patients tend to have a personal or family history of asthma, rhinitis, and various allergies. Primary skin lesions are not typically seen, but lichenification (an exaggeration of the skin folds) is common because of constant rubbing by the patient. Therapy involves avoiding wool or other irritating clothing. Antihistamines are used to treat pruritus in atopic dermatitis, although some physicians attribute their beneficial effects to their sedative properties.

15. What treatment should the physician consider if a patient presents with pruritus and "hives"?

Urticaria occurs as a consequence of histamine release. A history of wheals is usually associated with pruritus. A physical exam may reveal dermatographism, even if wheals are not present. Therapy includes antihistamines that have a peripheral antipruritic action when itch is due to histamine release.

16. What disease should the physician consider if the patient volunteers that his spouse also suffers from itching?

This history suggests an arthropod reaction, such as scabies or pediculosis pubis. Scabies commonly infects the entire family, especially if young children are present. The characteristic primary lesion is a burrow. Burrows may be difficult to visualize but are most commonly located on the flexor wrists, fingerwebs, and glans penis. Vesicles, papules, pustules, and excoriations are other skin lesions that may be present. Women often complain of pruritus about the nipples. Nocturnal itching is also characteristic of scabies.

If both members of the family have genital itching, the patient should be examined for pubic lice (*Phthirus pubis*) and nits attached to pubic hairs. Pediculosis pubis is one of the most infectious sexually transmitted diseases. Individuals have a 95% chance of becoming infected after a single exposure to an infected partner.

17. Is pruritus in HIV-infected patients common? What are the common causes of pruritus in these patients?

Pruritus is common in HIV-infected patients and is experienced with increasing frequency as the disease progresses. Occult HIV infection can present with generalized pruritus. Causes of pruritus secondary to skin disease in HIV-infected patients include 1) xerosis; 2) infectious etiologies, such as scabies; and 3) noninfectious etiologies, such as photoeruptions, eosinophilic pustular folliculitis, or pruritic papular eruption. Pruritus unassociated with skin disease is probably secondary to immune dysregulation of HIV disease. The physical exam will help identify specific causes of skin disease, but a significant number of HIV-infected patients have no demonstrable skin lesions.

Singh F, Rudikoff D: HIV-associated pruritus: etiology and management, *Am J Clin Dermatol* 4:177–188, 2003.

18. Which psychiatric disorder often presents with intractable pruritus?

Delusions of parasitosis is the fixed belief that a patient is infested with living organisms in the absence of evidence of such infestation. Delusions of parasitosis often occurs as a sole psychological disturbance, but it may be associated with an underlying personality disorder, such as the obsessive-compulsive type. A physician must take care not to miss a true infestation. A careful history, thorough examination of the skin, microscopic review of "bugs" brought in by the patient, and, occasionally, a biopsy of the "bite" sites is needed. Establishing a dermatology-psychiatry liaison is helpful in establishing a diagnosis and selecting therapy. The neuroleptic pimozide, a blocker of dopamine receptors, is considered an effective treatment but requires careful monitoring because of several potentially serious side effects.

Driscoll MS, Rothe MJ, Grant-Kels JM, Hale MS: Delusional parasitosis: a dermatologic, psychiatric, and pharmacologic approach, *J Am Acad Dermatol* 29:1023–1033, 1993.

19. Which patients with renal failure experience "renal itch"?

Pruritus reportedly affects 50% to 90% of patients undergoing peritoneal dialysis or hemodialysis. Pruritus usually starts 6 months after the start of dialysis and can be episodic, mild, and localized; or generalized, intractable, and severe. The etiology of uremic pruritus is poorly understood. Possibilities include secondary hyperparathyroidism, histamine release by mast cells, hypervitaminosis A, iron deficiency anemia, or some combination of these. The cornerstone of treatment is regular, intensive, efficient dialysis. Dietary restrictions, phosphate-binding therapy, and phototherapy (UVB) are alternative therapies.

Robertson KB, Meuller BA: Uremic pruritus, *Am J Health Syst Pharm* 53:2159–2170, 1996.

20. Which patients with liver disease are most likely to experience pruritus? What is the best screening laboratory test?

Cholestasis, or biliary obstruction, is the common denominator in pruritus due to liver disease. Although alanine aminotransferase, cholesterol, and bilirubin are usually elevated, the single best screening test for this is a serum alkaline phosphatase measurement.

21. What are the common causes of cholestic pruritus?

The three most common causes of cholestic pruritus are primary biliary cirrhosis, cholestasis of pregnancy, and cholestasis from drugs. Pruritus affects virtually 100% of all patients with primary biliary cirrhosis (PBC) and is the initial symptom in 50%. PBC is a disease of unknown etiology characterized by the destruction of small intrahepatic bile ducts by a granulomatous reaction. Approximately 90% of the patients are female. The serum antimitochondrial antibody test against M2, a component of the pyruvate dehydrogenase complex of mitochondrial enzymes, is 88% sensitive and 96% specific for PBC. Treatment is hepatic transplantation, and it completely eliminates the pruritus.

Benign cholestatic jaundice of pregnancy is a frequent cause of pruritus in pregnancy. The pruritus is most severe in the third trimester. The pruritus disappears and elevated liver function tests return to normal after delivery. Pruritus secondary to cholestasis frequently occurs with drug therapy. Common culprits include oral contraceptives, anabolic steroids, cephalosporins, chlorpropamide, cimetidine, erythromycin estolate, gold, nonsteroidal antiinflammatory drugs, nicotinic acid, penicillin, phenothiazine, phenytoin, progestin, and tolbutamide. Removal of the offending drug usually leads to resolution of symptoms. Other causes of cholestatic pruritus include primary sclerosing cholangitis, obstructive choledocholithiasis, carcinoma blocking the biliary tree, or chronic hepatitis C.

Mela M, Mancuso A, Burroughs AK: Review article: pruritus in cholestatic and other liver diseases, *Aliment Pharmacol Ther* 17:857–870, 2003.

Key Points: Pruritus

1. The initial approach in treating the pruritic patient should focus on identifying and treating a primary skin disorder.
2. Patients who do not have an obvious explanation for pruritus should undergo a physical examination and a laboratory evaluation to look for evidence of systemic disease.
3. All patients should be advised about appropriate skin care, which includes adequate nutrition and daily fluid intake, protection from the environment, and cleansing practices that do not dry the skin. In addition to the skin care factors, medications applied to the skin or taken by mouth may be necessary to treat pruritus.
4. All patients should be advised regarding the avoidance of scratching to focus on interrupting the itch-scratch-itch cycle.

22. Which hematologic disorders are known to present with pruritus?

Polycythemia rubra vera and Hodgkin's lymphoma are the two most common hematologic disorders known to cause pruritus. Between 14% and 52% of patients with polycythemia rubra vera suffer from pruritus. Pruritus is classically triggered by a sudden decrease in temperature (i.e., sudden cooling off after emerging from a warm bath). Treatment of the underlying disease is necessary to treat this symptom. A patient suffering from Hodgkin's lymphoma may present with a pruritus that precedes the diagnosis by as many as 5 years. The pruritus can be intolerably severe and continuous, or, less commonly, the patient may complain of a burning sensation. A review of 10 studies on Hodgkin's disease noted that 35% of patients suffered from pruritus sometime during the disease course, 15% presented with pruritus along with other symptoms, and 7% presented only with the symptom of pruritus. The significance of pruritus as a prognostic sign in Hodgkin's disease is unknown. Treatment of the lymphoma is the best therapy for pruritus of Hodgkin's disease.

Stadie V, Marsch WC: Itching attacks with generalized hyperhidrosis as initial symptoms in Hodgkin's disease, *J Eur Acad Dermatol Venereol* 17:559–561, 2003.

23. Is generalized pruritus a common symptom of endocrine disorders?

Generalized pruritus occurs in 4% to 11% of patients with thyrotoxicosis and occurs more commonly in patients with long-standing disease. No recent publications on the incidence of pruritus in patients with diabetes mellitus exist. Notwithstanding, patients are more likely to experience pruritus vulvae and pruritus ani secondary to candidiasis, dermatophyte infection, and bacterial infection.

24. Can itching cause skin disease?

Tissue damage caused by scratching may lead to chronic skin conditions such as lichen simplex chronicus or prurigo nodularis. Lichen simplex chronicus results from repeated scratching, which leads to a patch of chronic dermatitis that subsequently becomes lichenified, later becomes intensely pruritic, and leads to a perpetuation of the itch-scratch-itch cycle. Lichen simplex chronicus seems to be precipitated by stress, depression, and frustration. Prurigo nodularis, rather than lichenification, may result from persistent localized itching and scratching. Postinflammatory hypopigmentation and hyperpigmentation is often seen with chronic skin conditions and is a result of repeated scratching and associated inflammation.

25. What is the best symptomatic treatment for a patient with pruritus?

The best treatment for a patient with pruritus involves identifying an underlying dermatosis or systemic disorder responsible for the pruritus and treating that disease. All patients should be advised about appropriate skin care, which includes adequate nutrition and daily fluid intake, protection from the environment, and cleansing practices that do not dry the skin. In addition to the skin care factors, medications applied to the skin or taken by mouth may be necessary to treat pruritus. Topical agents containing menthol produce a cooling sensation. Topical agents containing phenol or camphor have local anesthetic effects. Pramoxine, another topical anesthetic, can provide relief. If appropriate, topical corticosteroids can be used for local control. Oral antihistamines, such as hydroxyzine or doxepin, are commonly used and often provide the first-line treatment for pruritus with no identifiable cause. Other less traditional therapies and techniques are reserved for refractory cases and are best reserved for the practicing clinical dermatologist to address (Table 67-3).

All patients should be advised regarding the avoidance of scratching to focus on interrupting the itch-scratch-itch cycle. Breaking the itch-scratch-itch cycle (an increase in itching that can result from the process of scratching) may also help to alleviate pruritus. The cycle may be broken by applying a cool washcloth or ice over the affected area.

Greece PJ, Ende J: Pruritus: a practical approach, *J Gen Intern Med* 7:340–349, 1992.

Table 67-3. Treatment of Pruritus

Topical	Cooling agents, emollients, topical corticosteroids, anesthetics
Systemic	Antihistamines, systemic corticosteroids, opioid receptor antagonists
Phototherapy	Ultraviolet B (UVB), narrowband UVB (NBUVB)
Miscellaneous	Transcutaneous electrical nerve stimulation (TENS), acupuncture, capsaicin

NAIL DISORDERS

Brian J. Gerondale, MD, and Daniel C. Dapprich, MD

CHAPTER 68

1. What functions do nails serve?

- Nails protect the terminal phalanx and fingertip from traumatic impact.
- They allow us to perform tasks that require manual dexterity.
- They are unparalleled in their ability to relieve itching.
- For many individuals they represent an extension of their esthetic beauty.

2. Why are nails important in medicine?

Nails are important because they are easily observable and serve as a window into the body. They are commonly affected by numerous internal (heart, liver, kidney) and external factors, including infectious agents, trauma, and drugs. Finally, nails may help in the differential diagnosis of closely related dermatologic disorders.

White GM, Cox NH: Disorders of nails. In White GM, Cox NH, editors: *Diseases of the skin*. Philadelphia, 2002, WB Saunders, pp 397–410.

3. Do any systemic diseases have specific nail findings?

Many systemic diseases have characteristic, but not mutually exclusive, nail findings. Most nail changes are part of a symptom complex or a reaction pattern that may be extremely helpful in making a particular diagnosis (Table 68-1).

Scher RK, Daniel CR: *Nails: therapy, diagnosis, surgery*, ed 3: Philadelphia, 2005, WB Saunders.

4. What are Beau's lines? How are they formed?

Beau's lines represent the most common but least specific nail changes seen with systemic diseases. They are a forward-pointing, wedge-shaped depression in the nail plate of variable depth and obliquity. They occur when there is temporary cessation of nail growth or decreased deposition of nail plate by the nail matrix. Frequently, Beau's lines are caused by mechanical trauma or diseases of the proximal nail fold. If all of the nails are affected at the same level, a systemic cause is indicated, while localized events (trauma) produce isolated lines.

Tosti A, Piraccini BM: Nail disorders. In Bolognia JL, Jorizzo JL, Rapini RP, editors: *Dermatology*, St Louis, 2003, Mosby, pp 1061–1078.

5. What is a splinter hemorrhage?

A splinter hemorrhage results from the extravasation of blood from the longitudinally oriented vessels of the nail bed. The blood usually attaches to the overlying nail plate and moves distally with it. The occurrence of a hemorrhage close to the lunula and, simultaneously, in multiple nails correlates more directly with systemic disease.

Saladi RN, Persaud AN, Rudikoff D, et al: Idiopathic splinter hemorrhages, *J Am Acad Dermatol* 50:289–292, 2004.

6. Are splinter hemorrhages always associated with subacute bacterial endocarditis?

A commonly held, almost "sacred teaching" in medical school but rarely true. There is a myriad of causes, with subacute bacterial endocarditis representing only a small fraction. By far, simple trauma is the most common cause. Other known entities include drug reactions, general illness, vasculitis, and trichinosis, to name a few.

Table 68-1. Nail Disorders in Systemic Disease

NAIL ABNORMALITY	AREA INVOLVED	ASSOCIATED DISEASE
Splinter hemorrhages	Bed	Bacterial endocarditis
Mees' lines	Plate	Arsenic exposure
Muehrcke's lines	Bed	Nephrotic syndrome
Terry's nails	Bed	Cirrhosis
Half-and-half nails	Bed	Chronic renal failure
Blue lunulae	Matrix	Wilson's disease
Red lunulae	Matrix	Rheumatoid arthritis
Clubbing	Plate/matrix	Pulmonary disorders
Spoon nails	Plate/matrix	Iron deficiency
Nail fold telangiectasias	Nailfold	Scleroderma, systemic lupus
Yellow nails	Plate	Pulmonary disorders, sinusitis

7. What is the difference between Mees' lines and Muehrcke's lines?

Mees' lines represent single or multiple transverse white lines that occur in the nail plate and move distally as the nail grows out. They are classically thought to be caused by arsenic intoxication, but many severe systemic insults may initiate them. **Muehrcke's lines** were described in 1956 by Robert C. Muehrcke in an article entitled "The Finger-nails in Chronic Hypoalbuminaemia." These represent transverse, double, white lines that are an abnormality of the vascular bed, probably a localized edematous state secondary to the hypoalbuminemia. The underlying causes of these lines include the nephrotic syndrome, liver disease, and malnutrition.

Muehrcke RC: The finger-nails in chronic hypoalbuminaemia, *Br Med J* 9:1327–1328, 1956.

8. What are "half-and-half" nails, and with what internal disease are they associated?

Half-and-half nails are characterized by apparent leukonychia (white color that disappears with pressure) that affects the proximal half of the nail (Fig. 68-1). Although it may be seen in normal individuals, it is associated with patients with chronic renal disease in approximately 10% of patients.

9. What is nail fold capillaroscopy? How is it useful?

It is the in vivo examination of nail fold and cuticle finger capillaries, with magnification, to detect variations in capillary patterns. Autoimmune connective tissue disorders can have subtle but distinct changes within these capillaries and the proximal nail fold. It can be useful in predicting which patients with Raynaud's syndrome will likely develop scleroderma. In those with scleroderma, the severity of capillary lesions may correlate with the degree of multisystem organ disease. Patients with dermatomyositis have capillary changes along with thickened, ragged cuticles. In systemic lupus, paronychial inflammation may be prominent with dilated tortuous capillaries distinctive.

Tosti A: The nail apparatus in collagen disorders, *Semin Dermatol* 10:71–76, 1991.

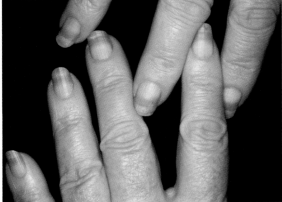

Figure 68-1. Half-and-half nails in a patient with chronic renal disease. (Courtesy of the Fitzsimons Army Medical Center teaching files.)

10. What is clubbing?

Clubbing refers to the increased bilateral curvature of the nails with proliferation of the soft tissues restricted to the distal phalanges (Fig. 68-2). It causes an increase in the emergence angle of the nail to equal or greater than 180 degrees. There are diverse causes of clubbing, including congenital or genetic factors, but 80% of clubbing is associated with respiratory ailments.

11. How is hypertrophic osteoarthropathy related to clubbing?

Clubbing may occur in association with hypertrophic osteoarthropathy, an uncommon but important entity. It consists of simple clubbing (including the toes), hypertrophy of the upper and lower extremities, peripheral neurovascular disease, acute burning bone pain, joint problems, and muscle weakness. More importantly, when complete, it is associated 90% of the time with malignant tumors of the chest.

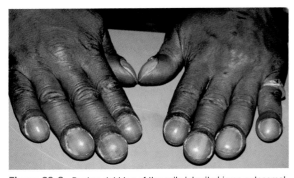

Figure 68-2. Benign clubbing of the nails inherited in an autosomal dominant fashion.

12. What is the yellow nail syndrome?

The yellow nail syndrome consists of the classic triad of lymphedema of the lower extremity, nail changes, and pleural effusion. The nails are thickened, yellowish, and curved side to side with absent lunulae and cuticles (Fig. 68-3). It is associated with a multitude of pulmonary diseases including tuberculosis, asthma, and respiratory tract cancers.

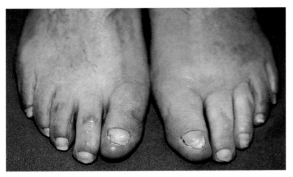

Figure 68-3. Yellow nail syndrome, demonstrating typical thick, yellow, and curved nails. (Courtesy of James E. Fitzpatrick, MD.)

Table 68-2. Dermatologic Disorders with Nail Changes

DISEASE	INCIDENCE	FINDINGS
Psoriasis	10%–50%	Pits, "oil spots"
Alopecia areata	20%–50%	Pits
Lichen planus	10%	Pterygium
Scleroderma	Frequent	Pterygium inversus unguium
Darier's disease	High	Wedge shaped, hyperkeratosis
Pityriasis rubra pilaris	Majority	Yellow-brown, hyperkeratotic

13. **Are there any characteristic nail changes in primarily dermatologic diseases?**

Unfortunately, because the nail unit has only limited ways of responding to pathologic insults, pathognomonic changes are seldom encountered. However, examination of the nails is imperative because there are certain changes that, viewed in context with the entire clinical picture, can help establish a diagnosis (Table 68-2).

Rich P: Nail disorders: diagnosis and treatment of infectious, inflammatory, and neoplastic nail conditions, *Med Clin North Am* 82:1171–1182, 1998.

14. **What are nail pits?**

Nail pits are shallow depressions in the nail plate that are the result of abnormally retained nuclei of the keratin-forming cells, which shed with growth (parakeratosis).

15. **Are there any differences between the nail pits of psoriasis and alopecia areata?**

Nail pits are the most common finding in psoriasis and are generally deep, large, and randomly placed. The nail pits in alopecia areata tend to be small and uniform and classically arranged in a "cross-hatched" or geometric pattern.

16. **What other nail findings are seen in psoriasis? What is the significance of nail changes?**

Psoriasis can affect all parts of the nail unit and, hence, causes a wide variety of changes in the nail that are characteristic and helpful diagnostic aids. Nail abnormalities may be the only manifestation of psoriasis. They are frequently associated with psoriatic arthropathy. In descending order of frequency, the nail findings in psoriasis are:

- Nail pits
- Oil spots (brownish-yellowish discolorations) (Fig. 68-4)
- Onycholysis (separation of the distal nail plate from the nail bed)
- Subungual hyperkeratosis
- Splinter hemorrhages

Baran R, Dawber R, Haneke E, Tosti A: *A text atlas of nail disorders*, St Louis, 1996, Mosby.

17. **How does a pterygium differ from pterygium inversus unguium?**

A **pterygium**, which is Greek for "wing," is classically associated with lichen planus. Lichen planus attacks the nail-forming unit, the matrix, and causes permanent scarring. Because the nail plate at that site is no longer made, the proximal nail fold attaches to the nail bed directly, and both grow out distally. This produces the "winglike" appearance.

Pterygium inversus unguium occurs when the nail plate distally does not separate from the underlying digital bed skin. The fingertip ulcerations and scarring also seen in scleroderma contribute to the inability of the nail to separate (Fig. 68-5).

18. **What is the most common cause and sequela of a subungual hematoma? How is it treated?**

By far, the most common cause is trauma to the nail bed. Most subungual hematomas are accompanied by a throbbing pain secondary to the accumulation of blood below the nail plate, which exerts pressure on the underlying bed (Fig. 68-6). An effective and simple treatment is to simply pass the tip of a heated paper clip through the nail into the hematoma. Pressure relief and lessening of pain rapidly ensue, making you an instant hero!

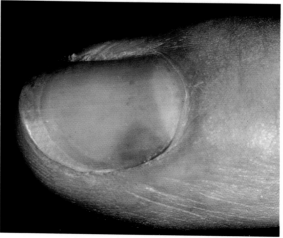

Figure 68-4. Typical "oil spot" on the nails of a patient with psoriasis. (Courtesy of James E. Fitzpatrick, MD.)

19. Do malignant melanomas occur in the nails?

Yes, although subungual melanomas account for only 1% to 4% of all melanomas in light-skinned individuals. However, they account for 25% of melanomas occurring in black individuals, and they tend to have a worse prognosis than melanomas elsewhere on the integument.

20. How do you tell the difference between a subungual hematoma and a malignant melanoma?

This is a very important distinction to make because a melanoma can have a high mortality rate if diagnosed late. One should have a high suspicion for a melanoma, if pigment develops in a single nail of a person aged 50 to 80 years old. Also, any band in the nail that is wider at the base or darkening is worrisome. Hutchinson's sign, the leaching of pigment into the surrounding nail fold, is considered pathognomonic. Hematoma pigment remains confined to the nail bed and gradually grows out with the nail. Melanonychia (longitudinal pigmented lines on nails) is also very common in individuals with darker skin and is a more likely diagnosis if multiple nails are affected, the lines are well demarcated laterally, they are not changing, and Hutchinson's sign is negative.

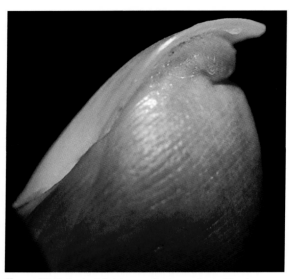

Figure 68-5. Lack of distal separation in a patient with scleroderma and pterygium inversus unguium. (Courtesy of James E. Fitzpatrick, MD.)

21. What nail changes are considered peculiar to human immunodeficiency virus (HIV) infection?

Patients with acquired immune deficiency syndrome may develop acromelanosis, in which hyperpigmented macules occur on the fingers, palms, soles, and nails. In the nails, they appear as longitudinal pigmentary bands (melanonychia). Hence, melanonychia of several nails with skin hyperpigmentation is a strong clue to HIV infection. Commonly, nail pigmentation is seen with the drug zidovudine. Proximal subungual onychomycosis and candidal onychomycosis are also considered a marker for HIV infection. Long-standing, treatment-resistant, periungual warts are common, and progression to squamous cell carcinoma is a distinct possibility.

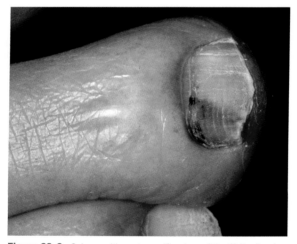

Figure 68-6. Subungual hematoma. (Courtesy of the Walter Reed Army Medical Center teaching files.)

22. What is onychocryptosis? Why does it occur?

Onychocryptosis represents an ingrown toenail. It occurs when the free edge of the nail plate penetrates through the soft tissue of the nail fold. Factors that are known to precipitate or secondarily cause this condition are excessive rotation of the toe, onycholysis along the nail margin, ill-fitting shoes, hyperhidrosis, and poor cutting (rounding the edges) of the nails. Infection is a secondary complication.

Cohen PR, Scher RK: Geriatric nail disorders: diagnosis and treatment, *J Am Acad Dermatol* 26:521–531, 1992.

23. What is a paronychia?

A paronychia is an inflammation of the nail fold surrounding the nail plate, which may occur in either an acute or chronic form. Acute forms are precipitated by some form of trauma or chemical damage and usually present as painful infections (Fig. 68-7). Chronic paronychias tend to occur in several fingers simultaneously and result from repeated wet activities. An exception to this rule is the chronic paronychia caused by the habitual sucking of a finger, which tends to favor only one finger! Primary skin conditions, eczema, and atypical infectious organisms may also contribute to chronic paronychias.

Jebson PJL: Infections of the fingertip: paronychias and felons, *Hand Clin* 14:547–555, 1998.

24. Which infectious organisms cause paronychia?

Typically, acute lesions are caused by bacteria such as *Staphylococcus, Streptococcus*, and *Escherichia coli*. Chronic infectious paronychia is more commonly due to *Candida* sp., molds (*Scytalidium* sp.), syphilis, tuberculosis, and leprosy.

25. How do you treat an acute paronychia?

A quick and easy method to relieve pain and hasten healing is to stab the purulent area with a no. 11 scalpel blade and discharge the pus. A topical refrigerant spray to temporarily numb the area prior to incision will make for a grateful patient. Antibiotics and soaks should then be instituted, starting with coverage for *Staphylococcus aureus* until the culture is back.

26. What is the most common cause of green nails?

The most common cause is *Pseudomonas aeruginosa*, which can colonize nail plates that are abnormally lifted up. This bacterium produces a pyocyanin pigment that imparts the green discoloration. After the nail is cut away, local therapy with a topical antiseptic or antibiotics is all that is needed for a cure (Fig. 68-8).

27. What is the difference between onychomycosis and tinea unguium? What organisms most commonly cause tinea unguium? Where does the infection typically start?

Whereas onychomycosis includes all fungal infections of the nail (dermatophytes and others), tinea unguium refers specifically to dermatophyte infection of the nail. The most common organisms are *Trichophyton rubrum* (most common), *T. mentagrophytes*, and *Epidermophyton floccosum*. The vast majority of infections start at the distal end of the nail. Proximal subungual infections are quite rare in people with normal immune systems.

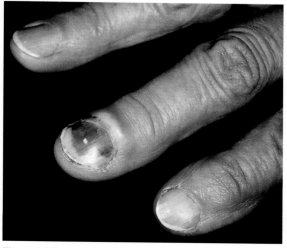

Figure 68-7. Acute paronychia demonstrating swelling, pus, and hemorrhage.

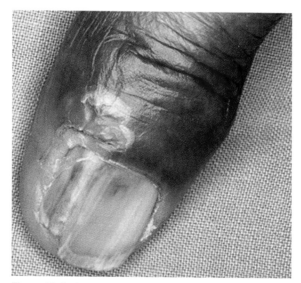

Figure 68-8. Green nail with onycholysis secondary to *Pseudomonas aeruginosa* infection. (Courtesy of the Fitzsimons Army Medical Center teaching files.)

Key Points: Nail Disorders

1. Nails serve as a window to the body.
2. Trauma is the most common cause of splinter hemorrhages.
3. Squamous cell carcinoma is the most common malignant tumor of the nail unit.
4. Diagnosis and prognosis of autoimmune connective tissue diseases may be enhanced by nail fold capillaroscopy.
5. X-ray any mass pushing up the nail plate.

---

28. List the antifungal medications most often used in the treatment of toenail onychomycosis.

See Table 68-3.

29. What should patients expect when undergoing treatment of onychomycosis?

The cure rate is 60% to 80% (*not* 100%). Fingernails grow 3 mm per month with complete replacement in about 6 months. Toenails grow 1 mm per month with replacement in 12 to 18 months. Therefore, at the end of a 6- to 12-week treatment course, the nails will not appear completely normal, but there usually is some healthy nail

Table 68-3. Antifungal Medications for Treatment of Toenail Onychomycosis

DRUG	BRAND NAME	DOSE
Itraconazole	Sporanox	Continuous: 200 mg qd for 12 weeks Pulse: 200 mg bid 1 week per month for 12 weeks
Terbinafine	Lamisil	Continuous: 250 mg qd for 12 weeks Pulse: 250 mg qd 1 week per q 3 months for 6–12 months
Fluconazole	Diflucan	150–200 mg every week for 12 months or until nails clear

Adapted from Zaias N, Rebell G: The successful treatment of *Trichophyton rubrum* nail bed (distal subungual) onychomycosis with intermittent pulse-dosed terbinafine, *Arch Dermatol* 140:691–695, 2004.

proximally. Of additional reassurance to patients is the fact that terbinafine and itraconazole reach maximum concentrations in the nail plate after discontinuing the medication, and they are present in the nail up to 9 months after treatment. There is a high risk of recurrence for toenail involvement, which can be mitigated by daily topical antifungal powders, creams, lacquers, and sprays.

Wolverton S: *Comprehensive dermatologic drug therapy*, Philadelphia, 2001, WB Saunders.

30. What is "habit tic" disorder? How is it different from median nail dystrophy?

This is a common self-induced nail condition of the thumb characterized by horizontal parallel ridges in the nail plate induced by constant manipulation of the cuticle and proximal nail fold. A closely related idiopathic condition, median nail dystrophy, can be easily confused with the above. Median nail dystrophy is marked by a normal cuticle and an inverted fir tree appearance to the central nail plate.

31. List the common benign "tumors" that occur in and around the nail unit.
- Acquired digital fibrokeratoma
- Exostosis
- Glomus tumor
- Periungual fibroma
- Pyogenic granuloma
- Myxoid (mucous) cyst

Salasche SJ, Orengo IF: Tumors of the nail unit, *J Dermatol Surg Oncol* 18:691–700, 1992.

32. What is an exostosis?

An exostosis is a common benign bony growth that occurs on the distal phalanx, usually of the great toe. It involves the bone first and secondarily the nail. Trauma is thought to play a role in its development, and it most commonly affects adolescent women. It presents as a slow-growing painful mass under the nail with frequent secondary infection (Fig. 68-9). Plain x-rays will easily delineate the pathology.

33. Name the four most common malignant tumors of the nail unit.

Squamous cell carcinoma (including Bowen's disease) is by far the most common malignant tumor of the nail unit and entire digit. The next most common is malignant melanoma, followed by basal cell carcinoma.

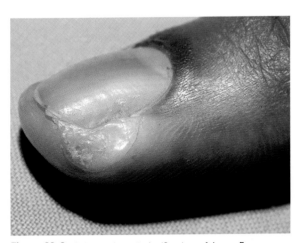

Figure 68-9. Subungual exostosis. (Courtesy of James E. Fitzpatrick, MD.)

DERMATOLOGIC TRIVIA

James E. Fitzpatrick, MD

There are three levels of knowledge: trivia, significa, and necessaria. Information that you consider to be trivial, your attending physician may regard as necessary.

1. What does the X in histiocytosis X mean?

It expresses the common etiologic link among the three clinical forms of the disease: eosinophilic granuloma, Hand-Schüller-Christian disease, and Letterer-Siwe disease. When Louis Lichtenstein coined the name *histiocytosis X* in 1953, he chose the X to represent the then-undetermined cause of the disorders. He wrote that the suffix X "has the advantage of brevity and, by implication, emphasizes the necessity for an intensive search for the etiologic agent." We now know that the common link is a proliferation of dendritic cells that are ultrastructurally and immunologically similar to Langerhans cells. Indeed, they probably are Langerhans cells, as reflected in the current name for histiocytosis X—Langerhans cell histiocytosis. Much about the disorder is still unknown, so perhaps Langerhans cell histiocytosis deserves to keep an X-designation.

Lichtenstein L: Histiocytosis X, *Arch Pathol* 56:84–102, 1953.

2. The suffix *-itis* has come to mean inflammation. What is inflamed in "pruritis"?

Nothing. The word is *pruritus*, not *pruritis*. It is derived from the Latin prurire, "to itch." Pruritus is commonly misspelled; please learn how to spell it correctly.

Bernhard JD: *Itch: mechanisms and management of pruritus*, New York, 1994, McGraw-Hill.

3. What is the difference between pruritus and itch?

There is none; the words are clinically interchangeable. Their ICD-9 codes are the same (698.9), so they are reimbursed equally, too.

4. Several names are used for the disease caused by *Bartonella bacilliformis*: bartonellosis, verruga peruana, Peruvian warts, Oroya fever, and Carrión's disease. Who was Carrión?

Daniel Carrión studied the relationship between the disfiguring, but seemingly benign, cutaneous disease verruga peruana, and the often-deadly disease Oroya fever. As part of a student research competition in 1885, the 26-year-old medical student inoculated himself with the blood of a patient with verruga peruana. Carrión soon developed the malignant form of *Bartonella* infection, Oroya fever, characterized by high fevers, severe myalgias, and profound hemolytic anemia. He postulated that the two conditions were related, but his experiment sadly ended fatally. A few decades later, his theory was proven correct, and now Carrión is the hero of the Peruvian medical profession.

Leonard J: Daniel Carrión and Carrión's disease, *Bull Pan Am Health Organ* 25:258–266, 1991.

5. What other illnesses are caused by *Bartonella* species?

Cat-scratch disease is caused by *B. henselae*, and trench fever is caused by *B. quintana*. Other conditions caused by various *Bartonella* species (including *B. henselae* and *B. quintana*) are most common in immunocompromised individuals, particularly those with HIV infection. These conditions include bacillary angiomatosis, peliosis hepatis, and a form of culture-negative endocarditis.

6. Sporotrichosis is also called "Schenck's disease," and the causative organism is named *Sporothrix schenckii*. Who was Schenck?

The disease is named after Bernard R. Schenck, who described the first definitive case of *sporotrichosis* (in an arm) in which the fungus was also isolated from the patient. Schenck was a second year medical student at Johns Hopkins Hospital when he made his famous discovery. The fungus could not be identified and was sent to Dr. E.F. Smith at the United States Department of Agriculture. Based on the colony appearance and microscopic morphology, Dr. Smith considered the fungus to be a species of *Sporotrichium*. In 1900, Hektoen and Perkins described a case of sporotrichosis in the finger of a boy who had struck his finger with a hammer. They reported the case as "Refractory subcutaneous abscesses caused by *Sporothrix schenckii*" and Dr. Schenck's name became forever associated with this fungal infection. Dr. Schenck did not become a dermatologist and reportedly specialized in obstetrics and gynecology after medical school.

7. What is the difference between Klippel-Trénaunay-Weber syndrome and Klippel-Trénaunay-Parkes-Weber syndrome?

There is no difference. They are examples of eponymy with synonymy; both refer to osteohypertrophic nevus flammeus or angioosteohypertrophy syndrome. The medical literature contains many reports, erroneous but oft-perpetuated, that distinguish the two as different syndromes on the basis of limb-length discrepancies. Weber and Parkes-Weber refer to the same person: Frederick Parkes Weber (1863–1962), an Englishman who was a consummate physician and erudite collector of unusual medical cases.

Gibbs DD: Rendu-Osler-Weber disease: a triple eponymous title lives on, *J R Soc Med* 79:742–743, 1986.

8. Which other eponymous dermatologic conditions include the name Weber?
- Rendu-Osler-Weber disease, or hereditary hemorrhagic telangiectasia
- Sturge-Weber syndrome (aka Sturge-Weber-Dimitri syndrome), or encephalomeningeal angiomatosis
- Weber-Cockayne syndrome, or epidermolysis bullosa (mild epidermal variant)
- Weber-Christian disease (nodular nonsuppurative panniculitis)

9. What is ciguatera poisoning?

Ciguatera poisoning is caused by ingestion of ciguatoxin, a tasteless toxin produced by dinoflagellates (*Gambierdiscus toxicus*). Humans are affected by eating carnivorous fish (such as barracuda or red snapper) that have accumulated the toxin as it is passed along the oceanic food chain. Ciguatera occurs along coral reefs in tropical or warm subtropical waters. Ciguatoxin interferes with sodium channels in mammalian cell membranes. There are a number of gastrointestinal symptoms, but the occasional fatality is usually due to cardiorespiratory involvement.

Lange WR: Ciguatera fish poisoning, *Am Fam Physician* 50:579–584, 1994.

10. What are the neurocutaneous manifestations of ciguatera poisoning?

Pruritus is noted in about half of the cases, often confined to palms and soles, and is exacerbated by exercise or alcohol consumption. There are often perioral and acral dysesthesias that most distinctively demonstrate a heat-cold reversal phenomenon. Dry mouth may also occur.

11. From what is cantharidin made?

Cantharidin ($C_{10}H_{12}O_4$), a vesicant therapy for molluscum contagiosum and warts, is a semipurified extract from blister beetles. The compound induces a blister at the epidermal–dermal junction. Blister beetles, mostly in the family Meloidae, have been used in Asian folk medicine for millennia. In the southern United States, horses are often afflicted with cantharidin toxicity after inadvertently eating the blister beetles that live in mowed alfalfa.

12. What is Spanish fly?

It is the legendary aphrodisiac powder made from crushed blister beetles (*Lytta* [syn. *Cantharis*] *vesicatoria*). Supposedly, it served as an excitatory rubefacient when applied to an uncooperative male appendage.

13. Seriously now, cantharidin has been confirmed as an aphrodisiac. Who uses it and how does it work?

Male beetles of the species *Neopyrochroa flabellata* secrete cantharidin from a gland on their heads as a courtship or prenuptial offering. Females prefer to mate with males who offer cantharidin, which the female then uses to protect her eggs from predacious grubs.

Eisner T, Smedley SR, Young DK, et al: Chemical basis of courtship in a beetle (*Neopyrochroa flabellata*): cantharidin as "nuptial gift," *Proc Natl Acad Sci U S A* 93:6499–6503, 1996.

14. Who is generally considered the father of modern dermatology?

Robert Willan (1757–1812), a Yorkshireman, was awarded the Fothergillian Gold Medal in 1790 for establishing a classification of skin disease that is still used today.

Clendening L: Robert Willan. In Clendening L, editor: *Source book of medical history*, New York, 1960, Dover, pp 560–563.

15. Name the eight orders in which Willan classified cutaneous disease.

Papules, scaling disorders, rashes (exanthems), bullae, vesicles, pustules, tubercles, and maculae. The terms are retained today in the daily parlance of the dermatologist.

16. What were Willan's four subtypes of pustules?

Phlyzacium, psydracium, achor, and cerion. Willan distinguished pustules by differences in size, characteristics of the pus, and quality of the scab. These terms have been abandoned. (Now *this* is trivia.)

17. What is a hunterian chancre?

It is the ulcer of primary syphilis, a syphilitic chancre.

18. Why does Jonathan Hunter's name grace this ulcer?

Jonathan Hunter was one of medicine's most influential practitioners. Among his works is the treatise "On the Venereal Disease," which addressed the then-unanswered question of whether gonorrhea and syphilis were different expressions of the same disease. Hunter attempted to settle the issue by inoculating himself in this manner: "Two punctures were made on [my] penis with a lancet dipped in venereal matter from a gonorrhea." Unfortunately, the donor of the "venereal matter" had both gonorrhea and syphilis. Hunter soon developed a chancre on his penis and later developed secondary syphilis. The mistaken conclusion of his little experiment was that gonorrhea and syphilis were the same disease. Incidentally, Dr. Hunter died 26 years after his self-inoculation from classic syphilitic heart disease.

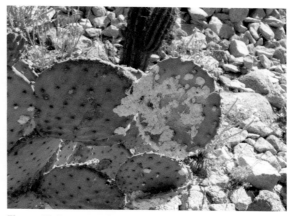

Figure 69-1. Prickly pear cactus demonstrating fluffy white wax secreted by the cochineal insect. The dye is produced from the dried crushed bodies of the actual insect.

19. Mucicarmine is a histologic stain used to detect mucin. From what natural source is mucicarmine obtained?

Cochineal, which is produced by a mealy buglike insect (*Dactylopius coccus*) that lives on several species of cacti (Fig. 69-1). The pigment's chemical properties serve as deterrents against predation by other insects. Cochineal dye is crimson and has long been used as a traditional textile dye in Mexico. Emily Dickinson described the colors of a ruby-throated hummingbird as "A resonance of Emerald/A rush of Cochineal." Check the ingredients on bottles of pink grapefruit juice and you're likely to discover that the pinkish-red color is conferred by cochineal-laden bug poop.

20. How does the Food and Drug Administration differentiate between an underarm deodorant and an underarm antiperspirant?

Deodorants are cosmetics that control, obscure, or mask body odor. As a cosmetic, it has no claim to alter the body's physiologic process of perspiring. Antiperspirants alter the natural process of sweating and are therefore considered an over-the-counter drug. Antiperspirants are often deodorants, too.

Schoen LA, Lazar P: *The look you like*, New York, 1990, Marcel Dekker.

21. What is Compound 606?

Also called *salvarsan*, Compound 606 was introduced to clinical medicine by future Nobel-laureate Paul Ehrlich in 1909. It was long considered the drug of choice for treponemal infections such as syphilis and yaws. The name reflects its place as the 606th compound tested by Ehrlich and his partner Sahachiro Hata. Ironically, salvarsan was developed not as a treatment for human syphilis but as part of an experiment on murine trypanosomiasis.

22. Who was James Lind?

James Lind (1716–1794), British naval surgeon, has received an inordinate share of credit in establishing the preventive and curative role of citrus products in the management of scurvy. Although Lind believed scurvy was caused by clogged skin pores, he conducted several shipboard trials of alleged antiscorbutic substances, leading to the use of citrus products (limes) by the Royal Navy during long voyages, hence, the moniker "limeys" for British sailors.

Carpenter KJ: *The history of scurvy and vitamin C*, New York, 1986, Cambridge University Press.

23. If citrus products prevent scurvy, why did the Royal Navy suffer from so many scurvy outbreaks a century after Lind?

Not all citrus fruits have high amounts of vitamin C. In the mid-1800s, long before Casimir Funk's theory of vital amines (vitamins), the Royal Navy changed its fruit supplier and started receiving a strain of Caribbean lime that has very little vitamin C. Several polar exploring expeditions used the nonprotective limes and suffered severe losses from scurvy. This led many to doubt the efficacy of citrus fruit in the management of scurvy. After the discoveries of Pasteur and Koch, a paradigm swept through medicine that most diseases were caused by bacteria, either by direct infection or by ptomaine, a bacteria-induced food poisoning. Indeed, several nutritional diseases had their "offending bacteria" identified, including scurvy, pellagra, and beriberi.

24. Hansen's disease (leprosy) is generally considered a tropical condition. Where was G.H. Armauer Hansen working when he discovered the causative bacillus of leprosy?

Norway. Leprosy was abundant in coastal Norway in the mid-1800s, so Hansen did not leave his country to study this "tropical" disease. Bergen, Norway, was the world's center for leprosy research. Leprosy may have been carried to Norway by Viking voyagers a millennium earlier.

Irgens LM: The discovery of *Mycobacterium leprae*, Am J Dermatopathol 6:337–343, 1984.

25. In the United States, most persons with newly diagnosed Hansen's disease are immigrants from Southeast Asia, but in one region of the country, Hansen's disease is endemic. Where is this region of endemic Hansen's disease?

Louisiana and eastern Texas. Individuals there can acquire the disease autochthonously, apparently with no contact with any other infected persons.

26. What seems to be the natural reservoir of Hansen's disease in these states?

In the past several decades, the nine-banded armadillo (*Dasypus novemcinctus*) has been found naturally infected with *Mycobacterium leprae* (Fig. 69-2). The disease manifests itself similarly to lepromatous leprosy. Persons who handle armadillos for work or sport are at increased risk for acquiring Hansen's disease. Curiously, the first reports of naturally occurring armadillo leprosy appeared several years after the animals started being used for experimental infections.

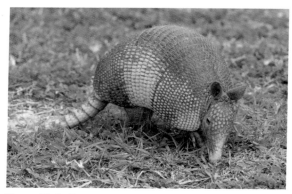

Figure 69-2. The nine-banded armadillo (*Dasypus novemcinctus*) that has been found to be a carrier of leprosy in the United States, especially in Texas. (From iStock_0000029548.)

27. Has there ever been a "leper colony" in the United States?

Yes. There have been two leprosariums in the United States, one in Carville, Louisiana and the other on Kalaupapa, Hawaii. Both leprosariums are closed; however, the National Hansen's Disease Museum is open to the public and still located in Carville.

28. Who was Father Damien?

Father Damien deVeuster was a Catholic missionary priest from Belgium who went to the leprosarium on Kalaupapa, Hawaii in 1873. At the time of his arrival, the leprosy colony did not have any buildings or potable water, and patients lived in caves and rudimentary shacks made of sticks and leaves. It was supplied by ships that would throw the supplies into the water and rely on either currents or leprosy victims to swim out to retrieve the supplies. Father Damien was responsible for building permanent structures, including churches, and organizing the leprosarium. Sadly, Father Damien developed leprosy and died in 1889.

29. Urology textbooks list about 50 causes of discolored urine. Several inherited metabolic disorders with cutaneous manifestations can cause discolored urine. If an infant's diapers have a black discoloration, what genodermatosis should you include in your differential diagnosis?

Alkaptonuria, or hereditary ochronosis. This is a rare, autosomal recessive disorder due to the absence of an enzyme, homogentisic acid oxidase, which normally helps metabolize tyrosine and phenylalanine. Much of the excess metabolite, homogentisic acid, is excreted in the urine. The urine turns dark on oxidation; hence, a freshly removed, urine-soaked diaper may have a normal color, but will quickly turn black upon exposure to air. Homogentisic acid is also accumulated in cartilage, leading to arthritis and to characteristic darkening of the sclera and pinnae.

30. If an infant's diapers have a reddish discoloration, what genodermatosis should you include in your differential diagnosis?

Erythropoietic porphyria. This is another very rare autosomal recessive disorder due to an absence in uroporphyrinogen III cosynthase, an enzyme required early in the heme synthesis pathway. Much of the excess substrate is excreted in the urine and may give diapers a distinctive reddish color. Patients develop a destructive, scarring photodermatitis and a variety of hematologic abnormalities. In acute intermittent porphyria, the urine of adolescents and adults may turn red upon standing also.

31. What is the eponymic name for erythropoietic porphyria?

Günther's disease. Some authorities believe that people with this disease are the basis for reports of "werewolves" in Europe. Individuals afflicted with this disorder avoid light, because it produces burning, and they demonstrate marked diffuse hypertrichosis, scarring, and erythrodontia (red-stained teeth).

32. What is "North Carolina spotless fever"?

The tickborne disease caused by *Rickettsia rickettsii* is usually called Rocky Mountain spotted fever. However, this name is a misnomer, because the disease rarely occurs today in the Rocky Mountain states but is common in the vicinity of North Carolina. Perhaps 20% of cases lack the petechial eruption at presentation. Each year, there are more cases of North Carolina spotless fever than there are of Rocky Mountain spotted fever—hence, the proposed name change.

Blythe WB: Lest we forget-Spring is here: North Carolina spotless fever in adults, *North Carolina Med J* 46:347–348, 1985.

33. What is the carrier protein of a hapten called?

Schlepper, from the German word for "drag" or "haul." The molecular weight of a hapten is too low to induce an allergenic response. The schlepper protein provides the molecular muscle to allow the hapten to serve as an antigen.

34. Do hair removal techniques (shaving, plucking, depilatories, waxing, electrolysis) cause new hair growth to be increasingly dark, coarse, or thick?

No, there is no scientific evidence to support this commonly held belief. The new growth is often sharp-tipped and stubbly, depending on the removal technique, and gives the illusion of bristliness.

35. Fifth disease is the common childhood exanthem also known as erythema infectiosum and is caused by parvovirus B19. (Everyone knows that.) But what is fourth disease?

It was a childhood exanthem described around 1900 that has been abandoned as a nosologic entity. A century ago, common childhood exanthems were assigned numbers one through six for ease of classification. Only fifth disease retains its numeric name. Fourth disease, also called *Dukes' disease* or *Filatow-Dukes disease*, purportedly consisted of a nonspecific febrile illness accompanied by a cutaneous eruption. It may have been a streptococcal toxin–mediated disease, but it is not considered a precise or specific disease description.

Bialecki C, Feder HM, Grant-Kels JM: The six classic childhood exanthems: a review and update, *J Am Acad Dermatol* 21:891–903, 1989.

36. Onchocerciasis is found in both Africa and South America. Where did the disease originate, and how did it cross the Atlantic?

It appears that disease caused by *Onchocerca volvulus* was originally endemic to tropical West Africa. The human cargo of the slave trade carried the disease to the Americas, where there were already native black flies and an awaiting ecological niche.

Hoeppli R: Parasitic disease in Africa and the Western hemisphere: early documentation and transmission by the slave trade, Basel, 1969, Verlag Recht Gesellschaft.

37. What skin disease does the sailor's curse, "I'll be jiggered" refer to?

It refers to parasitization by the jigger (*Tunga penetrans*). The gravid female flea burrows into the skin to where the eggs mature, and she passes them through an opening in the skin to the environment, where they mature in the soil. This flea is found in sandy shaded soil, and early sailors frequently took refuge in these areas, where they acquired this noxious pest. In most cases, only one or two jiggers are present, but some individuals have had hundreds of lesions at the same time. This parasitic disorder was first described by the Spanish conquerors and sailors of the *Santa Maria* that shipwrecked on the coast of Haiti at the end of the 15th century.

38. Tungiasis (jiggers) was originally confined to the subtropical and tropical regions of the New World. How did it get to Africa, where it is now extensively entrenched in the sub-Sahara region?

Ships returning from the New World sometimes took on sand for ballast. In 1872, a ship dropped infested sand ballast on the coast of West Africa introducing the noxious pest to this region. It is likely that it was introduced more than once, and it has also spread to Pakistan and parts of India on the Asian continent.

39. The first written account of poison ivy appeared in 1609 in the journal of this famous settler of the New World. Who wrote this account?

Poison ivy plant and its dermatitis were first described in Western literature by Captain John Smith of Princess Pocahontas fame. Captain Smith was the leader of the ill-fated mercantile colony at Jamestown, Virginia. His journal described this as "The poisonous weed, being in shape but little different from out English yvie; but being touched causeth redness, itchinge, and lastly blysters, the which howsoever, after a while they passe aveay of themselves without further harme. . . ." Modern dermatology textbooks can add little to his very accurate description!

Crissey JT, Parish LC, Holubar K: *Historical atlas of dermatology and dermatologists.* Boca Raton, FL, 2002, Parthenon Publishing Group.

40. What is the name of the dermatologist who invented adhesive tape?

We often take adhesive tape for granted, but it did not exist until it was invented by a German dermatologist, Paul Gerson Unna, the best known dermatologist in the world in the early decades of the 20th century. He was a brilliant dermatologist and produced many treatments including the Unna boot, which is still used today, and Unna's paste, eucerin and ichthyol (used for psoriasis and many forms of dermatitis). He was also a great dermatopathologist and teacher.

Crissey JT, Parish LC, Holubar K: *Historical atlas of dermatology and dermatologists.* Boca Raton, FL, 2002, Parthenon Publishing Group.

41. How many keratinocytes (skin cells) do you shed per minute?

It has been calculated that we shed about 35,000 skin cells per minute, which calculates to more than 50 million per day! In one year, the total number of shed keratinocytes would weigh almost 9 pounds. While this is truly trivia, it does highlight the fact that the skin is an amazingly active structure.

INDEX

A

Abrasions, child abuse-related, 449
Abscess, cutaneous, diabetes-related, 261-262
Acanthosis
    nigricans, 252, 253f, 261, 261f
        achrodons associated with, 253, 306f
        clinical disease states associated with, 253
        insulin resistance associated with, 253,
            259-260, 261
        malignant/paraneoplastic, 253, 259, 261,
            270-271, 271f
        obesity-related, 253, 288
        tretinoin treatment for, 394
    "sawtooth," 87
Acitretin, 53, 393t, 397-398, 397t
    anticarcinogenic activity of, 395
    use in phototherapy, 391
Acne and acneiform eruptions, 148-155
    acne conglobata, 148
    acne fulminans, 148, 154, 154f, 449
        as dermatologic emergency, 449
    acne mechanica, 148
    acne necrotica miliaris, 81
    acne rosacea, 148, 154-155, 155f
    acne vulgaris, 150
        cystic, inflammatory, 149f
        cystic, isotretinoin treatment for, 395-396
        differentiated from steroid acne, 153
        isotretinoin treatment for, 395-396
        light and laser therapy for, 152
        nodular, isotretinoin treatment for,
            395-396
        pediatric, 404, 407
        tretinoin treatment for, 394, 396
    androgenic, 264
    comedonal, 19
    cryosurgical treatment for, 372t
    in dialysis patients, 274-275
    dietary factors in, 149
    drug-induced/drug-aggravated, 148, 149f,
        152-153, 264
    excoriée, 148
    hormonal treatment for, 264
    keloidalis nuchae, 431, 434
    laser treatment for, 383
    lithium-related exacerbation of, 97
    neonatal, 82, 148, 152f
        differentiated from infantile acne, 152
    nutritional supplement-related, 264
    occupational exposure-related, 452
    pomade, 434
    Proprionibacterium acnes, 150
    pustular, drug-related, 81
    steroid, 81, 102, 153
    stress-related, 148-149
    subtypes of, 148
    in women, 264
Acne scars, laser therapy for, 381, 383-384, 384t
Acquired epidermolysis bullosa, collagen type VII
    antibodies in, 11
Acquired immunodeficiency virus syndrome
    (AIDS)

Acquired immunodeficiency virus syndrome
    (Continued)
    adverse drug reactions associated with, 98
    blastomycosis, 228
    coccidioidomycosis, 229
    cutaneous manifestations of, 98
    Merkel cell carcinoma associated with, 341
    Mycobacterium avium-intracellulare complex
        infections, 213
    sporotrichosis, 224-225
Acremonium, 219-220
Acroangiodermatitis, 304, 304f
Acrochordon, 15f, 305
    acanthosis nigricans-related, 252, 253f
    cryosurgical treatment for, 372
    diabetes-related, 262
    obesity-related, 288
Acrodermatitis
    continua of Hallopeau, 78, 80f
    enteropathica, 74-75, 77, 289-290, 291f
    papular, of childhood, 173, 173f
Acrokeratosis paraneoplastic, 255
Acromegaly, 266
Acropachy, 262
Acropustulosis, infantile, 82-83, 82f, 434
Actinic prurigo, 121, 122f
    phototherapy for, 387-388t
Actinic reticuloid, 120, 121f
Actinomycetoma, 226-227
Actinomycosis, as granuloma cause, 90t
Acupuncture, 435-436
Acyclovir
    as herpes simplex virus infection treatment,
        176, 177t
    as varicella-zoster virus infection treatment,
        179, 180t
Addison's disease, 126, 132, 263-264, 267
Adenocarcinoma, colonic, 270f, 270
Adenoma sebaceum, 39, 257, 309
Adenoviruses, 173
Adhesive tape, invention of, 477
Adolescents
    acne in, 149, 404
    guttate psoriasis in, 50
    papular acrodermatitis in, 173
    warts in, 182
Adrenocorticotropic hormone (ACTH)
    adverse cutaneous reactions to, 101t
    pigmentation effects of, 132, 263
African Americans. *See also* Skin of color
    alopecia in, 146-147
AGEP (acute generalized exanthematous), 81,
    103, 104f
Aging, cutaneous. *See* Dermatoheliosis
Ainhum, 434
Airway disease, atopic dermatitis-related, 58
Albinism, 126, 128, 129f
    ocular, 30
Albright's syndrome, 131
Alcohol abuse, as zinc deficiency cause, 290
Alitretinoin, 395
Alkaptonuria, 133-134, 476

Allergens, of the workplace, 454
Allergic contact dermatitis. *See* Contact dermatitis,
    allergic
Allergic reactions
    Churg-Strauss syndrome-related, 107, 107t
    to drugs, 97, 166
    to epinephrine, 365
    to local anesthetics, 364-365
    as urticaria cause, 166, 168
Allopurinol
    as alopecia cause, 103
    as ichthyosis cause, 34t
    as Stevens-Johnson syndrome cause, 99
    as toxic epidermal necrolysis cause, 98-99
    as vesiculobullous eruption cause, 73t
Alopecia, 143-147
    androgenic, 264
    areata, 144, 144f, 147, 407, 458-459
        nail findings in, 469, 469t
    central, centrifugal cicatricial, 144f, 146-147
    chemotherapy-related, 97
    in children, 407
    classification of, 143
    Darier's disease-related, 35
    discoid lupus erythematosus-related, 158
    drug-related, 103
    lichenoid, 85
    male pattern, 143
    moth-eaten, 143, 147, 147f, 198
    mucinosa, 147, 147f, 332
    myeloma-associated amyloidosis-related,
        112
    neoplastica, 339, 343f
    nonscarring (noncicatricial), 143, 458-459
    patchy, 143
    patchy nonscarring, differential diagnosis of,
        458-459
    in people of color, 432
    scarring (cicatricial), 143, 144f
    syphilis-related, 197-198
    tinea capititis-related, 217
    totalis, 144, 145f
    traction, 434, 458-459
    traumatic, child abuse-related, 450
    universalis, 144, 285-286
Alpha-1 antitrypsin deficiency, 139, 139f
Aluminum, as granuloma cause, 90t, 91t
Amebiasis, 235t, 238
Ameboma, 238
Amineptine, acne-exacerbating effect of, 153t
Amino acid metabolism disorders, as leukoderma
    cause, 128, 129t
para-Aminobenzoic acid, as sunscreen component,
    355-356, 355t
Amiodarone
    phototoxic reactions to, 103
    as pigmentation disorder cause, 101t, 133t,
        134, 134f
Amniocentesis pits, 436
Amoxicillin, adverse cutaneous reactions to, 98, 98t
    acute generalized exanthematous pustulosis,
        103, 104f

Amoxicillin, adverse cutaneous reactions to
    (Continued)
    in HIV-infected individuals, 283
    maculopapular skin eruptions, 98
    toxic epidermal necrolysis, 98-99
Amphetamines, as leukocytoclastic vasculitis
    cause, 105
Ampicillin, adverse cutaneous reactions to, 98, 98t
    leukocytoclastic vasculitis, 106f
    maculopapular skin eruptions, 98
    Stevens-Johnson syndrome, 99
Amyloid, 112
Amyloidosis, 115
    lichenoid, 112-113, 112f, 113t, 114f
    macular, 112-113, 113t, 133, 133t
    myeloma-associated, 112-113, 113t
    nodular, 112-113, 113t, 114f
    primary localized, 113t
    systemic, 112
        primary, 112-113, 113f, 113t, 256, 274, 278,
            278f, 279t
        secondary, 113, 113t, 279t
Anabolic steroids, acne-exacerbating effect of, 153t
Anagen effluvium, 145
Anaphylaxis
    arthropod sting-related, 243
    drug-related, 98
    systemic, 99-100
Anaplasmosis, 249-250t
Ancylostoma, as "creeping eruption" cause, 234
Androgens
    as acne cause, 264
    effect on sebaceous glands and hair, 264
Anemia, 222, 268-269
Angioedema
    C1 esterase deficiency associated with, 170
    with chronic urticaria, 168
    as dermatologic emergency, 449
    drug-related, 97, 100
    hereditary, 169-170
    treatment for, 170
    without urticaria, 168
Angiofibroma, 309, 408
    facial, tuberous sclerosis-related, 39, 40f
Angiokeratoma, 302-303, 302f
    corporis diffusum, 277-278
Angioma
    cherry, 302, 303f
    cryosurgical treatment of, 372
Angiomatosis
    bacillary, 281t, 284, 473
    bilateral retinal, von Hippel-Lindau
        disease-related, 41
    encephalomeningeal, 474
    homolateral leptomeningeal, 40-41
Angiomyolipoma, tuberous sclerosis-related, 40
Angiosarcoma, 313t, 339-340
Angiotensin-converting enzyme inhibitors
    as alopecia cause, 103
    as angioedema cause, 100
    as urticaria cause, 100
Annular skin lesions, 20
Anogenital area, warts of, 182t, 183-184, 183f,
    185, 186t, 187, 199
    HIV infection-related, 283-284
    prevention of, 184
Anosmia, 30
Ant stings, 243
Antibiotics. See also specific antibiotics
    as acne therapy, 148, 150
    as candidiasis risk factor, 97
    as lichen planus-like eruptions cause, 87t
    photoallergic/phototoxic reactions to, 119t
    as pustular eruption cause, 81
    as vesiculobullous eruption cause, 73t
Antibodies. See also specific antibodies
    in desmosome-damaging diseases, 9t
Anticoagulants, use in surgery patients, 369
Antidepressant drugs, acne-exacerbating effect
    of, 153t

Antiepileptic drugs
    acne-exacerbating effect of, 153t
    as alopecia cause, 147
    as lichen planus-like eruptions cause, 87t
    as vesiculobullous eruptions cause, 73t
Antifungal drugs, 222-223, 222t, 471, 472t
Antihemidesmosomal antibodies, 9-10
Antihistamines
    as atopic dermatitis treatment, 59
    as urticaria treatment, 168, 170
Antihypertensive drugs, as lichen planus-like
    eruptions cause, 87t
Anti-inflammatory drugs. See also Nonsteroidal
    anti-inflammatory drugs
    as lichen planus-like eruptions cause, 87t
Antimalarial drugs
    adverse cutaneous reactions to, 101
        lichen planus-like eruptions, 87t
        photoallergic/phototoxic reactions, 119t
        pigmentation disorder, 133t
        psoriasis-exacerbating effects, 53
    as granuloma annulare treatment, 94-95
    as sarcoidosis treatment, 93-94
Antimyeloperoxidase antibodies, as vasculitis
    markers, 105
Antineutrophil cytoplasmic antibodies, 108, 109
Antinuclear antibodies, 156
Antiperspirants, differentiated from deodorants,
    475
Antiphospholipid antibody syndrome, 163,
    163-164t
Antiretroviral therapy, cutaneous side effects of,
    73t, 285-286, 285f
Antiseptics, 366
Antisynthase syndrome, 162
Antituberculosis drugs, 211-212, 211t
    acne-exacerbating effect of, 153t
Anti-U1RNP ribonuclear protein antibodies,
    162-163, 163-164t
Aphrodisiacs, 474
Aphthosis, in HIV-infected individuals, 281t
Aplasia cutis congenita, 407
Arboviruses, 249-250t
Argyria, 134
Armadillo
    as Mycobacterium leprae (leprosy) reservoir,
        201, 476, 476f
    as sporotrichosis vector, 224
Armauer, G.H., 475
Arsenic
    as Mees' lines cause, 467t
    as pigmentation disorder cause, 128, 132,
        134
    as skin cancer cause, 312
    as squamous cell carcinoma cause, 290
Arteritis
    giant cell (temporal), 105t, 106, 125
    Takayasu, 105t, 110
Arthritis
    gouty, 116
    juvenile idiopathic, 163
    Lyme disease-related, 248
    mutilans, 52
    psoriatic, 50-51, 52, 52f
    reactive (Reiter's disease), 80-81
    rheumatoid
        nail changes associated with, 467t
    subcorneal pustular dermatosis-related, 79
Arthropod bites and stings, 73, 174, 464
Arthropods, classification of, 241
Arygria, 97
Ascites, 267-268
Ash-leaf hypopigmented macules, 39, 39f, 126
Aspergillosis, 219-220, 224, 230-231, 231t,
    232-233, 232f
Aspirin, adverse cutaneous reactions to, 100,
    105, 168
Assassin (kissing) bugs, 248, 249-250t
Astemizole, interaction with antifungal agents,
    223

Asthma
    atopic dermatitis-related, 57-58
    Churg-Strauss syndrome-related, 107, 107t,
        109t
Ataxia, cerebellar, 42
Ataxia-telangiectasia, 41-42, 258t
Atopic dermatitis, 57
    age-related phases of, 58-59, 58f, 404
    definition of, 57
    diagnostic criteria for, 57
    pediatric, steroid treatment for, 363
    phototherapy for, 387-388t, 389
    provoking or exacerbating factors of, 59,
        463-464
    treatment for, 59
    wool-related, 463-464
"Atopic march," 58
Atopy, 57
Atrophy, differentiated from lichenification, 19-20,
    20f
Auspitz sign, 52
Autoantibodies
    autoimmune connective tissue disease-related,
        160f, 163, 163-164t, 165t
    chronic urticaria-related, 166-167
Autoerythrocyte sensitization syndrome, 458
Autoimmune diseases, 10
    connective tissue diseases, 156-165, 468
    as dermatologic emergency, 442, 446-447
    lichen planus associated with, 86
    as lipodystrophy cause, 141
Autosomal dominant diseases, with skin findings
    and cancer, 256, 256t, 270
Autosomal recessive genodermatoses, photosensi-
    tivity-associated, 123-124t
Axon reflex, 167

B

Babesiosis, 248, 249-250t
Bacillus Calmette-Guérin, 207, 211
Bacterial infections, 188-194. See also specific
    bacteria
    as dermatologic emergency, 444-446
    in diabetic patients, 261
    diagnosis of, 27
    as granuloma cause, 90t
    in HIV-infected individuals, 280, 281t
    as leukocytoclastic vasculitis cause, 105
Bacterial skin cultures, 27
Bacterid, pustular, of Andrews, 78-79
Balanitis, circinate, Reiter's disease-related,
    80-81
Baldness. See Alopecia
Balneophototherapy, 389
Barbiturates, adverse cutaneous reactions to, 73t,
    99-100, 105
Bartonella bacilliformis, 473
Bartonella henselae, 473
Bartonella quintana, 473
Bartonellosis, 473
Basal cell carcinoma, 15f, 309, 312, 313t
    age factors in, 352
    clinical and histologic appearance of, 315
    cryosurgical treatment of, 372
    definition of, 315
    in HIV-infected individuals, 281t
    metastatic, 340
    Mohs surgery for, 374, 376, 376f
    of the nail unit, 472
    as nevoid basal cell carcinoma syndrome,
        316, 316f
    noduloulcerative, 18-19
    relationship to skin phototype, 352
    sporadic, 315
    sun exposure as risk factor for, 352
    treatment for, 314t
    variants of, 314t, 315f, 316f
Basal cell layer, of epidermis, 7f

Basement membrane zone, 6, 7f, 8f
  blistering diseases of, 9, 10t
  in bullous skin diseases, 9-10
  in epidermolysis bullosa, 9f
  hereditary diseases of, 8-9
  structural components of, 71f
Basic fibroblast growth factor, 132
Bat bugs, 248f
Bather's eruption, 239
Bazex syndrome, 255
BEAN SAP mnemonic, for Churg-Strauss syndrome, 110f
Beau's lines, 467
Bedbugs, 247, 247f, 248f
Bee stings, 241-243, 242f
Behçet's syndrome, 252, 254, 271
Benzocaine, phototoxicity of, 119t
Benzoyl peroxide, as acne therapy, 152
Beriberi, 288, 475
Beryllium, as granuloma cause, 91t
Beta-blocking agents, psoriasis-exacerbating effects of, 53
Beta-carotene, as pigmentation disorder cause, 101t
Beta-lactam antibiotics
  adverse cutaneous reactions to, 100
  as anaphylaxis cause, 100
Betel nut, 437
Bexarotene, 334, 393t, 395
Biliary tract disease, 267-268
Bilirubin, 271
Bindi, 437
Biologic agents, as psoriasis treatment, 53-54
Biologic response modifiers, as lichen planus-like eruptions cause, 87t
Biopsy, cutaneous
  for allergic contact dermatitis diagnosis, 73
  for dermatomyositis diagnosis, 162
  for epidermolysis bullosa diagnosis, 74
  for erythema nodosum diagnosis, 136, 137f
  incisional/excisional, 26
  indications for, 26
  for leprosy diagnosis, 206
  for melanoma diagnosis, 325
  punch, 26, 367-368
  sentinel lymph node, 326-327
  shave, 26, 368f
  for sporotrichosis diagnosis, 225
  for systemic amyloidosis diagnosis, 278
  for vesiculobullous disease diagnosis, 71
Bioterrorism, 233
Biotin deficiency, 288
Birthmarks, 294
Birt-Hogg-Dube syndrome, 279t
Bismuth, as pigmentation disorder cause, 133t, 134
Bites
  arthropod, 73, 174, 241
  human, child abuse-related, 450
Black flies, 241, 249-250t, 250, 477
Blackheads, 19
Blaschko lines, 129
Blastomycosis, 90t, 224, 227-228, 227f, 228f, 229-230, 231t
Bleomycin
  as pigmentation disorder cause, 101t, 132, 134
  as wart treatment, 185, 186t, 187
Blepharitis, 61-62
Blister beetles, 474
Blistering diseases. *See also* Mechanobullous disorders; Vesiculobullous disorders
  of the basement membrane zone, 9, 10t
  dermal involvement in, 9, 10t
  epidermal involvement in, 8
  hereditary, 8-9, 10
Blisters. *See also* Bullae; Vesicles
  in children, 406
  definition of, 70
  grouped configuration of, 20
  intraepidermal, 70, 70t
  subepidermal, 70, 70t
  viral exanthem-related, 172

Blood, adverse cutaneous reactions to, 98t
Bloom's syndrome, 123-124t, 258t
"Blueberry muffin baby," 401, 401f
Blue-gray dyspigmentation, 132-134, 134f
Body lice, 24, 245-246
Boils. *See* Furuncles
Bone disease, calcinosis cutis-related, 117
Borrelia burgdorferi, 140, 248
Bourneville disease. *See* Tuberous sclerosis
Boutonneuse fever, 249-250t
Bovine collagen injections, 92f
Bowen's disease. *See* Squamous cell carcinoma, in situ
BP antigens, 10t
Bradykinin, as vasodilatation and vascular permeability mediator, 167
Breast, fibrocystic disease of, 256-257
Breast cancer, 106, 253, 256f, 256t, 259, 269, 271, 395
Breastfeeding, leprosy transmission through, 201
Breslow's depth, of melanoma, 322, 323
Bromides
  as acne cause, 81, 153t
  as erythema nodosum cause, 135-136
  as pustular eruption cause, 81
Bronchospasm, beta-lactam antibiotics-related, 100
Brugia, 236
Bruising
  child abuse-related, 449, 450f
  chronic renal failure-related, 274t
"Buffalo hump," 264, 285
Bullae, 14
  causes of, 70
  differentiated from vesicles and pustules, 70, 78
  drug-related, 102, 102f
  grouped configuration of, 20
Bullous disease, of diabetes, 262
Bullous lupus erythematosus, 10t
Bullous pemphigoid. *See* Pemphigoid, bullous
Bullous pemphigoid antigen, 8-9
Bullous skin diseases. *See also specific diseases*
  basement membrane abnormalities in, 9-10
Bullous viral eruptions, 175-181
"Bull's-eye" lesions, 19, 19f
Burns
  child abuse-related, 449, 450f
  lightning strike-related, 450, 450f
  pseudomonal infections of, 192
Burrows, 18-19, 19f, 23-24, 244, 245f, 464
Buschke-Ollendorf syndrome, 308, 309
Busulfan, as pigmentation disorder cause, 132, 134
"Butterfly rash," 446
Butyrophenones, as ichthyosis cause, 32, 34t

C

C1 esterase deficiency, 170
Caduceus, 236, 237f
Café-au-lait macules (CALM), 15f, 300, 300f
  Albright's syndrome-related, 131
  Moynahan's syndrome-related, 131, 131f
  neurofibromatosis-related, 131, 256t, 299-300, 408
Calabar swelling, 235-236
Calcineurin inhibitors, 59, 87
Calcinosis cutis, 116
  chronic renal failure-related, 274t
  CREST syndrome-related, 160, 161f
  metastatic, 116-117
Calciphylaxis, 115, 117, 117f
Calcipotriene, as psoriasis treatment, 53
Cancer. *See also specific types of cancer*
  cutaneous manifestations of, 252-259, 312-318
    alopecia, 395
    calcinosis cutis, 117
    ichthyosis, 32, 34t
    leukocytoclastic vasculitis, 106
    lichen planus, 86

Cancer *(Continued)*
    multiple dermatofibromas, 310
    panniculitis-like lesions, 140-141, 141f
  dermatomyositis-related, 162
  retinoid prophylaxis and treatment for, 395
Candida, as panniculitis causal organism, 140
Candida albicans
  culture medium for, 22-23
  as cutaneous candidiasis causal organism, 221
  as diaper dermatitis causal organism, 404
  Hailey-Hailey disease-exacerbating effect of, 35
  as pustular bacterid causal organism, 78
Candidiasis, 221-222
  antibiotics as risk factor for, 97
  biologic therapy-related, 233
  clinical presentations of, 221, 221f, 221t
  diabetes-related, 262
  as granuloma cause, 90t
  in HIV-infected individuals, 226f, 231
  as leukocytoclastic vasculitis cause, 105
  mucocutaneous
    adult-onset chronic, 222
    in HIV-infected individuals, 280
  neonatal, 82
  as onychomycosis cause, 220
  in organ transplant recipients, 231
  oropharyngeal, in HIV-infected individuals, 282, 282f
Cantharidin, 185, 186f, 186t, 187, 474
Cao gió, 435
Capillaroscopy, nail fold, 468, 471
Captopril, 73t, 443f
Carbamazepine, 98-99, 147
Carbuncles, differentiated from furuncles, 189
Carcinoid/carcinoid syndromes, 253, 259, 259f
  metastatic, 341
Carcinoma
  erysipelatoides, 339, 342f
  metastatic, 15f
  telangiectaticum, 339
Carmustine, as mycosis fungoides treatment, 333
β-Carotene, as pigmentation disorder cause, 101t
Carotenemia, 262, 267
Carotenoderma, 290, 291f
Carpal tunnel syndrome, amyloidosis-related, 112-113
Carrión, Daniel, 473
Carrión's disease, 473
Casal's necklace, 288, 289f
Castration, culturally-sanctioned, 438
Cat hookworms, 234
Cataracts
  congenital, 402
  neurofibromatosis-related, 39
Cats
  mites of, 24, 246-247, 248
  as sporotrichosis vectors, 224
Cat-scratch disease/fever, 90t, 225, 231, 473
CD (cluster designation) nomenclature, in cell immunophenotyping, 336-337, 336t
Cell-mediated immunity, in lepromatous leprosy, 202
Cellophane tape preparations
  of animal mites, 24
  as tinea versicolor diagnostic test, 23, 24f
Cellulitis
  bacterial skin cultures of, 27
  coccidioidomycosis-related, 229
  dissecting, of the scalp, 434
  pseudomonal, 192
  staphylococcal, 188
  streptococcal, 188
Central nervous system tumors, neurofibromatosis-related, 38-39
Cephalosporins, adverse cutaneous reactions to, 81, 98t
Cervarix human papillomavirus vaccine, 184
Cervical cancer, 182, 184
Chagas' disease. *See* Trypanosomiasis, American
Chanarin-Dorfman syndrome, 33t

Chancre
  syphilitic (Hunterian), 24-25, 196-197, 196f, 282, 474-475
  tuberculous, 209
Chancroid, 434
Cheilitis
  actinic, 312, 314t, 318, 372
  angular, 282, 288
  granulomatous, 90t
Chemical peeling, 314t, 364
Chemokines, in urticaria, 167
Chemotherapy
  as alopecia cause, 97, 147
  contraindication during pregnancy, 185
  as mycosis fungoides treatment, 333-335
Cheyletiella mites, 24, 246-247, 247f, 248
Chickenpox (varicella), 178-179, 180t
Chiggers (sand fleas), 237, 237f
Chigoes, 237
Child abuse
  cutaneous signs of, 449-450, 450f
  misdiagnosis of, 408
CHILD syndrome, 33t
Children, 404-408. See also Infants; Neonates
  atopic dermatitis in, 58-59, 58f
  kwashiorkor in, 287, 288f
  leprosy in, 201
  molluscum contagiosum in, 187
  photodermatoses differential diagnosis in, 122
  roseola infantum in, 174, 174f
  seborrheic dermatitis in, 61, 61f
  sun exposure protection for, 354
  tinea capitis in, 217, 218f
  unilateral laterothoracic exanthem in, 173-174, 173f
  urticaria in, 166, 166f
  urticaria pigmentosa in, 169f
  wart treatment in, 187
  warts in, 182
Chimpanzee, as Mycobacterium leprae (leprosy) reservoir, 201
Chlorhexidine gluconate, 366
Chloroquine, as pigmentation disorder cause, 101t, 128, 134
Chlorpromazine, as blue-gray pigmentation cause, 134
Cholestasis, 464-465
Cholesterol emboli, 451
Chondrodermatitis nodularis helicis, 372
Chondrodysplasia punctata, 30, 33t
Chromium, as allergic contact dermatitis cause, 453f
Chromomycosis (chromoblastomycosis), 90t, 224-225, 226, 226f
Chronic suppressive therapy, for herpes simplex virus infections, 176-177
Chrysoderma, 134
Churg-Strauss syndrome, 105t, 107-109
  BEAN SAP mnemonic for, 110f
  differentiated from Wegener's granulomatosis, 108, 109t
Ciguatera poisoning, 474
Cimetidine, as ichthyosis cause, 32, 34t
Circumcision
  female, 438
  male, 438
Cirrhosis, 267, 467t
  primary biliary, 86, 464-465
Cisapride, interaction with antifungal agents, 223
Civatte bodies, 87
Clam digger's itch, 239
Clark's levels, of melanoma, 323
Clofazimine
  adverse cutaneous effects of, 34f, 34t, 101t, 134, 206
  as leprosy treatment, 205-206
Clonoorchis sinensis, 267
Clostridium perfringens, as gangrene causal organism, 445-446

Clothing
  as atopic dermatitis cause, 59
  sun-protective, 354
Clubbing, 467-468, 467t
Coagulation factor abnormalities, 444
  migratory superficial thrombophlebitis associated with, 254
Coal tar preparations, as psoriasis treatment, 53, 389-390
Cobalamin deficiency, 288
Coccidioidomycosis, 90t, 135-136, 224, 227, 229, 229f, 231, 432-433, 433f
  as bioterrorism agent, 233
Cochineal, 475, 475f
Cockayne's syndrome, 123-124t
Coin rubbing, 435
Colchicine, as alopecia cause, 147
Cold injury, as panniculitis cause, 139-140
"Cold sores," 175
Collagen
  congenital abnormalities of, 11, 11f
  type I, 11
  type III, 11
  type VII, 10t
  type VII antibodies, 11
  type XVII, 10t
Collagen vascular diseases, as dermatologic emergency, 446
Collagenoma, eruptive, 308, 308f
Collagenosis, reactive perforating, 274-275, 276, 394
"Collodion baby," 32, 35
Colloid milium, 114, 125
Colon cancer, 106, 257, 270, 339-340
Colorado tick fever, 241, 248, 249-250t
Columbus, Christopher, 195
Comedones, 18-19, 19f
Complement abnormalities, 141, 170
Compound 606, 475
Compulsions, 456
Condyloma acuminata, 182t, 183f
  differentiated from condylomata lata, 197-198
  HIV infection-related, 283-284
Condylomata lata, 197-198, 198f
C1 esterase deficiency, 170
Congenital bullous ichthyosiform erythroderma. See Hyperkeratosis, epidermolytic
Congenital ichthyosiform erythroderma, 30, 31t, 32, 32f
Congenital rubella syndrome, 402
Congenital varicella syndrome, 401
Congo floor maggots, 236
Conjunctivitis, Reiter's disease-related, 80-81
Connective tissue diseases
  autoimmune, 156-165, 468
  lichen planus associated with, 86
  mixed, 162-163
Conradi-Hünermann disease, 33t
Conradi's syndrome, 32
Contact dermatitis, 16f, 64-69
  allergic, 64-65, 73
    diagnosis of, 25, 66-68, 66f, 67t, 68f, 73
    differentiated from irritant contact dermatitis, 64t, 66, 67-68
    management of, 68-69
    occupational exposure-related, 452, 453f
    poison ivy-related, 20
    topical nitrogen mustard-related, 334
  differential diagnosis of, 68
  distribution of rash in, 65-66, 65t
  irritant, 64-65, 67
    differentiated from allergic contact dermatitis, 64t, 66
    management of, 68-69
    occupational exposure-related, 452, 452f, 454
  lichenoid, 87
  photoallergic, 119f
  topical steroids-related, 362
Coproporphyria, 102, 122

Corneocytes, 6
Corpuscular nerve receptors, 12
Corticosteroids
  acne-exacerbating effect of, 153t
  as Churg-Strauss syndrome treatment, 109
  as generalized pustular psoriasis cause, 78
  as gout treatment, 116
  as granuloma annulare treatment, 94-95
  as hypopigmentation cause, 128
  as mycosis fungoides treatment, 333
  as psoriasis treatment, 53
  as pustular acneiform eruption cause, 81
  topical, 358-363
    absorption of, 358-359
    addiction to, 362
    in combination with anti-infective products, 360
    potency of, 358, 359-360, 359t, 363
    side effects of, 360-362, 361f, 361t, 362f
  as urticaria treatment, 170
Cosmetic fillers, as granuloma cause, 90t, 91-92, 91t, 92f
Cosmetics, adverse cutaneous effects of, 65t, 435
Co-trimoxazole, as pustular eruption cause, 81
Cowden's syndrome, 256-257, 256t, 257f
Coxsackie viruses, 172-173, 174
Crabs (pubic lice), 245-246
"Cradle cap," 61, 61f
"Creeping eruption," 234, 234f, 235t
CREST syndrome, 160, 161f
Crohn's disease, 90t
Crowe's sign, 37
Crusts, 16, 17f
Cryoglobulinemia, mixed, 107
Cryoglobulins, 106-107
Cryosurgery, 314t, 364, 371-373
  for warts, 186t
"Cryptic bites," 247-248
Cryptococcosis, 140, 140f, 224, 230-232, 231t, 232f
Cultural dermatology, 435-439
Curettage, 314t
Curth's postulates, 252
Cushing's disease, 264, 264f
Cushing's syndrome, 261, 264f
Cyclophosphamide
  pigmentation effects of, 132
  as Wegener's granulomatosis treatment, 109
Cycloserine, as tuberculosis treatment, 211
Cyclosporine
  interaction with antifungal agents, 223
  as psoriasis treatment, 53
Cyproheptadine, as cold urticaria treatment, 170
Cysticercosis, 235t
Cysticercosis cutis, 446
Cysts, 14, 16f
  epidermoid, 256t
  in children, 406
  inclusion, 267, 270
  lymphatic, 304
  myxoid (mucous), 115-116, 372, 472
  trichilemmal, 16f
Cytochrome P-450 3A4, inhibition of, 222
Cytokeratins, 8
Cytomegalovirus infections, 172, 285-286
  in HIV-infected individuals, 281t
  neonatal/congenital, 400, 402

D

Dactylitis, blistering distal, 190-191, 191f
Danazol, as hereditary angioedema prophylaxis, 170
Dandruff, 55, 61
  "walking," 246-247
Dapsone
  as leprosy treatment, 205-206
  side effects of, 205-206
Darier's disease, 35-36, 36f, 54
  nail findings in, 469t
  as onychomycosis mimic, 220
  treatment for, 394, 395-396
Darier's sign, 168, 169f

Darier-White disease. *See* Darier's disease
Delusions
  definition of, 456
  of parasitosis, 240, 456-457, 457f, 464
Demeclocyline, phototoxic reactions to, 103, 103f
Demodex mites, 235t, 240, 240f
Dengue virus, 173, 249-250t
Denileukin diftitix, 335
Dental amalgrams, mercury-containing, 84-85
Deodorants
  as contact dermatitis cause, 65t
  differentiated from antiperspirants, 475
Depigmentation. *See also* Hypopigmentation
  albinism-related, 126
  chemical-related, 128
  definition of, 19
  leukoderma-related, 126-130
Deposition disorders, 112-117
Depression, isotretinoin-related, 151
Dermabrasion, 314t, 364
Dermal-epidermal junction, in epidermolysis
    bullosa, 9f
Dermatitis, 57-63
  actinic
    chronic, 120
    in HIV-infected individuals, 284
  artefacta/factitious, 457-458, 458f
  atopic. *See* Atopic dermatitis
  autosensitization, 62, 62f
  child abuse-related, 450
  contact. *See* Contact dermatitis
  cruris pustulosa et atrophicans, 434
  definition of, 57, 59
  diaper, 363, 404
  exfoliative, 59, 62-63
    adverse drug reaction-related, 97-98
  hand, 60, 60f, 219, 395, 452-453, 453f, 454
  herpetiformis, 73f, 76f, 257, 272-273, 273f
  nummular
    misdiagnosed as tinea corporis, 405
    phototherapy for, 387-388t
  papulosa nigra, 434
  pellagra-related, 288, 289f
  perioral, 148, 153, 291f
  periorificial, 362, 404, 407
  photocontact, 125
  radiation-related, 436
  seborrheic, 50, 54-55
    in adults, 61
    in children, 61, 61f
    differentiated from psoriasis of the scalp, 55
    in HIV-infected individuals, 280, 281t
    location of, 20-21
    phototherapy for, 387-388t
    in skin of color, 430
  secondary staphylococcal infections of, 188,
    190
  treatment for, 59
  "two-pajamas treatment," 60
Dermatofibroma, 309-310, 309f, 310f
  cryosurgical treatment for, 372
Dermatofibrosarcoma, 309
Dermatofibrosarcoma protuberans, 313t, 342,
  344, 374
Dermatographism, 464
Dermatoheliosis, 390, 394, 394t
Dermatology
  "father" of, 474
  terminology of, 14, 19
Dermatomal skin lesions, 20
Dermatomyopathies, inflammatory, autoantibodies
    associated with, 164-165t
Dermatomyositis, 161-162, 162f, 254,
  254f, 468
  amyopathic, 161, 162
  cancer associated with, 254, 259
  as dermatologic emergency, 446-447
  diseases associated with, 162
  as ichthyosis cause, 34t
  pediatric, 405, 405f

Dermatophyte infections. *See* Fungal infections
Dermatophyte Test Media (DTM), 22-23, 216
Dermatophytes. *See also* Fungal infections; Fungi
  culture media for, 22-23, 216
  definition of, 216
Dermatophytid reactions, 219, 219f
Dermatophytosis, in HIV-infected individuals, 281t
Dermatoses
  acquired perforating, of chronic renal failure,
    274-275, 276, 277f
  digital, 331
  HIV infection-related, 280
  plantar, juvenile, 404, 404f
  zoonotic, 247-248
Dermatosis papulosa nigra, 430
Dermis
  adventitial, 10
  blistering diseases of, 9, 10t
  effect of topical steroids on, 361
  in epidermolysis bullosa, 9f
  hereditary diseases of, 8-9
  papillary, 7f, 10
  periadnexal, 7f, 10
  reticular, 7f, 10
  structure and functions of, 6, 7f, 8f, 10-12
Dermographism, 16f, 166, 167f, 168
Dermopathy
  diabetic, 262
  nephrogenic fibrosing, 102
Dermoscopy, 322
Desmocollin, 9t, 71f
Desmoglein, 9t, 71f
Desmoid tumors, 256t, 270
Desmoplakin, 9t, 71f
Desmosomes (dense bodies), 6
  damage to, 9t
Dessication, epidermal prevention of, 8
deVeuster, Damien, 476
Diabetes mellitus
  acanthosis nigricans associated with, 260
  bacterial infections associated with, 261-262
  blastomycosis associated with, 228
  bullous eruption of, 74
  candidiasis associated with, 221-222
  fungal infections associated with, 262
  lichen planus associated with, 86
  lipodystrophy associated with, 141
  necrobiosis lipoidica associated with, 260,
    261f, 266
  as tuberculosis risk factor, 262
  xanthomas associated with, 265
Diabeticorum, bullous, 74
Diagnostic techniques, 22-27
Dialysis patients, 274-275, 275f, 277, 464
Diarrhea, pellagra-related, 288
Diazepam, adverse cutaneous reactions to, 100
"Dimple" (Fitzpatrick) sign, 309
Dirofilaria tenuis, 236
Diuretics, thiazide, 73t, 101
Dixyrazine, as ichthyosis cause, 32, 34t
Dog hookworms, 234
Dog tapeworms, 240
Dogs, mites of, 24, 246-247, 248
Down syndrome, as candidiasis risk factor, 221-222
Doxycycline, as vesiculobullous eruption cause, 73t
Dracunculiasis, 235t, 434
Dracunculus medinensis, 236
DRESS syndrome, 444
Dressings, contaminated, 233
Drowning, urticaria as risk factor for, 167
Drug eruptions, 97-104. *See also* specific drugs
  AIDS/HIV-related, 98
  allergic, 97, 166
  bullous, 73, 73t
  as dermatologic emergency, 442-444, 449
  exfoliative dermatitis, 63
  fixed, 97, 100, 133, 133t
  in HIV-infected individuals, 281t, 283
  immunologic, 97
  lichen planus-like, 87t

Drug eruptions *(Continued)*
  lichenoid, 87t, 88, 101
  life-threatening, 97
  morbilliform, 174
  nonimmunologic, 97
  photoallergic, 119f
  photosensitive, 125
  phototoxic, 103, 118f
  pustular, 81
  secondary syphilis as mimic of, 199
  serum sickness-like, 100
  as vesiculobullous disorders mimic, 75
Drug interactions, 97
Drug intolerance, 97
Drugs. *See also specific drugs*
  as alopecia cause, 147
  as ichthyosis cause, 32, 34t
  as leukocytoclastic vasculitis cause, 105
  photosensitive reactions to, 119t, 120
  with pigmentation-stimulating activity, 132
Dry lips, retinoid therapy-related, 397
Dry skin. *See* Xerosis
Dukes' disease (Fourth disease), 477
Dyskeratosis congenita, 258t
Dysmorphophobia, 457
Dysplasia
  ectodermal, 408
  osseous, 38
  sphenoid, 37

E

Ear piercing, 68, 307f, 431f, 438
Ecchymoses, acupuncture-related, 435-436
Echinococcosis, 235t
Echinococcus granulosus, 240
ECHO viruses, 173
Ecthyma
  bacterial skin cultures of, 27
  contagiosum (orf), 180, 181f
  differentiated from ecthyma gangrenosum,
    192-193
  gangrenosum, 192-193, 193f
  streptococcal, 190-191, 191f
Ectothrix infections, tinea capitis-related, 218
Eczema
  definition of, 57, 59
  differentiated from Hailey-Hailey disease, 35
  dyshidrotic, 16f
  herpeticum, 177-178
  as hypopigmentation cause, 129
  lesions of, 15f
  nummular, 60, 61f
  in skin of color, 430
Edema
  acute hemorrhagic of infancy, 106, 106f
  laryngeal, beta-lactam antibiotics-related, 100
  periorbital, 161
Ehlers-Danos syndrome, 11, 11f
Ehrlich, Paul, 475
Ehrlichiosis, 248, 249-250t
Ekbom syndrome, 457
Elastolysis, middermal, 125
Elastosis, solar, 125
Elderly persons, angiosarcoma in, 340, 340f
Electrocautery, 368
Electrocoagulation, 368
Electrodissection, 368
Electrofulguration, 368
Electrosurgery, 368-369
Elephantiasis, 236, 236f
Emboli, cholesterol, 451
Emergencies, dermatologic, 441-452
Enanthems, differentiated from exanthems, 172
Encephalitis, 249-250t
  equine, 172
  tick-borne, 248
Endocarditis, 467, 467t
  culture-negative, 473
  as leukocytoclastic vasculitis cause, 105

Endocrinologic disease, cutaneous manifestations of, 132, 465
Endometrial cancer, 269
Endothelin-1, 132
Endothrix infections, tinea capitis-related, 217, 218f
Entamoeba histolytica infections, 238
Enterobius vermicularis infections, 235
Enteropathy, gluten-sensitive, 76, 272-273, 273f
Enterovirus infections, 172-173, 174
  neonatal, 400, 402
Environmental disorders, as dermatologic emergency, 442, 449-451
Enzyme deficiencies, 97
Enzyme-linked immunosorbent assay (ELISA), 27, 73
Eosinophilia
  Churg-Strauss syndrome-related, 107, 107t, 109t
  DRESS syndrome-related, 444
Eosinophils, in chronic idiopathic urticaria, 169
Ephelides, 15f, 125, 299
  definition of, 128
  differentiated from lentigines/liver spots, 130, 299
  as melanoma risk factor, 320
  neurofibromatosis-related, 37, 126, 131
Epidermal inclusions, 16f
Epidermis
  in blistering diseases, 8
  effect of topical steroids on, 361
  structure and functions of, 6, 7f, 8, 8f
Epidermodysplasia verruciformis, 183, 184f, 185
Epidermolysis bullosa, 6, 43, 74, 474
  acquisita, 10t, 77
  in children, 406
  classification and inheritance of, 43
  congenital, 11
    recessive dystrophic, 11, 11f
  dermal epidermal junction in, 9f
  diagnosis of, 46-47, 47f
  dystrophic, 8-9, 9f, 43, 44f, 45-46, 46f, 74, 74t
  hemidesmosomal, 9f
  junctional, 9f, 43, 44-45, 44f, 45f, 74
    Herlitz type, 74t
    non-Herlitz type, 74t
    with pyloric atresia, 74t
  Kindler syndrome subtype of, 46
  simplex, 8, 9f, 43-44, 44f, 74, 74t
    Dowling-Meara type, 74t
    with muscular dystrophy, 74t
    Ogna type, 74t
    with pyloric atresia, 74t
  subtypes of, 74t
Epidermophyton, 216
Epidermophyton floccosum, 471
Epilepsy
  neurofibromatosis-related, 38
  Sturge-Weber syndrome-related, 41
  tuberous sclerosis-related, 39
Epiloia, 39. *See also* Tuberous sclerosis
Epinephrine, as local anesthetic, 365-366, 370
Epithelioma, 257
Epstein-Barr virus infections, 172-173, 174
  congenital/neonatal, 400, 402-403
  in HIV-infected individuals, 280, 281t
  as papular acrodermatitis of childhood cause, 173
Ergot poisoning, 444
Erosio interdigitalis blastomycetica, 221t
Erosio interdigitalis blastomycetica chronica, diabetes-related, 262
Erosions, 17, 17f
Erosive pustular dermatosis, of the scalp, 125
Erysipelas (St. Anthony's fire), 190-191, 191f, 192
Erythema
  ab igne, 133, 133t
  annular
    in children, 407
    as dermatologic emergency indicator, 445t

Erythema *(Continued)*
  chronicum migrans, 192f, 248
  in darker skin, 430
  diffuse, as dermatologic emergency indicator, 444-445
  dyschromicum perstans, 133, 133t
  elevatum diutinum, 110, 110f
  generalized pustular psoriasis-related, 80f
  gyratum repens, 20, 255
  induratum, 137f
    of Bazin, 136
    of Whitfield, 136
  infectiosum, 173, 173f, 477
  irritant contact dermatitis-related, 64
  marginatum, 20
  multiforme, 73t
    blastomycosis-related, 229
    coccidioidomycosis-related, 229
    drug-related, 97
    histoplasmosis-related, 229
    major, 99, 442
    secondary syphilis as mimic of, 199
    sporotrichosis-related, 224-225
  necrolytic, 74-75
    acral, 75
    migratory, 253, 253f
  nodosum, 15f, 135-136, 135t, 285-286
    biopsy of, 136, 137f
    blastomycosis-related, 229
    coccidioidomycosis-related, 229
    drug-related, 101
    histoplasmosis-related, 229
    leprosum, 201, 205f
    sarcoidosis-related, 92-93
    sporotrichosis-related, 224-225
    tinea pedis-related, 219
    treatment for, 136
    underlying conditions associated with, 135-136
  palmar, 267, 267t
  periungual, 447
  persistent, 257
  toxic, with pustules, 81
  toxicum neonatorum, 82
  violaceous, dermatomyositis-related, 161-162, 162f, 254, 254f
Erythematous, definition of, 19
Erythrasma, diagnostic techniques for, 22, 23f
Erythroblastosis fetalis, 401
Erythroderma, 62
  bullous congenital ichthyosiform, 74
  congenital bullous ichthyosiform. *See* Hyperkeratosis, epidermolytic
  diffuse exfoliative, 449
Erythromelalgia, 258
Erythromycin, 81, 119t
Erythropoietic protoporphyria, 114
Escherichia coli infections, as paronychia cause, 471
Esophageal dysfunction, CREST syndrome-related, 160
Estrogen therapy, as hyperpigmentation cause, 132
Estrogens, porphyria cutanea tarda-exacerbating effect of, 102
Ethambutol, as tuberculosis treatment, 211, 211t
Ethanol, porphyria cutanea tarda-exacerbating effect of, 102
Ethionamide, 205, 211
Etretinate, anticarcinogenic activity of, 395
Eumelanin, 127
Exanthems
  differentiated from enanthems, 172
  maculopapular, 97
  morbilliform, 97
  subitum, 174, 174f
  viral, 172-174, 477
    unilateral laterothoracic, 173-174, 173f
Excoriations, 17, 18f
  neurotic, 459, 459f
Exostosis, 472, 472f
Extracorporeal photochemotherapy, 391-392

F

Fabry's disease, 277, 302, 303
Facial nerve, temporal branch of, surgery-related injury to, 369-370, 369f, 370f
Facial paralysis, 61
Famciclovir, 176, 177t, 180t
Familial atypical multiple mole melanoma-pancreatic cancer (FAMM) syndrome, 259
Familial dysplastic mole syndrome (FDMS), as melanoma risk factor, 319-320
Fasciitis
  necrotizing, 190, 192, 444, 445-446, 446f, 447
  nodular, 308
Fat
  excess deposition of, 288
  subcutaneous (subcutis), 6, 7f, 10, 13
Fat deficiency, 288
Father Damien, 476
Favre-Racouchot syndrome, 125, 148, 155
Favus infections, 217-218
Fetus, harlequin, 30, 31t, 32, 33-34, 33f
Fibroblasts, 11
Fibroepithelioma of Pinkus, 315
Fibrokeratoma, digital, 307-308, 308f
  acquired, 472
Fibroma, periungual, 39-40, 40f, 408, 472
Fibromatosis, infantile digital, 308-309
Fibrosarcoma, 313t
Fibrosis, nephrogenic systemic, 102, 277-278
"Fibrous papule of the nose," 310
Fibrous tumors, of the skin, 305-310
Fibroxanthoma, atypical, 313t, 342-343
Fifth disease, 477
Filaggrin, 57-58
Filariasis/filarial infections, 235-236, 235t, 249-250t, 434
Filatow-Dukes disease, 477
Finger pebbles, 274t
Fingertip unit (FTU) application, of topical steroids, 360, 360f, 362
Fire ant stings, 243
Fissures, 17, 17f
Fitzpatrick ("dimple") sign, 309
Fitzpatrick skin type, as melanoma risk factor, 319-320
Fixed drug eruptions, 97, 100, 133, 133t
Fleas
  bites of, 241-242, 246f, 247, 250
  as disease vectors, 249-250t
  infestations of, 246, 477
"Flesh moles," 430
"Flesh-eating bacteria." *See* Fasciitis, necrotizing
Flour, as contact urticaria cause, 65f
Fluconazole, 218, 222, 222t
Fluke infection. *See* Schistosomiasis
Fluorescent antibody microscopy, for syphilis diagnosis, 24-25
Fluorescent treponemal antibody-absorption test, for syphilis diagnosis, 25
Fluorides, as pustular eruption cause, 81
Fluoroquinolones, as vesiculobullous eruption cause, 73t
5-Fluorouracil, 120, 132, 314t
Fluoxetine, 459
Folk medicine, 474
Follicular carcinoma, 313t
Folliculitis, 16f
  decalvans, 81
  eosinophilic, 285-286
    HIV infection-related, 281t, 283, 283f
    Malassezia-related, 220
    occupational exposure-related, 452
    pseudomonal, 190, 192-193
    staphylococcal, 261-262
Food allergens, 59, 65f
Forehead fibromatous plaques, 39, 40f
Foreign bodies, as granuloma cause, 90-91, 90t, 91t, 92
Fourth disease, 477
Fox-Fordyce disease, 394

Fragrances
    as contact dermatitis cause, 64t, 65t
    photoallergic reactions to, 119t
Freckles. *See Ephelides*
Freud, Sigmund, 62
Fundoscopic examination, in tuberous sclerosis
    patients, 40
Fungal infections. *See also specific fungi*
    deep, 224-233
        opportunistic, 224t, 228, 230-233
        subcutaneous, 224-227, 224t
        systemic or respiratory, 224t, 227-230
    as dermatologic emergencies, 444-446
    diabetes-associated, 262
    diagnostic techniques for, 22-27
    as erythema nodosum cause, 135-136
    as granuloma cause, 90t
    HIV infection-related, 280, 281t
    as leukocytoclastic vasculitis cause, 105
    superficial, 216-223
Fungi
    dematiaceous, 225, 231
    dimorphic, 224, 231
Furocoumarins, 132, 390, 391f
Furosemide, 73t, 87t, 102
Furuncles, 187f, 188-189, 189f
    differentiated from carbuncles, 189
Furunculosis, 214
Fusariosis, 224, 230, 231
Fusarium infections, 140, 219-220, 232-233
Futcher's lines, 428, 428f

G

Gamma-globulin, as urticaria cause, 100
Gangrene, 445-446
Gardasil, 184
Gardner-Diamond syndrome, 458
Gardner's syndrome, 256-257, 256t, 267, 270,
    270f
Garlic, 290
Gastrointestinal cancer, 253, 257, 269
Gastrointestinal disease, 267-273
Gatifloxacin, as tuberculosis treatment, 211
Gene therapy, for melanoma, 329-330
Generalized pustular psoriasis of von Zumbusch,
    78, 80f
Genitalia, culturally-sanctioned surgical alterations
    of, 438
Genitourinary cancer, 347
Geographic tongue, 405, 406f
Gianotti-Crosti syndrome, 173, 173f
Giant cell tumors, of the tendon sheath, 310,
    310f
Ginkgo, 290
Ginseng, 290
Glaucoma, Sturge-Weber syndrome-related, 41
Glioma, 38
    optic, 37-38
Glomerulonephritis, segmental necrotizing, 105
Glomus tumors, 472
    of Sucquet-Hoyer canal, 303
Glossitis, 253
Glossodynia, 460
Gloves
    for occupational skin disease prevention, 454
    rubber, as allergic contact dermatitis cause,
        454, 455f
Glucagonoma syndrome, 75, 253, 253f, 270
Glucocorticoids, excess of, 264
Gluten-sensitive enteropathy, 76, 272-273, 273f
Goeckerman therapy, 389-390
Gold, adverse cutaneous reactions to, 99-100,
    101, 101t, 133t, 134
Golgi-Mazzoni corpuscles, 12
Gonorrhea, 25, 199, 475
Gottron's papules, 161, 162, 254, 254f, 405,
    405f, 447
Gottron's sign, 161

Gout, 115, 116
gp100, as melanoma marker, 324
Graft-*versus*-host disease, lichenoid, 85, 88
Granuloma/granulomatous diseases, 90-96
    actinic (annular elastolytic), 90t, 95, 95f,
        125
    annulare, 20, 90t, 94-95, 94f, 96
        in HIV-infected individuals, 281t, 284-285
        misdiagnosed as tinea corporis, 405
    eosinophilic, 473
    faciale, 110-111, 110f
    foreign-body, 90-91, 90t, 92, 435-436
    gravidarum, 303
    immune, 90
    inguinale, 90t, 230, 434
    Majocchi's, 221
    multiforme, 434
    occupational exposure-related, 452
    pyogenic, 303, 303f, 406-407, 472
        cryosurgical treatment for, 372
    "swimming pool," 213, 213f
Granulomatous slack skin disease, 332, 332f
Graphite, as granuloma cause, 91f
Graves' disease, 262, 264, 285-286
    pretibial myxedema associated with, 114-115,
        262, 263f
Green nails, 471, 471f
Griseofulvin, 222t, 223
    interaction with cyclosporine, 223
    as tinea capitis treatment, 144-145, 218-219,
        405
Grouped skin lesions, 20
Guinea worm, 434
Gumma, 200, 209t
Günther's disease, 476
Gynecomastia, 267
Gyrate skin lesions, 20

H

Haber's syndrome, as ichthyosis cause, 34t
"Habit tic" disorder, 472
Hailey-Hailey disease, 34-35, 35f, 74
Hair
    depigmentation of, 127
    as granuloma cause, 90t, 91t
    in people of color, 432
Hair dye, as contact dermatitis cause, 64t,
    65t, 68
Hair follicles, 7f
Hair loss. *See Alopecia*
Hair removal techniques
    effect on hair growth, 477
    lasers, 383, 383t, 384-385, 384t
Hair shafts
    defects of, 408
    lice infestations on, 24, 25f
Hair transplantation, 143, 364, 436
Half-and-half nails, 274t, 275, 275f, 467t, 468,
    468f
Hallucinations, 456
Halogenoderma, 81
Halogens, acne-exacerbating effect of, 153t
Hamartoma
    miniliformis, 434
    retinal, tuberous sclerosis-related, 40
Hand
    adverse cutaneous drug reactions on, 102
    dermatitis of, 60, 60f, 452-453, 453f, 454
Hand, foot, and mouth disease, 172-173, 172f,
    180, 181f
Hand-Schüller-Christian disease, 473
Hansen, Gerhard Armeuer, 201
Hansen's disease. *See Leprosy*
Haptens, carrier proteins of, 477
Hartnup's disease, 75, 123-124t
Head and neck cancer, as leukocytoclastic
    vasculitis cause, 106
Head lice, 24, 25f, 245-246

Hearing loss, neurofibromatosis-related, 39
Heat stroke, 449
Heerfordt's syndrome, 93-94
Helicobacter pylori, 337-338
Heliotrope sign, 162, 162f, 254, 254f, 447
Helminthic infections, as leukocytoclastic vasculitis
    cause, 105
Hemangioblastoma, von Hippel-Lindau
    syndrome-related, 41
Hemangioma
    of infancy, 301, 301f, 303
    infantile capillary, 448, 449f
    lobular capillary, 406
    residua of, 301, 302f
    treatment for, 448
Hemangiopericytoma, 313t
Hematologic disorders, pruritus associated with,
    465
Hematoma
    acupuncture-related, 435-436
    Ehlers-Danlos syndrome-related, 11f
    subungual, 469-470, 470f
Hematuria, Hench-Schönlein purpura-related,
    106
Hemidesmosomes, 8f
    antibody-induced damage to, 9
Hemoptysis, Wegener's granulomatosus-related,
    108, 109t
Hemorrhage
    gastrointestinal, 268-270, 268t
    splinter, 274t, 467, 467t, 469
Hemorrhagic lesions, differential diagnosis of,
    444
Henna, 438-439, 439f
Henoch-Schönlein purpura, 27, 27f, 105t, 106,
    274, 278, 407
    PAPAH mnemonic for, 106
Hepatitis
    peliosis, 473
    transmission during laser therapy, 381
Hepatitis A, as leukocytoclastic vasculitis cause,
    105
Hepatitis B
    as leukocytoclastic vasculitis cause, 105
    as papular acrodermatitis of childhood cause,
        173
    as scarlet fever-like eruption cause, 173
Hepatitis C
    as leukocytoclastic vasculitis cause, 105
    as lichen planus cause, 86
    as nodular vasculitis cause, 136
    as scarlet fever-like eruption cause, 173
Hepatobiliary disease, 267-268
Hepatomegaly, amyloidosis-related, 112-113
Herbal remedies, cutaneous disorders associated
    with, 290
Hereditary leiomyomatosis/renal cell cancer
    syndrome, 256t, 279t
Hermansky-Pudlak syndrome, 126
Herpes genitalis, 175, 176f, 177
Herpes gestationis, 76-77
Herpes gladiatorum, 177-178
Herpes labialis, 175, 177-178
Herpes simplex virus infections, 16f, 20, 172, 175,
    177-178
    asymptomatic shedding in, 175-176
    diagnosis of, 23, 176
    in HIV-infected individuals, 280, 281t
    initial, 175
    neonatal, 82, 178, 400-401, 400f, 402
    primary, 175
    recurrent, 175, 176f
    treatment for, 176-177, 177t
Herpes simplex virus-1 infections, 175-176, 401
Herpes simplex virus-2 infections, 175-176, 177,
    401
Herpes zoster, 16f, 20, 172f, 178-179, 179f, 180t
    ophthalmicus, 180
Herpes zoster vaccine, 180
Herpesviruses, 172

Hidradenitis suppurativa, 154, 154f
Highly active antiretroviral therapy (HAART), cutaneous side effects of, 141, 285-286, 285f
"Highway 90 disease," 238
Hindi women, *bindi* of, 437
Hirsutism, 264
Histamine, 97, 167, 169
Histamine-releasing factor, 167
Histidinemia, 129t
Histiocytes
  in granulomas, 90
  parasitized, 230, 230t
Histiocytosis
  Langerhans cell, 406, 406f, 473
  malignant, 257
Histiocytosis X, 473
Histiocytoma, malignant fibrous, 343
Histone deactylase inhibitors, 335
Histoplasmosis, 224, 227-229, 229f, 230-231, 231t, 233
  African, 434
  as granuloma cause, 90t
  in HIV-infected individuals, 281t
Hives. See Urticaria
Hodgkin's disease, 257, 258, 271, 331, 336
  Ann Arbor classification staging system for, 335
  histologic classes of, 335-336
  pruritus associated with, 465
Homeopathic remedies, cutaneous disorders associated with, 290
Homocystinuria, 129t
Homogentisic acid deficiency, as dyspigmentation cause, 133-134
Hookworms, 19, 234, 234f
Hot flashes, 11-12
Hot tub folliculitis, 193, 193f
HTLV-1 virus, 337
Human herpesviruses, 172-173, 175
Human immunodeficiency virus (HIV) infection, 280-286
  fungal infections associated with, 231, 231t
  herpes genitalis as risk factor for, 177
  as ichthyosis cause, 34t
  as leukocytoclastic vasculitis cause, 105
  nail findings in, 470
  neonatal, 400, 402-403
  pruritus associated with, 464
  seborrheic dermatitis associated with, 55
  as skin cancer risk factor, 312
  as syphilis coinfection, 199
  transmission during laser therapy, 381
Human papillomavirus infections. See also Warts
  congenital/neonatal, 402-403
  in HIV-infected individuals, 280, 281t
  latent/subclinical, 184
  transmission during laser therapy, 381
Human papillomavirus vaccine, 184
Hunter, Jonathan, 475
Hutchinson's freckle, 327
Hutchinson's sign, 180, 327, 329, 470
Hutchinson's triad, 403
Hyacell, mycobacterial infections associated with, 214
Hyalinoses, 112
Hyalinosis cutis et mucosae, 114
Hyaluronic acid, as granuloma cause, 91-92
Hydatid disease, 240
Hydradenitis suppurativa, 264
Hydroa aestivale, 122, 125
Hydroa vacciniforme, 122, 125
Hydroxychloroquine
  as pigmentation disorder cause, 101t, 102f, 128
  as porphyria cutanea tarda treatment, 125
  as pustular eruption cause, 81
  as urticarial vasculitis treatment, 170
Hygroma, cystic, 304, 304f
Hyperglycemia, diabetic, 260
Hypergranulosis, "wedge-shaped," 87

Hyperkeratoses
  epidermolytic, 8, 30, 31t, 33-34, 74
  follicular, 289, 289f
  palmar, 32f
  plantar, obesity-related, 288
  subungual, 52, 80-81, 469
Hyperostosis, SAPHO syndrome-related, 152
Hyperparathyroidism, calcinosis cutis-related, 116
Hyperpigmentation
  adrenocorticotropic hormone-related, 263
  chemical-related, 133t
  chronic renal failure-related, 274t, 275t, 276
  definition of, 19
  discoid lupus erythematosus-related, 158, 158f
  drug-related, 101, 101t, 102f
  in HIV-infected individuals, 281t
  melanoderma, 130-132
  mottled facial, 394
  phototoxic, 120
  postinflammatory, 17, 127, 133, 133t, 134f, 428-429, 429f, 465
    topical tretinoin treatment of, 394-395
  racial variation in, 428
  syphilis-related, 199
  tinea versicolor-related, 220, 220f
Hyperplasia
  angiolymphoid, 303
  sebaceous, 372
Hypertension
  neurofibromatosis-related, 38
  portal venous, 267-268, 268f
Hyperthyroidism, 260, 263
Hypertrichosis
  lanuginosa, 253
  porphyra cutanea tarda-related, 75
Hypervitaminosis A, 289
Hyphae, fungal
  identification of, 22, 23f, 24f
  "mosaic," 216
Hypogonadism, 30, 38
Hypomelanosis of Ito, 129
Hypopigmentation
  chemical-related, 128
  definition of, 19
  discoid lupus erythematosus-related, 158, 158f
  leukoderma-related, 126-130
  postinflammatory, 127, 429, 465
  syphilis-related, 199
  tinea versicolor-related, 220, 220f, 430
Hypotension, beta-lactam antibiotics-related, 100
Hypothyroidism, 262-263, 264, 266, 334

I

Ibuprofen, as vesiculobullous eruption cause, 73t
Ice Man, 436
Ichthyosis, 257
  acquired, 32, 34, 34t, 93f
    in HIV-infected individuals, 281t
  cancer-related, 257
  inherited/congenital, 30, 31t, 32-34, 33t
    prenatal diagnosis of, 33-34
  kava-related, 437
  lamellar, 30, 31t, 32, 33-34, 35
  treatment for, 34-35, 394, 395-396, 397
  vulgaris, 30, 31t, 32f, 33, 35
  X-linked, 30, 31t, 32f, 33-34
"Id" reactions, 62, 62f
Ifluoperazine, as blue-gray pigmentation cause, 134
Immune restoration syndrome, 285-286
Immune surveillance, as epidermal function, 8
Immunobullous diseases, diagnostic tests for, 27
Immunocompromised patients. See also Acquired immunodeficeincy syndrome (AIDS); Human immunodeficiency virus (HIV) infection
  blastomycosis in, 228
  histoplasmosis in, 228, 232
  warts in, 182, 185, 187

Immunofluorescence tests
  direct, 26-27, 27f
    for subacute cutaneous lupus erythematosus diagnosis, 157
    for vesiculobullous disorders diagnosis, 72-73, 72t, 73f, 75
  indirect, 27, 73
Immunoglobulin A, in Henoch-Schönlein disease, 27f
Immunoglobulin E-mediated drug reactions, 27
Immunoglobulin G autoantibodies, detection of, 27
Immunophenotyping, of cells, 336
Immunosuppression. See also Acquired immunodeficiency syndrome (AIDS); Human immunodeficiency virus (HIV) infection; Immunocompromised patients
  photorelated, 125
Immunotherapy, for melanoma, 329
Impetigo, 16f
  bacterial skin cultures of, 27
  of Bockhart, 188
  bullous, 73, 188-189, 188f, 190
  contagiosum, 188
  differentiated from Hailey-Hailey disease, 35
  pediatric, 404
  staphylococcal, 183, 188-189, 188f, 190
  streptococcal, 188, 190, 191f
Incontinentia pigmenti, 74, 82
Infants
  hemangioma in, 301, 301f, 303
  herpes simplex virus infections in, 178
  photodermatoses differential diagnosis in, 122
  roseola infantum in, 174, 174f
  scurvy in, 289
Infection
  chronic renal failure-related, 274t
  as dermatologic emergency, 442
  as granuloma cause, 90t
  as leukocytoclastic vasculitis cause, 105
  as leukoderma cause, 129
  neonatal, 399-403
  occupational exposure-related, 452
  as panniculitis cause, 140, 140f
Infectious diseases, as dermatologic emergency, 444-446
Infestations. See Parasitic infestations
Inflammatory bowel disease, 135-136, 267
Inflammatory disorders, as dermatologic emergency, 442, 447-449
Infundibulofolliculitis, 434
Inherited disorders, 30-36
Injections
  of local anesthetics, 366
  as panniculitis cause, 139-140, 140f
Ink tattoos, 15f
Insect parts, as granuloma cause, 90t
Insect repellents, 250
Insect stings, as urticaria cause, 166, 168
Insects. See also specific insects
  as disease vectors, 248-250
Insulin resistance, 260-261
Insulin-like growth factor, 132
"Interface reaction," 87
Interferon
  contraindication during pregnancy, 185
  as mycosis fungoides treatment, 333-334
  as wart treatment, 186t
Intertrigo, 221t
  diabetes-related, 262
Iodides, 81, 135-136
Iodine, 81
Ipodate sodium, 98t
Iron deficiency, 467t
Irritants, in the workplace, 454
Isolated limb perfusion, as melanoma treatment, 330
Isomorphic response. See Koebner phenomenon
Isoniazid
  adverse cutaneous reactions to, 101
  acne-exacerbating effect, 153t

Isoniazid (Continued)
   lichen planus-like eruptions, 87t
   pustular acneiform eruptions, 81
   interaction with antifungal agents, 223
   as tuberculosis treatment, 211, 211t
Isotretinoin, 393t, 397
   as acne treatment, 150-151
   as alopecia cause, 103
   anticarcinogenic activity of, 395
   oral, 395-396
   photosensitizing effect of, 120
   side effects of, 102, 151-152
   teratogenicity of, 151-152
Itch. See Pruritus
Itraconazole, 218, 222-223, 222t, 225, 228

J

Jarisch-Herxheimer reaction, 97, 197
Jaundice, 267, 267t, 271
Jewelry, as contact dermatitis cause, 65t, 68
Jiggers, 477
Juxtaclavicular beaded lines, 434

K

Kala-azar. See Leishmaniasis
Kallman's syndrome, 30
Kaposi's sarcoma, 280-281, 281t, 282f, 313t, 395
   cryosurgical treatment for, 372
   cryptococcosis as mimic of, 232
   differentiated from acroangiodermatitis, 304
   endemic, 434
   ichthyosis associated with, 257
Kaposi's varicelliform eruption, 177-178
Kasabach-Merritt syndrome, 301-302, 303
Kava dermopathy, 437
Kawasaki disease, 105t, 449
   differentiated from polyarteritis nodosa, 109
Keloids, 305, 306-307, 307f, 434, 436
   cryosurgical treatment for, 372
   definition of, 431
   distinguished from hypertrophic scars, 306,
      307t
   ear piercing-related, 431f
   tretinoin treatment for, 394
Keratinization, disorders of, 29-36, 395-396, 397
Keratinocytes, 6, 8, 8f
   in epidermolysis bullosa, 9f
   multinucleated, 24f
   shedding of, 478
Keratoacanthoma, 257, 313t, 317, 317f
   treatment for, 314t, 372
Keratoderma, 54
Keratoma blennorrhagicum, Reiter's disease-
      related, 80-81
Keratosis
   actinic, 125, 312, 313t, 317-318, 318f
      treatment for, 314t, 318, 372, 394
   follicularis. See Darier's disease
   pilaris, 59, 394, 404
   sebaceous, cryosurgical treatment of, 372
   seborrheic, 306f, 430
      eruptive, 257
Keratotic pits, chronic renal failure-related, 274t
Kerion, 217, 218f, 405
Ketoacidosis, diabetic, 262
Ketoconazole, 222-223, 222t
KID (keratitis-ichthyosis-deafness) syndrome, 33t
Kidney cancer, cutaneous metastases of, 340
Kindler syndrome, 43, 46, 123-124t
Kissing bugs, 248, 249-250t
Klippel-Trénaunay-Parkes-Weber syndrome, 474
Klippel-Trénaunay-Weber syndrome, 302, 474
Koebner phenomenon, 20, 20f
   acupuncture-related, 435-436
   lichen planus-related, 85-86, 86f, 88
   psoriasis-related, 20, 20f, 52
   wart-related, 184

Koebnerization, 86
   Still's disease-related, 163
Koenen's tumors, 39-40, 40f
KOH examination. See Potassium hydroxide
      examination
Kohl, 435
Krause end bulbs, 12
Kwashiorkor, 128, 132, 287, 288f
   differentiated from marasmus, 287
Kyphoscoliosis, 38
Kyrle's disease, 274-275, 276

L

Labial lentigo, 300
Lacy eruptions, 173, 173f
Lamina lucida, 8-10, 44f
Laminin antibodies, 11
Langerhans cell histiocytosis, 406, 406f, 473
Langerhans cells, 6
Langota, 439
Larva currens, 234, 235f
Larva migrans, cutaneous, 234, 234f, 240
Lasers, use in dermatology, 364, 378-385
   for acne vulgaris, 152
   for actinic keratoses, 318
   carbon dioxide lasers, 378-379, 380-381, 380t
   for nevus of Ota, 296-297
   for skin cancer, 314t
   as targeted phototherapy, 389
   for warts, 185-186, 186t, 187
Leiomyomatosis, hereditary, 256t
Leiomyosarcoma, 257, 345
Leishmaniasis, 225, 230-231, 235t, 238, 238f,
      238t, 249-250t, 434
   as granuloma cause, 90t
Lenticular opacity, juvenile posterior subcapsular,
      38
Lentigines. See Lentigo
Lentigo, 299. See also Ephelides
   definition of, 130
   differentiated from freckles, 130
   labial, 300
   maligna, 313t
      cryosurgical treatment for, 372
      delineation of borders of, 22
      melanoma, 313t, 322, 325, 328f
   Moynahan's syndrome-related, 131, 131f
   Peutz-Jeghers syndrome-related, 126, 130,
      257
   simplex, cryosurgical treatment of, 372
   solar, 125, 128
      differentiated from ephelides, 299
      topical tretinoin treatment of, 395
LEOPARD mnemonic, for Moynahan's syndrome,
      131, 131f
Lepromin skin test, 203
Leprosy, 12, 201-206, 285-286, 434, 476
   causative bacillus of, 201-202, 203, 203f,
      205-206, 475
   as dermatologic emergency, 446
   diagnosis of, 203, 203f
   dimorphous (borderline), 201-202, 202f, 202t
   endemic, 476
   as hypopigmentation cause, 129-130
   as ichthyosis cause, 34t
   indeterminate, 201-202, 202f
   lepromatous, 201-202, 202f, 202t, 203,
      204-205, 204f
   as leukocytoclastic vasculitis cause, 105
   as leukoderma cause, 129
   natural reservoir of, 476
   as paronychia cause, 471
   reactional states of, 205-206
   tuberculoid, 201-202, 202f, 202t, 203
Leser-Trélat sign, 253, 257, 271
Letterer-Siwe disease, 473
Leukemia, 258t, 338, 338f
   as "blueberry muffin baby" cause, 401
   chronic lymphocytic, 338

Leukemia (Continued)
   as erythema nodosum cause, 135-136
   hairy cell, as leukocytoclastic vasculitis cause,
      106
   ichthyosis associated with, 257
   most common adult type of, 338
   as panniculitis mimic, 140-141
   retinoid treatment of, 395
   Sweet's syndrome-related, 252
Leukocytosis, Sweet's syndrome-related,
      252
Leukoderma, 127
   acquisitum centrifugum. See Nevus, halo
   amino acid metabolism disorders-related,
      128, 129t
   as pigmentation disorders cause, 126-130
Leukonychia, 468
Leukoplakia, 85f, 282, 282f
Leukotrichia, 127
Leukotriene D4 receptor antagonists, 170
Leukotrienes, 132, 167
Levofloxacin, as tuberculosis treatment, 211
Lice, 24, 25f, 245-246, 246f
   pubic, 24, 245-246, 464
Lichen myxedematosus, 113, 115
Lichen nitidus, 20, 88, 88f, 434
Lichen planopilaris, 85
Lichen planus, 20, 84
   isotretinoin treatment for, 395-396
   nail findings in, 469, 469t
   occupational exposure-related, 452
   as onychomycosis mimic, 220
   phototherapy for, 387-388t
   primary skin lesions of, 84
   pruritus associated with, 86
   in skin of color, 430, 430f
   tretinoin treatment for, 394
Lichen planus-systemic lupus erythematosus
      overlap syndrome, 87
Lichen sclerosis, 408
Lichen simplex chronicus, 20f, 88-89, 434,
      465
Lichen striatus, 88, 89f, 405, 405f
Lichenification, 88, 268
   differentiated from atrophy, 19-20, 20f
Lichenoid, definition of, 84
Lichenoid infiltrate, 87
Lichenoid skin eruptions, 84-89
   drug-related, 85, 87, 101
   photoeruptions, 120
   in HIV-infected patients, 284
Lichenoid-like skin eruptions, 87
Lidocaine, 364-365, 365t, 370
Lightning-strike injuries, 450, 450f
Limb perfusion, as melanoma treatment,
      330
Lind, James, 475
Linear immunoglobulin A bullous dermatosis,
      10t, 73t, 76, 76f
Linear skin lesions, 20
Linoleic acid deficiency, 288
Lipid-lowering agents, 87t, 223
Lipoatrophy, 135, 135t, 141-142, 141f
Lipodystrophy, 135, 135t, 141, 285, 285f
   acquired partial, 141f
   in HIV-infected individuals, 281t
Lipohypertrophy, 135t, 142
Lipoma, 15f
Liposarcoma, 313t
Liposuction, 364
Lips
   dry, retinoid therapy-related, 397
   macules on, 268-269
Lisch nodules, 37-38, 256t
Lithium
   acne-exacerbating effect of, 153t
   as pustular acneiform eruption cause, 81
   as vesiculobullous eruption cause, 73t
Liver disease, cutaneous manifestations of,
      267-268, 272, 272f, 464
"Liver palms," 267

Liver spots. *See* Lentigo, solar
Lobomycosis, 224
Local anesthetics, 364-365, 365t, 366, 370
  allergic reactions to, 364-365
Löfgren's syndrome, 93-94, 93f
Loiasis, 235-236, 235t, 249-250t
Louis-Bar syndrome. *See* Ataxia-telangiectasia
Lovastatin, interaction with antifungal agents, 223
Lumbar puncture, in syphilis patients, 199
Lung cancer, 106, 253-254, 269, 271
  metastatic, 339-340
  small cell, 341
Lunulae, red or blue, 467t
Lupus band test, 35, 160f
Lupus erythematosus. *See also* Systemic lupus
    erythematosus
  bullous, 10t
  cutaneous, 156, 156t
    acute, 156, 156t, 157f, 159t
    chronic, 156t, 158, 159t
    subacute, 156-157, 156t, 157f, 158, 158t,
      159t, 163-164t
  differentiated from lupus vulgaris, 210
  discoid, 129, 156t, 158-159, 158f
  drug-induced, 101, 101f, 158t, 159
  neonatal, 156t, 159-160, 159f, 407
    as dermatologic emergency, 446-447
  postinflammatory hyperpigmentation associated
    with, 429f
Lupus miliaris disseminatus faciei, 90t, 96, 96f
Lupus pernio, 92, 93f, 94, 210, 430-431
Lupus profundus, 137
Lupus vulgaris, 209-210, 209f, 210f
Lupus-nonspecific eruptions, 156
Lupus-specific eruptions, 159t
Lycopenemia, 267
Lyme disease, 140, 192, 248, 249-250t, 337-338,
    445
Lymph nodes, elective dissection of, 326
Lymphatic malformations, 304
Lymphedema, angiosarcoma associated with, 340
Lymphocutaneous disease, 225
Lymphoma, 258t, 341
  B-cell, 337
  definition of, 331
  in HIV-infected individuals, 281t
  as leukocytoclastic vasculitis cause, 106
  mucosa-associated lymphoid tissue (MALT),
    337-338
  as panniculitis mimic, 140-141, 141f
  pruritus associated with, 258
  T-cell, *129. See also* Mycosis fungoides
    as exfoliative dermatitis cause, 63
    ichthyosis associated with, 257
    phototherapy for, 387-388t
    relationship to Sézary's syndrome, 255
    Sweet's syndrome-related, 252
    treatment for, 335, 387-388t

M

Macrocephaly, 38
Macroglossia, amyloidosis-related, 112-113
Macules, 14, 15f
  café-au-lait (CALM), 15f, 300, 300f
    Albright's syndrome-related, 131
    Moynahan's syndrome-related, 131, 131f
    neurofibromatosis-related, 131, 256t,
      299-300, 408
  hypomelanotic, 129
    ash-leaf, 39, 39f, 126
    tuberous sclerosis-related, 37, 39, 39f
  on lips, 268-269
Maculopapular eruptions, 18
  as dermatologic emergency indicator, 444
  drug-related, 97-98
Madarosis, 204-205, 204f
Madura foot, 226-227, 227f, 434

Maggots, 236, 237f
Makeup, as contact dermatitis cause, 65t
Malabsorption syndromes, 128, 132, 289
Malaria, 249-250t
Malassezia infections, 23, 55, 61-62, 130, 153,
    220, 222, 430
Malingering, 457
Malnutrition, 221-222, 287
  child abuse-related, 450
Marasmus, 287
  differentiated from kwashiorkor, 287
MART1, as melanoma marker, 324
Mast cells
  in chronic idiopathic urticaria, 169
  in vasodilatation, 167
Mastocytosis, 387-388t, 406-407, 407f
Measles, 172-173
Mechanobullous disorders, 43-47
Median nail dystrophy, 472
Medlar bodies, 225, 226f
Mees' lines, 467t, 468
Mehndi, 438
Meissner corpuscles, 12
Melanin, 127
  dermal deposition of, 133, 133t
Melanocytes, 6, 127
  excess numbers of, 128, 132, 133t
  migration to skin, 294
  stimulation of, 132
Melanocyte-stimulating hormone, 132, 276
Melanocytic tumors, benign, 293-300
Melanocytosis, neurocutaneous, 42
Melanoderma, 127, 130-132
Melanoma, 313t, 319-330, 352
  ABCDEs of, 321-322
  acral lentiginous, 322, 323f, 328f, 352, 434
  age factors in, 352
  amelanotic, 323
  causes of, 319
  clinical appearance of, 321, 322f
  congenital melanocytic nevus-related, 296
  definition of, 319
  diagnosis and evaluation of, 323-324
  environmental factors in, 319-320
  genetic factors in, 319-320, 321
  host immune response to, 321
  incidence of, 319, 352
  in situ, 313t
    differentiated from atypical nevus, 298, 313t,
      322, 325, 326f, 328f
  metastatic, 325-326, 328, 339-340, 340f
  Mohs surgery for, 374-375
  of the nail unit, 470, 472
  nevus as risk factor for, 299
  nodular, 322, 323f
  ocular, 339
  recurrence of, 325-326
  relationship to skin phototype, 352
  sex factors in, 322, 352
  staging systems for, 323-324, 324t
  sunburn as risk factor for, 352
  superficial spreading, 322, 323f
  treatment for, 325-326, 328-330
Melanonychia, 470
  linear, 327, 327f, 329
  striata, 427-428, 434
Melanosis
  Becker's 131
Melanosomes, 6, 8
Melasma, 132, 133t, 384, 394-395
Meningioma, 38
Meningococcemia, 446f
Mental retardation, 38-39
Mercaptoethyl amines, as hypopigmentation
    cause, 128
Mercury, as pigmentation disorder cause, 133t,
    134
Merkel cell carcinoma, 313t, 340-341, 344, 374
Merkel cells, 6

Merlin protein, 39
Mesotherapy, 213-214
Metabolic disorders
  as ichthyosis cause, 32, 34t
  as pigmentation disorders cause, 132, 133-134
  as vesiculobullous disorders cause, 74
Metastatic skin lesions/tumors, 346-348. *See also*
    metastatic *under specific types of cancer*
  cryosurgical treatment for, 372
Methicillin, staphylococcal resistance to, 188,
    190, 280
Methotrexate, 53, 120
8-Methoxypsoralen, pigmentation effects of,
    132
Methylene blue, 24f
Microcomedones, 152
Microcystic adnexal carcinoma, 341-342, 374
Micrographic surgery. *See* Mohs surgery
Microhemagglutination-*Treponema pallidum*
    test, 25
Micronutrient supplements, 290
Microsporum, 216
Microsporum audoinii, 216, 218
Microsporum canis, 218, 404
Microsporum distortum, 218
Midazolam, interaction with antifungal agents,
    223
Miliaria
  crystallina, 73
  pustulosa, 81-82
Milk, as acne risk factor, 149
Milk-alkali syndrome, 117
Milkers' nodules, 180
Mineral oil, use in scabies diagnosis, 23-24
Mineral salt deposits, 112
Minimal erythema dose (MED), 388-389
Minimal phototoxic dose (MPD), 389
Minocycline
  as lupus erythematosus cause, 159
  as pigmentation disorder cause, 101t, 102f,
    133t, 134
Mites, 242, 250
  acquired from animals, 24
  chiggers (sand fleas), 237, 237f
  Demodex, 235t, 240, 240f
  as disease vectors, 249-250t
  infestations of, 246-247, 247f, 248, 250t
  as scabies cause, 19, 19f, 24, 244, 245f, 281t,
    464
  canine, 248
  diagnosis of, 23-24, 24f
  feline, 247
  Norwegian, 220, 244-245
  trombiculid, 237
"Mitten" deformities, 11
Mixed connective tissue disease, 162-163
Mohs surgery, 314t, 344-345, 364, 369,
    374-377
Moles. *See also* Nevus
  atypical, as skin cancer risk factor, 352
  definition of, 294
Molluscum contagiosum, 15f, 187, 187f
  cryptococcosis as mimic of, 232, 232f
  in HIV-infected individuals, 280, 281t,
    283-284
  treatment for, 283, 372t
Mongolian spot, 132, 133t, 296-297, 408, 408f,
    434
Monkeys, as *Mycobacterium leprae* (leprosy)
    reservoir, 201
Monobenzyl ether of hydroquinone, 128
Mononuclear cells, in chronic idiopathic urticaria,
    169
Moon facies, 264
Morbilliform eruptions, 172, 172f
  drug-related, 174
Morgellons, 240
Morphea, phototherapy for, 387-388t, 389
Mosquito bites, 241-242, 250

Mosquitoes, as disease vectors, 249-250t
Moxibustion, 435
Moxifloxacin, as tuberculosis treatment, 211
Moynahan's syndrome, 130-131
MRSA (methicillin-resistant *Staphylococcus aureus*), 188, 190, 280
Mucicarmine, 475
Mucinosis, 112-113, 114-116, 115f
   follicular, 147
   papular, 115
Mucormycosis, 224, 230, 231, 233
   diabetes-related, 262
   rhino-orbital-cerebral, 233
Mucous patches, 198, 198f
Muehrcke's lines/nails, 275, 467t, 468
Muir-Torre syndrome, 256t, 257, 344-345
Multiple hamartoma syndrome, 256-257, 256t, 257f
Multiple mucosal neuroma syndrome, 256t, 257
Multiple myeloma, 106, 115, 257, 271, 337
   as panniculitis mimic, 140-141
Multiple sulfatase deficiency, 33t
Mumps, 172
Munchausen syndrome, 458-459
Munchausen syndrome by proxy, 458
Mutilation, culturally-sanctioned, 438
Myasthenia gravis, 222, 310
Mycetoma, 224-225, 226-227, 227f
Mycobacteria
   atypical, 207, 212-215, 231
   classification of, 207, 208t
   staining characteristics of, 207
Mycobacterial infections, 207-215. *See also* Leprosy; Tuberculosis
   as dermatologic emergency, 446
   as granuloma cause, 90t
   as leukocytoclastic vasculitis cause, 105
Mycobacterium abscessus, 208t, 213-214
Mycobacterium africanum, 207, 208t
Mycobacterium asiaticum, 208t
Mycobacterium avium-intracellulare complex, 208t, 213, 285-286
Mycobacterium bovis, 207, 208t
   as tuberculosis vaccine, 211
Mycobacterium chelonei, 207f, 208t, 213-214, 214f
Mycobacterium fortuitum, 208t, 213-214, 214f, 225
Mycobacterium fredericksbergense, 213-214
Mycobacterium haemophilum, 208t
Mycobacterium intermedium, 208t
Mycobacterium kansasii, 208t, 214-215, 215f, 225
Mycobacterium leprae, 130, 201-202, 203, 203f, 205-206, 207, 208t, 476, 476f
Mycobacterium marinum, 140f, 208t, 213, 213f, 225
Mycobacterium mycoti, 208t
Mycobacterium scrofulaceum, 207f, 208t
Mycobacterium simae complex, 208t
Mycobacterium szulgai, 208t
Mycobacterium tuberculosis, 136-137, 203, 207, 208t, 209-210, 212
Mycobacterium ulcerans, 208t, 213
Mycobacterium xenopi, 208t
Mycobiotic agar, 216
Mycoplasma pneumoniae infections, 99
Mycosel agar, 216
Mycosis fungoides, 15f, 147, 331-335, 395
   subtypes of, 332
   TNM classification of, 333, 333t
   treatment for, 387-388t, 389, 395
Myiasis, 236, 237f
   furuncular, 236, 237f
Myositis, 222
Myxedema
   of hypothyroidism, 263, 263f
   pretibial, 114-115, 115f, 262-263, 263f, 266

N

Nafoxidine, as ichthyosis cause, 32
Nail changes,
   bleomycin-related, 185
   chronic renal failure-related, 274t, 275, 275f
   Darier's disease-related, 35
   diabetes-related, 262
   hyperthyroidism-related, 263
   hypothyroidism-related, 262
   lichen planus-related, 85-86, 86f
   nutritional disturbances-related, 287
   psoriasis-related, 52, 52f, 54
   psoriatic arthritis-related, 52f
   Reiter's disease-related, 80-81
   systemic disease-related, 467, 467t
Nail fold capillaroscopy, 468
Nail pits, 52, 469
Nail polish, as contact dermatitis cause, 65t, 66f
Nail-patella syndrome, 279t
Nails
   functions of, 467
   pigmentation of, 427-428
   tumors of, 472, 472f
Nalidixic acid, adverse cutaneous reactions to, 102
Naproxen, as vesiculobullous eruption cause, 73t
Native Americans, actinic prurigo in, 121, 122f
"Necklace of Venus," 129
Necrobiosis lipoidica, 260, 261f, 266
   as granuloma cause, 90t
Necrobiosis lipoidica diabeticorum, 260, 261f
Necrosis
   spider bite-related, 243-244
   warfarin-related, 103f
Neomycin, as pediatric allergic contact dermatitis cause, 404
Neonates. *See also* Infants
   acne vulgaris in, 404
   herpes simplex virus infections in, 178
   infections in, 399-401
   lupus erythematosus in, 407
   photodermatoses differential diagnosis in, 122
   pustular eruptions in, 82-83
   sclerema neonatorum in, 138-139, 450-451
   subcutaneous fat necrosis in, 138-139, 138f
Nephritic factor, C3, 141f
Nephritis, lupus, 163-164n
Nephrotic syndrome, 128, 467t
Nerve growth factor, 132
Netherton's syndrome, 32, 33t
Neuralgia, postherpetic, 179-180
Neuroblastoma, as "blueberry muffin baby" cause, 401
Neurocutaneous disorders, 37-42
Neurofibroma, 38
   peripheral, 37, 38f
   plexiform, 37-38, 38f
Neurofibromatosis, 256t, 407
   freckles associated with, 126
   type I, 37-38
      café-au-lait macules associated with, 37, 38f, 131, 299, 408
   type II, 37-38, 39
      café-au-lait macules associated with, 39
Neurofibromin, 37
Neurologic agents, as lichen planus-like eruptions cause, 87t
Neurologic disorders, amyloidosis-related, 112-113
Neuropathy
   Churg-Strauss syndrome-related, 107, 107t
   diabetic, 261-262
   differentiated from leprosy-related neuropathy, 203
Neurosyphilis, 197, 199
Neutral lipid storage disease, 33t
Nevoid basal cell carcinoma syndrome, 316, 316f
Nevus
   araneus, 407
   atypical, 299, 299f
      as melanoma risk factor, 319-320, 321

Nevus *(Continued)*
   Becker's, 131, 297, 297f
   comedonicus, 394
   compound, 294
   congenital, 131
      melanocytic/pigmented, 42, 408, 408f
      as melanoma risk factor, 319-320, 321
   connective tissue, 308, 408
   definition of, 294
   depigmentosa, 129
   epidermal, 294
      linear, 394t
   halo, 294-295, 295f
   intradermal, 294, 295f
   of Ito, 132, 133t, 296, 434
      differentiated from nevus of Ota, 132-133, 296
   junctional, 15f, 294
   melanocytic, 294
      acquired, 294
      atypical, 297-298, 299
      blue, 294, 296, 332f
      combined, 296
      congenital, 42, 294-295, 296
      extracutaneous, 300
      multiple, 270
      as melanoma risk factor, 321-322
   of Ota, 132, 133f, 133t, 296-297, 434
      differentiated from nevus of Ito, 132-133, 296
   sebaceous, 294, 407
   spilus, 131, 300, 300f
   spindle cell, 294
   Spitz, 294, 297, 297f
   Sutton's. *See* Nevus, halo
Niacin
   deficiency of, 75, 437
   as ichthyosis cause, 32, 34t
Nickel
   as common allergen, 68
   as contact dermatitis cause, 64t, 68, 68f, 404, 453f
Nikolsky's sign, 443-444
Nitrogen mustard, topical
   as mycosis fungoides treatment, 333-334
   pigmentation effects of, 132
Nits, 24, 246f
Nocardiosis, 90t, 136, 140, 225, 231
Nodules, 14, 15f
   "apple-jelly hue," 91
   benign pseudorheumatoid, 96
   in children, 406, 406f
   hemorrhagic, in children, 406
   Lisch, 37-38, 256t
   milkers', 180
   rheumatoid, 15f, 90t, 95-96, 95f
   sarcoid, 92
   Sister Mary Joseph's, 270f, 340, 344f
   subependmal, 40
Nodulosis, accelerated, 95-96
Nonsteroidal anti-inflammatory drugs
   adverse cutaneous reactions to, 102
      alopecia, 103
      lichen planus-like eruptions, 87t
      photoallergic/phototoxic reactions, 119t
      Stevens-Johnson syndrome, 99
      toxic epidermal necrolysis, 98-99
      urticaria, 100, 166
      vesiculobullous eruptions, 73t
   as urticaria treatment, 170
North Carolina spotless fever, 476-477
Nose
   fibrous papule of, 310
   herpes zoster of, 180
Notalgia paresthetica, 462
Nutritional disturbances, cutaneous manifestations of, 289-292
   hyperpigmentation, 132
   ichthyosis, 32, 34t
   leukoderma, 128
Nutritional supplements, as acne cause, 264
Nystatin, 222t, 223

O

Obesity
  cutaneous manifestations of, 253, 288
  truncal, Cushing's disease-related, 264, 264f
Obsession, 456
Obsessive-compulsive disorders, 457-458, 459
Occupational dermatology, 451-455
Ochronosis, 133-134, 133t
Ocular disorders
  albinism-related, 128
  pseudoxanthoma elasticum-related, 270
  seborrheic dermatitis-related, 55
  Sturge-Weber syndrome-related, 41
Odland bodies, 6
"Oil spots," 469, 469f
Oils, exposure to, as skin cancer cause, 312
Omega brand, 437
Onchocerciasis, 129, 235, 235t, 240, 249-250t,
  434, 477
Onychocryptosis, 470
Onychodystrophy, lichen planus-related, 85
Onycholysis, 192, 469
  hyperthyroidism-related, 263
  psoriasis-related, 52
  Reiter's disease-related, 80-81
Onychomycosis, 219-220, 219f, 470-472, 472t
  chronic renal failure-related, 274t
  diabetes-related, 262
  differentiated from tinea unguium, 471
  in HIV-infected individuals, 280
  mimics of, 220
Opera glass deformity, 52
Ophiasis, 143
Opiates, as urticaria cause, 166
Opportunistic infections
  definition of, 230
  fungal, 230-233
Oral cancer, 258t
Oral contraceptives
  as acne cause, 264
  as acne treatment, 151t, 264
  adverse cutaneous reactions to, 100, 101t, 102,
    135-136
  interaction with acne treatment, 150
Oral mucosa, pigmentation of, in people of color,
  428
Orange skin, jaundice-related, 271
Orf (ecthyma contagiosum), 180, 181f
Organ transplant patients
  fungal infections in, 228, 231
  Merkel cell carcinoma in, 341
  skin cancer in, 312
Oroya fever, 473
Osler-Weber-Rendu syndrome, 268-269, 269f, 303
Osteitis, SAPHO syndrome-related, 152
Osteoarthropathy, hypertrophic, 468
Osteoma, 256, 256t, 267, 270
Osteoma cutis, 117
Otitis media, external, 192
Ovarian cancer, 162, 259, 269, 339
Overdosage, 97

P

Pacemakers, implication for electrosurgery,
  368-369
Pachyonychia congenita, as onychomycosis
  mimic, 220
Pacinian corpuscles, 12
Pagetoid growth, 343-344
Pagetoid reticulosis, 332
Paget's disease, 255, 256f, 259, 313t, 374
Pain, differentiated from pruritus, 461
Pallor, chronic renal failure-related, 274t, 275t, 276
Palpation, of skin lesions, 14, 21
Pancreatic cancer, 253-254, 259, 269
Pancreatic fat necrosis, 139, 139f
Pancreatitis, 265, 271-272, 272f
Panhypopituitarism, 266

Panniculitis, 135-142
  alpha-1 antitrypsin deficiency-related, 139, 139f
  diagnosis of, 142
  lobular, 135, 135t, 137
  lupus, 137-138, 138f, 156t, 159
  mixed, 135t
  pancreatic disease-related, 271-272, 272f
  septal, 135, 135t
  subacute nodular migratory, 135
  trauma-related, 135t, 139-140
PAPAH mnemonic, for Henoch-Schönlein purpura,
  106
Papilla, 7f
Papular eruption of blacks, 434
Papules, 14, 15f
  blue-black hyperkeratotic, 302, 302f
  as dermatologic emergency indicator, 444
  grouped configuration of, 20
  lichen planus-related, 84-85, 85f, 86f
  lichenoid, 88
  sarcoid, 92, 92f
  Wegener's granulomatosis-related, 108
Papulosis
  Bowenoid, 182
  lymphomatoid, 336-337, 337f
Papulosquamous dermatoses/skin eruptions,
  50-56
  HIV infection-associated, 281f
  in skin of color, 430
Paracoccidioidomycosis, 224, 227, 229-230, 230f
Paraffin, as granuloma cause, 90t, 91t, 92
Paraproteinemia, immunoglobulin G lambda, 115
Parapsoriasis, 50, 56, 331, 332f
  phototherapy for, 387-388t
Parasitic diseases, as dermatologic emergencies,
  446
Parasitic infestations, 235-240, 244-246
Parasitosis
  delusions associated with, 240, 456-457,
    457f, 464
  differential diagnosis of, 456
Para-substituted phenols, as hypopigmentation
  cause, 128
Parkinson's disease, 55, 61
Paronychia, 192, 221t, 262, 470-471, 471f
Parvovirus B19 infections, 173-174, 477
  as leukocytoclastic vasculitis cause, 105
  neonatal, 400, 402
  as papular acrodermatitis of childhood cause,
    173
  during pregnancy, 402
Patch test, 26
  for allergic contact dermatitis diagnosis, 25,
    66-68, 66f, 67t, 68f, 453, 455f
Patches, 14
  hypomelanotic, 129
  Shagreen, 39-40, 408
Pathergy, 252
Pautrier's microabscesses, 331
"Peau de orange" appearance, of granola faciale,
  110-111
Pediatric dermatology, 404-408. See also Children;
  Infants; Neonates
Pediculosis pubis, 245-246, 464
Pediculus humanus capitis, 24, 245-246
Pediculus humanus corporis, 24, 245-246
Pellagra, 74-75, 290, 437, 475
  four "Ds" of, 288, 289f
  as hyperpigmentation cause, 132
Pemphigoid
  bullous, 10t, 73, 73t, 76f, 257
    antigen of, 8-9
    antihemidesmosomal antibodies in, 9-10
    diagnostic tests for, 27
    differentiated from cicatricial pemphigoid,
      75
    relationship to lichen planus, 87
  cicatricial, differentiated from bullous
    pemphigoid, 75
Pemphigoid (herpes) gestations, 10t

Pemphigus
  definition of, 8
  erythematosus, 9t
  familial. See Hailey-Hailey disease
  foliaceus, 9t, 54
    differentiated from pemphigus vulgaris, 75-76
    immunoglobulin A, 9t, 80
    paraneoplastic, 9t, 255, 255f, 259
  vegetans, 9t
    differentiated from Hailey-Hailey disease, 35
  vulgaris, 9t, 73, 257, 443-444, 443f
    differentiated from Hailey-Hailey disease, 35
    differentiated from pemphigus foliaceus,
      75-76
Penicillamine, as vesiculobullous eruption cause, 73t
Penicillins, adverse cutaneous reactions to,
  100-101, 105, 135-136
Penicilliosis, 224, 224t, 227, 230-231
Penile nodules, artifical, 438
Penis
  condyloma acuminatum of, 183f
  lichen planus of, 86f
  syphilitic chancre of, 24-25
  tinea cruris of, 439
Perforating disorders, acquired, phototherapy for,
  387-388t
Peripheral nerve sheath tumors, malignant, 313t
Perlèche, 221t
  in diabetic patients, 262
Permethrin, 244-245, 246
Persistent light reactivity, 120
Petechiae, 18
  acupuncture-related, 435-436
  as dermatologic emergency indicator, 444, 445t
  differentiated from purpura, 19
  viral exanthem-related, 173
  Wegener's granulomatosis-related, 108
Peutz-Jeghers syndrome, 126, 130, 131f, 256t,
  257, 267, 269
Phaeoanellomyces (Exophiala) werneckii, 221
Phaeohyphomycosis, 224-225, 226
Pharyngitis, psoriasis-exacerbating effect of, 53
Phenobarbital, 98-99
Phenothiazines, 101t, 103, 119t, 133t
Phenylketonuria, 129t
Phenytoin
  acne-exacerbating effect of, 153t
  as alopecia cause, 103, 147
  interaction with antifungal agents, 223
  as lichen planus-like eruptions cause, 87t
  as pustular acneiform eruption cause, 81
  as Stevens-Johnson syndrome cause, 99
  as toxic epidermal necrolysis cause, 98-99
Phenytoin hypersensitivity syndrome, 97
Pheochromocytoma, 38, 41, 256t
Pheomelanin, 127
Phlebotomy, as porphyria cutanea tarda treatment,
  125
Phobias, 456
Photoaging. See Dermatoheliosis
Photoallergic reactions
  differentiated from phototoxic reactions, 118
  drug-related, 97, 103, 119f
Photodistributed eruptions, 118
Photodynamic therapy, 152, 314t, 389, 391-392
Photomedicine, therapeutic. See Phototherapy
Photoonycholysis, 120
Photopheresis, 391-392
  extracorporeal, 335
Photosensitive dermatoses, 118-125
  drug-related, 98
  facial, differentiated from acute lupus
    erythematosus, 156
  genodermatoses, 122, 123-124t
  in HIV-infected individuals, 281t, 284
  occupational exposure-related, 452
  viral exanthems as, 174
Photosensitivity
  definition of, 118
  predisposing factors for, 120

Phototherapy, 386-392
blue-light, 386
for mycosis fungoides, 333
for pruritus, 466t
Photothermolysis, selective, 378-379
Phototoxic reactions, 73t, 120
differentiated from photoallergic reactions, 118
drug-related, 97, 103, 118f
Phthirus pubis, 24, 245-246
Phytophotodermatitis, 120
Piebaldism, 128
Piedra, 221
Pigmentation
normal, pigment components of, 127
racial differences in, 127
stimulation of, 132
terminology of, 19
Pigmentation disorders, 126-134. *See also*
Hyperpigmentation; Hypopigmentation
blue-gray dyspigmentation, 132-134
chronic renal failure-related, 274t, 275t, 276
diagnosis of, 126
leukoderma, 126-130
occupational exposure-related, 452
Pilomatricoma, 406, 406f
Pimozide, 457
Pinkus tumors, 315
Pinta, 129-130
Pinworms, 235
Pityriasis
alba, 59, 429, 429f
lichenoides et varioliformis acuta, 50, 56, 56f, 199
rosea, 50, 54-55, 55f
misdiagnosed as tinea corporis, 405
morbilliform, 174
phototherapy for, 387-388t
secondary syphilis as mimic of, 55-56, 199
in skin of color, 430
rotunda, 434
rubra pilaris, 50, 54
isotretinoin treatment for, 395-396
nail findings in, 469t
rash of, 54, 54f
retinoid treatment for, 397
versicolor. *See* Tinea versicolor
Plague, 249-250t
Plant dermatitis, as pediatric allergic contact
dermatitis cause, 404
Plaques, 14, 15f
angiolupoid sarcoidal, 92
sarcoid, 92, 93f
Platelet-activating factor, as vasodilatation and
vascular permeability mediator, 167
Plectin, 44
Pneumonia, *Pneumocystis carinii,* 283
Poikiloderma
atrophicans vasculare, 331
of Civatte, 125
Poison ivy, 20, 68, 73, 404, 477
Poliomyelitis, 61
Polyangiitis, microscopic, 105, 105t
differentiated from polyarteritis nodosa, 109
Polyarteritis, microscopic, 109, 278
Polyarteritis nodosa, 105t, 278
classic (systemic), 109
differentiated from
microscopic polyangiitis, 109
nodular vasculitis, 137
primary cutaneous, 109, 110f
Polycythemia
as ichthyosis cause, 34t
rubra vera, 465
Polymorphous light eruptions, 120-121, 121f, 125,
156, 405, 406f
phototherapy for, 387-388t
Polyposis syndromes, 269
hereditary, 268t
Polyps, intestinal, 256t, 269-270, 305

Pompholyx, 60, 60f
"Popsicle panniculitis," 139-140
Pork tapeworms, 240
Porokeratosis, tretinoin treatment for, 394
Porphyria, 115, 156
chronic renal failure-related, 274t
eosinophilic deposits associated with, 114
erythropoietic, 476
photodermatoses-related, 122
variegate
differentiated from porphyria cutanea tarda, 124
photodermatoses-associated, 122
Porphyria cutanea tarda, 74, 75f, 102, 122-124,
272, 272f, 434
diagnostic test for, 23f
differentiated from
pseudoporphyria, 75
variegate porphyria, 124
drug-induced exacerbation of, 102
in HIV-infected patients, 284
as hyperpigmentation cause, 132
photodermatoses-related, 122
treatment for, 124-125
Porphyria-like eruptions
dialysis-related, 277
drug-related, 73t
Port-wine stain, 302
Sturge-Weber syndrome-related, 40-41, 41f
von Hippel-Lindau disease-related, 41
Potassium dichromate, as pediatric allergic contact
dermatitis cause, 404
Potassium hydroxide examination, 22, 23f
for superficial fungal infection diagnosis, 216
for tinea capitis diagnosis, 22
Potassium iodide, as sporotrichosis treatment, 225
Povidone-iodine (Betadine), 366
Pox, rickettsial, 249-250t
"Prayer marks," 439
Prednisone, as sarcoidosis treatment, 93-94
Pregnancy, 416-421
candidiasis during, 221-222
erythema nodosum during, 135-136
generalized pustular psoriasis during, 78
granuloma gravidarum of, 303
hyperpigmentation during, 132
isotretinoin use during, 151
local anesthesia use during, 366
neurofibromatosis during, 37
oral isotretinoin use during, 396
pruritus during, 464-465
tretinoin use during, 395
wart treatment during, 185
Prenatal diagnosis
of congenital ichthyosis, 33-34
of epidermolysis bullosa, 43, 47
Progestins, acne-exacerbating effect of, 153t
Propioniacterium acnes, 148
Propylthiouracil
as leukocytoclastic vasculitis cause, 105
as nodular vasculitis cause, 136
Prostaglandin D2, as vasodilatation and vascular
permeability mediator, 167
Prostate cancer, 106, 341f
Protease inhibitors, as lipodystrophy cause, 141
Protein deficiencies, 97, 128, 287
Proteinosis, lipoid, 114
Protoporphyria, 114
erythropoietic, 122, 125, 125f
Prototheosis, as granuloma cause, 90t
Protozoan infections, as leukocytoclastic vasculitis
cause, 105
Prurigo
actinic, 121, 122f, 387-388t
nodularis, 465
Pruritus, 461-466
atopic dermatitis-related, 57-58, 59
brachioradial, 125
cancer-related, 258
cholestic, 464-465

Pruritus *(Continued)*
definition of, 461, 473
drug-related, 97
generalized, 461-462, 463, 463t
in HIV-infected individuals, 281t, 387-388t
irritant contact dermatitis-related, 64
lichen planus-related, 86
liver disease-related, 268
localized, 461, 462t
misspelling of, 473
renal failure-related, 276-277, 387-388t
scabies-related, 244
scratching response to, 58
syphilis-related, 197
treatment for, 465, 466t
Pseudofolliculitis barbae, 431-432, 434
Pseudohypoparathyroidism, calcinosis
cutis-related, 116
Pseudolymphoma, 337, 337f
Pseudomonas aeruginosa infections, 192-193
in diabetic patients, 261-262
as green nail cause, 471, 471f
"Pseudomonas hot hand-foot syndrome,"
193
Pseudomonas infections
diagnostic techniques for, 22
of the toe web, 434
Pseudoporphyria, 75, 102, 102f, 120, 122,
274t
Pseudoxanthoma elasticum, 269-270
Psoralen and ultraviolet light, type A (PUVA),
388, 390f
acne-exacerbating effect of, 153t
bath, 391
comparison with ultraviolet radiation B therapy,
388-389
contraindications to, 391
definition of, 390-391
as granuloma annulare treatment, 94-95
as lichen planus treatment, 87
as mycosis fungoides treatment, 333-334
retinoid (RePUVA), 391
Psoralens
action mechanisms of, 390-391
definition of, 390
phototoxicity of, 103, 119t
pigmentation effects of, 132
as vesiculobullous eruption cause, 73t
Psoriasis, 15f, 50
definition of, 50
drug-related, 53
erythrodermic, 50
exacerbating factors in, 53
as exfoliative dermatitis cause, 63
genetic factors in, 50-51
guttate, 50-51, 51f
morbilliform, 174
pediatric, 407
in HIV-infected individuals, 281t
as hypopigmentation cause, 129
incidence of, 50
inverse, 50, 51f
Koebner phenomenon of, 20, 20f
lithium-related exacerbation of, 97
location of, 20-21
locational variants of, 50
morphologic variants of, 50
nail findings in, 50, 469t, 469t
non-cutaneous manifestations of, 52
as onychomycosis mimic, 220
palmoplantar, 50
plaques of, 50, 51f, 54
pustular, 16f, 50, 53, 78-79
of scalp, 50, 55
seborrheic distribution of, 54
secondary syphilis as mimic of, 199
in skin of color, 430
treatment for, 53, 389-390, 397-398
phototherapy, 387-388t
tretinoin, 394

Psychocutaneous disorders, 456-460
Pterygium
    differentiated from pterygium inversus unguium,
        469, 470f
    lichen planus-related, 85
Ptosis, ipsilateral brow, 370, 370f
Puberty, precocious, neurofibromatosis-related, 38
Pubic lice, 24, 245-246, 464
Purpura, 18
    "cockade," 106
    differentiated from petechiae, 19
    gastrointestinal disease-related, 267
    Henoch-Schönlein, 27, 27f, 105t, 106, 274,
        278, 407
    PAPAH mnemonic for, 106
    myeloma-associated amyloidosis-related, 112
    palpable, as dermatologic emergency, 445t,
        446f
    "postprotoscopic," 112
    psychogenic, 458
    Wegener's granulomatosis-related, 108
Purpuric gloves and socks syndrome, 173
Pustular bacterid of Andrews, 78-79
Pustular eruptions. See Pustules
Pustules, 14, 16f, 78-83
    classification of, 78, 79t
    as dermatologic emergency indicator, 444, 445t
    differentiated from vesicles and bullae, 78
    grouped configuration of, 20
    in neonates, 82-83
    Willan's classification of, 474
Pustulosis
    acute generalized exanthematous (AGEP), 81,
        103, 104f
    neonatal cephalic, 153
    palmar/plantar, 79
    SAPHO syndrome-related, 152
Pyoderma
    acupuncture-related, 435-436
    faciale, 148, 153-154, 153f
    gangrenosum, 252, 258f, 267-268, 269f
        cryptococcosis as mimic of, 232
        as dermatologic emergency, 447, 448f
        internal cancer-related, 258
        leukemia associated with, 338
        Wegener's granulomatosus-related, 108
Pyrazinamide, as tuberculosis treatment, 211, 211t
Pyroxidine deficiency, 288

Q
Q fever, 249-250t
Q-switching, of laser radiation, 379, 382-383, 383t
Quadriplegia, 61
Quinacrine, as pigmentation disorder cause, 101t
Quinquaud's disease, 81

R
Rabbits, mites of, 24
"Raccoon eyes," 159f
"Racing larva," 234
Radiation. See also Ultraviolet radiation
    infrared, as hyperpigmentation cause, 132
    ionizing, as hyperpigmentation cause, 132
    solar
        acute effects of, 353
        chronic effects of, 353
        health benefits of, 354
        protection from, 354, 355-356, 355t
        as skin cancer cause, 312-313
        stimulated emission of, 378
Radiation recall reaction, 120
Radiation therapy
    as alopecia cause, 145
    ineffectiveness as melanoma treatment, 328
    for mycosis fungoides, 333
    for skin cancer, 314t

Radiation therapy (Continued)
    as skin cancer cause, 312
    for warts, 185
Radiocontrast media, as urticaria cause, 166
Ramsay Hunt syndrome, 180
Rapid plasma reagin test, for syphilis diagnosis,
    25, 55-56, 197
Raynaud's disease, 444
Raynaud's phenomenon, 160-161, 185
Raynaud's syndrome, 162-163, 444, 468
"Razor bumps," 431
Recessively-inherited diseases, with skin findings
    and internal cancer, 257, 258t
Red man syndrome, 449
Reed-Sternberg cells, 335
Refsum's disease, 33-34, 33t
Reiter's syndrome, 281t
Relapsing fever, 248, 249-250t
Relaxed skin tension lines (RSTLs), 369-370, 369f
Renal cancer, cutaneous metastases of, 340
Renal cell carcinoma, 41, 106
Renal disease, cutaneous manifestations of,
    274-279
Renal failure, chronic
    calcinosis cutis-related, 117
    nail changes associated with, 467t, 468, 468f
    pruritus associated with, 387-388t, 464
Renal transplantation, 276
Rendu-Osler-Weber disease, 474
Repeated open application test (ROAT), 68, 68f
RePUVA, 391
Respiratory disorders, nail changes associated
    with, 467t
Respiratory infections, fungal, 224t, 227-230
Respiratory syncytial virus, 172-173
Rete ridge, 7f
Reticulohistiocytosis, multicentric, 259
Retinoic acid, adverse cutaneous reactions to, 101
Retinoids, 393-398
    as acne treatment, 152
    anticarcinogenic activity of, 395
    contraindication during pregnancy, 185
    as Darier's disease treatment, 36
    as ichthyosis treatment, 35
    as lichen planus treatment, 87
    as mycosis fungoides treatment, 333-334
    as psoriasis treatment, 53
    side effects of, 396-397, 397t
        ichthyosis, 32, 34t
        photosensitiziing effect, 120
    use in phototherapy, 391
    as wart therapy, 186t
Rhabdomyoma, congenital, tuberous sclerosis-
    related, 40
Rheumatoid arthritis. See Arthritis, rheumatoid
Rheumatoid factor, 163-164t
Rheumatoid nodules, 15f
Rhinisporidiosis, 224
Rhinitis
    allergic, atopic dermatitis-related, 58
    syphilitic, 403
Rhinoscleroma, 230t
Rhinosporidiosis, 224
Riboflavin deficiency, 288
RICE mnemonic, for brown recluse spider bites, 244
Rickettsial infections, 271
    as dermatologic emergency, 444-446
Rocky Mountain spotted fever, 241, 248, 249-250t,
    476-477
Rifabutin, as tuberculosis treatment, 211, 211t
Rifampin
    interaction with antifungal agents, 223
    as leprosy treatment, 205-206
    side effects of, 205-206
    as tuberculosis treatment, 211, 211t
Rifapentine, as tuberculosis treatment, 211, 211t
Ringworm. See Tinea
River blindness (onchocerciasis), 235, 235t
Rocky Mountain spotted fever, 241, 248, 249-250t,
    476-477

Rosacea, 240
    differentiated from acute cutaneous lupus
        erythematosus, 156
    granulomatous, 90t, 96
Roseola infantum, 174, 174f
Rothmund-Thomson syndrome, 123-124t
ROUGH mnemonic, for Wegener's granulomatosis
    diagnosis, 106
Royal Navy, scurvy outbreaks in, 475
Rubella, 172-173, 174
    neonatal, 400-401, 402
Ruffini corpuscles, 12

S
Sabouraud's dextrose agar, 22-23, 216, 219
"Saddle nose" deformity, 200, 204f
"Sago-grain" vesicles, 60f
Sailors, tattoos on, 436, 436f
Sailor's curse, 477
St. Anthony's fire (erysipelas), 190-192, 191f
Salvarsan, 475
San Joaquin Valley fever. See Coccidioidomycosis
Sand fleas (chiggers), 237, 237f
Sandworms, 234
SAPHO syndrome, 152
Sarcoidosis, 92-93, 92f, 285-286, 430-431,
    431f, 434
    calcinosis cutis-related, 117
    definition of, 92
    as erythema nodosum cause, 135-136
    as granuloma cause, 90t
    as hypopigmentation cause, 129
    as ichthyosis cause, 34t
    presenting as
        Heerfordt's syndrome, 93
        Löfgren's syndrome, 93, 93f
        lupus pernio, 92, 93f
    treatment for, 93-94
Sarcoma
    epitheloid, 339, 344
    Ewing's, 341
    Kaposi's, 280-281, 281t, 282f, 313t, 395
        cryosurgical treatment for, 372
        cryptococcosis as mimic of, 232
        differentiated from acroangiodermatitis,
            304
        endemic, 434
        ichthyosis associated with, 257
Sarcoptes scabiei, 19
Sarcoptes scabiei var. hominis, 244
Scabies, 19, 19f, 24, 244, 245f, 281t, 464
    canine, 248
    diagnosis of, 23-24, 24f
    feline, 247
    Norwegian, 220, 244-245
Scales, 16, 18f
Scalp
    angiosarcoma of, 340, 340f
    erosive pustular dermatosis of, 125
    seborrheic dermatitis of, 61-62, 61f
Scalp conditions, in people of color, 432, 432f
Scarification, 437
Scarlet fever, staphylococcal, 188
Scarlet fever-like eruptions, 173
Scars, 17, 18f
    acne-related, laser therapy for, 381, 383-384,
        384t
    distinguished from keloids, 306, 307t
    hypertrophic, 305, 306-307, 372
    as skin cancer cause, 312
    surgical, 369, 384, 436
"Schenck's disease," 473
Schistosomiasis, 235t, 239
Schlepper protein, 477
Schwannoma, vestibular, 37-38, 39
Schwannomin, 39
Schwann's cells, 12
Scleredema, 115

Sclerema neonatorum, 138-139, 450-451
Sclerodactyly, 160-161, 161f
Scleroderma, 160, 160f, 257
    autoantibodies associated with, 165t
    nail findings in, 467t, 468, 469t, 470f
    phototherapy for, 387-388t, 389
Scleromyxedema, 115
Sclerosis
    progressive systemic, 160-161
    systemic, 165t, 279t
    tuberous, 37, 129, 279t, 407-408
Sclerotherapy, 364
Scratching, as pruritus response, 58
Scrofuloderma, 208, 209t, 210-211, 211f
Scrotum, elephantiasis of, 236, 236f
Scurvy, 289, 289f, 475
Scutula, 217
Scytalidium, 471
Scytalidium dimidiatum, 219
Sebaceous carcinoma, 344-345, 374
Sebaceous glands
    effect of hormones on, 264
    function of, 10
    hyperplasia of, 148
Sebaceous skin tumors, Torre's syndrome-related, 257
Seborrheic areas, distribution of, 54
Sebum, 10, 148
Secrets, Top 100, 1-4
See Cats and Dogs Fight mnemonic, for fluorescent tinea capitis diagnosis, 218
Self-examination, of skin, 353
Self-inflicted skin lesions, 457-458, 458f
Sentinel lymph node biopsy, 326-327
Septicemia
    staphylococcal, 188
    streptococcal, 190
Serum sickness-like drug eruptions, 100
Sézary's syndrome, 252, 332, 333f, 335
Shagreen patches, 39-40, 408
Shaving, as pseudofolliculitis barbae cause, 431
Shingles, 20
Shock, anaphylactic, solar urticaria-related, 122
Short stature, 30, 38
Silica, as granuloma cause, 90t, 91t
Silicone, as granuloma cause, 90t, 91-92, 91t
Silver, as pigmentation disorder cause, 133t, 134
Simulium, 235, 236f
Sinus abnormalities, Churg-Strauss syndrome-related, 107, 107t
Sinusitis, 467t
Sister Mary Joseph's nodules, 270f, 340, 344f
Sixth disease, 174, 174f
Sjögren-Larsson syndrome, 33-34, 33t
Sjögren's syndrome, 157-160, 162-165
    in mothers of neonatal lupus erythematosus patients, 407
Sjögren's syndrome antibodies, as lupus erythematosus markers, 157, 160, 407
Skin
    aging-related changes in, 390, 394
    ashy, 427
    dry scaly. See Ichthyosis
    innervation of, 11-12
    loss of, 12
    self-examination of, 353
    structure and functions of, 6-13
    thick
        diabetes-related, 262
        hypothyroidism-related, 263, 266
    vasculature of, 11-12, 12f
Skin cancer, nonmelanoma, 125. See also Basal cell carcinoma; Skin lesions/tumors; Squamous cell carcinoma
    age factors in, 352-353
    classification of, 312, 313t
    common, 312-318
    genetic factors in, 352
    phototherapy-related, 390-391
    prevalence of, 352

Skin cancer, nonmelanoma (Continued)
    prevention of, 313, 353
    risk factors for, 352
    sex factors in, 352-353
    in skin of color, 433
    sun exposure-related, 352
    treatment for, 313, 314t
        cryosurgery, 372t, 373
        Mohs surgery, 374-377
    uncommon, 339-345
Skin care products, as allergic contact dermatitis cause, 68
Skin diseases, Willan's classification of, 474
Skin lesions/tumors, 14-21
    arrangements and configurations of, 20
    diagnosis of, 21
    flat differentiated from raised, 14
    location of, 20-21
    neurofibromatosis-related, 39
    pigmentation disorders-related, 126
    primary
        definition of, 14, 15-16t
        differentiated from secondary, 16-17
    palpation of, 14
    secondary, 17, 17t
        differentiated from primary, 16-17
    self-inflicted, 457-458, 458f
Skin of color, 427-434
Skin phototypes, relationship to skin cancer risk, 352, 352t
Skin resurfacing, with lasers, 381-382, 383, 384-385, 384t
Skin tag. See Acrochordon
"Slapped cheek" rash, 173
Sleeping sickness. See Trypanosomiasis, African
Sneddon-Wilkinson disease. See Subcorneal pustular dermatosis
Soap, as dermatitis cause, 59, 64t
Soft tissue augmentation, 364
Soft tissue fillers, mycobacterial infections associated with, 214
S100, as melanoma marker, 323
Soret band, 386, 389
Sousa, John Phillip, 58
Spanish fly, 474
Sparganosis, 235t, 239, 239f
Spider angioma, 267, 267t
Spider bites, 241-242, 243-244, 243f, 244
Spider telangiectasia, 407
Spitz, Sophie, 297
Spoon nails, 467t
Sporotrichoid disease pattern, 225, 231
Sporotrichosis, 90t, 224-225, 224t, 225f, 231, 231t, 473
Squamous cell carcinoma, 271, 313t
    actinic keratosis-related, 318
    age factors in, 352
    arsenic ingestion-related, 290
    chromomycosis-related, 226
    epidermolysis bullosa-related, 46
    in HIV-infected individuals, 281t
    in situ (Bowen's disease), 15f, 312, 313t, 317f
        arsenicism-related, 290, 372, 471
        cryosurgical treatment for, 314t
        of the nail unit, 473
    keratoacanthoma type, 317
    lichen planus-related, 86
    metastatic, 316-317
    oral, cutaneous metastases of, 340
    relationship to skin phototype, 352
    sun exposure as risk factor for, 352
    treatment for, 314t
        cryosurgery, 372
        Mohs surgery, 374
    wart-related, 470
Stanozolol, as hereditary angioedema prophylaxis, 170
Staphylococcal carriage
    elimination of, 189
    in HIV-infected individuals, 280

Staphylococcal infections, 188-190
    neonatal, 82
    as paronychia cause, 471
Staphylococcal scalded skin syndrome, 188-189, 190f
Staphylococcus aureus infections, 188
    as atopic dermatitis cause, 59
    gangrene, 445
    Hailey-Hailey disease-exacerbating effect of, 35
    in HIV-infected individuals, 280, 284
    methicillin-resistant, 188, 190, 280
    as nummmular eczema cause, 60
    recurrent, 189
    STAR complex, 174
Starch, as granuloma cause, 90t, 91t
Statins, interaction with antifungal agents, 223
Stem cell factor, 132
Stem cells, cancer, 320
Steroids. See also Corticosteroids
    topical, 358-363
        as periorificial dermatitis cause, 404
Stevens-Johnson syndrome, 73t, 97, 99, 283
    differentiated from toxic epidermal necrolysis, 99, 442, 442t, 443f
    drugs associated with, 99
    treatment for, 443
Stewart-Treves syndrome, 340
Still's disease, 163, 446-447
Stings. See Arthropod bites and stings
Stomatitis, 80-81, 84
    vesicular, with exanthem. See Hand, foot, and mouth disease
Stratum basalis, 6
Stratum corneum, 6, 7f, 8
    in epidermolysis bullosa, 44f
    in lichen planus, 87
Stratum granulosum, 6, 7f
Stratum spinosum, 6, 7f, 8f
Streptococcal infections, 190-192
    as erythema nodosum cause, 135-136
    as leukocytoclastic vasculitis cause, 105
    as panniculitis cause, 140
    as paronychia cause, 471
Streptomycin
    as pustular eruption cause, 81
    as tuberculosis treatment, 211
Stress, as dermatologic disorder exacerbating factor, 58, 148-149, 460
Stretch marks, 394t
Striae
    of Cushing's syndrome, 264, 264f
    distensae (stretch marks), 394
    topical steroids-related, 361f
Strongyloides, 234, 235f
Sturge-Weber syndrome, 37, 40-41, 474
Subcorneal pustular dermatoses, 79-80
    lithium-related exacerbation of, 97
Subcutaneous fat necrosis of the newborn, 138-139, 138f
Subcutis, structure and function of, 6, 13
Sucquet-Hoyer canal, glomus tumors of, 303
Suicide, isotretinoin-related, 151
Sulfonamides, adverse cutaneous reactions to, 100-101, 101f, 102
    erythema nodosum, 135-136
    in HIV-infected individuals, 283
    leukocytoclastic vasculitis, 105
    photoallergic reactions, 103
    Stevens-Johnson syndrome, 99
    toxic epidermal necrolysis, 98-99
    urticaria, 100
    vesiculobullous eruptions, 73t
Sulfur-containing medications, 119t
Sun exposure. See Radiation, solar
Sun protection. See also Sunglasses; Sunscreens
    during phototherapy, 388f
Sunburn, 125, 353, 353t
    in children, 405
    as melanoma risk factor, 320
    as skin cancer risk factor, 352
    treatment for, 357

Sun-damaged skin. *See* Dermatoheliosis
Sunglasses, 356, 388f
Sunscreens, 313, 351-357
   as photoallergic reaction cause, 119t
   as polymorphous light eruption treatment, 121
   sun protection factor (SPF) of, 355-356
   use by children, 354, 356
   use by vitiligo patients, 127
Superantigens, bacterial, 78
Superficial muscular aponeuritic system (SMAS),
   369
Surgery, dermatologic, 364-370
   on patients with skin of color, 433
Surma, 435
Sutures and suturing, 367
Swallow bug, 248f
Sweat glands
   apocrine, 10
   carcinoma of, 313t, 341
   eccrine, 7f, 10
Sweet's syndrome, 229, 252, 252f, 259
Swimmer's itch, 239
"Swimming pool" granuloma, 213, 213f
Synovitis, SAPHO syndrome-related, 152
Syphilis, 195-200, 475
   causal organism of, 195
   chancres of, 24-25, 196-197, 196f, 282,
      474-475
   congenital, 82, 403, 403f
   diagnosis of, 24-25, 196-197, 199
   as granuloma cause, 90t
   in HIV-infected individuals, 281-282, 281t
   late benign, 200
   latent, 199
   neonatal, 400, 402
   as paronychia cause, 471
   primary, 195-197, 196f
   secondary, 25, 195, 195f, 197-198, 198f, 199
      as leukoderma cause, 129
      pigmentation disorders associated with, 129
      as pityriasis rosea mimic, 55-56
   tertiary, 199, 200f
   treatment for, 475
Syphiloderm, 197
Syringomyelia, 61
Systemic diseases
   pigmentation disorders as markers for, 126
   pruritus associated with, 463
Systemic lupus erythematosus
   acute, as dermatologic emergency, 446
   autoantibodies associated with, 163-164t
   bullous, 11, 77, 156t, 159
   as dermatologic emergency, 446
   as discoid lupus erythematosus risk factor, 158
   drug-induced, 163-164t
   as ichthyosis cause, 34t
   idiopathic, 101
   multiple dermatofibromas associated with, 310
   nail changes associated with, 467t
   relationship to lichen planus, 87
   rheumatoid nodules associated with, 96
   subacute cutaneous lupus erythematosus
      associated with, 157

T

Tabes dorsalis, 199
Tachyphylaxis, 360-361, 362
Tacrolimus, 59, 87
Taenia solium, 240, 446
Talc, as granuloma cause, 90t, 91t
"Tan-in-a-bottle" lotions, 356
Tanning, 128
Tanning pills, 356
Tapeworm infections, 239-240, 239f, 446
"Tapioca" vesicles, 60f
Tar
   phototoxicity of, 120
   as skin cancer cause, 312

Tardive dyskinesia, 457
Targeted therapy, for melanoma, 330
Targetoid (target) lesions, 18-19, 19f
Tattoos/tattooing
   cultural factors in, 436, 436f
   as granuloma cause, 92, 90t
   henna-related, 439f
   mycobacterial infections of, 214
   radiation-port, 436
Tazarotene, 395
Telangiectasia, 18-19, 18f
   acquired facial, most common cause of, 303
   CREST syndrome-related, 160, 161f
   Cushing's syndrome-related, 264
   cuticular, 254
   hemangioma-related, 302f
   hereditary hemorrhagic. *See* Osler-Weber-
      Rendu syndrome
   nail fold, 467t
   periungual, diabetes-related, 262
   progressive systemic sclerosis-related,
      160-161
   spider, 407
Telogen effluvium, 145-146
Tendon sheath, giant cell tumors of, 310, 310f
Tendon xanthoma, 15f
Terbinafine, 222t
   interaction with cyclosporine, 223
   as pustular eruption cause, 81
   as sporotrichosis treatment, 225
   as tinea capitis treatment, 219
Terry's nails, 467t
Testicular cancer, 269
Testosterone, acne-exacerbating effect of, 153t
Tetracyclines
   as acne necrotica miliaris treatment, 81
   adverse cutaneous reactions to, 73t, 100-101,
      102-103, 102f, 119t
   contraindication in children, 153, 404
   as sarcoidosis treatment, 93-94
Thallium, as alopecia cause, 147
Thermoregulation, cutaneous, 13
   dermal vasculature in, 11-12
Thiamine deficiency, 288
Thibierge-Weisenbach syndrome. *See* CREST
   syndrome
Thioridazine, as blue-gray pigmentation cause, 134
Thiouracil, acne-exacerbating effect of, 153t
Thiourea, acne-exacerbating effect of, 153t
Thorns, as granuloma cause, 91f, 91t
Thrombophlebitis, superficial
   differentiated from nodular vasculitis, 137
   migratory, 253-254, 270-271
Thrush, 221t, 262
Thymoma, 222
Thyroid cancer, 270
Thyrotoxicosis, 465
Tick-bite fever, 249-250t
Ticks
   bites of, 242, 248-249, 249f
   as disease vectors, 192, 241, 248, 249-250t,
      476-477
   prevention of, 249-250
   removal from skin, 249
Tinea
   barbae, 217t
   capitis, 144-145, 144f, 147, 216, 217-218,
      217t, 222, 458
      carrier state in, 219
      in children, 404-405, 407
      clinical patterns of, 217, 218f
      diagnostic techniques/tests for, 22
      fluorescent, 218
      hypersensitivity reaction to, 405
      treatment for, 218-219, 405, 407
      "TVs are in houses" mnemonic for, 217
   corporis, 15f, 20, 217f, 217t, 405
   cruris, 217f, 217t
      HIV infection-related, 280
   faciei, 217f, 217t

Tinea *(Continued)*
   incognito, 361t
   manuum, 217t, 280
   nigra, 221
   pedis, 217t, 219, 274t, 280
   penile, 439
   unguium, 217t, 471
   versicolor, 220, 220f, 430, 430f
      diagnostic techniques for, 22-23, 24f
      as hypopigmentation cause, 129-130, 130f
Tinnitus, neurofibromatosis-related, 37, 39
Toads, as wart cause, 187
Toe webs, pseudomonal infections of, 192
Tongue, geographic, 405, 406f
Tonofilaments, 8, 8f
Top 100 Secrets, 1-4
Tophi, gouty, 116, 116f
Topical medications. *See also* Corticosteroids,
   topical
   as acne treatment, 150
   causing photoallergic/phototoxic reactions, 119t
   retinoids, 393-394, 393t, 394t
TORCHES infections, 400, 402
Torre's syndrome, 256t, 257
Total body surface area (TBSA), in topical steroid
   application, 360, 362
Toxic epidermal necrolysis, 73t, 283, 442, 444,
   447, 449
   differentiated from Stevens-Johnson syndrome,
      99, 442, 442t, 443f
   drug-related, 98-99
Toxic shock syndrome, 188, 190, 445
Toxocara, as panniculitis cause, 140
Toxoplasmosis, 230
   neonatal, 400-401, 402
Transepidermal elimination, 276
Transient bullous dermolysis, 45
Transient neonatal pustular melanosis, 82
Trauma
   as Koebner phenomenon cause, 20, 20f
   as panniculitis cause, 135t, 139-140
Trench fever, 473
Treponema carateum, 130
Treponema pallidum, 24-25, 129-130, 195,
   196-197, 199
Treponematoses, pigmentation disorders associ-
   ated with, 129-130
Tretinoin
   as ichthyosis treatment, 34
   topical, 393t, 394-395
      side effects of, 395
   as wart treatment, 186, 186t
Triatomids, 248
Triazolam, interaction with antifungal agents, 223
Trichilemmoma, 256-257
Trichinella spiralis, 235, 446
Trichinosis, 235
Trichomycosis axillaris, 194, 194f
Trichophyton, 216
Trichophyton ferrugineum, 218
Trichophyton mentagrophytes, 219-220, 221, 471
Trichophyton rubrum, 216, 219, 221, 471
Trichophyton schoenleinii, 218
Trichophyton soudanense, 217
Trichophyton tonsurans, 22, 216-217, 218, 222, 404
Trichophyton violaceum, 217
Trichorrhexis nodosa, 146, 146f
Trichosporon, as piedra causal organism, 221
Trichotemnomania, 459
Trichothiodystrophy (PIBIDS), 33t
Trichotillomania, 145, 145f, 147, 407, 458-459, 459f
Trichotiodystrophy, 123-124t
Trimethadione, acne-exacerbating effect of, 153t
Trimethoprim-sulfamethoxazole, 98, 98t
Triparanol, as ichthyosis cause, 32, 34t
Tripe palms, 253, 271
"Triple response," 167
Triva, dermatologic, 473-478
Trousseau's sign, 253-254
Trypanosoma, as panniculitis cause, 140

Trypanosomiasis, 230, 240, 434
  African, 235t, 238, 239f, 249-250t261
  American, 235t, 238, 248, 249-250t
Tsetse flies, 241, 249-250t
Tubercles, 212
Tuberculosis, 207-212
  cutis orficialis, 209-210, 210f
  diabetes as risk factor for, 262
  as leukocytoclastic vasculitis cause, 105
  multidrug-resistant, 211-212
  as nodular vasculitis cause, 136-137
  as paronychia cause, 471
  verrucosa cutis, 208, 209-210, 209t
Tuberculosis vaccine, 211
Tuberculoid reactions, 209-210
Tuberous sclerosis, 37, 129, 279t, 407-408
Tubers, 40
Tularemia, 90t, 193-194, 194f, 225, 231, 241, 248
Tumor d'emblee, 332
Tumor necrosis factor-α, 135
Tumor necrosis factor-α agonists, 233
Tumor necrosis factor-α inhibitors, 53-54, 212
Tunga penetrans, 477
Tungiasis, 237, 237f, 477
Tuskegee Study, 200
"20-nail dystrophy," 85-86, 86f
Twin transfusion syndrome, 401
"Two-pajamas treatment," 60
Tyndall effect, 296
Typhus, 248
  epidemic, 241, 249-250t
  murine, 249-250t
  scrub, 237, 249-250t
Tzanck preparation/smear, 23, 24f, 176, 179

U

Ulcers, 16
  Buruli, 213, 434
  definition of, 17f
  erythema induratum-related, 137f
  factitial, 459f
  hemangioma-related, 301, 301f
  infected, bacterial skin cultures of, 27
  leprosy-related (mal perforans), 204-205, 204f
  pyoderma gangrenosum-related, 268, 269f
  sickle cell, 434
  as skin cancer cause, 312
  tropical, 434
Ultraviolet booths, 388, 388f
Ultraviolet radiation (UV)
  electromagnetic spectrum of, 128, 386, 386f, 388
  epidermal blockage of, 8
  as facial telangiectasia cause, 303
  as psoriasis treatment, 53
  sensitivity to. *See* Photosensitivity
  as telangiectasia cause, 18-19
Ultraviolet radiation A
  biologic effects of, 353
  as melanoma cause, 319-320
  phototherapeutic use of, 388-389, 391
Ultraviolet radiation A-1, as atopic dermatitis treatment, 59
Ultraviolet radiation B
  biologic effects of, 353
  comparison with PUVA, 388-389
  as melanoma cause, 319-320
  phototherapeutic use of, 388
    as atopic dermatitis treatment, 59
    as lichen planus treatment, 87
    as pruritus treatment, 466t
    side effects of, 390
    as vitiligo treatment, 127
Ultraviolet radiation B phototest sites, 121f
Ultraviolet radiation C, 353
Ultraviolet-sensitive syndrome, 123-124t
Urbach-Wiethe disease, 114
Uremic frost, 274t, 275, 275t, 277

Urethritis
  gonococcal, 25
  Reiter's disease-related, 80-81
Uric acid, in gout, 116
Urine, discoloration of, 476
Urticaria, 16f, 166-170
  acute, 166
  autoimmune, 163
  beta-lactam antibiotics-related, 100
  cholinergic, 166, 168
  chronic, 166-167, 168
    treatment for, 170
  cold, acquired, 100, 166, 167, 167f, 170
  contact, 65
    allergic, 65, 65f
    nonimmunologic, 65
    occupational exposure-related, 452
  delayed pressure, 170
  as dermatologic emergency, 449
  drug-related, 97, 100, 168
  idiopathic, 166
    chronic, 169
  morbilliform, 174
  physical, 166, 167, 168
  pigmentosa, 16f, 406-407, 407f
    pediatric, 169f
  as pruritus cause, 464
  solar, 122, 168, 168f
    phototherapy for, 387-388t
  tinea pedis-related, 219
  treatment for, 170
  Wegener's granulomatosis-related, 108
  wheals of, 464
Usage test, 68, 68f
Uveitis, Heerfordt's syndrome-related, 93
Uvulectomy, perinatal, 439

V

Vacciniforme scars, 122
Vaginitis, lichen planus-related, 85
Valacyclovir, 176, 177t, 180t
Valproic acid, as alopecia cause, 147
Vancomycin, 73t, 166
Varicella-zoster virus infections, 172, 175, 178-179, 179f
  diagnosis of, 23, 179
  in HIV-infected individuals, 280, 281t, 284
  neonatal, 400-401
Varices, esophageal, 268f
Vascular anomalies/malformations, 302
  childhood, 448
Vascular lesions, laser therapy for, 383, 384t
Vascular neoplasms, 379-382
Vascular permeability, mediators of, 167
Vasculature, cutaneous, 11-12, 12f
  dermal, thermoregulatory function of, 11-12
Vasculitides, 444
Vasculitis, 105-111, 257
  cancer-related, 259
  in children, 407
  cryoglobulinemic, 107
    definition and classification of, 105, 105t
    essential cryoglobulinemic, 105t
  leukocytoclastic, 105-106, 105t, 107, 278, 447, 449
    as dermatologic emergency, 446
    Henoch-Schönlein purpura variant of, 105t, 106
    Wegener's granulomatosis-related, 108
  nodular, 136-137
  septic, 192
  urticarial, 102, 163-164t, 169-170, 169f
Vasodilatation, mediators of, 167
Vasovagal response, to local anesthesia, 365
Venereal Disease Research Laboratory (VDRL) test, for syphilis diagnosis, 25, 55-56, 197
Venous lakes, 303
Verruca plana. *See* Warts, flat

Verruca vulgaris. *See* Warts, common
Verruga peruana, 473
Vesicles, 14
  causes of, 70
  as dermatologic emergency indicator, 444-445
  differentiated from pustules and bullae, 70, 78
  grouped configuration of, 20
Vesiculobullous disorders, 70-77
  acute, 70, 71t
  chronic, 71t
  as dermatologic emergency, 442-444
  diagnostic tests for, 71-73, 72t
  drug-related, 97
  external agents-related, 73, 73t
  genetic/inherited, 74
Vilanova's disease, 135
Viral exanthems, 172-174
Viral infections. *See also specific viruses*
  as dermatologic emergencies, 444-446
  in HIV-infected individuals, 280, 281t
  as leukocytoclastic vasculitis cause, 105
  as skin cancer cause, 312
Viral vaccinations, as papular acrodermatitis of childhood cause, 173
Virchow cells, 203
Vitamin A. *See also* Retinoids
  deficiency of, 289
  physiological effects of, 393
  toxicity of, 289
Vitamin B-complex deficiencies, 288
Vitamin C deficiency. *See* Scurvy
Vitamin D
  calcinosis cutis-related toxicity of, 117
  deficiency of, 289
  metabolism of, relationship to sun exposure, 354, 356
Vitamin deficiencies
  of fat-soluble vitamins, 289
  of water-soluble vitamins, 288
Vitamin K deficiency, 289
Vitiligo, 15f, 126-127, 128, 128f, 262, 429
  phototherapy for, 387-388t
Voigt's lines, 428, 428f
von Hippel-Lindau disease, 41
von Recklinghausen's disease. *See* Neurofibromatosis, type I
Vulvar disorders, 422-426

W

Waardenburg's syndrome, 126
Waldenström's macroglobulinemia, 115
Warble, 236
Warfarin
  drug interactions of, 222
  as necrosis cause, 97, 103f
Warts, 182-187
  anogenital, 182t, 183-184, 183f, 185, 186t, 187, 199
    cryosurgical treatment for, 372
    in HIV-infected individuals, 283-284
    prevention of, 184
  as cancer risk factor, 182
  common, 182, 182t, 183f, 186t
    in HIV-infected individuals, 283-284
  cryosurgical treatment for, 372
  "fairy ring," 185, 186f
  flat, 182, 182t, 183f, 186t, 394
  in HIV-infected individuals, 283-284
  "kissing," 184f
  laryngeal, 185
  neonatal perianal, 403f
  palmar, 182, 182t
  periungual, 182, 184, 187, 380, 470
  Peruvian, 473
  plantar, 182, 182t, 185, 186t, 187, 380
  prevention of, 184
  treatment for, 184-185, 186-187, 186f
Wasp stings, 242-243

Weber-Cockayne syndrome, 474
Wegener's granulomatosis, 105t, 106-107, 108-109, 108f, 278
  differentiated from Churg-Strauss syndrome, 108, 109t
Werewolves, 476
West Nile fever, 249-250t
West Nile virus, 241
Wheals, 14, 16f, 464
  urticaria-related, 167-168, 167f
Wheat, as contact urticaria cause, 65f
Whiteheads, 19
Wickham's striae, 84, 85f
Willan, Robert, 474
Wilson's disease, 467t
"Winter itch," 463
Wiskott-Aldrich syndrome, 258t
Wood's lamp examination, 22, 23f, 272
  for pigmentation diagnosis, 126
  for Pseudomonas infection diagnosis, 193
  for tinea capitis diagnosis, 22, 218
Wool, as atopic dermatitis cause, 59, 463-464
Woringer-Kolopp disease, 332

Wound infections, 188, 190, 192
Wound myiasis, 236
Wrinkles
  photoinduced, 394
  treatment for, 381-382
Wuchereia bancrofti, 236

X

Xanthelasma (palpebra), 265-266, 265f
Xanthoma, 266
  eruptive, 265-266, 265f
  tendinous, 15f, 265-266
  tuberous, 265-266
Xeroderma pigmentosum, 123-124t, 319-320, 321, 352
Xerosis, 274t, 463
  atopic dermatitis-related, 59
  chronic renal failure-related, 274t
  in HIV-infected individuals, 280, 281t
  retinoid therapy-related, 397

Y

Yaws, 129-130, 475
Yellow fever, 249-250t
Yellow nail syndrome, 468, 468f
Yellow nails, 467t
Yellow skin
  carotenoderma-related, 290, 291f
  chronic renal failure-related, 274t
  diabetes-related, 262
  hypothyroidism-related, 262, 263f
  jaundice-related, 271
Yersinia infections, 135-136, 249-250t

Z

Zidovudine, adverse cutaneous reactions to, 101t, 134
Zinc deficiency, 289-290
Zirconium, as granuloma cause, 91t
Zoonotic infestations, 246-248
Zygomycosis, 224t